AF538310

ALLERGY
Theory and Practice

ALLERGY
Theory and Practice

Edited By

Phillip E. Korenblat, M.D.

Associate Professor of Medicine
Department of Internal Medicine
Washington University School of Medicine
Co-Director, Allergy Clinics
Jewish Hospital of St. Louis
St. Louis, Missouri

H. James Wedner, M.D.

Associate Professor of Medicine
Department of Internal Medicine
Division of Allergy and Immunology
Director, Allergy Clinics
Washington University School of Medicine
St. Louis, Missouri

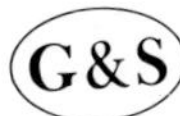

GRUNE & STRATTON, INC.

(Harcourt Brace Jovanovich, Publishers)

Orlando San Diego New York
London Toronto Montreal Sydney Tokyo

Library of Congress Cataloging in Publication Data
Main entry under title:

Allergy—theory and practice.

Bibliography
Includes index.
1. Allergy. I. Korenblat, Phillip E. II. Wedner, H. James. [DNLM: 1. Hypersensitivity—Diagnosis. 2. Hypersensitivity—Therapy. WD 300 A4349]
RC584.A45 1984 616.97 83-22607
ISBN 0-8089-1619-X

Grune & Stratton, Inc.
Orlando, Florida 32887

Distributed in the United Kingdom by
Grune & Stratton, Ltd.
24/28 Oval Road, London NW 1

Library of Congress Catalog Number 83-22607
International Standard Book Number 0-8089-1619-X
Printed in the United States of America

85 86 87 10 9 8 7 6 5 4 3 2

Contents

Acknowledgments

The editors are indebted to all the contributors for the effort they have put into making this a worthwhile publication.

We wish to acknowledge the contributions of Mamie Tomich, whose secretarial and editorial assistance has been invaluable, and those of Scott Frankel, whose hours spent in the library cross-checking many of the references are greatly appreciated. Finally, we must thank our families for their encouragement in this undertaking and their understanding when time that should have been spent with them was devoted to the completion of this volume.

Preface

It is a rare physician who has never been confronted with an allergic problem. The spectrum of allergic diseases is so broad and the number of potentially allergic individuals so great that no physician can ignore the question, "Do you think I could be allergic to that?" This is particularly true for physicians who specialize in the primary care of children or adults, who encounter potential allergic reactions on an almost daily basis. Nevertheless, the teaching of theory, diagnosis, and treatment of allergic diseases in medical schools is largely nonexistent. Because of insufficient training, many physicians feel ill at ease when confronted with anything beyond a minor allergic reaction. In some instances, this lack of knowledge may lead to failure to identify accurately an allergy, thereby denying the patient what may be a very simple and effective treatment.

Our understanding of the atopic state has grown exponentially in recent years. As it is a major purpose of this volume to provide practicing physicians with information on the diagnosis and therapy of allergy, it is both necessary and appropriate that the volume begin with a discussion of the immunologic basis of the allergic state and a description of mediators released and how they result in symptoms associated with allergy.

The rest of the book is divided into sections on the evaluation of the allergic patient, manifestations of the allergic state, treatment, allergic lung disease, specific allergies, and pediatric allergies. In each section, the contributors have included pertinent theory along with the more practical aspects of treatment. For readers who wish a more detailed, basically orientational, or theoretical view of the allergic state, carefully selected volumes are listed at the end of each chapter.

In closing, we note with sorrow the untimely death of Donald Strominger, a contributor to this book and prominent St. Louis allergy specialist. His presence will surely be missed.

Contributors

John P. Atkinson, M.D. Investigator, Howard Hughes Medical Institute; Head, Division of Rheumatology, Department of Internal Medicine, Washington University School of Medicine, St. Louis, Missouri

Jack Barrow, M.D. Associate Professor of Clinical Medicine, Washington University School of Medicine, St. Louis, Missouri

Leonard Cohen, M.D., Ph.D. Assistant in Medicine, Division of Allergy and Immunology, Department of Medicine, Washington School of Medicine, St. Louis, Missouri

James M. Corry, M.D. Assistant Professor of Pediatrics, Department of Pediatrics, Washington University School of Medicine, St. Louis, Missouri

Arnold Dankner, M.D. Associate Professor of Clinical Medicine, Department of Internal Medicine, Washington University School of Medicine; Co-Director, Allergy Clinic, Jewish Hospital of St. Louis, St. Louis, Missouri

Rand Dankner, M.D. Instructor, Clinical Medicine, Division of Allergy and Immunology, Department of Internal Medicine, Washington University School of Medicine, St. Louis, Missouri

James H. Day, M.D., F.R.C.P.(C), F.A.C.P Head, Division of Allergy and Clinical Immunology, Department of Medicine, Queens University; Head, Department of Immunology, Kingston General Hospital, Kingston, Ontario, Canada

Robert J. Dockhorn, M.D. Chief, Allergy–Immunology, University of Kansas School of Medicine/Children's Mercy Hospital; Professor of Pediatrics, University of Missouri, Kansas City, Missouri

Joel A. Goebel, M.D. Fourth-year Resident, Department of Otolaryngology, Washington University School of Medicine, St. Louis, Missouri

J. Andrew Grant, M.D. Chief, Division of Adult Allergy, University of Texas Medical Branch, Galveston, Texas

Peter Konig, M.D., Ph.D. Professor of Pediatrics, Department of Child Health, University of Missouri Health Sciences Center; Chief, Division of Pediatric Allergy, University of Missouri School of Medicine, Columbia, Missouri

Phillip E. Korenblat, M.D. Associate Professor of Medicine (Clinical), Department of Internal Medicine, Washington University School of Medicine; Co-Director, Allergy Clinic, Jewish Hospital of St. Louis, St. Louis, Missouri

Anthony Kulczycki, Jr., M.D. Associate Professor of Medicine and Assistant Professor of Microbiology and Immunology, Howard Hughes Medical Institute Laboratory and Department of Internal Medicine; Division of Allergy and Immunology, Washington University School of Medicine, St. Louis, Missouri

Stephen S. LeFrak, M.D. Associate Professor of Medicine, Department of Medicine, Washington University School of Medicine; Co-Director, Respiratory and Clinical Care Division, Department of Medicine, Jewish Hospital of St. Louis, St. Louis Missouri

Walter H. Lewis, M.D. Professor of Biology, Division of Botany, Washington University, St. Louis, Missouri

Kenneth P. Mathews, M.D. Professor of Medicine, Chief, Division of Allergy, University of Michigan Medical School; University Hospital, Ann Arbor, Michigan

David A. Mathison, M.D. Division of Allergy and Immunology, Department of Clinical Research, Scripps Clinic and Research Foundation, La Jolla, California

Charles W. Parker, M.D. Director, Howard Hughes Institute Laboratory and Professor of Medicine, Microbiology, and Immunology, Department of Internal Medicine, Division of Allergy and Immunology, Washington University School of Medicine, St. Louis, Missouri

Warren W. Pleskow, M.D. Clinical Instructor, Dept. of Internal Medicine and Allergy, Scripps Memorial Hospitals, University of California at San Diego, La Jolla, California

Scott Sale, M.D. Chief Resident, Internal Medicine, The Jewish Hospital of St. Louis; Clinical Instructor, Washington University Medicial Center, St. Louis, Missouri

Lawrence Samuels, M.D. Assistant Professor of Medicine (Clinical–Dermatology), Department of Internal Medicine, Division of Dermatology, Washington University School of Medicine, St. Louis, Missouri

Susan Bromberg Schneider, M.D. Clinical Instructor in Internal Medicine, Washington University School of Medicine; Department of Internal Medicine, St. Luke's Hospital, St. Louis, Missouri

Jeffrey Schulman, M.D. Clinical Instructor, Department of Pediatrics, Washington University School of Medicine, St. Louis, Missouri

Robert M. Senior, M.D. Professor of Medicine, Co-Director, Respiratory and Critical Care Division, Department of Medicine, Jewish Hospital of St. Louis, St. Louis, Missouri

Donald G. Sessions, M.D. Professor of Otolaryngology, Department of Otolaryngology, Washington University School of Medicine, St. Louis, Missouri

Gerald Shatz, M.D. Assistant Professor of Medicine (Clinical), Division of Allergy and Immunology, Washington University School of Medicine, St. Louis, Missouri

Ronald A. Simon, M.D. Division of Allergy and Immunology, Department of Clinical Research, Scripps Clinic and Research Foundation, La Jolla, California

Raymond Slavin, M.D. Professor of Medicine, Chief, Division of Allergy, St. Louis University School of Medicine, St. Louis, Missouri

Donald D. Stevenson, M.D. Division of Allergy and Immunology, Department of Clinical Research, Scripps Clinic and Research Foundation, La Jolla, California

Donald B. Strominger, M.D. Professor of Pediatrics (Clinical), Department of Pediatrics, Washington University School of Medicine, St. Louis, Missouri

Timothy J. Sullivan, M.D. Associate Professor of Medicine; Chief, Division of Allergy and Immunology, Department of Internal Medicine and Microbiology, University of Texas Health Science Center, Dallas, Texas

J. Allen Thiel, M.D. Associate Professor of Clinical Medicine, Department of Internal Medicine Division of Allergy and Immunology, Washington University School of Medicine; Director, Department of Allergy, St. John's Mercy Medical Center, St. Louis, Missouri

H. James Wedner, M.D. Associate Professor of Medicine, Department of Medicine, Division of Allergy and Immunology; Director, Allergy Clinics, Washington Unviversity School of Medicine, St. Louis, Missouri

John A. Wood, M.D. Assistant Professor of Medicine (Clinical), Department of Medicine, Washington University School of Medicine, St. Louis, Missouri

H. James Wedner
Phillip Korenblat

1

Introduction: Allergy Past and Future

Allergic reactions were described in the earliest writings. Egyptian hieroglyphs suggested the death of a pharaoh as the result of an allergic reaction to a bee sting. Even earlier, Chinese writings accurately described asthma and its treatment. Interestingly, the herbal medicine suggested in these writings, Mah-Huang, is derived from an extract of the bark of trees of the genus *Ephedra,* thus making ephedrine, still a common constituent of some asthma preparations, the oldest known drug for the treatment of any allergic disease. Both Hippocrates and Galen accurately described allergic reactions and other atopic states in their writings and even suggested that some of these might be the result of environmental factors. The first accurate description of hay fever was provided by Bostock in 1819, and 50 years later Blakley was the first to prove that pollen caused the allergic reaction by performing the first skin test. In 1906 the term "allergy" was coined by von Pirquet, who derived the term from the Greek word "allol," meaning "change in the original state." This represented von Pirquet's theory that substances were capable of inducing an alteration in an individual's specific responsiveness. Von Pirquet and Schick suggested that the alteration could be one of increase (hypersensitivity) or decrease (immunity). Interestingly, the term "anaphylaxis," the most potent of the allergic responses, antedates that of allergy by several years. It was first coined by Richet in 1902.

The actual practice of allergy probably can be related to the work of Noon, who was the first to inject extracts of pollen into patients in the hope of altering their allergic state. Interestingly, Noon, following the work of Erlich and Semmleweise, believed that allergies were the result of toxins contained in pollen. His hope was that by injecting increasing amounts of the toxin containing extracts he would be able to reduce or desensitize the patient to these toxins. Although this idea seems outlandish in light of current knowledge, it should be remembered that it was fully 50 years following Noon's original report that the real nature of the allergic response was described with the discovery by Ishizaka and Ishizaka that reagenic antibody

ALLERGY: THEORY AND PRACTICE
ISBN 0-8089-1619-X

was Immunoglobulin E (IgE). Nonetheless, the desensitization procedure of Noon was an effective therapeutic modality providing another example in medicine where the treatment of a disease antedated knowledge of the nature of that disease by many years.

Cook and Cocca were the first to recognize that there was a class of diseases with similar characteristics and coined the term "atopy" (from the Greek "atopos" meaning "strangeness") for this class of diseases. Later Sulzberger added atopic dermatitis (infantile eczema) to the list of atopic diseases. Our current understanding of the atopic state has grown literally by leaps and bounds. We now recognize that atopy represents a genetically inherited ability to form IgE antibodies against a variety of foreign substances and that the IgE binds to tissue mast cells or circulating basophils and on subsequent interaction with the offending antigens results in the release of the mediators of the allergic state. The immunology of the allergic state and a description of the mediators released and how they result in the symptoms associated with the allergic state are described by Drs. Grant and Parker in Chapters 2 and 3.

As our understanding of immunology in general and atopic immunology in particular, as well as the mediators of the allergic response, has grown rapidly in the last decade, so has the development of therapeutic modalities for the treatment of allergic diseases. It might be interesting to speculate on some of these newer therapeutic modalities that might soon become available to the practicing physician. These developments can be divided into three broad categories: (1) new drugs for the treatment of allergic disorders, (2) new preparations for desensitization, and (3) modalities for turning off an allergic response (the production of IgE) or preventing its production from ever taking place.

As described in detail in the subsequent chapters, a broad variety of therapeutic agents are available for the treatment of allergic disorders. These include antihistaminics, beta-adrenergic agonists, membrane stabilizing agents such as disodium cromoglycate, theophylline, and corticosteroids. Strides are being taken in each of these areas. The most exciting new therapeutic agent in the area of antihistaminics is a new class of drugs that are incapable of penetrating the blood–brain barrier. These agents avoid the major side effect of antihistaminic therapy, drowsiness, and allow the use of significantly higher dosages, which should serve to prevent some allergic reactions that are unresponsive to antihistaminics with the use of conventional therapeutic agents. A large number of new $beta_2$-specific agonists have recently been synthesized, and many of these are currently in clinical testing in Europe or this country. The most promising of these, fenoterol, is currently under consideration by the U.S. Food and Drug Administration (FDA) for licensure in the United States and may be available by the time this volume is published. The major disadvantage of disodium cromoglycate (cromolyn sodium, Intal, elegantly described by Peter Konig in Chapter 17), is that this agent is not effective for asthma or rhinitis in oral form. A whole class of oral cromolyn-like drugs have been synthesized and are currently undergoing testing. The most promising of these is ketotifen (Zatiden). This drug not only has cromolyn-like properties, but is also a potent antihistaminic agent and is currently being considered for licensure by the FDA. This will probably be the first in a large class of drugs with the property of "membrane stabilization." In the area of corticosteroid therapy one new drug is presently on the horizon. This is a steroid that is fluorinated at the 21 position, thereby conferring the property of fat insolubility. As a result, it seems to have significantly less potential for causing the major side effects associated with corticosteroid therapy, particularly bone demineralization, while maintaining its anti-inflammatory and antiallergic potential. This drug, fluocortalone, is currently in use in Europe and should be available in this country within the relatively near future. Finally, as pointed out by Phillip E. Korenblat in Chapter 21, atropine or atropine-like agents have a significant place as therapeutic modalities in the treatment of asthma. A number of atropine-like agents have been synthesized, and one of these ipotroprium (SCH 1000, Atrovent) has been licensed for use in aerosolized form in a number of European countries and has proved quite beneficial. One would anticipate that this drug should be available as a therapeutic agent for the treatment of asthma in this country within the next few years.

In the field of agents for immunotherapy two broad categories should be considered as being on the horizon. First, the use of highly purified allergenic substances. As pointed out by J. Allen Thiel in Chapter 27 on hymenoptera sensitivity, the major advance in clinical medicine to date in this area has been the use of purified venom preparations. Work is now under way on the identification of the actual antigens responsible for allergic reactions to a variety of pollens. Examples are the identification of antigen E as the major offending agent in ragweed pollen or the identification of a single protein that is responsible almost entirely for sensitivity to the mountain cedar. Clearly, it would seem to be beneficial to be able to hyposensitize patients to the actual proteins responsible for allergy to that particular pollen. On the other hand, it should be pointed out that in some cases the extract of the whole pollen may be preferable to the purified proteins. This has been demonstrated, for example, in the situation of timothy pollen where use of the purified timothy pollen proteins was of significantly less benefit than the use of a whole extract of timothy pollen. The explanation for this apparent paradoxic occurrence can most probably be derived from the assumption that the minor proteins within the whole pollen extract are of major importance in the production of allergy to this substance and its treatment by hyposensitization immunotherapy. In other instances the number of proteins that can be extracted and shown to have allergenic potential may be so great that it will be impossible to compound a catalog of the purified proteins. This is particularly true for mold antigens. Work by Salvaggio and his coworkers has demonstrated that at least 56 individual proteins in Alternaria are capable of inducing IgE production. Regardless of these exceptions, continued advancement in the delineation of purified antigens will provide for the clinician an additional edge in the administration of immunotherapy. The second important advancement in IT has been the development of alternate methods for increasing the potency of immunotherapy extracts in such a way that they become more tolleragenic. Efforts along these lines have taken three different approaches: (1) the use of highly denatured preparations to form an allergoid, by analogy similar to the production of a toxoid such as tetanus toxoid; (2) polimerization of the allergy extract with glutaraldehyde, a process developed because it has been widely shown that polymers tend to be less immunogenic and more tolleragenic than are native proteins; and (3) the linking of relevant allergenic proteins to backbones that render them relatively tolleragenic such as the linking of ragweed antigen E to a polyethylene glycol backbone. Work on these three methods has been carried out largely with ragweed antigen E, and each one has been shown to confer a high degree of tolleragenicity to the antigen E molecule. This allows one to use greater amounts of antigen over shorter periods of time to produce the same degree of hyposensitization. Several of these preparations are undergoing clinical trials, and presumably one or more of them will be available for use in the treatment of human disease in the relatively near future.

As our knowledge of the control mechanisms involved in the generation of an allergic response increases, our ability to modulate atopic sensitivity specifically or nonspecifically may emerge. One example is the recent discovery of a relatively nonspecific suppressor of the allergic response. This substance, originally described by Katz, has been shown to be an effective nonspecific inhibitor of any IgE response in the mouse. More recently, this same group has presented evidence for a similar substance in humans. Interestingly, this substance, called suppressor factor of anaphylaxis (SFA), appears to be capable of decreasing IgE synthesis regardless of whether it is injected prior to antigenic stimulation or following the antigenic challenge. Clearly, the availability of such a product would allow one to decrease dramatically overall sensitivity in atopic individuals. This would, of course, represent the ultimate treatment of the allergic state.

Our understanding of the mechanisms involved in the generation of an allergic sensitivity and of the appropriate methods for the diagnosis and treatment of the allergic state have increased greatly over the past 5–10 years, and we anticipate that our knowledge will continue to expand at a rapid rate. Some of these newer methods for the diagnosis and treatment of allergies are now available and are the focus of this volume.

Others are in the wings ready to come on stage. It is our hope that the brief discussion in this chapter will make readers aware of "things to look for" so that when available, they may be incorporated in the care of the allergic patient. It is not our intention to convert physicians engaged in the practice of primary medical care into allergists; however, we do hope that it will allow them to approach the allergic patient with a degree of confidence so that they can accurately evaluate and adequately treat many allergic disease states. In addition, the information provided in this volume will enhance the physicians ability to identify those patients who might benefit by referral for more sophisticated forms of allergic therapy.

PART 1

Basic Allergic Mechanisms

J. Andrew Grant

2

Fundamentals of the Immune System and Hypersensitivity Reactions

The allergic diseases are a major cause of illness in people of all ages. One survey revealed that allergies were the second most frequent complaint in the population (Table 2-1). In 1975 about 35 million people in the United States suffered from allergic diseases (Table 2-2). Thus community physicians must maintain their skills in the proper management of these illnesses.

The immune system, which consists of a series of complex cellular and humoral elements, can interact specifically with many different types of molecular structures (antigens) to distinguish self from nonself (foreign). The functions of the system are to protect the body against harm that can be caused by external microorganisms and toxins and to eliminate internal threats, such as neoplastic cells. The immune system can also respond inappropriately, however, and cause hypersensitive (allergic) disorders.

The science of immunology is an outgrowth of microbiology (historical developments are summarized in Table 2-3). This chapter reviews the basic principles of immunology, examines mechanisms of the allergic response, and describes some clinical allergic syndromes.

FUNDAMENTALS OF THE IMMUNE SYSTEM

In the last century it was discovered that defense of the host could be mounted by both cellular and humoral elements (Table 2-3). Although each element of the defense system has been found to have unique functions (Table 2-4), considerable interdependence does exist. For example, macrophages and T lymphocytes regulate the synthesis of specific antibodies by B lymphocytes, and antibodies and complement fragments are necessary for normal phagocytosis by neutrophils.

ALLERGY: THEORY AND PRACTICE
ISBN 0-8089-1619-X

Table 2-1 *Prevalence Rate of the 10 Leading Conditions Occurring During the Past Year*

Condition	Prevalence Rate per 100 Persons
Dental conditions	11.1
Allergies	9.4
Overweight	7.8
Strep throat or sore throat	7.2
Hypertension	7.0
Colds	5.8
Arthritis or rheumatism	5.5
Headches	5.3
Bronchitis or coughing	4.1
Sinus trouble	4.0

Taken from a survey of 7945 individuals in suburban Cook and DuPage Counties in Illinois. Cited in *Asthma and the other allergic diseases*, National Institute of Allergy and Infectious Diseases (NIAID) Task Force Report, 1979. Reproduced with permission.

Table 2-2 *Estimated Prevalence of Allergic Disorders in the United States in 1975*

	Population Affected (Millions)
Total	35.3
Asthma	8.9
Hay fever	14.6
Other allergic conditions	11.8
Eczema	
Urticaria	
Angioedema	
Allergic reaction to	
Foods	
Drugs	
Insect stings	

Cited in *Asthma and the other allergic diseases*, NIAID Task Force Report, 1979. Reproduced with permission.

Table 2-3 *Milestones in Development of Immunology*

Year	Observation	Importance
1796	Cowpox vaccination	First immunization by Jenner
1879	Mesenchymal cells with staining with basic dyes	Identification of mast cells (and later basophils) by Ehrlich
1880	Attenuated vaccines	Immunization with bacteria of low virulence by Pasteur
1882	Macrophage response to foreign bodies	Recognition of cellular immunity by Mitchnikoff
1890	Antitoxic effect of serum from immunized animals	Origin of humoral immunity and antibody by Behring
1894	Heat-labile serum bacteriolytic factor	Description of complement by Bordet
1902	Lethal shock during immunization of dogs	First report of anaphylaxis by Richet and Portier
1905	Serum sickness described	Von Pirquet introduced the terms hypersensitivity and allergy for altered reactivity
1910	Tissue response to histamine	Role of histamine in allergy described by Dale
1911	Pollen injections for rhinitis	First use of immunotherapy for allergic disorders by Freeman & Noon
1921	Passive transfer of cutaneous response to an antigen	Description by Prausnitz and Kustner of a serum factor (reagin) responsible for allergy
1938	Antibodies present in gamma globulins	Initial chemical characterization of antibodies by Tiselius & Kabat
1942	Passive transfer of immunity by cells	Confirmation of the role of lymphocytes in immunity by Landsteiner & Chase
1952	Histamine in mast cells	Description of the cells triggering certain allergic reactions by Riley & West
1963	Identification of four types of hypersensitivity reaction	Systematic analysis of the etiologies for allergic disorders by Gell & Coombs
1966	Isolation of IgE	Identification of the reaginic antibody by Ishizaka & Ishizaka
1966	Migration inhibition factor	First lymphokine described by David, Bloom, & Bennett

Table 2-4 *Fundamental Features of the Immune System*

Humoral Immunity	Cellular Immunity
Mediated by antibodies, complement, etc.	Mediated by T lymphocytes and/or secreted lymphokines
Passively transferred by serum	Passively transferred by T cells
Antibodies made by B-cell-derived plasma cells	Host defense against most intracellular organisms, viruses, fungi, tumor cells
Host defense against most bacteria	

Cellular Elements

The normal development of the immune system is outlined in Figure 2-1. Stem cells that arise in the fetal liver are the precursors of lymphocytes, granulocytes, erythrocytes, and thrombocytes. Subsequently, stem cells are found in the bone marrow.

Lymphocytes

Lymphocytes are the antigen-specific components of the cellular immune system. These cells have highly specific receptors that can distinguish between the antigens of *normal* host origin and those that are foreign. The lymphocytes tolerate the antigens of the normal cells, but foreign antigens, such as those on bacteria, induce a vigorous defense reaction.

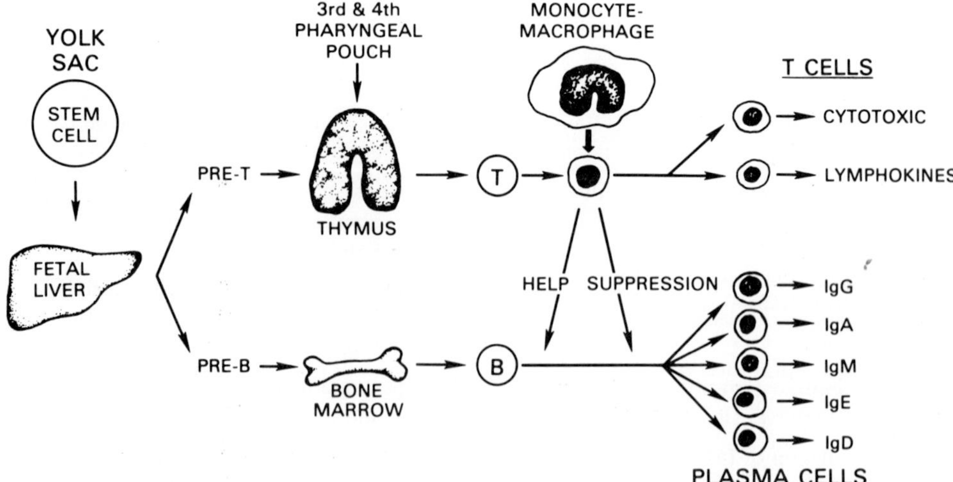

Fig. 2-1. Development of the immune system. The lymphoid stem cells arise in the yolk sac and then pass into the fetal liver. Stem cells can be found in the bone marrow late in gestation and after birth. Stem cells may develop either into T cells or B cells. Macrophages are essential for normal function of lymphocytes. Helper and suppressor cells arising from T lymphocytes control the maturation of B cells to plasma cells.

T CELLS. The thymus of the fetus, which develops from the third and fourth pharyngeal pouches during the sixth week of gestation, influences the differentiation of immature lymphocytes into thymus-derived cells (T cells). These cells are the most abundant type of circulating lymphocytes in the adult. T Cells can be distinguished clinically by their ability to bind sheep erythrocytes (the E-rosette test). Recently, monoclonal antibodies (such as OKT3) have been developed that identify unique antigens on T cells. Within the lymph nodes, T cells predominate in the medullary and paracortical areas. Removal of the thymus from the fetus results in severe depletion of cells from the paracortical and medullary regions and in impairment of normal T-cell functions.

The thymus secretes hormones (such as thymosin) that are partly responsible for its effect on the immune system. These hormones have been isolated and used clinically to restore T-cell responses.

T Lymphocytes are essential for proper regulation of the immune response. The two types of regulatory T cell that can be recognized are helper cells and suppressor cells (Figure 2-1 and Table 2-5). Also, these cells can be identified by monoclonal antibodies, which bind to unique membrane structures: helper cells by OKT4 antibody and suppressor cells by OKT5 and OKT8 antibodies. Helper cells are important for normal antibody production and for T effector cell response. In contrast, suppressor cells retard both of these functions. An increase or decrease in the numbers of either cell type can be harmful. For example, too many suppressor cells or too few helper cells may be seen in hypogammaglobulinemia. Reduction in suppressor cells has been reported in patients with multiple sclerosis, eczema, and

Table 2-5 *Functions of T Lymphocytes*

Regulation of immune response
- Helper cells
- Suppressor cells

Killing of foreign cells by cytotoxic lymphocytes

Immunologic modulation by release of soluble products (lymphokines) affecting
- Macrophages
  - Migration inhibition factor
  - Macrophage activating factor
  - Monocyte chemotactic factor
- Neutrophils
  - Leukocyte inhibition factor
- Basophils
  - Basophil chemotactic factor
  - Histamine releasing activity
- Eosinophils
  - Eosinophil chemotactic factor
- Lymphocytes
  - Lymphocyte chemotactic factor
  - Interleukin 2 that stimulates lymphocyte responses

systemic lupus erythematosus (SLE). Increased numbers of suppressor cells are seen after viral infections such as infectious mononucleosis.

Another important function of T cells is the destruction of foreign cells, including mycobacteria, fungi, and viruses. Cytotoxic T cells are activated by antigen from these pathogens. Other lymphocytes, called "natural killer" cells, do not require specific antigen stimulation to initiate their function. Both cytotoxic T cells and natural killer cells participate in defense against tumor cells arising within the host. T Cells are also involved in the rejection of transplanted tissues.

The third function of T cells is the production of mediators that influence the response of other cell types (Table 2-5). T Cells, activated by exposure to specific antigens, secrete molecules called *lymphokines*. Mycobacteria induce the formation of lymphokines that attract and activate macrophages. Antigens from poison ivy stimulate release of lymphokines that attract basophils. Also, eosinophils, lymphocytes, and neutrophils may be recruited by lymphokines. All of these cells may play a fundamental role in host defense and in hypersensitivity reactions.

Exposure to a number of microorganisms causes development of permanent T-cell sensitization. Examples include mycobacteria, *Histoplasma, Candida*, and a number of viruses such as mumps. Skin tests of normal individuals with antigens from these pathogens causes induration, which is maximal after about 2 days. Anergy, which is the absence of response to any of these antigens, is found in patients with many chronic diseases.

B CELLS AND PLASMA CELLS. In birds, removal of the bursa of Fabricius, an organ near the cloaca, results in depletion of cells in the germinal centers of lymph nodes and in reduced antibody levels. The germinal centers of nodes, therefore, are said to be populated by bursa-derived cells (B cells). No organ that is equivalent to the bursa of Fabricius has been identified in mammals; the term "B cell" in mammals refers to "bursa-equivalent" or "bone-marrow-derived" cells. In the mammalian fetus, B cells appear first in the liver and then the marrow. Removal of the thymus does not affect the formation of B cells but may influence their function because of the lack of helper and suppressor T cells. B Cells can be identified by the presence of antibodies on their surfaces. About 25% of the peripheral blood lymphocytes in adults are B cells.

B Cells are precursors of the plasma cells that synthesize antibodies. The differentiation of B cells to plasma cells is controlled by helper and suppressor T cells (Fig. 2-1). Each clone of plasma cells makes only one type of immunoglobulin. The many different clones of plasma cells that are found in an individual are responsible for the diversity of antibody response necessary for recognition of the many antigens present in the environment.

Phagocytes

The circulating phagocytic cells are monocytes, neutrophils, and eosinophils. These cells migrate into areas of inflammation in response to specific chemotactic factors such as the complement-derived anaphylatoxin C3a and C5a, lymphokines, bacterial products, and collagen fragments and become localized at sites of invasion by microorganisms. Foreign cells are recognized specifically by circulating antibody and the complement system. The deposition of antibody and/or complement fragments on the surface of foreign cells is called *opsonization*, a process that facilitates ingestion by the phagocytes. Subsequently, a series of metabolic processes are activated that enable the phagocytes to kill the foreign cell.

MONOCYTES AND MACROPHAGES. Macrophages may arise from circulating monocytes or may be confined to specific organs. Both blood monocytes and fixed macrophages are essential participants in the inflammatory response. Macrophages are especially important in defense against intracellular parasites such as mycobacteria, *Histoplasma*, *Toxoplasma*, and viruses. Macrophages are recruited and activated by lymphokines produced in response to these microorganisms. Macrophages also respond to other causes of tissue injury and to inorganic material.

In addition to their role as phagocytes, macrophages regulate the actions of lymphocytes. Antigens are first ingested by macrophages before the antigens interact with receptors on the lymphocyte surface. In addition, macrophages secrete factors that facilitate the response of both B and T cells. Macrophages and lymphocytes are the predominant cells at sites of chronic inflammation, and their interaction seems essential for defense.

NEUTROPHILS. The first cells to appear in an acute inflammatory reaction are polymorphonuclear neutrophils. These cells contain specific lysosomal granules that can fuse with ingested material or be extruded into the extracellular environment. The granules contain a variety of degradative enzymes, including acid hydrolases, neutral proteases, and lysozyme. Activated neutrophils produce the high-energy intermediates dyroxyl radical, superoxide, and hydrogen peroxide, which aid in the killing of microbes. Inherited defects in neutrophilic migration, phagocytosis, granule function, or peroxide formation are responsible for recurrent and often fatal infections.

EOSINOPHILS. The function of eosinophils has not been determined with certainty; however, their association with parasitic infections is now clear. Mast cells, basophils, and lymphocytes secrete factors that attract eosinophils. These cells accumulate frequently at sites of parasitic infections, neoplasms, and allergic reactions. Eosinophils contain enzymes that may limit the response of other inflammatory cells, especially basophils and mast cells. Evidence accumulated over the last 5 years indicates additional roles for eosinophils. A major basic protein that is released from eosinophilic granules is toxic to schistosomula and other parasites. This protein can be recovered from the bronchial secretions of asthmatic patients and is toxic to respiratory epithelial cells. The eosinophil may thus be important in defense against helminth infections, but also may contribute to the pathogenesis of bronchial asthma.

Mast Cells and Basophils

Histamine, a substance that regulates the permeability of capillaries, is found principally in the lysosomes of tissue mast cells and circulating basophils. These cells also are distinguished by membrane receptors for IgE antibodies. Allergic reactions are initiated when antigens bind to the IgE on basophils and mast cells and cause a release of histamine and other mediators (described in Chapter 3), which cause leakage of fluid into the extravascular spaces, spasm of smooth muscle, attraction of neutrophilic and eosinophilic granulocytes, and activation of platelets.

Degranulation of basophils or mast cells can also result from interaction with fragments generated by complement activation or by factors released from lymphocytes. These mechanisms are discussed later.

Humoral Elements

The bactericidal properties of serum were recognized at the end of the nineteenth century (Table 2-1). The humoral factor that appears after the host is exposed to a microbe or other foreign substance was called an *antibody*. Antibodies interact specifically with antigens. Another humoral element, the complement system, may enhance the effects of antibodies or may directly interact with microbes.

Antibodies

Immunoglobulins that can bind to a given antigen are called *antibodies*. These proteins have a unique structure (Fig. 2-2). Each antibody has at least two heavy (H) and two light (L) chains that are bound together. An antibody consists of three compact units linked together by hinge regions. Because the linkages between the three units are highly susceptible to cleavage by certain enzymes, it has been possible to separate the units and identify the functions of the different parts of the immunoglobulin molecule. Papain digestion will produce two Fab fragments and one Fc fragment (Fig. 2-2). The Fab (antigen-binding) fragment has the ability to bind to antigens and so incorporate the antibody properties of the immunoglobulin. The Fc or "crystallizable" fragment is responsible for the unique biological properties of the five different classes of immunoglobulin.

The five different classes of immunoglobulin each have a different type of heavy

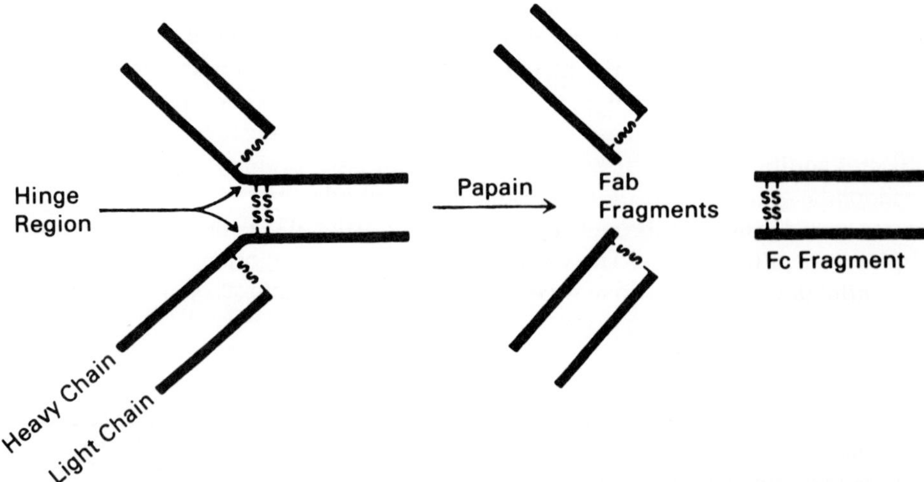

Fig. 2-2. Basic structure of immunoglobulins. These molecules can be cleaved by papain into three separate fragments. The two Fab fragments contain the antigen-binding activity of the original molecule. The Fc fragment has most of the class-specific properties of the intact immunoglobulins such as binding to complement or to specific cell types.

chain. The classes and their H chains are IgG, gamma (γ); IgA, alpha (α); IgM, mu (μ); IgD, delta (δ); and IgE, epsilon (ε). The structure of the H chains determines both the structure and the function of each class of immunoglobulin. Immunoglobulins also have two types of L chain, kappa (κ) and lambda (λ). The basic properties of each class are outlined in Table 2-6).

All immunoglobulins have at least two identical H and L chains (e.g., $\gamma_2\kappa_2$ or $\gamma_2\lambda_2$). All classes of immunoglobulin share the same structure of four chains (Fig. 2-2). The IgA type may contain two or more of these structures linked together, and IgM is normally a pentamer (Fig. 2-3).

Genetic, congenital, or acquired defects in B-cell function may cause reduced synthesis of the immunoglobulins of one or more class. These immunodeficiencies are often associated with recurrent infections, especially with pyogenic bacteria (see Chapter 31).

Increased serum concentrations of immunoglobulins are produced by chronic stimulation of the immune system. Because antibodies are formed by many different plasma cell clones, they are heterogenous. Chronic infections, liver diseases, and collagen-vascular disorders may cause polyclonal gammopathy, a heterogeneous increase in immunoglobulins. One plasma cell clone can also occasionally be responsible for an increase in immunoglobulin level. This condition is called *monoclonal gammopathy* and may be a benign condition or a plasma cell malignancy termed *multiple myeloma* or *Waldenstrom's macroglobulinemia*.

Serum protein electrophoresis (SPE) is generally used to evaluate overall immunoglobulin concentrations. A broad increase in the gamma region is typically seen in polyclonal gammopathy, whereas monoclonal gammopathy is diagnosed by a sharp spike (Fig. 2-4). If the results of SPE suggest a monoclonal gammopathy, the diagnosis is confirmed by immunoelectrophoresis. The concentrations of four of the individual

Table 2-6 *Properties of the Immunoglobulin Classes*

	IgG	IgA	IgM	IgD	IgE
Heavy chain	γ	α	μ	δ	ε
Light chain	K or λ	K or λ	K or λ	K or λ	K or λ
Subclasses	1,2,3,4	1,2	1,2		
Normal adult serum concentration (mg/dl)	800–1800	90–450	60–280	0.3–40	0.001–0.05
Serum half-life (days)	23	6	5	3	2.5
Complement activation through C_1	All but IgG_4	– –	+ +	– –	– –
Exocrine secretions	+	+ + +	+	?	±
Crosses placenta	+	– –	– –	– –	– –
Binds to mast cells and basophils	Possibly IgG_4	– –	– –	– –	+ + +
Binds to macrophages	+ +	– –	– –	– –	– –
Secretory component	– –	+	– –	– –	– –

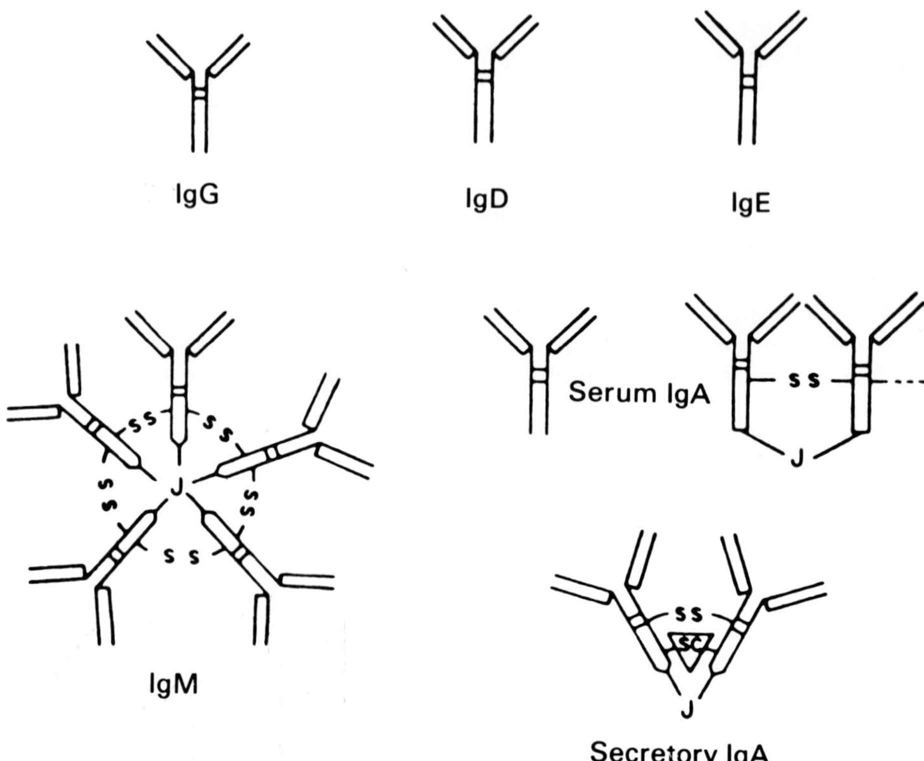

Fig. 2-3. Structure of the five classes of immunoglobulins. The IgG, IgD, and IgE types exist as monomers of the basic four-chain subunit structure shown in Figure 2-2, whereas IgM is usually a pentamer. Serum IgA can be a monomer or a polymer, and secretory IgA is a dimer. The IgM and IgA subunits are joined by disulfide bonds and by a J chain. Secretory IgA also is found by secretory component that retards the destruction of the immunoglobulin.

classes can be determined by radial immunodiffusion. A more sensitive radioimmunoassay is required to determine the concentration of IgE (see Chapter 5).

IgG. The most abundant immunoglobulin in the circulation and interstitial fluids is IgG (Table 2-6). Most serum antibodies against bacteria, viruses, and exogenous toxins are IgG immunoglobulins. Antibodies of the IgG class can adhere to macrophages and neutrophils via Fc receptors on these cells to facilitate phagocytosis. Maternal IgG crosses the placenta to become the principal antibody of the neonate. The first component of the complement system (C1) may be activated by IgG after the antibody binds to an antigen.

IgM. Antibodies of the IgM class theoretically have 10 antigen-binding sites. These antibodies bind to antigens and to C1 more efficiently than do other immunoglobulin classes. Beause of its size, IgM is generally confined to the vascular compartment, and does not cross the placenta. Because IgM is usually the first antibody that is produced after exposure to an antigen, it provides early protection against infection.

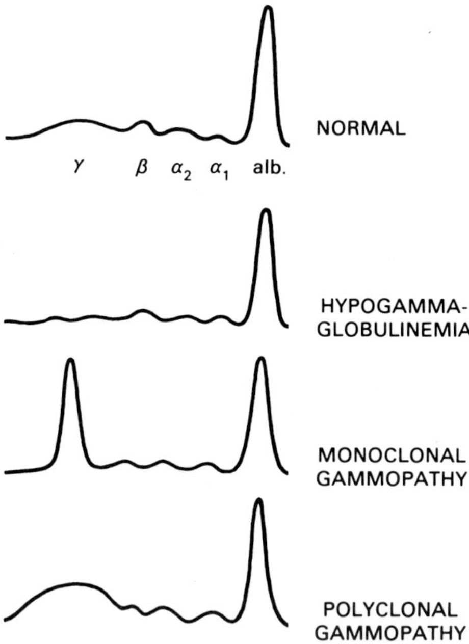

Fig. 2-4. Serum protein electrophoresis patterns. The albumin, α_1, α_2, β, and γ globulin regions are noted.

IgD. IgD is found on B cells and in small quantities in serum. The function of IgD is unknown.

IgE. In 1921 Prausnitz and Kustner discovered that serum could transfer cutaneous sensitivity to antigens and predicted the discovery of a unique class of reaginic antibodies. This class was finally isolated in 1966 and named *IgE*. Most IgE is found not in the serum, but on the surface of basophils and mast cells. Antigens that bind to IgE on these cells are called *allergens;* examples include windblown pollens, fungi, and animal danders.

Complement

The primary humoral response to the binding of antigen and antibody is activation of the complement system, which consists of approximately 20 different proteins that bind to antibodies, other complement proteins, and cell membranes and that regulate complement activation. The complement system is one of the principal effector systems of inflammation that is induced by the immune system. The complement system can also be activated by proteolytic enzymes and by bacterial cell walls without the aid of immune mechanisms. The major functions of the system in the killing of bacteria are the attraction (chemotaxis) of phagocytes, the increased adherence of phagocytes to antigens (opsonization), and cell lysis (Fig. 2-5).

The factors C1 through C9 were named in the order in which they were discovered (Fig. 2-5). Fragments formed by complement activation are indicated by small letters (for example, C5a). An important part of host defense is the binding of

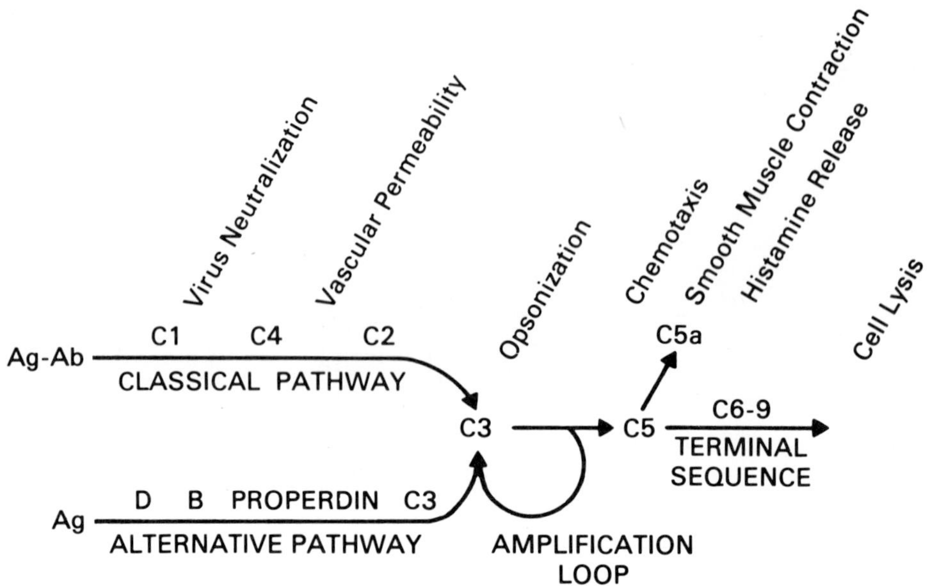

Fig. 2-5. The complement system. The two pathways for activation are illustrated. In the classic pathway, C1 binds to the Fc portion of antibodies (Ab) that have linked to appropriate antigens (Ag) to form immune complexes. In the alternative pathway, antigens on the surface of certain microorganisms permit activation of factors D, B, C3, and properdin in the absence of antibodies; C3 is the junction point of the two pathways. An amplification loop provides a positive feedback to increase the activation of later components. Subsequently, factors C5 through C9 are activated in a cascade fashion to release C5a and to form holes in cell membranes (resulting in cell lysis). The fragments and complexes formed during complement activation have multiple roles in inflammation and host defense; the major actions of complement are listed diagonally at the top of the figure.

antibodies to invading microorganisms with a secondary linkage to C1. The classic pathway is activated when C1 binds to the Fc portion of antibodies of the IgG or IgM classes. Subsequently, C4, C2, C3, and C5 through C9 are activated.

Serum can kill certain microbes even in the absence of specific antibodies because of the existence of an alternative pathway for complement activation (Fig. 2-5). Components of the cell wall of bacteria interact directly with complement factors D, B, and properdin to achieve activation of C3 and subequently C5 through C9. An amplification loop allows positive feedback, which increases the number of the molecules of C3 and C5 through C9 that are activated through either the classic or alternative pathways.

If the complement system were allowed to operate in an uncontrolled fashion, the effects would be harmful. As with most biological systems, a series of natural inhibitors regulate activation and ensure that the complement system is "turned off" most of the time. With some diseases, however, these inhibitors are overcome, and the continual activation of complement contributes to the pathologic process. An example is hereditary angioedema, in which an inhibitor of C1 is deficient. This syndrome is characterized by recurrent swelling of subcutaneous tissues, gastrointestinal (GI) tract, and respiratory system. Laryngeal obstruction secondary to edema may prove fatal.

Serum normally contains additional humoral effector mechanisms such as the coagulation, fibrinolysis, plasmin, and kallikrein systems.

HYPERSENSITIVITY REACTIONS

During the nineteenth century researchers discovered the protective role of the immune system; early in the present century the potentially harmful elements of immunity were identified. When Bordet and Richet attempted to protect dogs against a sea anemone toxin by immunizing them repeatedly with small doses of the toxin, the animals unexpectedly died of shock. Bordet and Richet coined the term "anaphylaxis" (which means "the opposite of protection") to describe this reaction. At about the same time, other researchers were investigating the protective value of serum from animals that had been immunized with diphtheria and tetanus toxins. Although most human recipients responded favorably to immunization with the serum, some developed fever, arthralgias, and rash a few weeks after they received the animal serum. This illness was called *serum sickness*. In 1906, von Pirquet defined the altered reactivity of the host after exposure to a foreign substance (allergen) as an allergy. He also distinguished the protective and harmful potential of immune responses.

Since von Pirquet's time, the elements of the immune system have been defined. The immune pathways that function as the protective mechanisms can also cause injury. Various models have been developed to investigate allergic or hypersensitivity reactions and to correlate these reactions with specific diseases. The most widely used classification, which was introduced by Gel and Coombs (1969) describes four types of hypersensitivity illustrated in Figure 2-6.

Type I Immediate Hypersensitivity

Allergic reactions that are manifest within seconds or minutes after exposure to an allergen usually involve IgE, mast cells and basophils, and several mediators. The bridging of two adjacent IgE antibodies on the cell surface triggers a series of intracellular events: increased phospholipid turnover, increased flux of calcium across the plasma membrane, and decreased cyclic-AMP (cAMP) levels. Although the precise relationships between these events are unknown, the result is release of numerous preformed mediators, such as histamine, and the synthesis of new mediators, such as slow-reacting substances (the leukotrienes), platelet activating factor, and prostaglandins (see Chapter 3). These substances cause edema, spasm of smooth muscle, granulocyte attraction, activation of platelets, and increased production of mucus. Immunoglobulin antibodies are also on the surface of basophils and mast cells. It has been suggested that these antibodies, in addition to IgE, may initiate allergic reactions.

Clinical Correlation

A typical patient with a type I reaction visits a physician because of rhinorrhea, nasal congestion and obstruction, sneezing, and conjunctivitis. Symptoms typically are worse during periods of peak pollination, which are generally the fall and spring months. Besides pollen, other substances that may provide this condition are molds,

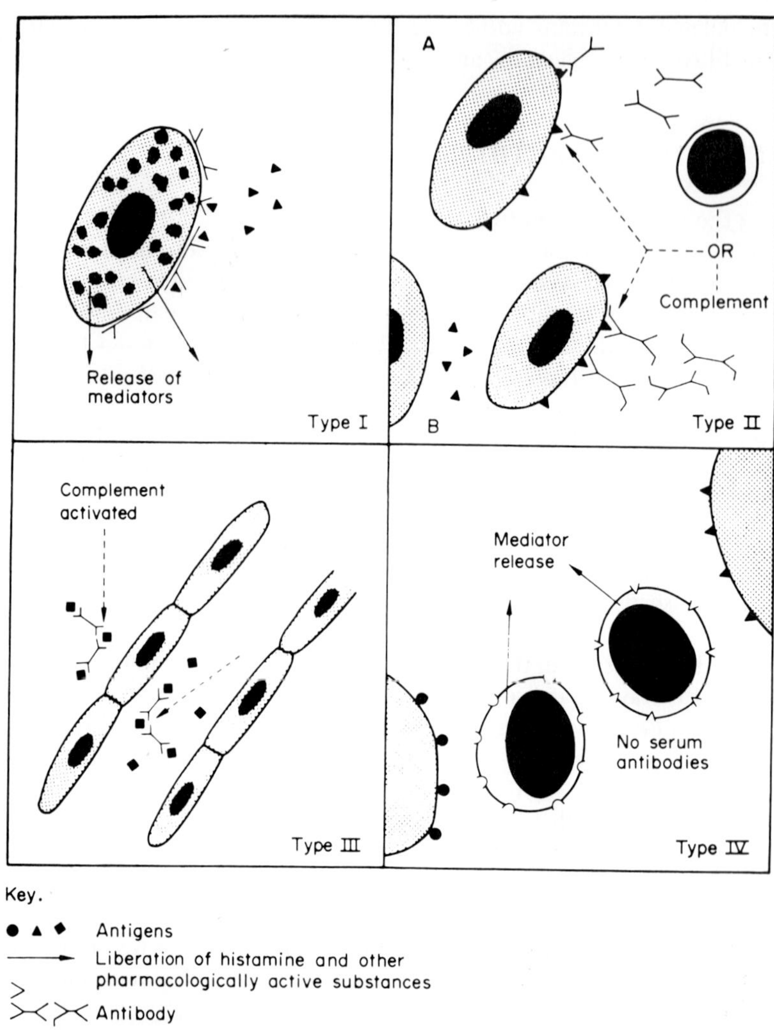

Fig. 2-6. Mechanisms of hypersensitivity reactions. From Gell, P. H., Coombs, R. R. A., & Lachmann, P. J. (Eds.), *Clinical aspects of immunology* (ed. 3). Oxford: Blackwell, 1975, p. 765. With permission.

animal danders, house dust, and (less frequently) foods. Complications of this condition include otitis and sinusitis.

Allergic rhinitis is the most common allergic condition. Although this disorder is never fatal, it impairs the normal functions of its victims significantly and often causes absences from work and school.

Nasal tissues contain a great number of mast cells. Activation of these cells by inhaled allergens results in the release of histamine, which produces edema and increased mucus production. During this process, chemotactic factors attract eosinophils, the principal cell type found in nasal secretions of patients with allergic rhinitis. As discussed previously, the role of eosinophils in the pathogenesis of allergic conditions is uncertain.

Other disorders that result from type I reactions include bronchial asthma, anaphylaxis, and urticaria.

Diagnostic Procedures

Skin testing is most frequently used to demonstrate immediate hypersensitivity. In this test, a drop of concentrated antigen is placed on the skin, which is then pricked with a needle. The wheal-and-flare response is recorded in about 15 minutes and is correlated with the degree of sensitivity to that antigen. If the prick test is negative, sensitivity may be demonstrated by intradermal injection of antigen. Another technique is measurement of IgE concentrations in serum, although total IgE is not a precise indicator of allergic conditions. The measurement of specific IgE antibodies by the radioallergosorbent test (RAST) is more helpful.

Type II Cytotoxic Hypersensitivity

Circulating antibodies may develop against antigens on the surface of cells. For example, antibodies to red cells are found in autoimmune hemolytic anemias. Penicillin binds to the red cell surface to serve as an antigen in penicillin-induced anemia. A similar process causes Rh hemolytic disease of newborn infants. Antibodies of the IgG or IgM class usually activate complement. Red cell survival is shortened by direct complement lysis or by opsonization and phagocytosis.

Other drugs may induce the formation of antibodies. Quinidine, for example, becomes attached to platelets and binds an antibody against the drug. Complement activation causes platelet destruction and thrombocytopenia.

In Goodpasture's syndrome, antibodies form against basement membrane antigens, and pulmonary and renal lesions usually develop. Immunofluorescent studies of biopsy specimens from these organs reveal a linear deposit of complement fragments and antibodies. In this syndrome, chemotactic complement products (especially C5a) attract neutrophils, which later release destructive enzymes from cellular granules.

In vitro studies have demonstrated that target cells, coated with antibody, can activate cytotoxic lymphocytes directly. This reaction may be associated with the rejection of tumors and organs that have been transplanted.

Type III Immune Complex Hypersensitivity

When antibodies combine with soluble antigens in blood, immune complexes are formed. C1 binds to the Fc portion of antibodies and complement is activated. Then C5a anaphylatoxin is generated, which can trigger release of histamine from basophils and mast cells. Histamine induces increased vascular permeability and allows immune complexes to pass easily into the extravascular space. Here again, complement activation causes the formation of chemotactic factors that attract neutrophils. Enzymes from neutrophils can then produce severe tissue damage.

Serum sickness is one example of a condition that is produced by immune complexes. In this disorder, foreign proteins that are combined with host antibodies are deposited in the skin and joints and then produce the characteristic cutaneous and arthritic symptoms.

Immune complex nephritis is another example. When this condition develops shortly following a streptococcal infection, the antigen in the complex may be derived from the streptococcus. Nephritis is also seen in SLE. In this disease, antibodies are formed against endogenous DNA and other nuclear antigens. The degree of renal impairment can be correlated with the quantity of the circulating complex. Because of continual activation of complement by the complexes, the severity of lupus can also be monitored by measuring the depression of serum complement.

Type IV Delayed Hypersensitivity

The reaction of T cells to microbes is extremely important for suppression of chronic fungal, tuberculous, and viral infections; however, an excessive response can lead to extensive formation of granulomas by macrophages and lymphocytes. The enzymes from macrophages may produce necrosis. An extensive reaction in the lung may cause cavitation and further impairment of respiration.

Many substances can induce delayed hypersensitivity, which is often manifest as contact dermatitis. Antigens (e.g., urushiol from poison ivy and other organic and inorganic chemicals) combine with skin proteins to produce a complete antigen. A mononuclear reaction develops with infiltration of cells into the upper dermis within 4–6 hours. Later, the infiltration extends into the epidermis. Erythema and edema occur, and epithelial vesicles may form. Within 1–2 days following antigen exposure, basophilic infiltration is often noted. Factors are released by lymphocytes that attract basophils and induce degranulation with the release of histamine. In this reaction, histamine may be responsible for some of the symptoms of erythema and pruritus.

The etiology of contact dermatitis can often be determined by patch testing with antigens. The cutaneous response is noted in 2 days and may be correlated with allergic sensitivity. The use of intradermal testing with mycobacterial and fungal antigens to establish that cellular immune mechanisms are intact was discussed earlier.

REFERENCES

Gell, P. H. H. and Coombs, R. R. A. (Eds.) *Clinical aspects of immunology*. 2nd ed. Philadelphia: F. A. Davis Co., 1969.

Prausnitz, C., and Kustner, H. *Bakteriol*. 1921, *86*, 160.

Richet, C. *Anaphylaxis*. London: University Press, Constable, 1913.

Von Pirquet, C. *Munch. Med. Worcenschr*, 1906, *53*, 1457.

SUGGESTED READINGS

Barrett, J. T. *Basic immunology and its medical application*. St. Louis: Mosby, 1980.

Middleton, E., Reed, C. E., and Ellis, E. F. *Allergy Principles and Practice*. St. Louis: Mosby, 1978.

Parker, C. W. *Clinical immunology*. Philadelphia: Saunders, 1980.

QUESTIONS

For each type of cell (1–3), select the most closely associated function (a–e).

1. Basophil
2. Macrophage
3. Eosinophil

   a. ingests antigens prior to presentation to lymphoid cells
   b. produces superoxide and hydrogen peroxide
   c. releases a major basic protein that is toxic to certain parasites
   d. secretes antibodies
   e. has receptors for IgE

4. True statements concerning typical laboratory findings in allergic asthma include

   a. circulating immune complexes
   b. positive immediate skin tests
   c. positive patch tests
   d. positive lung biopsy for complement fragments in the basement membrane
   e. increased serum IgE

5. Complement functions include

   a. releasing histamine from mast cells
   b. attracting neutrophils
   c. increasing neutrophil phagocytosis of bacteria
   d. cytolysis of microorganisms
   e. red cell lysis

Answers can be found in Appendix B at the end of the book.

Charles W. Parker

3

Allergic Mediators

Broadly speaking, the allergic diseases constitute a diverse group of clinical syndromes. These include classic allergic respiratory diseases, allergic pneumonitis, anaphylaxis, serum sickness, autoimmunity, systemic and organ-directed reactions including contact skin sensitivity, transplantation rejection, and various types of allergic response to infectious agents and neoplasms. The pathophysiology of this diverse group of diseases involves a complex array of mediators that vary with the type and stage of the reaction. These mediators may be classified as (a) low-molecular-weight mediators of acute allergic reactions such as histamine, platelet activating factor (PAF), slow reacting substance (SRS), leukotriene B, and other arachidonate metabolites; (b) polypeptide mediators such as bradykinin and the biologically active complement fragments C3a and C5a; and (c) protein and glycoprotein mediators released from lymphoid cells that help in regulating the immune response and are generally designated as monokines (from monocytes), lymphokines (from lymphocytes), or neutrokines (from neutrophils), depending on the cell type in which they originate. Since this book is concerned primarily with allergic responses of the immediate hypersensitivity type (type I), particular emphasis is given to the mediators involved in these reactions.

MEDIATOR FORMATION AND RELEASE

The mediators that are known or suspected to be important in immediate hypersensitivity generally are capable of inducing smooth-muscle contraction and increased vascular permeability, accounting for the changes in the skin, nose, and lower respiratory tract that characterize most acute allergic reactions in humans. If a short-lived allergic stimulus is involved, the mediators are released acutely at the time of the stimulus and act for relatively short periods (often less than 1 hour), and the response subsides with little or no inflammatory residue. The rapidly appearing

ALLERGY: THEORY AND PRACTICE
ISBN 0-8089-1619-X

wheal-and-flare response seen in skin during immediate type hypersensitivity testing with environmental antigens is an example of this type of response. When the stimulus is more marked and prolonged, the response may continue for many hours. In addition, the spectrum of mediators may change during this time, and an inflammatory exudate will almost certainly form. Even apparently pure IgE responses may persist for many hours, particularly in highly sensitive individuals who are challenged with large amounts of antigen.

Mediators may either exist preformed or be generated de novo at the time the response is initiated. Most of the important mediators in IgE-mediated allergic reactions are produced primarily by mast cells and basophils. Other leukocytes may share this capability or even be more important sources depending on the mediator and the type of stimulus. The particular cell involved in mediator release depends on the tissue. Mast cells are prominent in small blood vessels and connective tissue throughout the body, including the skin and lung. Basophils are primarily circulating cells but under special circumstances may secondarily infiltrate the skin, kidney, and nasal and bronchial secretions and participate in allergic responses locally. Despite the ability of basophils to infiltrate tissues, the cells involved in allergic reactions in the skin and lung presumably are primarily mast cells.

The importance of mast cells and basophils in allergy is due to the presence of high-affinity IgE receptors on their surfaces that permit them to bind IgE antibodies and become sensitized. When reexposure to an antigen that has produced IgE antibodies occurs, cell-bound IgE molecules become bridgd by the antigen and there is an acute biochemical response on the part of the cell that leads to the appearance of mediators outside the cell. The release of mediators may involve the actual extrusion of granules outside the cell or the formation of communications from the cell surface into granules still inside in the cell. The exact nature of this biochemical signal is still poorly understood but probably involves changes in phospholipid metabolism, the release of free arachidonic acid (AA) and formation of AA metabolites, cellular uptake of Ca^{2+}, and the introduction of phosphate groups on the IgE receptor and other intracellular proteins (protein phosphorylation). Regardless of the mechanism, there appear to be close parallels between secretion from mast cells and basophils and other cell types with a major secretory function such as the beta cells in pancreatic inlets.

In addition to IgE antibodies, there are a variety of other known or suspected mechanisms for triggering mast cells and basophils to release their mediators, including (a) sensitization and immunologic activation through minor reagenic antibodies (in humans, probably mainly IgG_4); (b) exposure to C3a and C5a, which are activated complement fragments with histamine releasing and other biologic activities; (c) stimulation with polybasic molecules such as polymyxin B and cationic polypeptides from neutrophils; (d) stimulation with kinins (basic oligopeptides released enzymatically from high-molecular-weight protein substrates in plasma during clotting); (e) hyperosmolar media (radiopaque contrast media and hypertonic glucose solutions); and (f) lymphokines. These stimuli provide alternative mechanisms for releasing allergic mediators when IgE antibodies are not available or are no longer operative. For example, production of C3a and C5a may be the basis for classic anaphylactic symptoms such as urticaria during otherwise typical serum sickness reactions where complement-fixing antibodies primarily of the IgG type appear to be involved and IgE antibodies may not be demonstrable. The availability of non-

IgE-dependent systems for mediator release can also explain why apparently nonimmunologic stimuli such as the radiopaque contrast media produce reactions that are clinically very similar or identical to acute anaphylaxis.

There are many individuals with chronic urticaria, rhinitis, or asthma in whom proof of IgE-mediated allergy is not obtainable, and it is suspected that the usual allergic mediators are released by some other immunologic or nonimmunologic mechanism. At this time, however, there is little direct evidence that mast cell or basophil products are involved, and other explanations for their symptoms need to be considered.

Clearly, the major factor in environmental allergy is an increased production of IgE antibodies; however, it is possible that other factors may significantly influence the allergic response. For instance, there is still much to be learned about possible differences between individuals in the lung and skin content of histamine and other mediators and their roles in the provocation of allergic symptoms, and it is also possible that some individuals more readily release their mast cell or basophil mediators than do others, resulting in a greater response to the same stimulus. Moreover, there may be differences in tissue responsiveness to histamine and other mediators, as suggested by the increased responsiveness of the airway in allergic individuals to inhalation challenge with histamine or methacholine. Studies in inbred guinea pigs have suggested that real differences may exist in the content and releasability of allergic mediators in lung between different strains. These differences appear to be correlated with the susceptibility of the animals to systemic anaphylaxis and bronchospasm. In this connection allergic and nonallergic individuals appear to differ from one another in pupillary response to adrenergic and cholinergic agents, suggesting that the changes in pharmacologic reactivity are not necessarily limited to areas of increased allergic reactivity. Subgroups of patients with chronic idiopathic urticaria and nonallergic asthma whose basophils release histamine spontaneously have been described, but much additional study is needed before it can be concluded that the *in vitro* results have relevance for their symptoms.

Our present knowledge of the mediators involved in human hypersensitivity is based on a number of different experimental approaches, including direct measurements of the mediators or their metabolites in tissues, blood, serosal fluid or urine at various times during hypersensitivity reactions *in vivo* and study of isolated cells, tissues, and cultured cell lines for the type and quantity of mediators produced. The most useful *in vitro* systems for the study of IgE-mediated allergy in humans have been peripheral blood leukocytes (with basophils as the responding cell) and chopped surgical or autopsy lung specimens (with mast cells as the responding cell). These systems are generally used as crude cell mixtures in which the vast majority of cells are not directly involved in the response, but with special efforts nearly homogenous responding cell preparations can be obtained. Other experimental approaches involve study of the pure mediators or mixtures of mediators with isolated smooth-muscle and blood vessel preparations, other tissue systems or isolated cells for determination of their potency and spectrum of action, and susceptibility to pharmacologic inhibition; analysis of pathologic and physiologic changes after inhalation or injection of the mediators *in vivo;* evaluation with selective inhibitors of mediator biosynthesis (e.g., inhibitors of prostaglandin synthesis) or end organ action (e.g., the antihistamines) *in vivo* in terms of their effectiveness in reducing the symptoms and physiologic or pathologic manifestations of allergy; and analysis of individuals with proliferative disorders involving mediator-producing cells (mastocytosis, basophilic, leukemia). Approaches such as these have provided important insights into the major mediators involved in human allergy.

Despite the availability of these and a number of useful animal systems to study hypersensitivity and the role of mediators, there are still significant gaps in our knowledge. Although measurements of mediators in skin biopsy specimens and special skin chambers are acceptable research techniques in human beings, ethical considerations obviously preclude similar studies in critical immunologic target organs such as the lung. Measurements in sputum and nasal secretions pose no ethical difficulties but have proved to be difficult to interpret because of sampling and standardization problems. Many immunologic reactions are primarily localized to a single organ such as the lung. For allergic mediators produced in a variety of tissues such as histamine, measurements in blood and urine have not been particularly informative because of the background of mediator synthesis outside the target organ. Even if mediators are not produced elsewhere in the body the mediators may be so potent and biologically labile that negative results in blood or urine are meaningless. Administration of pure mediators by aerosol or injection does not deliver the mediators into the precise areas where release occurs during ongoing allergic reactions *in vivo*, and the results may thus be misleading. Life-threatening allergic reactions such as systemic anaphylaxis cannot be deliberately induced experimentally in humans. Whereas anaphylactic reactions do occur in medical practice, particularly in response to drugs, because of their unexpected and catastrophic nature and the marked lability of many of the suspected mediators, they do not lend themselves readily to systematic study. None of the mediator inhibitors used to block allergic responses is absolutely specific or completely effective in its action. Animal systems have provided important insights in terms of different types of allergic mediators and the spectrum of allergic tissue responses in which they participate. There are marked interspecies differences in allergic mechanisms, however, making extrapolations from one species to another very difficult. Knowledge as to the local concentrations of mediators achieved during hypersensitivity reactions *in vivo* is limited.

INDIVIDUAL MEDIATORS

Histamine

The existence of histamine (5-β-imidazolylethylamine) and its importance in allergic responses has been recognized for many years. The overall potential of histamine as an immunologic regulatory molecule has been recognized only within the past decade, suggesting important functions for histamine in addition to its role in immediate hypersensitivity. Since other allergic mediators may subserve similar regulatory functions, this information for histamine is discussed in some detail.

Most or all of the histamine in the tissues involved in hypersensitivity responses is present in either mast cells or basophils. The primary mode of synthesis of histamine is through the action of the enzyme, histidine decarboxylase. Histamine is stored in mast cell and basophil granules in a preformed state, probably in the form of a complex with heparin. Since mast cells contain relatively large quantities of histamine, it has been estimated that extracellular histamine concentrations as high as

100 μM may occur transiently in tissues in areas where mast cells are abundant. Histamine acts on small blood vessels, primarily at postcapillary venules to increase their permeability. Histamine also produces smooth-muscle contraction. Bronchospasm is induced when histamine is given by aerosol to allergic individuals, although there is little or no response in normals. These actions are blocked by conventional (H_1) antihistamines such as pyrilamine and involve cellular receptors with most of their specificity directed toward the ethylamine side chain of histamine. Effects of histamine on acid production on the stomach and its anti-inflammatory effects on leukocytes are blocked by H_2-type antagonists such as cymetidine and involve receptors that primarily recognize the imidazole ring of histamine. The H_2 effects of histamine appear to be exerted through increases in intracellular cAMP and are frequently similar to those of β-adrenergic agents. The early wheal-and-flare responses in the skin involving IgE antibodies reach a maximum after 15–30 minutes and are blocked almost entirely by H_1-type antihistamines. However, some of the late cutaneous responses involving IgE antibodies referred to previously require a combination of H_1 and H_2 antihistamines for effective suppression.

Attempts to follow allergic reactions in the lungs through measurements of serum or urinary histamine or its metabolites have almost always been unsuccessful. Increases in blood or urinary histamine have been reported only under special circumstances such as in acute asthma induced by deliberate antigen challenge or vigorous exercise, and even here, the changes have been inconsistent. The failure to observe consistent increases in histamine levels relates to the existence in blood and tissues of enzymes that rapidly metabolize histamine. In addition, histamine is filtered at the glomerulus and is rapidly excreted in the urine when systemic levels are elevated. Larger changes are seen during urticarial skin lesions involving an entire extremity in subjects with cold urticaria. Rises in blood histamine have been also described during acute systemic anaphylaxis. Attempts to distinguish between allergic and nonallergic asthma or other forms of chronic respiratory disease by measurement of histamine metabolites in the urine have not been useful. In addition to its effects as an allergic mediator, histamine can affect immune function in a number of other ways:

INHIBITION OF LEUKOCYTE FUNCTION. Histamine produces a variety of inhibitory effects on leukocyte function *in vitro*. In general, these actions appear to be mediated through H_2 receptors and increases in cAMP. Histamine is capable of inhibiting T-cell proliferation, lymphokine production by T and B lymphocytes, lymphocyte-mediated cytotoxicity, and enzyme secretion by neutrophils. Histamine may also regulate its own secretion since human peripheral blood basophils secrete less histamine when the histamine concentration in the medium is above 0.1 mM. These observations suggest the possibility of unexpected effects of antihistamines, particularly the H_2 blockers on immune responsiveness *in vivo*. Relatively high concentrations of histamine are required for these effects *in vitro*, however, raising questions about the physiologic importance of leukocyte modulation by histamine *in vivo*. Even with the extensive use of histamine H_2 receptor antagonists such as cimetidine for peptic ulcer, effects on circulating lymphocyte numbers, antibody synthesis, and delayed hypersensitivity reactions *in vivo* have been relatively unimpressive.

DELAYED HYPERSENSITIVITY. Histamine and other mast cell mediators may play a role in some forms of delayed-type hypersensitivity responses (DTH) in the skin.

Certain DTH responses in humans and guinea pigs, particularly those with erytherma but no induration, may be associated with basophilic infiltration in the skin, and partial basophilic degranulation is frequently observed in these areas. It can thus be assumed that mediator release is occurring locally. In rodents, which have very few basophils and are often resistant to histamine, cutaneous mast cells undergo similar changes during DTH responses and serotonin antagonists are markedly inhibitory. Histamine and serotonin are also apparently important in experimental models for multiple sclerosis in mice. The available evidence is that they act by promoting the migration of sensitized lymphocytes into the nervous system.

SERUM SICKNESS–VASCULITIS. Still another general action of vasoactive mediators is to condition the walls of small blood vessels to the local deposition of the immune complexes. It has been known for some time that immune complex glomerulonephritis in rabbits is markedly inhibited by histamine and serotonin antagonists, and there is some evidence that H_1 antihistamines may exert a similar effect in preventing serum sickness in humans.

CHEMOTAXIS. Histamine is also chemotactic for eosinophils, which may help to explain the association of eosinophilic tissue infiltration with allergy.

PROTEIN BIOSYNTHESIS. Histamine regulates complement synthesis in monocytes and the production of suppressor lymphokines by T cells.

One of the questions that remains partially unanswered is the extent to which histamine continues to contribute to allergic reactions *in vivo* when the response has been in progress for hours or days. What is known is that histamine can be resynthesized *in vivo* in mast cells over a several-week period following granule release from these cells. Histamine synthesis has been demonstrable in isolated mast cells or organ cultures containing mast cells. Recently a lymphokine produced by T cells has been described in mice that induces increases in histidine decarboxylase activity and promotes histamine formation in immature or even apparently mature lymphoid cell preparations containing mast cells. It has also been recently shown that activated T lymphocytes produce products that directly stimulate the growth and replication of mast cell and basophil precursors in the bone marrow, thymus, and peripheral lymphoid tissue. This provides a potential mechanism for expanding the number of mast cells and basophils available for participation in immediate hypersensitivity reactions. In addition, there are lymphocyte products that directly stimulate or potentiate histamine release, including immune interferon, a protein with other interesting properties that is presently undergoing intensive study for its possible therapeutic value in preventing viral infections or slowing tumor growth. Such lymphokines provide possible mechanisms for helping sustain allergic responses by ensuring a further source of mediators and by promoting mediator release through non-IgE-dependent mechanisms following the initial IgE-dependent phase of the response.

Arachidonate Metabolites

Arachidonic acid (AA) is a polyunsaturated C-20 fatty acid. It is usually numbered from the carboxy end of the molecule. Thus the carboxyl carbon is number 1 and the final carbon is number 20 (Fig. 3-1). The double bonds of AA are at the 5, 8,

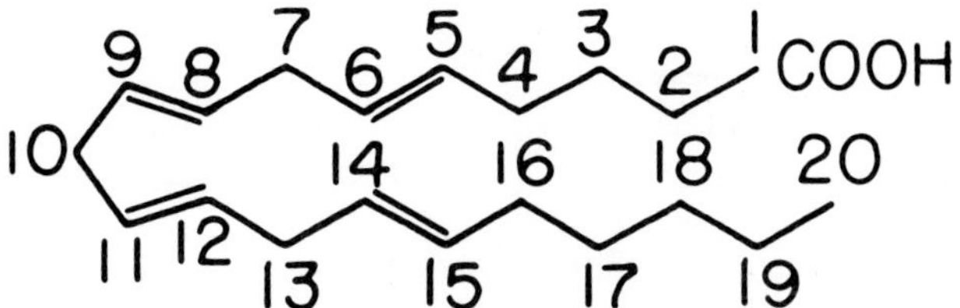

Fig. 3-1. Structure of arachidonic acid. From Snider, D. E. and Parker, C. W. Prostaglandins. In *Allergy: Principles and Practice*. edited by E. Middleton, C. E. Reed and E. F. Ellis. St. Louis: C. V. Mosby Company, 1978, p. 531, Fig. 30-1.

11, and 14 positions. The four double bonds make AA very flexible biosynthetic precursor, partially explaining why it is metabolized to so many biologically important products. The two major pathways of AA metabolism in mammalian cells are the cyclooxygenase and lipoxygenase pathways (Fig. 3-2).

Lipoxygenase products of known or suspected importance in allergy are produced through the 5-lipoxygenase pathway and include the leukotrienes [SRS and leukotriene B (LTB_4)] and 5-hydroxyeicosatetraenoic acid (5-HETE). The major cyclooxygenase products are the primary prostaglandins (especially PGE_2, PGD_2, and $PGF_{2\alpha}$), thromboxane A_2 (TxA_2), and prostacyclin (PGI_2) (Fig. 3-3). These various AA metabolites differ in their cells of origin, stability, and biologic actions frequently demonstrating antagonistic effects.

For AA to be metabolized, it must be released from its cellular stores in phospholipids and triglycerides. The mechanism of this release is still not completely understood. One enzyme that may be involved is phospholipase A_2 which removes

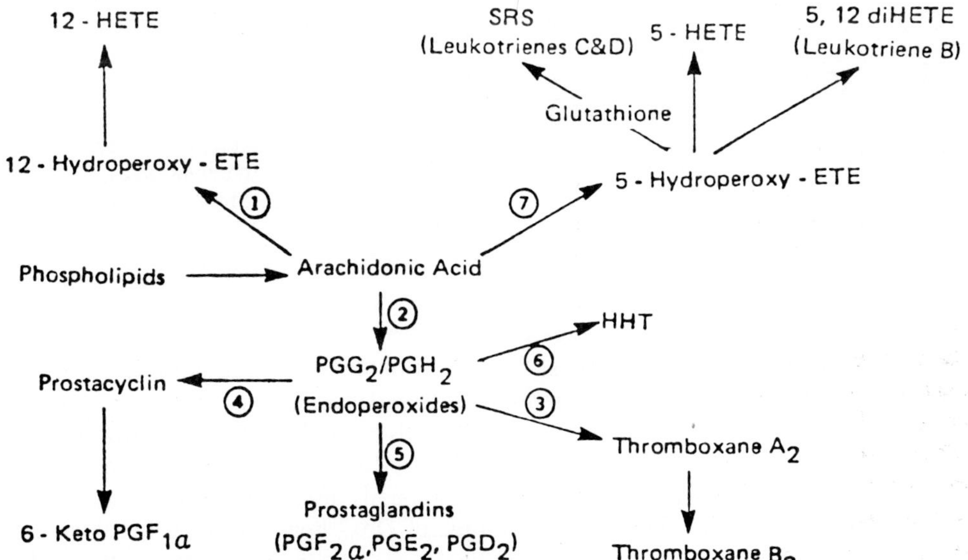

Fig. 3-2. Pathways of arachidonic metabolism.

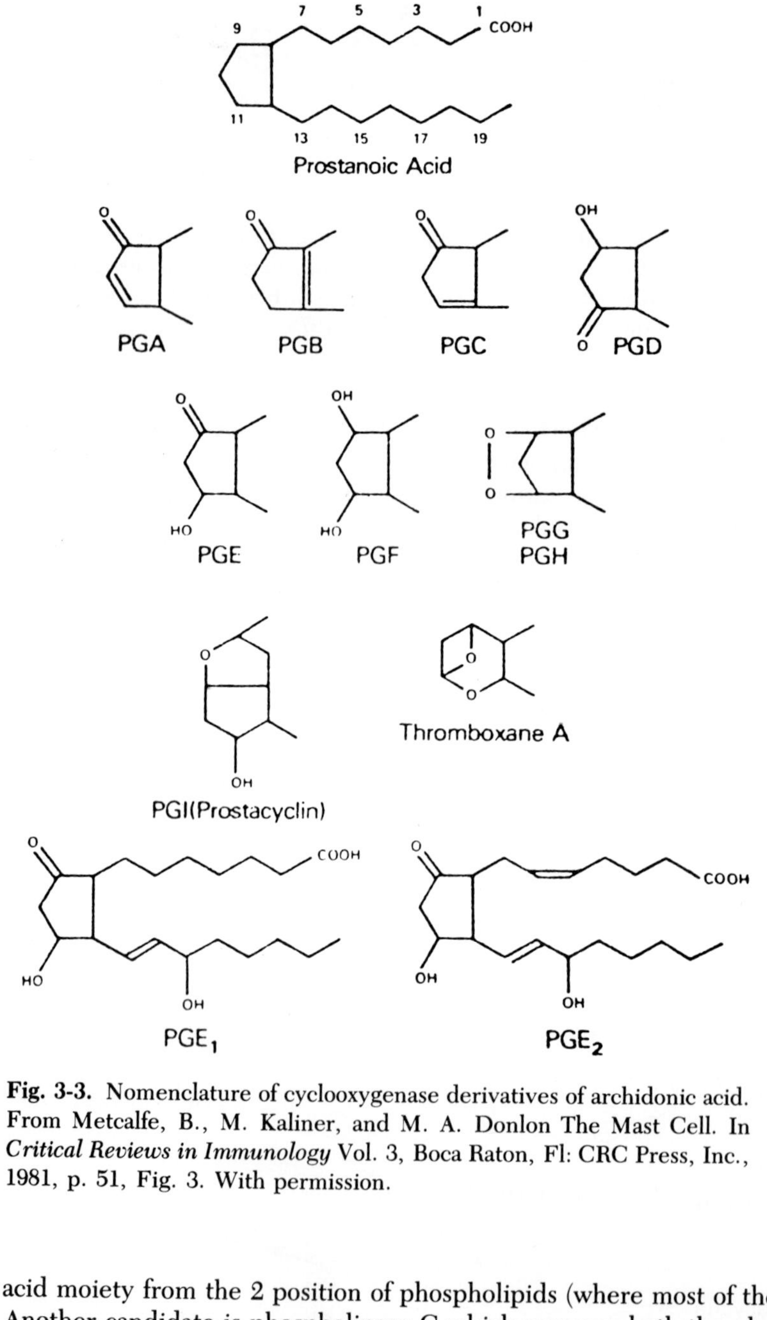

Fig. 3-3. Nomenclature of cyclooxygenase derivatives of archidonic acid. From Metcalfe, B., M. Kaliner, and M. A. Donlon The Mast Cell. In *Critical Reviews in Immunology* Vol. 3, Boca Raton, Fl: CRC Press, Inc., 1981, p. 51, Fig. 3. With permission.

the fatty acid moiety from the 2 position of phospholipids (where most of the AA is located). Another candidate is phospholipase C which removes both the phosphate group and the polar side chains from phospholipids to produce diacylglycerol (DAG). Diacylglycerol is further degraded by DAG lipase to produce monoacyglycerol and free fatty acids. It accumulates rapidly in mast cells after stimulation of mediator release and these cells contain large amounts of DAG lipase activity. Involvement of this enzyme can explain the rapid incorporation of radioactivity into phosphatidic acid and back into phosphatidyl inositol in $^{32}PO_4^{2-}$-labeled cells that occurs in many different cell types deriving activation at the cell surface since both of these products are rapidly synthesized from DAG. Both phospholipase A_2 and phospholipase-C activation probably occur through calcium-dependent mechanisms. Further elucidation of the mechanism of AA release is of some importance since pharmacologic suppression of release represents one possible approach to the control of AA metabolite formation. In this connection, it is of interest that a protein with a molecular weight of about 40,000 has recently been described that promotes the release of AA in crude lung systems stimulated with antigen. Interestingly, the release of this protein is apparently inhibited by corticosteroids, suggesting one possible level of action of corticosteroids in the treatment of ongoing allergic responses involving the lung.

The 5-lipoxygenase involved in leukotriene biosynthesis differs from the other enzymes of the AA pathway in that it is largely inactive until the cells are stimulated. Since the enzyme is Ca^{2+}-dependent, this activation may be due to an influx of Ca^{2+} into the cytoplasm.

Lipoxygenases metabolize fatty acid with at least two double bonds separated by three carbons inserting a hydroperoxy group and producing a new arrangement of double bonds. In addition to 5-lipoxygenase, lipoxygenases exist that act elsewhere in the AA molecule, the most notable of which is the 12-lipoxygenase in platelets that produce 12-HETE. Possible sources of 5-lipoxygenase products in tissue include mast cells, basophils, macrophages, polymorphonuclear lymphocytes, and possibly lymphocytes.

The cyclooxygenase produces a nine-membered ring structure (cyclopentane ring) that utilizes the 8, 9, 10, 11, and 12 carbons of the original AA molecule. The initial products produced, PGG_2 and PGH_2, differ from one another as to whether a peroxy or hydroxy group is present at the 15 position. The PGH_2 product can be used for prostaglandin, TxA_2 or PGI_2 synthesis. Anti-inflammatory agents such as aspirin and indomethacin block the cycloxygenase enzyme itself, reducing PGG_2 and PGH_2 formation and inhibiting the production of all of these products, although not necessarily to the same extent.

Slow-Reacting Substance

Slow-reacting substance was originally described in 1940 by Kellaway and Trethewie as a factor produced in lungs perfused with antigens. It produced a characteristic slow but exceptionally sustained contractile response in appropriate smooth-muscle preparations. In contrast to histamine, SRS is not preformed but is generated acutely at the time that mast cells or basophils are stimulated. It is not stored in granules either before or after the response. In 1977 our laboratory reported that SRS was a metabolite of AA through the lipoxygenase pathway (Jakschik et al, 1977). We subsequently showed that the molecule contains sulfur bound in thioether linkage. Once the precursors of the molecule became known, it was soon possible to identify SRS as a family of C-20 fatty acids with glutathione, cysteinyl-glycine, or cysteine in their side chains. The glutathionyl form of the SRS molecule (also termed *leukotriene C*) is produced first and subsequently metabolized to cysteinyl-glycine SRS, leukotriene D, and finally to cysteinyl SRS (leukotriene E) (Fig. 3-4). These different SRS species differ in their relative activities in various smooth-muscle preparations, but they all are more potent than histamine in both rat and isolated

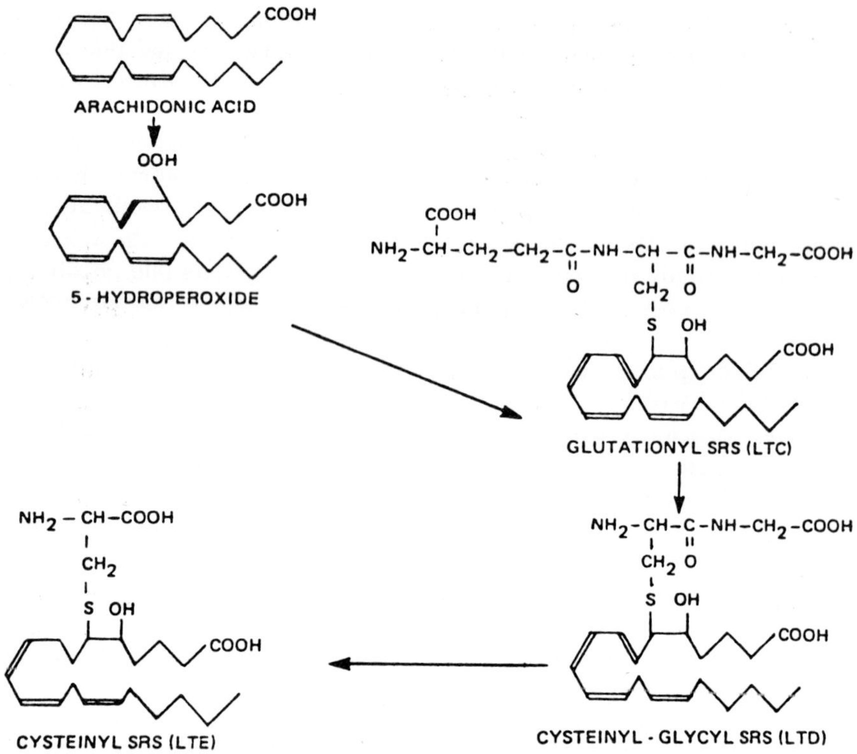

Fig. 3-4. Proposed sequence for the formation of several major SRS species beginning with glutathionyl SRS with subsequent conversion to cysteinyl-glycyl SRS. From C. W. Parker SRS-A of rat basophil leukemia and rat mast cells in 4th Symposium on Biochemistry of Allergic Reactions, 1980.

guinea pig intestinal smooth muscle and in human and guinea pig trachobronchial smooth-muscle preparations. They decay sufficiently rapidly that very little, if any, of the original SRS is still available after 15 minutes, and by 1 hour almost all is in the cysteinyl form. LTC is degraded to LTD by enzymes that catalyze the transfer of gamma glutamyl groups. The conversion of LTD to LTE is promoted by amino or carboxypeptides peptidases that remove the glycine moiety from the SRS molecule. These degradations occur in both tissues and blood. Slow-reacting substance may also be active in peripheral airways. It has been identified in human sputum and lung and is produced during IgE-dependent stimulation of sensitized lung fragments. Since inhibitors of the cycloxygenase pathway and antihistamines are seldom helpful in asthma, this has suggested the possible importance of SRS in the bronchospasm of asthma. Slow-reacting substance also alters vascular permeability and produces wheal and erythema response in the skin. The presence of SRS receptors in the ileum suggests a role for SRS in IgE-mediated expulsion of parasites from the intestine. Slow-reacting substance also affects nerve impulses in the central nervous system (CNS), producing a very long sustained effect, not unlike its effect on smooth muscle contractility in the intestine.

The source of SRS in IgE-mediated reactions in lung and skin remains to be clearly defined. It has been difficult to stimulate isolated rat peritoneal mast cells to produce SRS in IgE-dependent systems. Since it now appears that macrophages have IgE receptors, they must be considered as another possible source of SRS during allergic reactions. On the other hand, mast cells clearly have the biosynthetic capabilities to produce SRS and remain an important possibility as biosynthetic sourses of SRS as shown by their responses to some immunologic stimuli. Moreover, it has recently been reported that isolated human lung mast cells produce SRS (MacGlashan, 1982).

At present, there are no therapeutic agents available for clinical use that selectively inhibit SRS biosynthesis or end organ action. The Fisons compound, FPL55712, has been useful in investigational work. It is a selective end organ antagonist for SRS but is unstable *in vivo* and is not itself a practical candidate as a pharmacologically useful SRS inhibitor.

Agents that lower intracellular glutathione levels in SRS-producing cells with 25% or less of the original levels profoundly inhibit SRS biosynthesis. It remains to be seen, however, whether this approach could be used on a long-term basis in the absence of serious toxicity. Several long-chain fatty acids with triple instead of double bonds selectively inhibit the 5-lipoxygenase pathway; however, it remains to be shown that these agents are sufficiently nontoxic *in vivo.* Any antagonists of the 5-lipoxygenase itself, of course, will affect the formation of two other potential mediators of the 5-lipoxygenase pathway—5-HETE and 5,12-dihydroxyeicosatetraenoic acid (5,12-di-HETE).

In contrast to the cyclooxygenase pathway, the lipoxygenase pathway is not inhibited by anti-inflammatory agents such as aspirin and indomethacin. Indeed, some of the anti-inflammatory agents may inhibit the peroxidase enzyme that converts the 5-hydroperoxide to 5-HETE. The formation of 5,12-di-HETE and SRS may thus be promoted by these agents as well as by the increased availability of AA due to inhibition of the cycloxygenase. This is a possible explanation for the enhancing effect of aspirin and indomethacin in individuals with aspirin-sensitive asthma.

Leukotriene B

Leukotriene B (5,12-di-HETE or LTB_4) is another product of the 5-lipoxygenase pathway that may be important in allergic inflammation. It has potent chemotactic and chemokinetic activity on neutrophils and probably other leukocytes, including eosinophils, producing effects at concentrations as low as 10^{-11} *M*. It also aggregates neutrophils and promotes the release of lysosomal enzymes from these cells. It is much less active in its effect on smooth-muscle contractility and vascular permeability than is SRS. It is rapidly degraded by neutrophils to products that are hydroxylated or carboxylated at the 20 position, and it may be an important regulator of leukocyte chemotaxis *in vivo,* although much further work is needed to substantiate this possibility.

Under ordinary circumstances, 5-HETE is quantitatively the most prominent of the 5-lipoxygenase products. It is active in stimulating chemotaxis at concentrations of 1×10^{-6} *M* and higher and also promotes the release of granule enzymes or histamine from neutrophils or mast cells. Interestingly, 5-HETE can be incorporated covalently into phospholipids and triglycerides, providing a means of altering membrane structure and perhaps contributing to the changes in membrane function that accomplish these stimulatory effects.

Thromboxanes

The thromboxane TxA_2 is produced from the cyclooxygenase product PGH_2 by the enzyme thromboxane synthease. It is produced primarily by platelets and macrophages. It is a potent constrictor of vascular and airway smooth muscle. It also aggregates platelets and leukocytes and produces granule enzyme release in platelets. Although the mechanism of action of TxA_2 is not known, it has been shown to lower cAMP in platelets. At 37°C TxA_2 is rapidly hydrolyzed nonenzymatically to thromboxane B_2 (TxB_2), which is biologically inactive. Estimates of TxA_2 formation are usually made by measuring TxB_2. Substituted imidazoles selectively inhibit thromboxane synthesis, but their use has been limited to experimental animals. Stable and selective agonists and antagonists of TxA_2 are not available.

Prostacyclin (PGI_2)

Prostacyclin, another cyclooxygenase product, is also very labile chemically. It is produced by vascular endothelial cells and macrophages. It dilates airway smooth muscle and blood vessels apparently through its ability to elevate the intracellular cAMP levels. Because of its lability, PGI_2 formation is determined by measurements of 6-keto PGF, its inactive hydrolyses product.

Prostaglandins

Prostaglandin E_2 (PGE_2) is another cAMP agonist that dilates smooth muscle and blood vessels and, like PGI_2, may suppress acute allergic responses. It is produced by virtually all cells. It is produced in very substantial quantities by macrophages and to a lesser extent by polymorphonuclear leukocytes. It induces maturation of immature T and B lymphocytes. In mature leukocytes it is ordinarily inhibitory, decreasing mitogenesis and lymphokine release both in T and B lymphocytes and macrophages. Neutrophil-mediated cytotoxicity as well as enzyme and mediator release from mast cells, neutrophils, and macrophages are also inhibited. Prostaglandin E_2 has been suspected to be involved in the reduction of cellular immunity associated with Hodgkin's lymphomas in humans. Long-acting PGE_2 analogs suppress allograft rejection and immune complex gloneurolonephritis in animals but cause side reactions such as diarrhea in humans, making it uncertain whether this pharmacologic action will be really useful clinically. Prostaglandin E_2 is rapidly destroyed in the circulation by enzymes that convert its 15-*OH* group to a keto group, making it unlikely that it acts as a circulating hormone as was originally postulated.

In contrast to PGE_2, PGD_2, $PDF_{2\alpha}$, and its metabolite 15-keto $PGF_{2\alpha}$ all constrict bronchial smooth muscle, suggesting the possibility of their involvement in the bronchoconstriction associated with asthma. The compound PGD_2 is primarily a product of mast cells, which produce it in very considerable quantities; thus it is likely to be present during acute allergic reactions in the skin and lung. These cells produce much less $PGF_{2\alpha}$ than PGD_2; however, histamine-stimulated $PGF_{2\alpha}$ formation in chopped human lung fragments has been demonstrated, suggesting an alternative source of $PGF_{2\alpha}$. Moreover, the lower respiratory tract in asthmatics is highly susceptible to aerosolized $PGF_{2\alpha}$. The major argument against the importance of PGD_2 and $PGF_{2\alpha}$ in asthma is the failure of aspirin and indomethacin to help most asthmatics. Although it is possible that the cells producing these products in lung are unusually resistant to these agents, the available evidence does not support this.

Platelet Activating Factor (PAF)

Platelet activating factor is a family of structurally closely related, stable neutral lipids with a glyceryl core, a phosphorylcholine head group at the 3 position, one of several long-chain alkyl ethers at the 1 position, and esterified acetyl group at the 2 position (Fig. 3-5). It is produced by basophils, neutrophils, and macrophages in response to immunologic or nonimmunologic stimuli. It produces platelet and neutrophil aggregation and secretion, increases vascular permeability, and has moderately potent effects on smooth-muscle contraction. With rabbit platelets, concentrations as low as 10^{-11} *M* are effective in producing aggregation. In rabbits, PAF appears to play a major role in the shock and acute pulmonary hypertension associated with acute anaphylaxis. The role of PAF in acute allergic reaction in humans is uncertain. It is rapidly destroyed by deacytylases present in blood and tissues.

Anaphylotoxins

The anaphylotoxins C5a, C3a, and C4a are activated fragments of the complement proteins C5, C3, and C4, respectively, which release histamine from mast cells and basophils. They also stimulate smooth muscle contraction and increase vascular permeability and aggregate polymorphonuclear leukocytes. C5a also stimulates chemotaxis.

Toxic Metabolites of Oxygen

During acute stimulation of mast cells and leuckocytes, there is an acute increase in O_2 consumption and the concurrent formation of toxic metabolites of O_2, including superoxide, H_2O_2, hydroxy radicals, and possibly singlet oxygen. These products are capable of damaging microorganisms in normal tissues either alone or in combination with other products of these cells such as myeloperoxidase, which uses H_2O_2 for

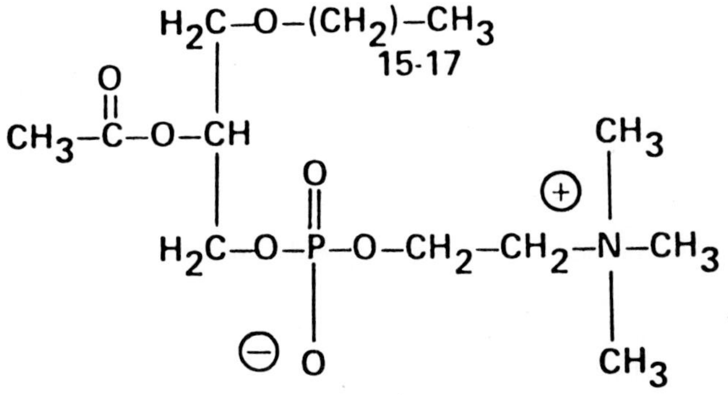

```
                 H2C—O—(CH2)—CH3
                  |        15-17
        O         |
        ||        |
  CH3—C—O—CH                           CH3
                  |      O          ⊕   |
                  |      ||             |
                 H2C—O—P—O—CH2—CH2—N—CH3
                         |              |
                  ⊖      O             CH3
```

Fig. 3-5. Structure of AGEPC. (1-0-hexadecyl/octadecyl-2-acetyl-sn-glyceryl-3-phosphorylcholine).

activation. Involvement of these O_2 metabolites in allergic inflammation is suggested by studies with enzymes such as catalase and superoxide dismutase that respectively catabolize H_2O_2 and superoxides.

Serotonin

Although serotonin can contract smooth muscle and increase vascular permeability, it is not particularly potent. Moreover, in humans mast cells and basophils appear to contain little or no serotonin. It is, therefore, doubtful that serotonin plays a major role as an allergic mediator in humans.

REFERENCES

Dy, M., Lebel, B., Kamoun, P. and Hamburger, J. *J.E.M.*, 1981, *153*, 293.

Jakschik, B. A., Falkenhein, S., and Parker, C. W. *Proc. Natl. Acad. Sci.*, 1977, *74*, 4577–4581.

Kellaway, C. H. and Trethewie, E. R. *Quart. J. Exp. Physiol.*, 1940, *30*, 121.

MacGlashan, D. W., Schleimer, R. P., Peters, S. P., Schluman, E. S., Adams, G. K., Newball, M. H. and Lichtenstein, L. M. *J. Clin. Invest.* 1982, *70*, 747.

Parker, C. W. *Clinical Immunology*. Philadelphia: W. B. Saunders, 1980, pp. 753–773.

Parker, C. W. In *Immunopharmacology*. New York: Marcel Dekker, Inc., 1983.

Parker, C. W. In *Fundamental Immunology*. New York: Raven Press, in press.

Schrader, J. W., Lewis, S. J., Clark-Lewis, I. and Culvenor, J. G. *Proc. Natl. Acad. Sci. USA* 1981, *78*, 323.

Stenson, W., Snyder, D. E., and Parker, C. W. In *Allergy: Principals and Practice*. St. Louis: C. V. Mosby Company, 1981, pp. 531–547.

Sullivan, T. J. and Kulczycki, A. Jr. In *Clinical Immunology*. Philadelphia: W. B. Saunders, 1980, pp. 115–142.

QUESTIONS

1. All of the following are important actions of histamine except:
   a. inhibition of T & B cell function.
   b. smooth muscle contraction.
   c. increased vascular permeability.
   d. chemotaxis for neutrophils.
   e. inhibition of monokine production.

2. Each of the following is a lipoxygenase product of arachidonic acid except:
   a. 5,12 dihydroxyeicosatetraenoic acid.
   b. leukotriene C_4.
   c. platelet activating factor.
   d. 5-HETE.
   e. leukotriene D_4.

3. Each of the following is a cyclooxygenase product of arachidonic acid except:
   a. cyclic endoperoxides PGG_2 and PGH_2.
   b. thromboxane A_2.
   c. prostacyclin (PGI_2).
   d. prostaglandin D_2.
   e. 5-hydroperoxyeicosatetraenoic acid.
4. Slow-reacting substances LTC_4 and LTD_4 may cause all of the following except:
   a. inhibition of lymphokine secretion.
   b. a wheal and flare reaction when injected into the skin.
   c. bronchial smooth muscle contraction.
   d. alterations in vascular premeability.
   e. increased ileal contractions.
5. All of the following cause smooth muscle contraction except:
   a. histamine.
   b. Prostaglandin E_2.
   c. $PGF_{2\alpha}$.
   d. platelet activating factor.
   e. PGD_2.

Answers can be found in Appendix B at the end of the book.

PART 2

Evaluation of the Allergic Patient

Kenneth P. Mathews

4

Historic Interview and Examination

This discussion focuses particularly on patients with atopic diseases, since these are the preponderant types of allergy seen by primary care physicians. More limited reference is made to other forms of hypersensitivity states that also are "allergy" according to the original definition of this term (von Pirquet, 1906).

GENERAL MEDICAL OR PEDIATRIC HISTORY

It is of utmost importance to begin with a thorough, perceptive general medical history. Just because the patient complains of "asthma," for example, is no assurance that this is in fact the proper diagnosis. After all, it is just as important to determine that the cause of the patient's complaints is *not* allergy as it is to establish an allergic etiology. The general medical history also provides clues about possible complications of an allergic problem (e.g., adverse effects of drugs).

The usual identifying information about the patient's occupation and place of residence is of more importance in assessing allergic patients than in most other cases. For example, as one develops the history, it makes quite a bit of difference at times to appreciate whether the patient lives in a rural environment or is a factory worker living in the inner city. Then the chief complaint and present illnesses are elicited as in the usual medical or pediatric evaluation. This is the time to ask questions that help to differentiate allergic diseases from the many other conditions that may simulate them. For example, has the "asthmatic" patient had hemoptysis, chest pain, fever, edema, palpitations, chronic cough productive of purulent sputum, or failure to grow normally? Has the rhinitic patient had frequent headaches, sore throat, fever, lymphadenopathy, anosmia, epistaxis, or only unilateral nasal stuffiness? In short, a broad consideration of the differential diagnosis of the patient's chief complaints must precede focusing on an allergic etiology thereof.

The past medical history and family history obviously should include specific

ALLERGY: THEORY AND PRACTICE
ISBN 0-8089-1619-X

inquiry about the atopic diseases: allergic rhinitis, allergic asthma, atopic dermatitis, and allergic urticaria. In recording the review of systems, emphasis again should be placed on questions relevant to the differential diagnosis of the patient's chief complaint.

ALLERGY HISTORY

If the general history suggests an allergic disease, one must ascertain what factors are important in producing the difficulty in the individual patient (see Fig. 4-1 for outline). The history is the major approach in making this assessment, and the most important clinical skill to be learned in evaluating allergic patients is to acquire facility at asking discerning questions so that logical deductions can be made about the causes of the patient's difficulty. Note that "causes" is referred to in the plural, since in the large majority of patients more than one factor causes the patient to react. The procedure is much like detective work, and there are a variety of ways to proceed. The following method has been used for many years and has the virtue of being easy to remember. It involves asking three basic questions relevant to when the patient experiences (and does not experience) trouble, where the patient experiences (and does not experience) trouble, and what agents has the patient personally noted to cause difficulty. Let us consider these three basic issues in detail since they form the backbone of the etiologic allergic workup.

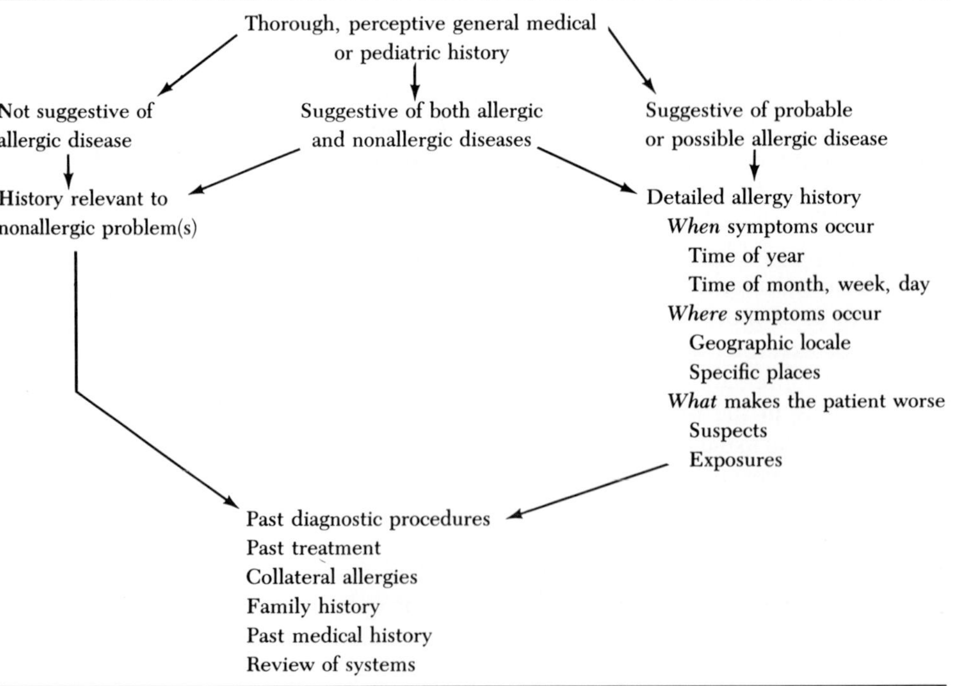

Fig. 4-1. History taking for evaluation of allergies.

WHEN. First it is desirable to get an overview of the patient's lifelong problem. One wishes to know whether the disease is progressively worsening, gradually improving, or remaining at a stationary level over a long period of time. It also is well to determine how frequently the patient has been having trouble lately and establish the time of year when symptoms occur; namely, is the difficulty seasonal, perennial, or perennial with seasonal exacerbations? If there is a seasonal component, as precise information as possible as to the exact dates of the season is needed.

Given an observant and accurate patient living in the northeastern or north-central United States where pollen seasons are quite sharply defined, one often can deduce the causative allergen(s) from the history, although these conclusions should be confirmed by objective data (see Chapter 5). In areas with longer pollen seasons, such as Southern California, it is more difficult to draw conclusions about pollen allergens from the history alone, but the latter can exclude a number of possibilities. Of course, pollen seasons vary markedly with the latitude, and there can be minor year-to-year variations in the onset of the tree pollen seasons as a result of weather conditions in late winter. In any case, one should be familiar with the dates of exposure to the common tree, grass, and weed pollens and mold spores in one's areas of practice.

When seasonal mold allergies are important, the dates of onset and offset of symptoms are more variable depending on the threshold of the patient's sensitivity. For example, a patient living in the Chicago area who is mildly sensitive to *Alternaria* and *Cladosporium* may experience seasonal symptoms from perhaps early June to mid-October, but highly sensitive patients can have trouble from April until there have been snowfalls in November or December. There also is the problem of deciding whether prolonged seasonal symptoms are due to a succession of pollen allergies, fungus allergy, or both. Relating to patients living in northern states, two or three points in the history are helpful in making this distinction. One is that the observant patient who has trouble from grass and weed pollen will recall that there is a period in midsummer, approximately from mid-July to early August, when less severe difficulty is experienced then either before or after this time. On the other hand, this is the very time of year when mold spores tend to be at their peak. Another point concerns the time of offset of symptoms in the fall. Typically the patient with weed pollen hay fever has pretty well cleared up by mid-October in northern states unless there is an additional allergy to house dust or mold spores. Persistence further into fall is compatible with mold spore allergy. Finally, a number of the most important mold spores grow on dead vegetation, such as hay and straw. Marked difficulty around hay, as in barns or hay rides, would thus suggest mold allergy, as would also difficulty with fallen leaves.

After assessing yearly patterns of symptomatology, one should consider both the time of month and time of week. A few women are worse premenstrually, but this is a conspicuous feature only in occasional cases of urticaria. Of more importance is whether the schoolchild or worker is better or worse over the weekend than during school days or workdays. This information can provide clues about potential etiology, particularly when occupational exposures are important. It is also worth noting the time of day or night when the patient tends to experience maximal trouble. It should be mentioned, however, that many patients with asthma tend to have trouble especially during the night regardless of etiology, and thus a history of nocturnal difficulty in asthmatics does not necessarily implicate something in the patient's bedroom. Likewise, many patients with rhinitis tend to feel stuffiness when they first get up in the morning regardless of the cause of trouble. Probably this is largely postural, relating to increased venous and lymphatic pressure in the head on recumbency, and again this does not necessarily implicate allergy to something in the bedroom.

WHERE. Regarding where the patient experiences trouble, it should first be determined where the patient was living at the time symptoms initially began. Particularly in asthmatics, it often is of interest to ascertain whether patients can recall the circumstances of their very first asthmatic attacks. Then the patients are asked where they have lived during the intervening years and whether moves had any effect on the severity of the allergic symptoms. If they have not moved about very much, similar information can be obtained by asking them whether they have left the area on vacation at a time when they would expect to have symptoms. Taken in conjunction with the time of year the patient has symptoms, such information can be almost diagnostic.

In addition to major changes in locale, one also is interested in knowing the effect of minor changes in such. Are there any placed where the patients know that they are likely to be worse or better? What about damp places? Air-conditioned places? In general, is the patient worse outdoors or indoors? What about getting away from home to nearby places? For example, what happens if the child spends the weekend at a grandmother's house on the other side of town? Or with a neighbor in the next block? If the patient has been hospitalized, have symptoms remitted promptly, almost before much treatment was instituted, or did it take a week or two of intensive therapy before the patient improved? Questions along these lines may lead one to the deduction that almost the only place where the patient has symptoms is in the home. In such an instance one would suspect pets in the home, molds growing in the basement, the emotional climate in the home, and so forth.

WHAT. What does the patient suspect to have worsened the condition? It is well to frame questions along these lines in such a manner that one will get the patient's own observations and not a recital based on information from previous physicians or friends or the patient's knowledge about previous skin tests. It may thus be well worth prefacing one's questions with "Try not to be prejudiced by what you know about previous skin tests or what other doctors or other people have told you. What do *you* think makes you worse?" Of course, the patients often mention irritants, which undoubtedly are important but are probably secondary factors in aggravating the difficulty, such as cigarette smoke, soap powder, cold air, and so forth. If, however, patients also mention substances that are potential allergens, considerable weight should be given to these observations under these conditions. Of course, patients may forget to mention some things they have noted to make them worse unless they are specifically reminded of them. In addition, patients do not always suspect things that are making them worse, and one does want to know whether they are being exposed to potentially important allergens regardless of suspicions about them. Because of these considerations, it is desirable to inventory the patient's environment with respect to both the presence of potential allergens and the patient's suspicions as to whether they cause symptoms. Since it may be difficult to keep in mind the items of information desired, it may be helpful to develop a checklist.

Furthermore, since obtaining this data is tedious and time-consuming, it is attractive to develop a form that can be filled out by patients or their parents. In fact, if it is known that this questionnaire is relevant to the patient's problem, it is ideal to mail it to the patient in advance of this appointment so that the information will be available when the physician takes the history. It should be noted that a number of the items querried about are irritants rather than allergens, but nevertheless they can be important sources of difficulty. Also included are a number of stimuli that are important in precipitating symptoms of vasomotor rhinitis. It probably is not directly relevant to ask atopic patients about suspected contactants (except occasionally in urticaria), since there is no positive correlation between allergic contact dermititis and atopic disease, but this is included for completeness. The extent of inquiry about the potential role of emotional factors is variable and is influenced by whether the history that has been developed up to this point suggests that the patient's symptoms are likely to be explicable on the basis of environmental allergens or infections, as well as one's initial impression of the patient's personality. It is true that in certain cases tension, anxiety, and other forms of emotional stress may precipitate symptoms of allergic disease, but it is erroneous to assume that there is a major psychogenic component requiring extensive evaluation in many or most cases of allergy.

In cases of urticaria or angioedema there is less emphasis on potential inhalant allergen exposures than in cases of respiratory allergy. Here it is appropriate to emphasize drugs, food, food additives, infection, physical agents (trauma, cold, heat, and sunlight), symptoms of connective tissue disease or neoplasms, insect bites, emotional stress, or items in contact with or penetrating the skin (see Chapter 9).

PREVIOUS DIAGNOSTIC STUDIES AND TREATMENT

Since many allergic disease are chronic conditions, patients frequently have had a number of previous diagnostic studies. Depending on when and where these were done, one may or may not wish to accept their results at face value or as being currently valid, but at the least it is worth noting such information as results of previous sinus or chest roentgenograms, examinations of secretions, blood counts, previous skin tests, pulmonary function tests, sweat tests, and so on. Summaries of any previous hospitalizations should be perused, if available. Sometimes this information enables one to avoid wasting resources in repeating previously unproductive procedures.

Information about previous treatment and the results obtained is also of major interest, of course. A common error is failure to inquire about past use of nose drops and nasal sprays, which will lead to missing diagnoses of rhinitis medicamentosa. In rhinitis cases one also would like to know what antihistamines have been tried, whether they were helpful, and whether they produced side effects. One also should inquire about proprietary rhinitis and cold tablets, other types of decongestant, and antibiotics. Similarly, in asthmatics information regarding the usual oral drugs taken for asthma as well as the use of nebulizers is important. If the patient has used aerosol therapy, some detail about the frequency of its use or how quickly a pressurized nebulizer has been used up is important information to obtain. Of course, one also wants to obtain information about any previous corticosteroid therapy, either local or systemic. If the patient has taken these drugs, it is necessary to know how often they have used them, how long they were taken, and how recently they were taken and to have some idea about dosage. If patients have been treated by hyposensitization therapy, information as to how long they had the injections, how frequently they had the injections, whether they had any reactions, and whether they improved following the course of injections should be obtained. In addition, it is important to know the composition of the allergy extract and the maximal dosage reached—information that the patient seldom has. Often it is desirable to obtain this information by telephone, particularly if the patient is not doing well and changes in the hyposensitization program are contemplated. One should be especially alert to the possibility that the patient is being treated with very dilute extracts that would be unlikely to have a therapeutic effect.

PHYSICAL EXAMINATION

Because allergic processes often occur intermittently, a negative examination at one point in time should not lead one to discount the validity of the patient's complaints. When the diagnosis is obscure, however, it is very helpful to have the patient return to be seen promptly when experiencing symptoms. This is particularly valuable in assessing patients with intermittent skin rashes. Recording the height and weight on graphs showing percentiles of the predicted value is particularly indicated in children with severe asthma, especially if they are taking corticosteroid drugs chronically. The respiratory rate is an often neglected observation of value in assessing the severity of asthma (Fischl et al., 1981). The degree of pulsus paradoxus also should be noted in such patients, and marked tachycardia, unless due to medications, also correlates with the parameters of asthma severity (Fischl et al., 1981). Simple spirometric measurements should be a routine part of the examination in asthmatics.

Noteworthy observations on inspecting the patient include the presence of orthopnea, mouth breathing, "adenoid" facies, "allergic shiners" (discoloration under the eyes), or a cushingoid appearance due to previous therapy. In addition to inspecting any skin lesions, it is worth noting whether there is seborrhea in the scalp, Dennie's folds radiating outward and slightly downward from the inner canthus of the eyes, and the appearance of the nails—length, cleanliness, and whether presenting a buffed appearance indicative of rubbing of the skin. Patients with urticaria should be checked for dermographism, with the back being more responsive than the extremities, and any lesions suggestive of urticaria pigmentosa should be rubbed to see if they urticate.

A sound ears, nose, and throat examination, preferably with the aid of a head mirror in adults, is of obvious importance in patients with complaints relating to these organs. A pneumatic otoscope should be used to confirm suspected loss of tympanic membrane mobility. Particularly in boys with conjunctivitis, the tarsal plates and limbal areas should be inspected closely for evidence of lesions suggestive of vernal conjunctivitis. Needless to say, a careful nasal examination is a central part of the evaluation of many allergic patients, and one may wish to collect secretions (by blowing onto wax paper) for staining for eosinophils at that time. Typically the mucosa appears pale and swollen in allergic rhinitis cases, but this is quite variable. Having the patient sniff through each nostril gives a gross estimate of nasal obstruction. Checking for sinus tenderness should be routine, and occasionally transillumination of the sinus may be helpful. If there is poor visualization of the nasal airway, repetition of the examination after applying a vasoconstrictor may be useful in excluding polyps or other obstructions farther back in the nose. On oral examination, the presence of marked overbite, dental malocclusion, and a highly arched, narrow palate may be due to childhood nasal obstruction. Prominent cervical lymphadenopathy may suggest infection of the upper respiratory tract. A deviated trachea cannot be accounted for by asthma, nor can the presence of supraclavicular nodes.

Inspection of the thorax may show pseudorachitic deformities simulating Harrison's grooves at the sites of diaphragmatic attachment, especially in children, and chronic asthmatics of all ages may display increased anteroposterior diameter of the chest; chest expansion may be decreased. Percussion of the chest should include an estimate of diaphragmatic excursion by change in the level of dullness from full inspiration to expiration, and the chest in general may be hyperresonant in asthmatics. On auscultation one looks for prolonged expiratory phase and diffuse inspiratory and expiratory wheezing, more prominently the latter. Wheezes often can be brought out in quiescent asthmatics by listening anteriorly during deep expiration with the patient sitting up and leaning forward and with compression of the chest (especially in children). However, one should be wary of confusing sounds arising from the larynx or upper airways. Conversely, the very severe asthmatic may have a silent chest, without wheezing, but such patients are in obvious respiratory distress. One should especially note whether the ausculatory findings are similar bilaterally. It may be difficult to determine the left border of cardiac dullness in the hyperinflated patient, and evidence of an arrythmia, S_3, S_4, or other cardiac abnormality needs to be evaluated with special care in the older, dyspneic patient. The same may be said of liver enlargement or dependent edema. Assessment of splenomegaly and careful examination of the joints and muscles are especially indicated in chronic urticaria cases where an underlying connective tissue disease needs to be excluded. Clubbing of the digits is very important in that it *does not* occur in uncomplicated asthma. Hyporeflexia and slow return of the ankle reflexes may be present in the hypothyroid patient with a stuffy nose, whereas hyperflexia might suggest hyperthyroidism in the patient with urticaria. It is desirable to test rhinitis patients for anosmia.

SUMMARY

A thorough and perceptive general medical and pediatric history and examination are the necessary cornerstones for the evaluation of allergic patients. In addition to providing a valuable assessment of the patient's general health, they help to prevent errors of assuming an allergic basis for nonallergic problems and of ascribing unwarranted clinical significance to positive skin tests and other diagnostic procedures. A discerning allergy history based especially on the time and place of occurrence of symptoms often can provide major clues regarding the causes of patients' allergic problems. Some of the most relevant observations to be made in examining such patients also have been reviewed.

Case History

Eric is a 9-year-old boy from St. Louis presenting with a history of coughing and wheezing for the past 6 years. His "asthma" now is occurring daily throughout the year and is progressing in severity. He is the same on weekends as on school days and did not improve on trips to New Orleans and Dallas. Road dust, house dust, and chalk dust exacerbate his cough. Intradermal skin tests 2 years ago are reported to have shown numerous positive reactions to house dust, fungi, and a variety of foods. He has been receiving hyposensitization treatment with house dust and fungus allergens since then. Previous chest roentgenograms have shown transient areas of atelectasis and hyperinflation. Treatment with theophylline and aerosol albuterol has given only modest improvement. The maternal grandmother had asthma in her later years. Past medical history and review of systems revealed no gastrointestinal (GI) complaints, but increasing nasal congestion and mouth breathing the past 2 years. Eric always has been small for his age.

Examination revealed a small, thin boy at the fifth percentile of his expected height and weight. Abnormal findings were bilateral nasal polyps, hyperinflation of the chest, and generalized inspiratory and expiratory course rales and wheezes. The level of sweat chloride was 90 mEq/l.

In general, the continuous, progressive nature of the respiratory difficulty should raise doubts about the diagnosis of "asthma," and its occurrence at a variety of times and places is not suggestive of an allergic component. The suspected agents can act as irritants, and inexperienced observers not infrequently overread intradermal skin test reactions and/or test with too large volumes. Subnormal growth would suggest cystic fibrosis in this setting (even in the absence of GI symptoms), and since nasal polyps are most often associated with cystic fibrosis at this age, a sweat test obviously is called for. There are other patients who have both cystic fibrosis and asthma.

REFERENCES

Fischl, M. D., Pitshenik, A., and Gardner, L. B. *New Engl. J. Med.*, 1981, *305*, 783–789.

Von Pirquet, C. *Munch med. Wochenschr.*, 1906, *53*, 1457.

Appendix 4-A *University of Michigan Medical Center Patient's Allergy Survey Sheet*

NAME ______________________ REG. NUMBER ______________
DATE ______________________ OCCUPATION ______________

Please fill in blanks and circle other applicable answers. Feel free to make additional comments. Base your answers on *your own observations,* and not on what you have been told by others or what you may already know about previous skin test results. Although these questions are rather detailed, the information provided will be of major assistance to the doctor in helping you.

Circle answers

I. Inhalants

A. *Dust*

Does exposure to house dust make your symptoms worse? Yes No

What symptoms? ______________________

Location of home?	*Type of house?*	*Heating system?*
Country	Frame	Hot air
Surburban	Brick	Hot water
City	Other_____	Steam
		Space heater

Aproximate age of house?_____ years

How long have you lived there?_____ years

Bedroom (yours)

Floor covering?	*Mattress*	*Pillow(s)*
Carpeting with pad	Age_____ years	Age_____ years
Carpeting without pad	Type:	Type:
Rug with pad	Inner-spring, cotton,	Feather
Rug	foam rubber, feather,	Foam rubber
Throw rug	other_______	Other_______
Linoleum	Other mattresses in	Other pillows in
Other_______	room?	room?
None	Yes No	Yes No
	Plastic cover on	What type? _______
	mattress?	
	Yes No	

Window coverings?	*Closet?*	*Walls?*
Washable curtains	None	Wall paper
Unwashable	Door kept open	Pictures
curtains or drapes	Door kept closed	Pennants
Other __________	No door (recessed)	Tapestries
__________	Used for storage?	Others __________
__________	Seasonal clothes only?	__________

Beds and bedding
Comforters, quilts?
Chenille bedspreads?

Furniture
None upholstered?

Living room?
Carpeting
Rug
Matting under carpet or rug
Throw rug
Drapes
Curtains

Furniture?
Average age?_____ years
Oldest upholstered piece?
Type?__________
Age?__________

Basement? Dry Damp None Finished

Basement Use? Storage only Washing area Playroom Other _______

Place of work? Location?____________________
Worse symptoms there? Yes No

B. *Molds*

Do you have worse symptoms after exposure to the following?

Hay	Yes	No	Raking leaves	Yes	No
Barns	Yes	No	Eating cheese	Yes	No
Circuses	Yes	No	Eating mushrooms	Yes	No
Damp basements	Yes	No	Drinking beer	Yes	No
Cutting grass	Yes	No	Drinking wine	Yes	No

C. *Danders*

What pets do you have?

Cat(s)	Horse
Dog(s)	Hamsters
Parakeet(s)	Other _____
Carnaries	___________

Are the following near your home?

Stables	Yes	No
Dairies	Yes	No
Barns	Yes	No
None of these		

Are you exposed to animal hair? Mohair, rabbit fur-lined gloves, none.
other ________________________________

Are you exposed to animals in your work? Yes No
If so, what animals? ________________________________

What animals, if any, aggravate your symptoms? ____________________
Or none? ____________________

D. *Miscellaneous*: Do you have worse symptoms after exposure to the following?

Cosmetics	Yes	No	Cotton lint	Yes	No	Paint, varnish	Yes	No
Perfumes	Yes	No	Newspaper	Yes	No	Kapok lint	Yes	No
Wave sets	Yes	No	Dentrifices	Yes	No	Wool	Yes	No
Chemicals	Yes	No	Insecticides	Yes	No	Food cooking	Yes	No

II. Foods Do any foods make you worse? Yes No

If so, please name them: ____________________
Symptoms produced? ____________________
Have any special allergy diets been tried in the past? ____________________

____

None?
Type of diet: ____________________
Conclusions reached ____________________
Please indicate approximately how often you eat the following foods:

Bread	_____	slices per day	Turkey	_____	servings per month
Wheat cereal	_____	servings per week	Fish	_____	servings per month
Pie	_____	servings per week	Beef	_____	servings per week
Cookies	_____	servings per week	Pork	_____	servings per month
Pastries	_____	servings per week	Broccoli	_____	servings per month
Spaghetti	_____	servings per month	Peas	_____	servings per month
Macaroni	_____	servings per month	Peanut	_____	servings per month
Noodles	_____	servings per month	Peanut butter	_____	servings per month
Oats	_____	servings per month	Nuts	_____	servings per month
Rice	_____	servings per month	Cocoa	_____	servings per month
Rye	_____	servings per month	Chocolate candy	_____	servings per month
Corn	_____	servings per month	Chocolate pudding	_____	servings per month
Corn bread	_____	servings per month	Chocolate sauce	_____	servings per month
Popcorn	_____	servings per month	Chocolate ice cream	_____	servings per month
Hominy	_____	servings per month	Cokes & colas	_____	servings per month
Milk	_____	servings per day	Orange juice	_____	servings per month
Ice cream	_____	servings per week	Grapefruit or juice	_____	servings per month
Buttermilk	_____	glasses per month	Strawberries	_____	servings per month
Coffee	_____	cups per day	Raspberries	_____	servings per month
Tea	_____	cups per day	Tomato	_____	servings per week
Eggs	_____	number per week	Peaches	_____	servings per month
Potato	_____	servings per week	Pear	_____	servings per month
String beans	_____	servings per month	Apricots	_____	servings per month
Lima beans	_____	servings per month	Banana	_____	servings per month
Soy beans	_____	servings per month			
Cauliflower	_____	servings per month			
Cabbage	_____	servings per month			
Chicken	_____	servings per month			
Lamb	_____	servings per month			

III. Drugs Did you take any medications in the last 12 hours? Yes No

Have you ever had an adverse reaction to any of the following drugs:

Aspirin	Yes	No	Nerve medicines	Yes	No	Other antibiotics	Yes	No
Nose drops	Yes	No	Vitamins	Yes	No	Hormones	Yes	No
Laxatives	Yes	No	Sulfa drugs	Yes	No	Antitoxins	Yes	No
Sedatives	Yes	No	Penicillin	Yes	No	Antihistamines	Yes	No
Tonics	Yes	No	"Mycins"	Yes	No	Cortisone-like steroid drugs	Yes	No
						Others ____________		

IV. Physical agents Do you have worse symptoms after exposure to the following?

Heat	Yes	No	Weather changes	Yes	No
Cold	Yes	No	Dampness	Yes	No
Exercise	Yes	No	Air conditioning	Yes	No
Drafts	Yes	No			
Sunlight	Yes	No			

V. Hobbies Please circle your hobbies. Double circle any that seem to aggrevate your symptoms.

Bird study	Gardening	Sewing
Botany	Golfing	Stamp collecting
Camping	Knitting	Swimming
Bowling	Movies	Television
Cooking	Painting	Wood working
Carpeting	Photography	Other ________
Farming	Reading	____________

VI. Habits

Average hours of sleep: _____ hours

Smoking: None, or _____ packs of cigarettes per day
_____ cigars per day
_____ pipefuls per day

Drinking: _____ bottles of beer per week
_____ other alcoholic drinks per week
_____ no alcoholic drinks

VII. Immunization

Smallpox	received	adverse reaction
Diphtheria	received	adverse reaction
Tetanus	received	adverse reaction
Whooping cough	received	adverse reaction
Polio	received	adverse reaction
Typhoid	received	adverse reaction
Influenza	received	adverse reaction
Measles	received	adverse reaction
Adenovirus	received	adverse reaction
Others: ____________		
	received	adverse reaction

VIII. Rashes from contactants

Poison ivy	Yes	Never	Rashes from cosmetics	Yes	Never
Poison sumac	Yes	Never	Rashes from clothing	Yes	Never
Poison oak	Yes	Never	Rashes from metals	Yes	Never
Rashes from other plants	Yes	Never	Rashes from hobbies	Yes	Never
Rashes from work	Yes	Never	Rashes from household agents	Yes	Never
Rashes from ointments	Yes	Never			

IX. Psychological factors

Financial problems:	______	Major	______	Little
Nervous tension:	______	Considerable	______	Little
Work adjustment:	______	Easy	______	Difficult
School adjustment:	______	Easy	______	Difficult
Married:	______	Yes	______	No
Marital adjustment:	______	Easy	______	Difficult

X. Insect stings

Have you ever had an unusual reaction from an insect sting or bite? ______

Type of insect ______
Type of reaction ______
Nothing unusual ______

XI. Is there other pertinent information about exposure to environmental allergens that you can give us? ______

______

______

______

______

XII. Flare-up of symptoms with upper respiratory infections? ______

General Medical or Pediatric History

Allergy History

When symptoms occur
Where symptoms occur
What the patient suspects
Environmental survey
Previous diagnostic studies and treatment
Allergic contact dermatitis

Physical Examination ______

______

______

QUESTIONS

1. Which of the following suggest(s) that a patient's rhinitis is not due to allergy?

   a. Fever
   b. Sneezing
   c. Cervical lymphadenopathy
   d. Itching of the nose
   e. Prominent sore throat

2. Which of the following suggest(s) that a patient's rhinitis is due to inhalant seasonal mold allergy?

   a. Seasonal occurrence in April and May (in Chicago)
   b. Seasonal occurrence June to October (in Chicago)
   c. Improvement after ground is covered with snow
   d. Symptoms on exposure to hay
   e. History of an allergic reaction to penicillin

3. Which *one* of the following is most likely to provide a useful clue about the cause of allergic contact dermatitis?

   a. Dietary history
   b. Time of year when rash occurs
   c. Distribution of the skin lesions
   d. Immunization history
   e. Geographic location where the rash developed

4. Physical examination of an asthmatic patient is *least* likely to reveal:

   a. Increased respiratory rate
   b. Inspiratory wheezing
   c. Absent wheezing
   d. Pulsus paradoxus
   e. Clubbing of the digits

5. Examination of a child with allergic rhinitis is likely to reveal:

   a. Conjunctival injection
   b. Cobblestoning of the conjunctivae
   c. Sinus tenderness
   d. Nasal polyps
   e. Pale nasal mucosa

Answers can be found in Appendix B at the end of the book.

Robert J. Dockhorn

5

Diagnostic Tests for Allergic Disease

SKIN TESTING

Charles Blackley reported in 1873 that allergy skin testing could identify the cause of hay fever (Blackley, 1873). Application of grass pollen to an abrasion on his forearm was followed by whealing. Skin testing done in much the same way has continued to be the most useful method of establishing specific allergens responsible for atopic symptoms. Three methods are currently in use: scratch, prick, and intradermal testing.

Scratch Testing

The skin over the back or volar surfaces of the forearms is suitable for scratch testing. A larger number of tests can be applied to the back, and small children may tolerate the procedure with less anxiety if they are unable to see the maneuver that produces the scratches. Any sharp instrument such as a sharp needle or lancet can be used for scratching. Scratches should be uniform in depth. Pressure must be sufficient to interrupt the epidermis, but the scratch should not be deep enough to draw blood. If a linear scratch is made, scratches should be short and of the same length.

Aqueous solutions of extracts at concentrations of 1:10–1:20 weight for volume (w/v) [2500–5000 protein nitrogen units (PNU)/ml] are generally used for scratch testing. House dust extracts are often used at concentrations of 1:2 (w/v, 25,000). The choice of allergens for testing will depend on the medical history, environment, aeroallergens common to the particular locality, and possibly diet. Use of mite extract is also helpful. Use of a control containing diluent without allergen is essential, and a histamine control (1:1000 histamine acid phosphate) facilitates interpretation when there are no other positive reactions.

ALLERGY: THEORY AND PRACTICE
ISBN 0-8089-1619-X

Reactions are ready at 15–20 minutes after gentle removal of all extracts by blotting. Excessive rubbing may cause false-positive reactions and should be avoided.

Advantages of scratch testing over intradermal testing include safety, the speed with which a number of tests can be done, and the readiness with which it is accepted by most patients. Scratch testing is probably more specific but is less sensitive than intradermal testing. Important allergens will often remain unrecognized if scratch testing is not supplemented with intradermal testing to some of the most important inhalant allergens, particularly where there is a significant history.

Prick Testing

Prick tests are done by placing drops of aqueous extracts of allergens on the skin first and then pricking the skin through the drops with the point of a small needle such as a 26-gauge disposable needle or a sharp darning needle. Prick testing causes less discomfort than scratch testing and less nonspecific reactivity as a result of trauma. Consequently results of testing are read more easily with prick testing. Like scratch testing, however, prick testing lacks sensitivity and should be supplanted by intradermal testing where historically indicated.

Intradermal Testing

The skin over the outer aspect of the arm is most suitable for intradermal testing. Tests should be done low enough to permit application of a tourniquet above them if necessary because of a systemic reaction, and because of this possibility the back should not be used for intradermal testing.

Intradermal testing is much more sensitive than scratch or prick testing, and systemic reactions are more likely to follow intradermal testing. This hazard is minimized by testing initially by the scratch or prick method to obviate the need for intradermal testing with those allergens to which the patient has the most extreme hypersensitivity. Only allergens that have elicited negative or 1+ reactions with scratch or prick testing are used in intradermal testing. If this precaution is observed, 1:400–1:4000 w/v (1000–100 PNU/ml) concentration of aqueous extracts can safely be used for intradermal testing. Epidermoid concentrations of 1:400 or 1:500 are often used for intradermal testing, whereas concentrations of 1:1000 are suitable for pollens and molds. If previous scratch or prick testing has not been done, it is safest to use only more highly dilute extracts for initial intradermal testing.

The needle is introduced into the epidermis and 0.01–0.02 ml is injected to produce a very small wheal. Approximately the same volume should be injected for each test. A dilutent control is necessary, as is a control with 1:10,000 histamine acid phosphate, which facilitates interpretation if all other tests are negative.

Reactions to intradermal tests are read at 10–15 minutes. Intradermal testing is usually limited to 20–30 tests at a time to minimize the risk of systemic reactions. Other disadvantages include some discomfort to the patient, although intradermal testing can be almost painless when properly done and the greater amount of time required for applying tests. The major disadvantage is frequent nonspecific reactions due to irritants in allergen extracts, which are more frequent with feathers, dust, and molds than with pollens.

Interpretation of Skin Tests

There is no uniformly accepted method of reading allergy skin tests. One method of grading reactions as compared to the diluent control follows:

−	Same as control
+	Erythema (with control negative)
+ +	Wheal (3–5 mm or twice as large as control)
+ + +	Large wheal (8 mm or three times as large as control)
+ + + +	Wheal with pseudopods

Distinctions based on small differences in the size of wheals resulting from testing with extracts with no reliable standard of potency cannot be justified. It has been suggested that reactions could be compared to the histamine controls that might be graded as 3+ reactions, but this has not gained wide acceptance.

Use of this grading system and extracts of suitable composition and concentration 2+ reactions are considered significant. Occasional 1+ reactions may be significant if correlated closely with the history, however, and 2+ reactions may lack clinical significance if not correlated with the history.

False-positive reactions may be due to the presence of histamine or histamine-releasing agents in the extract, intradermal testing with too large a volume or an extract that is too concentrated, intradermal testing with extracts containing more than 5% glycerin, intradermal injection of air, or mechanical trauma from too much pressure during application of the scratch. Dermographism may prevent accurate reading of tests despite comparison with controls, necessitating other methods of evaluation.

False-negative reactions may be due to testing with inactive extracts. Some loss of potency of pollen extracts at concentrations of 1:1000 stored at 4°C has been reported to occur within 4 months. Concentrated extracts (1:20) in 50% glycerol are stable for at least 1 year and possibly much longer.

Antihistamines have a suppressive effect on skin reactivity that may last for as long as 5–8 days after administration. The suppressive effects of hydroxyzine hydrochloride (Atarax) and hydroxyzine pamoate (Vistaril) or tricyclic antidepressant is especially potent and long-lasting. Neither oral aminophylline nor ephedrine inhibits responses to allergy skin testing in adults. Intravenous isoproterenol, subcutaneous or intravenous epinephrine, and intravenous aminophylline have been reported to inhibit skin reactivity to allergy testing, but terbutaline has no inhibitory effect after oral administration or following intracutaneous injection in combination with the antigens.

Although adrenal corticosteroids have definite suppressive effects on delayed hypersensitivity, they apparently have no significant effect on responses to allergy skin testing for immediate, type I hypersensitivity. Recent reports have demonstrated that steroids may inhibit basophil histamine release to secific allergens, however, and this should be borne in mind (Schleimer, 1982).

Another cause of false-negative reactions is testing during the refractory period following systemic anaphylaxis. Testing should be deferred for 2–4 weeks following such a reaction.

False-negative reactions also may occur with testing for foods and certain drugs, possibly due to allergy to haptens, metabolites, or digestive products of foods. Reliable, clinically significant skin reactions can also follow testing with foods.

Scratches that are either too superficial or too deep and intradermal tests that are too deep can also cause false-negative reactions.

Testing with groups of allergens in a single extract may cause a false-negative reaction when allergy to only one component is present. The number of different allergens in such mixtures should be kept to a minimum, therefore, and the dilutional effect of other allergens should be considered in determining the concentrations to be used in the mixture.

Positive skin tests are sometimes elicited before a particular allergen has caused clinical symptoms, and skin reactivity to allergens of previous clinical significance may persist despite clinical tolerance. These are not false-positive reactions, but they are reactions that lack immediate clinical significance.

Despite these discrepancies, skin testing is still regarded as the most useful and most practical method of evaluation for most atopic subjects, although other techniques may be helpful in further evaluation of some patients.

LABORATORY EVALUATION

Assays for Total IgE

Radioimmunosorbent Tests

Two radioimmunoassays for IgE currently in use are the radioimmunosorbent test (RIST) and the double antibody radioimmunoassay. Both procedures depend on the inhibition of binding of radioiodinated purified IgE myeloma protein to specific IgE antibody. A commercially available kit utilizing the RIST principle, the Phadebas IgE test, is available from Pharmacia Laboratories (Fig. 5-1). Standards of known IgE concentration and the unknown serum are incubated with Sephadex-anti-IgE and purified ^{125}I-IgE. The unlabeled IgE in the standard or unknown competes with ^{125}I-IgE for anti-IgE binding sites. Reaction mixtures then are washed by centrifugation and the insoluble Sephadex–anti-IgE-^{125}I complexes are counted in a gamma spectrometer. The higher the concentration of unlabeled IgE in the standard or unknown, the lower the radioactivity of the Sephadex complexes. The limit of sen-

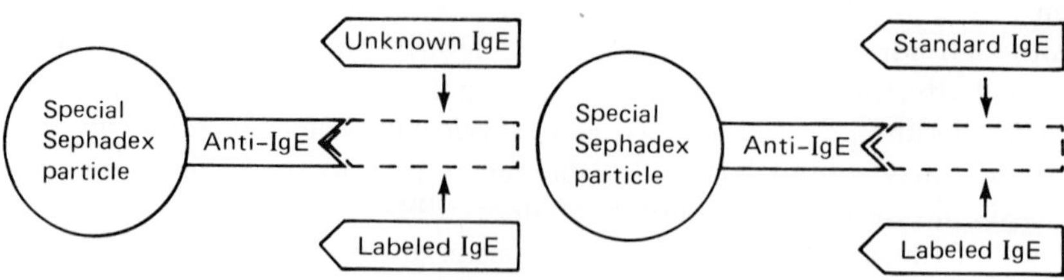

Fig. 5-1. Phadebas IgE test—RIST. From Dockhorn, R. J. *Ann. Allergy*, 1982, *49*(1), p. 2. With permission.

Table 5-1 *Normal IgE Values as Determined by RIST*

Age (Years)	*n*	Geometric Mean (U/ml)	+1 SD* (U/ml)	+2 SD (U/ml)
1	12	7	21	58
2	18	11	26	61
3	6	11	21	40
4	7	20	37	70
7	19	26	75	221
10	17	39	115	337
14	19	32	78	187

From Dockhorn, R. J. *Ann. Allergy*, 1982, *49*(1), 2. With permission.
*Degrees of standard deviation.

sitivity of this assay is approximately 2–5 ng/ml (Wide & Porath, 1966). Normal IgE values as determined by RIST are shown in Table 5-1.

Double Antibody Radioimmunoassay

The double antibody radioimmunoassay for total IgE, known commercially as the Phadebas IgE PRIST [paper radioimmunosorbent test (PRIST)] (Fig. 5-2), is a "sandwich"-type modification of the solid-phase radioimmunoassay. This test is a

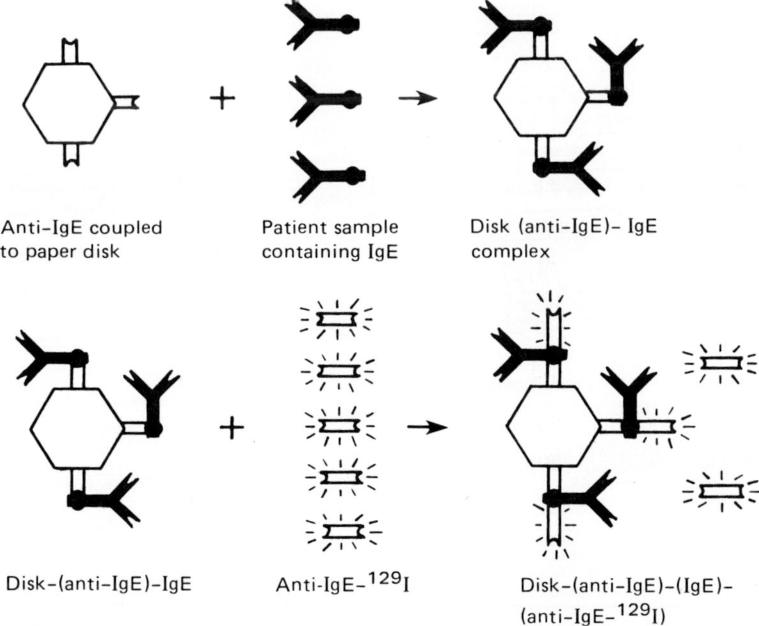

Fig. 5-2. Principle of Phadebas IgE PRIST. From Dockhorn, R. J. *Ann. Allergy*, 1982, *49*(1), p. 2. With permission.

direct radioimmunoassay using paper disks as a solid phase. Anti-IgE covalently coupled in the paper disk reacts during the first incubation with the IgE in the serum sample. After washing, radioactively labeled immunosorbent-purified antibodies against IgE are added, forming a complex. The radioactivity of this complex is measured in a gamma counter. The more bound radioactivity found, the more IgE is present in the serum sample (Ceska & Lundkvist, 1972). Normal IgE levels as determined by PRIST are shown in Table 5-2.

The correlation between serum IgE levels and atopic disease in older children and adults has been confirmed in a large number of studies. In infants and children under 1 year of age, total IgE has predictive value. In the older age group, measurement of total serum IgE levels has not contributed significantly to the diagnosis, predictive value, or treatment of atopic disorders. Only about 60% of patients with allergic rhinitis and 75% of patients with allergic asthma have elevated total serum IgE levels. Radioimmunoassays for total IgE lack the necessary specificity. They may be valuable, however, in screening for other diseases associated with abnormal IgE levels.

Serum IgE levels are elevated in a number of parasitic infections, including

Table 5-2 *Normal IgE Levels as Determined by PRIST*

Age	*N*	Geometric Mean (kU/l)	+1 SD (kU/l)	+2 SD (kU/l)
Newborn	37	0.5	1.0	2.0
1–11 months	51	2	12	56
1 year	22	3	15	83
2 years	26	6	29	132
3 years	33	2	35	101
4 years	27	7	33	144
5 years	30	21	56	148
6 years	31	16	95	573
7 years	30	14	88	552
8 years	32	19	71	270
9 years	35	17	88	464
10 years	40	28	110	421
11–14 years	98	27	111	456
15–19 years	50	24	96	384
20–30 years	52	14	59	239
31–50 years	52	19	79	324
51–80 years	34	12	48	197

From Dockhorn, R. J. *Ann. Allergy*, 1982, *49* (1), 2. With permission.

paragonimiasis, visceral larva migrans, capillariasis, ascariasis, fascioliasis, and bronchopulmonary aspergillosis. Elevated serum IgE levels also have been reported in some dermatologic conditions, including chronic acral dermatitis, bullous pemphigoid, and the dermatitis associated with the Wiskott-Aldrich syndrome. Low levels of IgE have been reported in conjunction with variable or combined immunodeficiency states; hypogammaglobulinemias, macroglobulinemia, and multiple myeloma; isolated IgA deficiency; and ataxia telangiectasia. It has also been shown that healthy individuals may exist with an isolated serum IgE deficiency (Yunginger & Gleich, 1975).

Tests of Specific IgE

Radioallergosorbent Test

A large number of the IgE of atopic individuals are specifically reactive with identifiable environmental allergens. Measurement of these antigen-specific IgE antibodies is essential for the diagnosis of atopic disorders, but a suitable test must be able to handle the minute quantities involved and the wide variation among patients. Two methods are currently in use: skin testing that is an *in vivo* bioassay in the allergic individual and *in vitro* assays of specific IgE. The radioallergosorbent test (RAST), which fulfills these requirements, was described first in 1967 (Wide et al., 1967). The suspected allergen is coupled to solid-phase particles, such as Sephadex or cellulose, or to filter-paper disks. Antigen-specific IgE antibodies, as well as other antibodies, react with the allergen and are bound to the allergen-polymer complex. When excess serum protein is washed away, the presence of bound IgE antibody is determined by addition of ^{125}I-labeled anti-IgE. The radioactive anti-IgE bound to the antigen-polymer complex is measured in a gamma scintillation counter after excess labeled antiserum has been removed.

The concentration of IgE antibody in the serum sample tested is proportional to the radioactivity of the processed complex. The gamma count rate is expressed as a percentage of a reaginic reference serum, as a numeric score related to the IgE allergen-polymer complex, or in terms of the amount of radioactivity initially added to each test tube. The introduction of antigen-coupled filter-paper disks by Pharmacia Laboratories is a practical implementation of this technique (Fig. 5-3). The RAST is used in conjunction with histories, skin tests, and provocative challenge tests to diagnose a variety of allergies. Specifically, the RAST has been adapted to measure serum IgE antibodies to pollens, animal danders, house dust and house dust mites, foods, stinging insects, molds, and recently penicillin. Results from RAST testing have been correlated with findings from bronchial and rhinoconjunctival provocative challenge tests for a variety of allergens. Agreement between these procedures has ranged from 59% for allergies to house dust to 93% for fish allergies. High correlations have also been obtained between the RAST and measures of leukocyte sensitivity, such as the leukocyte histamine-release test, and between the RAST and symptom indices of patients who are highly sensitive to ragweed and who have hay fever (Fig. 5-4). A positive RAST in healthy, nonallergic individuals is very rare, probably less than 1 in 200 (Johansson, 1975).

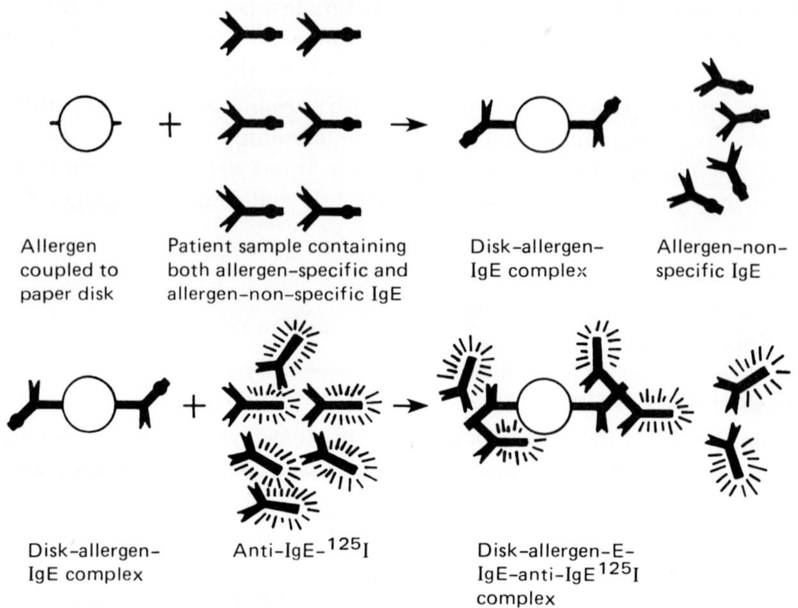

Fig. 5-3. Principle of Phadebas RAST. From Dockhorn, R. J. *Ann. Allergy*, 1982, *49*(1), p. 3. With permission.

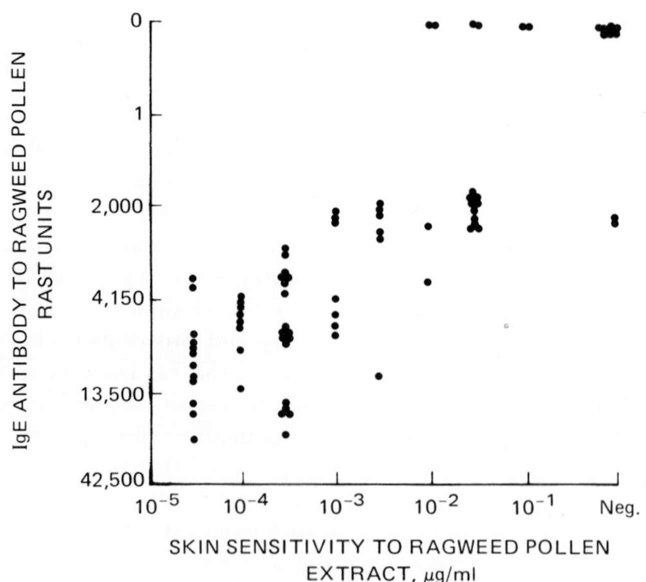

Fig. 5-4. Correlation between RAST and skin test reactivity to ragweed pollen. From Dockhorn, R. J. *Ann. Allergy*, 1982, *49*(1), p. 3. With permission.

Interpretation of RAST Results

Results of RAST testing are influenced by the degree of patient exposure to allergenic stimulation. In patients with hay fever, the level of IgE antibody to the offending pollen is lowest just before the pollen season. The titer increases fairly rapidly during the season and then decreases slowly over a period of many months. On rare occasions, patients have presented with a negative RAST before the pollen season and then become positive during the season (Johansson, 1975). A similar increase in IgE antibody level occurs during the initial phase of specific immunotherapy. This increase occurs regularly and has been used to monitor treatment programs. It has been suggested that a diminished seasonal IgE antibody response is a good criterion for measurement of the efficacy of preseasonal immunotherapy (Levy et al., 1973).

Although the RAST is not as sensitive as intradermal skin testing, it has several advantages when used in conjunction with or as an alternative to conventional test procedures. Results of the RAST are not affected by the presence of allergic symptoms or depressed by the medications used for symptomatic treatment of allergic disease. The small serum samples can be saved for follow-up study.

RAST Scoring System

One of the greatest difficulties with the RAST has been with the confusing scoring systems that have been set up for determining the results of the RAST test. The Phadebas RAST scoring system utilizes four reaginic reference standards: Standard A, which is pooled serum from patients highly sensitive to Birch pollen allergen; Standard B, which is a fivefold dilution of Standard A; Standard C, which is a fivefold dilution of Standard B; and Standard D, which is a twofold dilution of Standard C. Each of these reference standards has been assigned an arbitrary number of Phadebas RAST units known as *PRU*. The Phadebas RAST units are based on the observation that the Phadebas Standard B had binding ability similar to 10 units of IgE in the PRIST system and thus was assigned 10 Phadebas RAST units. The PRU is only a relative term and does not quantitate specific IgE.

The major difficulty in RAST scoring seems to be what is known as the "cut-off level." At the present time the cut-off point for the Phadebas RAST is 0.35 PRUs. The selection of a cut-off level or the separation of positive from negative results in any laboratory test is an arbitrary and difficult matter. Because of concerns over cut-off points in scoring systems, a modified RAST scoring system has been suggested by Fadal and Nalebuff. The original modified RAST consisted of utilizing an initial incubation period of 18 hours rather than the 3 hours utilized in the original RAST. Further, it increased the test serum volume from 50 to 100 μl, and the disks are removed from the original tubes and placed in fresh tubes before counting. Then to develop the modified scoring system, the fivefold changes in serum concentration were maintained; however, in order to keep counts constant from day to day despite variations in temperature and isotope decay, a time control was incorporated using 25 units of IgE reacted with the RAST isotope and determining the time required to reach 25,000 counts. In this type of scoring system the low limit of detectable levels of allergen-specific IgE or the cut-off level is 1.5 times the binding of negative control; therefore, the cut-off point is 750 counts. Sera with counts between 250 and 750 counts are thus recorded as negative indicating allergen-specific IgE antibody below detectable levels. This system would then have the cut-off point at levels as low as 0.02 or 0.04 PRUs. From this information one can see that the physician is presented with a dilemma when it comes to determining the significance of the test in relationship to the clinical condition of the patient. It would seem that all of these RAST classes, cut-off points, PRUs, and arbitrary scores tend basically to confuse the physician and also tend to indicate that one particular procedure is superior to another. It must be remembered, however, that the bottom line of all of these tests is a radioimmunoassay for detection of allergen-specific IgE antibody. It is also quite clear that the most important aspect of scoring is the fact that the greater the number of counts the more allergen-specific IgE antibody is present in the patient's sera. It still seems plausible the physician should be considered sufficiently intelligent to determine the severity of the patient's problems by a careful history and physical examination and by having the radioactive counts for a specific allergen on a specific patient without having to worry about scoring systems and other factors. If the physician is furnished with a positive and negative control from that run, and if the test is based on a specific amount of IgE, the physician should be able to determine the significance of the laboratory test without all the scoring systems that have been devised.

Enzyme-Linked Immunosorbent Assay

In another *in vitro* test, the enzyme-linked immunosorbent assay (ELISA) described by Engvall & Perlmann (1972), the allergens are absorbed onto the inside surface of a plastic tube. Antibodies in the patient's serum bind to the allergen on the tube wall, and reagins are then detected by adding enzyme-labeled anti-IgE. In a preliminary study in a selected material, Ahlstedt, Eriksson, & Hanson (1974) found rather good agreement between results obtained with the ELISA and clinical allergy.

The ultimate place of the various new diagnostic tests in clinical allergy is still being established. Factors such as cost, convenience, safety, and diagnostic precision have to be taken into consideration when choosing among the methods of diagnosis.

CONCLUSION

The first step in the diagnosis of an allergic condition is a thorough history regarding the patient's own observations of the allergens eliciting the symptoms and a careful physical examination. The testing that is done, either skin testing or laboratory testing, should be used to confirm clinical observations. The measurement of total circulating IgE may or may not be helpful. Total IgE levels may be elevated in conditions other than allergic conditions, and those individuals suffering from allergic reactions to single or only a few allergens may have fairly low total IgE levels. Antigen-specific tests, such as the RAST and ELISA are more specific than skin testing, even though it has been stated in the past that the laboratory tests are not as sensitive as skin tests.

REFERENCES

Ahlstedt, S., Eriksson, N. E., & Hanson, L. A. *Abstr. Acta Allergol.*, 1974, *29*, 137.

Blackley, C. H. In *Experimental researches on the causes and nature of catarrhus aestivus (hay fever and asthma)*. London: Balliere, Tindall and Cox, 1873.

Ceska, M., & Lundkvist, U. *Immunochemistry*, 1972, *9*, 1021–1030.

Engvall, E., & Perlmann, P. *J. Immunol.*, 1972, *109*, 129–135.

Johansson, S. G. O. In G. N. Vyas, D. O. Stites, & G. Brecher (Eds.), *Laboratory diagnosis of immunologic disorders*. New York: Grune & Stratton, 1975, p. 231.

Levy, D. A., Ishizaka, K., & Goldstein, O. What happens to allergic symptoms and IgE antibody when immunization is stopped? Presented at VIII International Congress on Allergology, Excerpta Medica International Congress Series 300, 1973, p. 80.

Nalebuff, D. J. and Fadal, R. G. The modified RAST assay: An aid in the diagnosis and management of allergy disorders. *Cont. Educ. Fam. Physician*, 1979, *10*, 64.

Schleimer, R. P., Mac Glashan, D. W., Gillespie, E., Lichtenstein, L. M. Inhalation of basophil histamine release by anti-inflammatory steroids. *J. Immunol*, 1982, *129*, 1632.

Wide, L., Bennich, H., & Johansson, S. G. O. *Lancet*, 1967, *2*, 1105–1107.

Wide, L., & Porath, J. *Biochem. Biophys. Acta.*, 1966, *130*, 257–259.

Yalow, R. S., & Berson, S. A. *Gastroenterology*, 1970, *58*, 1–14.

Yunginger, J. W., and Gleich, G. J. *Pediatr. Clin. N. Am.*, 1975, *22*, 3–15.

SUGGESTED READINGS

Bazaral, M., Orgel, H. A., & Hamburger, R. N. *J. Immunol.*, 1971, *107*, 794–801.

Bennich, H., & Johansson, S. G. O. *Vox Sang.*, 1970, *19*, 1.

Bennich, H., & Johansson, S. G. O. *Adv. Immunol.*, 1971, *13*, 1–55.

Coombs, R. R. A., et al. *Lancet*, 1968, *1*, 1115–1118.

Coombs, R. R. A., Howard, A. N., & Mynors, L. S. *Br. J. Exp. Pathol.*, 1953, *34*, 525–534.

Eriksson, N. E. Diagnostic methods in reaginic allergy. Goteborg, Sweden: University of Goteborg, 1977, p. 26.

Gleich, G. J., Averbeck, A. K., & Swedlund, H. A. *J. Lab. Clin. Med.*, 1971, *77*, 690–698.

Ishizaka, K., Ishizaka, T., & Hornbrook, M. M. *J. Immunol.*, 1966, *97*, 75–85.

Johansson, S. G. O. In G. N. Vyas, D. O. Stites, & G. Brecher (Eds.), *Laboratory diagnosis of immunologic disorders*. New York: Grune & Stratton, 1975, p. 231.

Johansson, S. G. O., Bennich, H., & Wide, L. *Immunology*, 1968, *14*, 265–272.

McGuigan, J. E. *Mayo Clin. Proc.*, 1973, *48*, 637–639.

Orange, R. P., & Austen K. F. In B. Amos (Ed.), *Progress in immunology*. New York: Academic Press, 1971, p. 173.

Prausnitz, C., & Kustner, H. *Centrabl. Bakteriol. 1 Abt. Orig.*, 1921, *86*, 160.

Tapay, N. J., In F. Speer & R. J. Dockhorn (Eds.), *Allergy and immunology in children*. Springfield, IL: Thomas, 1973, p. 363.

QUESTIONS

1. Each of the following is an advantage of scratch testing over intradermal testing except:

    a. Safer
    b. Speed at which tests can be done
    c. Patient acceptance

d. More sensitive
e. More specific

2. Each of the following is an advantage of prick testing over scratch testing except:

a. More sensitive
b. Easier to read
c. Less discomfort
d. Less nonspecific trauma
e. More specific

3. The major advantage of intradermal skin testing is

a. Fewer systemic reactions
b. Less expensive
c. Greater sensitivity
d. Greater specificity
e. Easier to perform

4. The following drugs will block skin test reactivity:

a. Systemic steroids
b. Antihistaminics
c. Beta-adrenergic agonists
d. Theophylline
e. Cromolyn sodium

5. RAST tests may be used in each of the following situations except:

a. Severe dermatographism
b. Extremely potent antigens
c. Extensive eczema
d. Patients who have had a recent anaphylactic reaction
e. To confirm a 3+ positive prick test

6. A PRIST to measure total IgE would be elevated in each of the following except:

a. Wiskolt-Aldrich syndrome
b. Bronchopulmonary aspergillosis
c. Bullous pemphigoid
d. Chronic intrinsic asthma
e. Parasitic infections

Answers can be found in Appendix B at the end of the book.

PART 3

Manifestations of the Allergic State

Leonard Cohen

6

Rhinitis

"Rhinitis" is the term for an inflammation of the nasal mucosa. It is often thought to be a trival affliction, but only by those who have never suffered with it. Rhinitis will affect nearly 20% of the American population at some point in their lives. A survey done in 1975 estimated that there were 3 million lost work days and 2 million lost school days each year from allergic rhinitis alone. It was also estimated that $500 million is spent annually on physicians' care and drugs.

PHYSIOLOGY

The nose serves many functions besides being the organ of the sense of smell. It filters 10,000 liters of inspired air daily, removing all particles greater than 100 μm and 80% of particles as small as 5–10 μm in size. Contact with the rich blood supply of the nasal mucosa helps to regulate the temperature and humidity of inspired air. Transudation of fluid through the nose's extensive fenestrated capillary network provides the moisture for the humidification process.

The quantity of nasal secretions is dependent on the pressure and flow of blood entering the capillaries, which in turn is controlled by the tone of the nasal arteries. The pseudostratified ciliated columnar epithelium, which makes up the posterior two-thirds of the nasal passages, is rich in goblet cells that secrete approximately a liter of mucus per day. This mucus is carried backward through the choanae by the beating action of the cilia lubricating the nasal, pharyngeal, and laryngeal mucosal surfaces before it is swallowed. This mucus blanket flows at a rate of 0.5 cm/min and is probably the most effective means of filtering particles from the inspired air.

Nasal mucosal tissue has the properties of erectile tissue because of the porosity of the endothelial basement membrane and the fact that its capillary bed is in parallel with an arteriovenous anastomosis and large venous sinusoids (Ritter, 1978). Nasal vasculature is innervated by both parasympathetic (cholinergic) efferents that dilate

ALLERGY: THEORY AND PRACTICE
ISBN 0-8089-1619-X

and sympathetic (primarily alpha-adrenergic) efferents that constrict the blood vessels. As expected, under cholinergic dominance the nasal tissue swells and obstructs the airway, whereas alpha-adrenergic predominance shrinks the nasal tissue and restores the airway. Glandular secretions are predominately under cholinergic influence.

The terms "nasal" and "turbinate cycle" refer to the alternating constriction and dilatation of the right and left turbinate sinusoids every 0.5–4 hours. As one nasal chamber opens and the mucosal glands secrete, the erectile tissue of the opposite nares fills with blood and partially obstructs the airflow. In normal individuals this turbinate cycle can be detected by rhinometric flow–volume measurements. This cycle is exaggerated in patients with vasomotor instability.

Swelling of the turbinates by any mechanism can occlude the orifices of the sinuses leading to secondary sinus symptoms. The eustachian tubes open in the posterior nasopharnyx, and their blockage may lead to serous otitis media, infection, or hearing loss.

DIFFERENTIAL DIAGNOSIS

Rhinitis can be divided into three broad categories: allergic, nonallergic, and infectious. As illustrated graphically in Figure 6-1, there is some overlap as patients may have two or more simultaneous causes of rhinitis. A common clinical observation is that patients with a classic seasonal inhalent allergy often have symptoms of perennial nonallergic rhinitis at other times of the year. Very commonly, rhinitis medicamentosa is superimposed on other forms of rhinitis when patients abuse alpha-adrenergic topical decongestants.

Differential Diagnosis in Young Children

Congenital nasal malformations must be considered in the differential diagnosis of nasal obstruction in very young children (Sakowitz & Berman, 1981). Choanal atresia can be confirmed when a metal probe or catheter cannot be inserted more than 32 mm from the edge of the nostril. Congenital dermoid cysts of the nose are

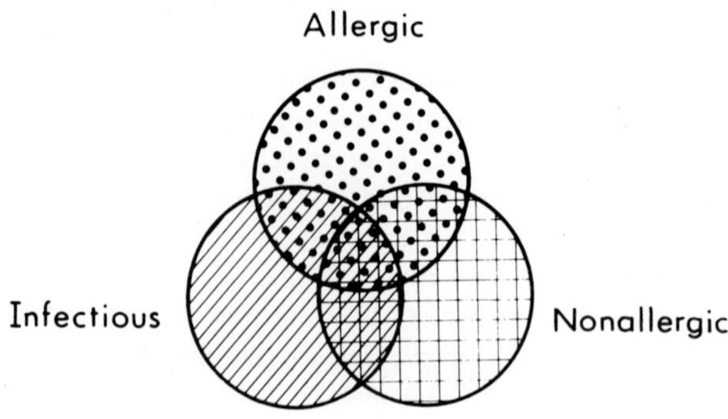

Fig. 6-1. Spectrum of rhinitis.

very rare but surgically correctible. Benign and malignant tumors have been reported in children as well as adults. In congenital syphilis, the profuse rhinorrhea labeled "snuffles" often results in marked excoriation of the upper lip. Of particular importance is the finding of nasal polyps in children, since cystic fibrosis may be the cause. A properly performed sweat test is indicated in all children with nasal polyps. There is also the possibility of a foreign body that has been inserted by either the child or an older sibling as the cause of nasal obstruction and/or a foul-smelling discharge.

Although reported, pollen allergy is very unusual during the first 3 years of life. The more common allergies in this age group are house dust, animal allergens (danders, feathers, hairs), and foods. Selected skin tests may be helpful in identifying the specific antigen. The history may be corroborating in this age group by an elevated serum IgE level.

Differential Diagnosis in Adults

The diagnosis of classic seasonal allergic rhinitis (hay fever) is not difficult. However, the differential diagnosis for chronic perennial rhinitis is more challenging. A good medical and environmental history (see Chapter 4) may reveal evidence for rhinitis brought on by pregnancy, hypothyroidism, aspirin sensitivity, cockroach infestation, quaternary ammonium compound fabric softeners, house dust, furry or feathery pets, or a moldy humidifier.

Table 6-1 shows a comparison of the diagnostic tests that are currently available to identify specific causative allergens. Properly performed skin testing through prick and/or intradermal injection of an appropriate concentration of allergic extract remains today the best laboratory confirmation of allergic rhinitis.

Nasal provocation testing should be available only for experimental purposes. It can be used to study the effect of drugs on symptoms brought on by antigen

Table 6-1 *Comparison of Diagnostic Tests for Aeroallergens*

Variable*	Prick Test	Intradermal Test	RAST	Nasal Challenge
Sensitivity	+	+ +	+	±
Specificity	+ +	+	+ +	±
Lack of risk	+ +	+	+ +	0
Ease of performance	+ +	+ +	$	±
Ease of evaluation	+ +	+ +	+	0
Objectivity	+	+	+ +	0
Reproducibility	+ +	+ +	+ +	0
Lack of seasonal variability	+	+	0	0
Can test patient on antihistamine	0	0	+ +	0

*Key: + + high, + moderate, ± low, 0 almost never, $ = costly.

Table 6-2 *Differential Diagnosis of Rhinitis*

History of	Allergic*	Nonallergic†	Vasomotor	Infectious
Sneezing	+ + +	+ +	±	±
Rhinorrhea	+ + + Watery	+ + Watery	± Mucoid	+ + Greenish
Pruritus	+ + +	+ +	0	0
Nasal congestion	+ +	+	+ + +	+ + +
Postnasal drip	+	+	+ + +	+ + +
Fever	0	0	0	+ +
Family history	+ + +	?	0	0
Worsening with emotions or change in temperature	±	0	+ + +	0

*Key (in this and other columns here and in Tables 6-3 and 6-4): + + + almost always, + + often, + occasional, ± rare, 0 almost never.
†Nonallergic rhinitis can be subdivided into cases with and without nasal eosinophils.

exposure. Its clinical usefulness is limited because of a low degree of sensitivity, specificity, and a relatively high risk of laryngeal edema or anaphaylaxis. However, cases have been reported in which allergic rhinitis was diagnosed from a nasal challenge with house dust mite (*Dermatophagoides* species) antigen in patients with negative RAST and skin tests.

The differential diagnosis of rhinitis is summarized in Table 6-2. Historic evidence for sneezing, rhinorrhea, pruritus, conjunctivitis, and a positive family history

Table 6-3 *Differential Diagnosis of Rhinitis*

History of	Allergic	Nonallergic*	Vasomotor	Infectious
Physical examination				
Nasal mucosa	Pale	Pale	Pink	Red
Nasal polyps	+	0	+	±
Inflamed conjunctiva	+ +	+ +	0	0
Laboratory				
Nasal eosinophils	+ +	*	+	0
Nasal neutrophils	0	0	±	+ +
Blood eosinophils	+ +	±	±	±
Elevated total IgE	+ +	±	±	±
Positive skin test	+ + +	0	0	0

*Nonallergic rhinitis can be subdivided into cases with and without nasal eosinophils.

suggest that the patient's rhinitis has an allergic component. On the other hand, nasal obstruction with a postnasal drip, worsened by emotions or changes in the weather, without a family history suggest vasomotor instability.

Physical examination of the nose is invaluable. A good nasal examination with a lighted speculum or headlamp is paramount in the diagnosis of structural deformities, cysts, polyps, tumors, or Wegener's granulomatosis. The color and degree of edema of the turbinates may help in the discrimination between infectious, allergic or nonallergic rhinitis. As Table 6-3 illustrates, in adults as in children, confirmatory tests for allergic rhinitis include nasal or peripheral eosinophilia and an elevated IgE level. The sine qua non for allergic rhinitis remains the corroboration of a good atopic history by the relevant positive skin tests. Neutrophils may be present in nasal secretions in infectious rhinitis.

TYPES OF RHINITIS

Allergic Rhinitis

The incidence of allergic rhinitis is estimated to include up to 10% of all children, but is quite rare under the age of 5. Rackeman & Edwards (1952) did a retrospective study of 700 children with rhinitis and found that 80% still had rhinitis after 20 years. In general, patients with seasonal allergic rhinitis have a greater chance of spontaneous remission than those with perennial symptoms. Many allergic rhinitis sufferers have hyperresponsive bronchial airways during methacholine challenges; however, epidemiologic studies have been unable to prove that allergic rhinitis precedes the development of extrinsic asthma to the same antigen.

Nonallergic Rhinitis

In spite of innumerable articles in the literature discussing perennial nonallergic rhinitis, this area remains one of the most confusing subjects in medicine. Twelve possible causes of nonallergic rhinitis have been identified, yet the exact cause is never elucidated in the majority of patients:

- NARES syndrome
- Aspirin sensitivity (pseudoallergy)
- Rhinitis medicamentosa
- Atrophic rhinitis
- Hormonal imbalance (hypothroidism, pregnancy)
- Vasomotor rhinitis
- Structurally induced rhinitis (septal deviation, cysts, etc.)
- Primary nasal mastocytosis
- Neoplasm
- Wegener's granulomatosis
- Midline granuloma
- Sarcoidosis

The term "vasomotor rhinitis" has been used by some authors to include any nonimmunologic, noninfectious chronic type of rhinitis. The present author prefers a more restricted definition and has separated classic vasomotor rhinitis from the other causes of nonallergic, noninfectious rhinitis (see Tables 6-2–6-4).

Vasomotor rhinitis causes intermittent nasal obstruction with postnasal drip and a minimum of pruritus, sneezing, and conjunctival symptoms. It is aggravated by factors that include strong emotions, odors, and changes in temperature or weather. Laboratory testing usually reveals no nasal eosinophils, normal IgE levels and normal absolute eosinophil counts (Tables 6-2 and 6-3). It is postulated that the pathophysiology is in the vasomotor fibers efferent to the nasal vasculature.

On the basis of this suspected pathology attempts at surgical denervation, by division of the Vidian nerve (which supplies most parasympathetic fibers to the nasal mucosa) has been attempted in severe cases unresponsive to medical treatment. This denervation is felt to increase responsiveness of the nasal mucosa to circulating catecholamines. Needless to say, this procedure is controversial at best.

Some recent studies have reported on the efficacy of cryosurgery on the inferior turbinate as a means of treating obstructive vasomotor rhinitis (Moore and Bicknell, 1980; Bicknell, 1979). Submucus diathermy, repeated local applications of silver nitrate, zinc ionization, and injections of hydrocortisone into the inferior turbinates have all been suggested as treatments for this chronic debilitating condition. Each of these techniques has its own supporters. Other techniques including acupuncture and phonostimulation have been shown to work no better than placebo. To date, no therapy seems to work in all patients.

Some clinicians support the concept that since vascular tone can be increased by a regular exercise program, this may help patients suffering with vasomotor rhinitis. Many patients claim significant improvement, but a controlled study has not yet been performed. Finally, many patients obtain some relief from intranasal saline irrigation using a special nasal adaptor (Anthony Products, Inc., Indianapolis, Indiana) on a "Water-Pik" appliance.

Table 6-4 *Effective Therapy for Rhinitis*

History of	Allergic	Nonallergic*	Vasomotor	Infectious
Avoidance	+ + +	0	0	0
Antihistamines	+ + +	+ +	+	+
Decongestants	+ +	+ +	+	+ +
Topical steroids	+ + +	*	0	?
Topical cromolyn	+	+	±	?
Topical ipratropium	+ +	?	?	+
Immunotherapy	+ + +	0	0	0
Antibiotics	0	0	0	+ + +
Exercise program	0	0	+ +	0
Water-Pik saline lavage	+	?	+ +	+ +

*Nonallergic rhinitis can be subdivided into cases with and without nasal eosinophils.

Rhinitis Medicamentosa

Rhinitis medicamentosa should always be considered in the differential diagnosis of obstructive rhinitis. Typically, a history of alpha-adrenergic nasal decongestant abuse is obtained. The mechanism for the observed rebound nasal congestion is unknown, but it may be that the topical alpha-adrenergic agents have a small amount of beta-adrenergic effect that outlasts the alpha effect and thereby causes vasodilitation and tissue congestion.

Oxymetazoline (Afrin) and xylometazoline (Otrivin) have less tendency to cause rebound than epinephrine, ephedrine, or phenylephrine topical decongestants. Even so, the use of such agents should be strictly limited to less than 5 days unless needed in the preparation for nasal operations, or as an adjunct for treating serous otitis media or sinusitis.

Treatment for the underlying disorder that lead to the decongestant abuse is needed, but first the patient must be weaned from the decongestant. One technique that helps the patient get through the miserable first 4–7 days is discontinuance in only one nostril initially and the use of a nonabsorbable steroid nasal inhaler such as beclomethasone (Vancenase or Beconase) or flunisolide (Nasalide). After the rebound congestion in the first nostril clears, the alpha-adrenergic decongestant is thrown away for good. When this method fails, systemic therapy with oral decongestants and corticosteroids is needed.

Other medications that may be the cause of rhinitis medicamentosa include the alpha-adrenergic blockers used in the treatment of hypertension and oral contraceptives.

Infectious Rhinitis

Infectious rhinitis can cause symptoms that are episodic as in the common cold or persistent as in chronic bacterial nasopharyngitis or sinusitis. Greenish-yellow mucus production with nasal congestion and postnasal drip are common complaints. The nasal mucosa appears red and swollen. Neutrophils with intracellular bacteria are commonly seen on nasal smears. Oral decongestants or the sparing use of topical decongestants and appropriate antibiotics are the mainstay of treatment. Sinus x-rays are needed to diagnose sinusitis. Once diagnosed, mild, acute sinusitis can be treated with appropriate antibiotics in combination with oral and nasal decongestants and warm compresses. However, more severe or chronic sinusitis must be treated for a minimum of 3–4 weeks to effect a cure.

Aspirin Sensitivity

Aspirin sensitivity usually occurs in young adults, but it has been reported in children and older adults. Nasal manifestations of aspirin sensitivity are characterized by profuse watery rhinorrhea usually followed by severe persistent nasal congestion, secondary to bilateral nasal polyps and to massive eosinophilic infiltration of the nasal and sinus mucosa. Chronic sinusitis and asthma frequently occur in these individuals. Nearly all these individuals are also sensitive to the other nonsteroidal anti-inflammatory agents. Recent studies report that less than 5% of aspirin-sensitive individuals are also tartrazine (F.D.&C. Yellow 5)-sensitive (Chapter 29).

Therapy involves avoidance of aspirin (naturally occurring dietary salycilates do not have to be avoided), other nonsteroidal anti-inflammatory agents and if proved by challenge testing, tartrazine. Intranasal corticosteroids often help control the rhinorrhea and polyposis.

Nonallergic Rhinitis with Eosinophils

Two recent papers have tried to characterize nonallergic rhinitis by the presence or absence of nasal eosinophils. Such eosinophils are found in approximately 50% of cases of allergic rhinitis. Mullarkey et al. (1980) described 21 patients with nasal eosinophils with symptoms similar to vasomotor rhinitis (nasal congestion and/or rhinorrhea, low IgE levels and negative skin tests). Some of these patients had polyps and sinusitis. More than 90% of these patients responded to either antihistamines or corticosteroids (intranasal or systemic). They postulated that this group of patients may represent early aspirin sensitivity.

Jacobs et al. (1981) described 52 patients with nasal eosinophils and symptoms similar to those seen in perennial allergic rhinitis (sneezing, watery rhinorrhea and pruritus) except for an "on-again, off-again" pattern. Again, no allergies could be documented in this group of patients. The term "NARE (nonallergic rhinitis with eosinophils) syndrome" was coined for these patients. Total IgE levels were normal, and no nasal polyps or aspirin sensitivity was detected. They unfortunately did not comment on the patients' responses to antihistamines or corticosteroids.

A bias in patient selection may account for the differences in symptomatology of the patients in each of the two articles. However, the presence of nasal eosinophils mandates a trial of intranasal corticosteroids in patients with nonallergic rhinitis.

CURRENT THERAPIES

Table 6-4 summarizes the currently available therapeutic modalities for rhinitis.

Avoidance

Avoidance techniques are useful in managing allergic rhinitis. Something as simple as a pollen mask may give your patient enormous benefit when mowing the lawn, or cleaning a dusty, moldy home. An electrostatic or high-efficiency particulate air (HEPA) filter can create a dust-free, pollen-free environment, conducive to a good night's sleep.

Antihistamines

Antihistamines are very useful in the treatment of allergic rhinitis by reducing the rhinorrhea, pruritus, and sneezing. They are also helpful in controlling the accompanying allergic conjunctivitis. By the nature of their competitive H_1 blockade, they work best when given before histamine attaches to its receptor. They have very little effect on nasal obstruction and hence are not very useful in vasomotor rhinitis. Some antihistamines have an antiseratonin effect [cyproheptadine (Periactin)], and cinnarizine [Dimitron (experimental)] is thought to be a calcium slow channel blocking agent. Most antihistamines have anticholinergic and sedative effects as well.

Intranasal Corticosteroids

The use of topical steroid treatment for rhinitis has been recently reviewed (Cockcroft et al., 1980; Okuda & Mygind, 1980). In some studies up to 85% of the patients with seasonal allergic rhinitis had excellent relief of nasal symptoms with 400 μg of beclomethasone dipropionate (BDP) intranasally each day. The lack of control of eye symptoms supports the interpetation of a strict local action of BDP. The response rate in perennial allergic rhinitis is slightly less than that of seasonal rhinitis, and studies on perennial nonallergic rhinitis showed even less of a dramatic improvement, but BDP was still subjectively and objectively better than a placebo inhaler. It may take as long as 2 weeks before perennial allergic or nonallergic rhinitis respond to BDP therapy, unlike seasonal allergic rhinitis, which often improves within hours to days.

Intranasal flunisolide (at doses of 20 μg/day) is probably as effective as BDP (at doses of 400 μg/day) and has the added advantage of a longer duration of action allowing for a convenient twice daily (bid) dosing schedule (Sahay et al., 1980). However, the package insert warns that at only twice the recommended daily dosage, some patients developed adrenal suppression as indicated by lowered A.M. cortisol levels.

Similar studies with intranasal BDP reveal that approximately 4 times the recommended dosage (1600–2000 μg/day) was necessary to induce adrenal suppression. Thus BDP has an extra margin of safety.

Cromolyn Sodium

Cromolyn sodium was first described in 1967 as a "mast cell stabilizing drug"; however, the exact mechanism for its action in inhibiting the release of the mediators of immediate hypersensitivity remains unknown. Nasalcrom (cromolyn sodium) is available for use in the nose as a powder or as a 4% solution. Although several studies have shown it to be more efficacious than a placebo, the degree of improvement is not as good as one would have expected.

Immunotherapy

Clinical improvement in allergic rhinitis by high-dose immunotherapy with allergic extracts has been demonstrated in many well-controlled studies. Several immunologic mechanisms for the beneficial effects of immunotherapy have been suggested (see Chapter 13). By whatever mechanism, approximately 75% of patients have a marked reduction in the symptoms of seasonal allergic rhinitis with appropriate immunotherapy using currently available pollen extracts. The data on the efficacy of immunotherapy with mold and house dust extracts are less impressive.

NEW AND FUTURE DEVELOPMENTS

Beta-adrenergic agonists such as terbutaline or fenoterol, when used intranasally, have been shown to exert a potent inhibitory effect on allergen-induced mediator release from mast cells.

The compound ICI 74,917 is postulated to have a mode of action similar to that of cromolyn sodium, but when used topically, it is several hundred times more potent, allowing it to be administered by a pressurized aerosol. In one study, it worked better than placebo or cromolyn sodium in patients with hay fever.

Ipratropium is a parasympatholytic agent with high topical activity and very few systemic side effects. It has been used in many studies for the treatment of asthma. It causes bronchial dilatation without tachyphylaxis. There is at least one double-blind crossover placebo controlled study of ipratropium with 20 patients who had severe rhinitis and watery rhinorrhea. Fourteen patients preferred ipratropium, and six patients either had no preference or preferred the placebo. Another study showed that this topical agent can even reduce the rhinorrhea associated with the early days of the common cold. Further studies are needed to determine the extent of benefit to patients by blocking local cholinergic receptors in the nose.

The effect of prostaglandins E_1 and $F_{2\alpha}$ in increasing nasal patency has been known for years. Their use has been clinically limited by severe local irritation, headache, nasal throbbing, and sore throat. Recently, no such side effects were seen when 17 phenyl trinor $PGF_{2\alpha}$ was tried in a few patients with vasomotor rhinitis. This prostaglandin derivative increased nasal patency for 3–7 hours (Karim et al., 1979). Much more work is needed before this can be considered an accepted form of therapy for nasal obstruction.

CONCLUSION

Patients with rhinitis should be approached with the same open mind as used to diagnose chest pain or abdominal pain. Their history should be carefully evaluated for clues, questions regarding the appropriate historic and environmental data should be asked, a thorough nasal exam should be performed, and skin testing and other confirmatory studies should be done if indicated. Therapy can then be chosen with confidence.

Case History

A 38-year-old white female presented complaining of 4 years of "a constant cold." She uses up to 35 tissues per day, sneezes occasionally in a staccato fashion, and has both nasal and mild conjunctival pruritus. She has symptoms year round, which are worse in spring and fall. She also reports staccato sneezing while doing housework, dusting, and changing her bed. Her rhinorrhea usually worsens when she has a cold; in fact, almost all of her upper respiratory infections (URIs) in the last 2 years end with profuse embarrassing rhinorrhea. She has had several severe episodes of sinus pressure and headaches in the last few months, always accompanied by a postnasal drip and rhinorrhea that was not purulent.

She denies asthma and allergies to food, medication, or stinging insects. She has had only mild relief with over-the-counter antihistamines and does not use topical decongestants. Significant family history includes an asthmatic father, a mother with hay fever, and a sister who had childhood eczema. Her daughter, age 2, has asthma. The patient presently lives in a single-family home with forced-air heat and a central humidifier. There is moderate cockroach infestation. Her mattress is 10 years old, and the bedroom has shag rugs, venetian blinds, and a 10-year-old foam rubber pillow that is now shredded.

Physical examination reveals pale boggy turbinates and two large polyps. Laboratory findings include 4+ nasal eosinophils, 500 eosinophils/mm^3, and a total IgE of 250 IU/dl. She has significantly positive skin tests for house dust, molds, cats, dogs, cockroaches, ragweed, timothy pollen, and oak and maple trees. Sinus films demonstrated mucosal thickening in the maxillary sinuses without air fluid levels.

Therapy includes strict house dust avoidance, and new Dacron polyester pillow and rubberized mattress covers have been instituted. The venetian blinds and shag rugs were allowed to remain but were to be vacuumed 2–3 times a week. She was advised to wear a pollen mask while doing her housework. Professional insect extermination for cockroach infestation was recommended, as was cleaning of the humidifiers in her furnace. Therapy included a long-acting combination antihistamine-decongestant and intranasal beclomethasone dipropionate to control nasal polyps and pollenosis; on this regimen the patient did well. She will be observed for one pollen season and, if the seasonal component of her rhinitis is not improved, will be started on appropriate pollen immunotherapy.

REFERENCES

Bicknell, P. G. Cryosurgery for allergic and vasomotor rhinitis. A new probe, 1979, *J. Laryngology and Otology 93*, 143.

Cockcroft, D. W., Hargreave, F. E., & Dolovich, J. In N. Mygind & T. J. H. Clark (Eds.), *Topical steroid treatment for asthma and rhinitis*. London: Bailliere Tindall, 1980, pp. 143–154.

Jacobs, R. L., Freedman, P. M., & Boswell, R. N. *J. Allergy Clin. Immunol.*, 1981, *67*, 253–262.

Karim, S. M. M., Aclaikan, P. G., Kunaratnam, N. Effect of 17-phenol PHF$_{2\alpha}$ on nasal patency in man, 1979, *Prostaglandins and Medicine* 3, 33.

Moore, J. R., Bicknell, P. G. A comparison of cryosurgery and submucous diathermy in vasomotor rhinitis. *J. Laryngology and Otology*, 1908, *94*, 1411.

Mullarkey, M. F., Hill, J. S., & Webb, D. R. *J. Allergy Clin. Immunol. 65*, 1980, 122–126.

Okuda, M., & Mygind, N. In N. Mygind & T. J. H. Clark (Eds.), *Topical steroid treatment for asthma and rhinitis*, London: Bailliere Tindall, 1980, pp. 22–33.

Rackeman, F. M., & Edwards, M. C. *New Engl. J. Med.*, 1952, *246*, 815, 823, 858–863.

Ritter, F. N. In E. Middleton, C. E. Reed, & E. F. Ellis (Eds.), *Allergy: Principles and Practice*. St. Louis: Mosby, 1978, p. 359.

Sahay, J. N., Chatterjee, S. S., & Engler, C. *Clin. Allergy*, 1980, *10*, 65–70.

Sakowitz, S. R., & Berman, B. A. In B. A. Berman and K. F. MacDonnell (Eds.), *Differential diagnosis in treatment of pediatric allergy*. Boston: Little, Brown, 1981, pp. 335–345.

SUGGESTED READING

Hillas, J., Booth, R. J., Somerfield, S., Morton, R., Avery, J., & Wilson, J. D. *Clin. Allergy*, 1980, *10*, 253–258.

Tandon, M. K., & Strahan, E. G. *Clin. Allergy*, 1980, *10*, 459–462.

QUESTIONS

1. Eosinophils in nasal secretions

   a. are usually found in vasomotor rhinitis
   b. are the sine qua non of allergic rhinitis
   c. eliminate from consideration the diagnosis of nonallergic rhinitis
   d. suggest a trial of intranasal corticosteroids

2. The most efficacious therapy for relieving all symptoms of ragweed pollinosis is

   a. avoidance of ragweed
   b. antihistamine-decongestant
   c. corticosteroids
   d. immunotherapy with ragweed extract

3. The most cost-effective means of identifying the causative allergen in allergic rhinitis is

   a. RAST
   b. nasal provocation tests
   c. skin testing
   d. PRIST

4. A 40-year-old white male complains of persistent watery rhinorrhea and a chronic postnasal drip of several months' duration. Conjunctivitis and serous otitis media are also revealed on physical examination. The differential diagnosis includes all of the following except

   a. perennial allergic rhinitis
   b. nonallergic rhinitis with nasal eosinophils
   c. Wegener's granulomatosis
   d. vasomotor rhinitis
   e. early aspirin sensitivity

5. The component of the autonomic nervous system that causes nasal tissue swelling and mucus secretion is

   a. parasympathetic
   b. $beta_1$-adrenergic
   c. alpha-adrenergic
   d. $beta_2$-adrenergic

Answers can be found in Appendix B at the end of the book.

Joel A. Goebel
Donald G. Sessions

7

Serous Otitis Media and Sinusitis

The human respiratory system comprises an integrated system lined with ciliated columnar (respiratory) epithelium. This lining is present in the mastoid air cells, the eustachian tube, the paranasal sinuses, the trachea, and the bronchial tree and is studded with goblet cells in all locations except the mastoid cells. Otitis media (OM) and sinusitis are diseases that reflect the response of respiratory epithelium to insult from either bacteria, fungi, viruses, antigens, or chemical irritants. This chapter discusses serous otitis media and sinusitis with respect to clinical presentation, diagnosis, and medical and surgical management. Emphasis is placed on approaching the differential diagnosis and therapeutic alternatives with certainty.

SEROUS OTITIS MEDIA

General Considerations

The middle-ear space communicates freely with the nasopharynx through the eustachian tube. This predominantly cartilaginous passage is horizontal at birth and assumes a 45° inferomedial angle with further development normally by age 7. This tube serves as the sole equalizer of atmospheric pressure for the middle-ear and mastoid space. Because of its sharp angle and small radius, the eustachian tube is susceptible to inflammation and obstruction leading to transudation of fluid in the middle ear. Insults such as nasopharyngitis, antigenic irritation of the tubal mucosa, adenoiditis, and mechanical obstruction by tumor result in negative pressure changes within the middle-ear space. This promotes increased capillary transudation and microhemorrhage within the enclosed cavity. Continued inflammation leads to increased mucus production with resultant collection of fluid in the middle ear. An allergic response may result in greater dysfunction since histamine, released from the sensitized mast cell, causes capillary leakage leading to tubal swelling and increased fluid production.

ALLERGY: THEORY AND PRACTICE
ISBN 0-8089-1619-X

Under these circumstances, ciliary action is impaired, and the fluid—ranging from a thin transudate to a more tenacious mucoid exudate—cannot be cleared or resorbed. This situation promotes coexisting or secondary bacterial colonization and results in the onset of infectious OM and its complications—chronic nonsuppurative OM, hearing loss, and progressive epithelial cysts with great destructive potential (e.g., cholesteatoma).

Epidemiology

Serous otitis is mainly a disease of younger children, especially those less than 7 years of age (Oppenheimer, 1976). The more horizontally situated tube of the young child is prone to contamination and conduction of inflammation and infection into the middle ear. Lymphoid hyperplasia seen in Waldeyer's ring around each tubal orifice also predisposes to mechanical obstruction and inflammation.

There is no sexual predisposition to OM. Children with cleft palates are particularly susceptible to OM. These individuals lack proper opening mechanics of their eustachian tubes due to poor tensor veli palatini function. Coupled with their increased tendency for upper-respiratory infections (URIs) and nasopharyngitis, these children suffer from chronic eustachian tube obstruction and retrograde middle-ear contamination.

Etiology

Serous OM is a clinical indication of eustachian tube dysfunction. Whatever the insult to the mucosa of the system may be, the end result is the accumulation of fluid and resultant impairment of hearing. A major cause is nasopharyngitis with rhinitis, which results in inflammation and induration of the eustachian tube. This, in turn, impedes middle-ear ventilation to the point that negative pressures created by absorption of gases into the bloodstream promote transudation of fluid. Direct infection of the middle-ear mucosa via retrograde contamination may precede or follow this process. Hence middle-ear effusion can precede an acute otitis media by providing a suitable culture medium for infection or may present only as transudation of fluid due to tubal dysfunction *without* purulence.

Hypertrophied adenoids with repeated adenoiditis may cause serous OM by mechanical obstruction and contiguous contamination of the nearby tube orifices. Adenoidectomy is still performed for repeated serous effusion of the middle ear.

Barotrauma triggers a series of mechanical events that may result in serous effusion. The eustachian tube normally opens with swallowing or yawning to momentarily ventilate the middle ear and equalize the pressure gradient across the tympanic membrane. A pressure of about 25 mm Hg is required to open the eustachian tube voluntarily; if the gradient reaches 90 mm Hg or greater, even muscular action cannot open the tube. Therefore, rapid changes in pressure as in diving or airplane descents create negative middle-ear pressures that can trigger eustachian tube dysfunction and subsequent serous OM. For this reason, chewing gum, frequent yawning, or swallowing is recommended during flying to minimize pressure gradients within the middle-ear cavity.

Allergic responses of the tubal and nasal mucosa account for a significant portion of cases that are refractory to medical treatment and surgical manipulation (Dees & Lefkowitz, 1972; Ishikawa, Bernstein, Reisman, 1972). Mucosal metaplasia with increased mucus production produces a persistent, tenacious effusion that resists treatment until the allergic component is diagnosed and adequately treated.

Nasopharyngeal tumors should be suspected in any adult presenting with unilateral serous otitis media. Since the eardrum is easier to inspect than the nasopharynx, the otoscopic finding of middle-ear effusion is frequently the first clue to nasopharyngeal neoplasm.

Other causes include metabolic and immunodeficient states that extend beyond the scope of this discussion. Table 7-1 lists these diseases for reference.

Table 7-1 *Etiology of Serous Otitis Media*

- Eustachian tube obstruction
  - Nasopharyngeal obstruction
    - Adenoid hypertrophy
    - Neoplasm
    - Fibrous scarring (adenoidectomy)
  - Intratubal obstruction
    - Tubal edema
      - Upper respiratory infection
      - Sinusitis
      - Allergy
    - Congenitally narrow eustachian tube
  - Middle-ear orifice obstruction
    - Chronic suppurative otitis media
      - Polyps
      - Cholesteatoma
      - Fibrosis
    - Residual mucoid transdate from acute suppurative otitis media
  - Failure of physiologic opening of eustachian tube
    - Cleft palate
    - Submucous cleft of palate
    - Neurologic disease
- Middle-ear mucosal metaplasia
  - Recurrent acute suppurative otitis media
  - Chronic suppurative otitis media
- Systemic factors
  - Hypothyroidism
  - Hypogammaglobulinemia
  - Diabetes mellitus

From English, G. N. *Otolaryngology, a textbook*. New York: Harper & Row, 1976, p. 158. With permission.

Clinical Presentation

The most common presentation of serous effusion is a mild conductive hearing loss. In children, this may result in a change in school performance, increased volume of the television or radio, or unexplained inattentiveness. An abnormal screening audiogram warrants further investigation, but hearing sensitivity losses of less than 20 dB are rarely detected, and a "normal" screening test does not rule out a clinically significant effusion.

Accompanying URI symptoms, pain or stuffiness in one or both ears, *autophony* (hearing one's own voice louder in the involved ear), tinnitus, and dizziness are consistent with middle-ear effusion. The discomfort of a nonsuppurative fluid accumulation is different from the severe, sharp, throbbing pain of an acute infectious otitis.

Diagnosis

Findings on otoscopy are variable. Minimal retraction of the tympanic membrane and decreased mobility on insufflation are early signs of tubal dysfunction. Serous fluid, if present, is usually golden yellow or may or may not contain air bubbles (evidence of partial tubal function). There is minimal injection of the eardrum itself, and bony landmarks are notable. This is in contrast to the bulging, inflamed, opaque, dull tympanic membrane seen in an acute OM.

Audiometric tests demonstrate a mild conductive component in the involved ear with typical air–bone gaps of 15–20 dB (Fig. 7-1). Larger air–bone gaps suggest additional mechanical disturbances.

Tympanometry or impedance audiometry reveals varying degrees of decreased compliance at ambient pressures (usually negative) and a flatter response to positive and negative pressure readings, indicating stiffness of the middle-ear conduction system (Fig. 7-2).

Although allergy has been shown to produce middle-ear mucosa changes, its role in eustachian tube dysfunction and serous OM remains controversial.

Differential Diagnosis

Middle-ear effusion has been classified in many different ways—serous, mucoid, mucopurulent, tympanic hydrops, and tubotympanic catarrh. This chapter deals with typical serous fluid resulting from uncomplicated eustachian tube dysfunction and transudation of fluid. It is important, therefore, to decide whether the process has either an acute infectious or a chronic exudative component.

Acute mastoiditis with middle-ear effusion clinically progresses through five stages: (a) hyperemia, (b) exudation, (c) suppuration, (d) coalescence, and (e) complication (Shambaugh & Glasscock, 1980). The tympanic membrane is progressively altered in each stage with increasing erythema, injection, loss of landmarks, and bulging or spontaneous perforation. Other signs and symptoms include mastoid tenderness and erythema, severe throbbing, ear pain, increased leukocyte count with a left shift, and persistent elevated temperature.

Acute otitis media likewise presents with similar tympanic membrane changes and evidence of an acute purulent process. Spontaneous perforation or tympanocentesis yields thick purulent drainage.

HEARING RECORD

NAME

ADDRESS

INITIAL TEST DATE

AGE 11 SEX MALE

M.D., HOSP., CLINIC NO.

AUDIOLOGIST

AUDIOMETER

AUDIOGRAM
PLOTTED TO ANSI 1969 VALUES

Frequency in HZ

	125	250	500	1000		2000		4000		8000
(Difference in dB ANSI vs. ASA)	9	15	14	10	10	8.5	8.5	6	9.5	11.5

HEARING THRESHOLD LEVEL IN dB: -10, 0, 10, 20, 30, 40, 50, 60, 70, 80, 90, 100, 110

MASKING
AIR / BONE

KEY TO AUDIOGRAM

MODALITY		LEFT	RIGHT
AIR CONDUCTION	UNMASKED	X	O
	MASKED	□	△
BONE CONDUCTION	UNMASKED	>	<
	MASKED	]	[
AIRCONDUCTION - SOUND FIELD		S	

Test Reliability: fair

EAR	P/T AVE	SRT	SL PB%	SL PB%	SL PB%
RIGHT		20			
LEFT		35			
Discrimination List					

Speech tests via (Circle) MLV Phono Tape

Fig. 7-1. Pure tone audiogram of 11-year-old white male with serous effusion bilaterally. Note 20–30-dB air-bone gap in lower frequencies with less effect at higher frequencies.

Chronic otitis media, on the other hand, usually presents as a long-standing thick drainage commonly referred to as "mucoid." Although some patients will develop this picture earlier in the course of disease, this finding usually represents long-standing effusion secondary to repeated attacks of acute otitis media, persistent tubal dysfunction, or chronic bacterial inflammation of the middle-ear mucosa.

Medical Management

The major goal in treating serous otitis media is to restore drainage and ventilation to the middle-ear cavity. Medical management is geared toward reducing mucosal injection and membrane leakage, removing concurrent URI, and mechanically promoting tubal patency.

Antihistamines and Decongestants

Patients exhibiting tubal dysfunction with serous effusion are routinely placed on a regimen of antihistamine and/or decongestant therapy. Peritubal edema has been implicated as a cause for dysfunction, and hence such therapy is aimed at

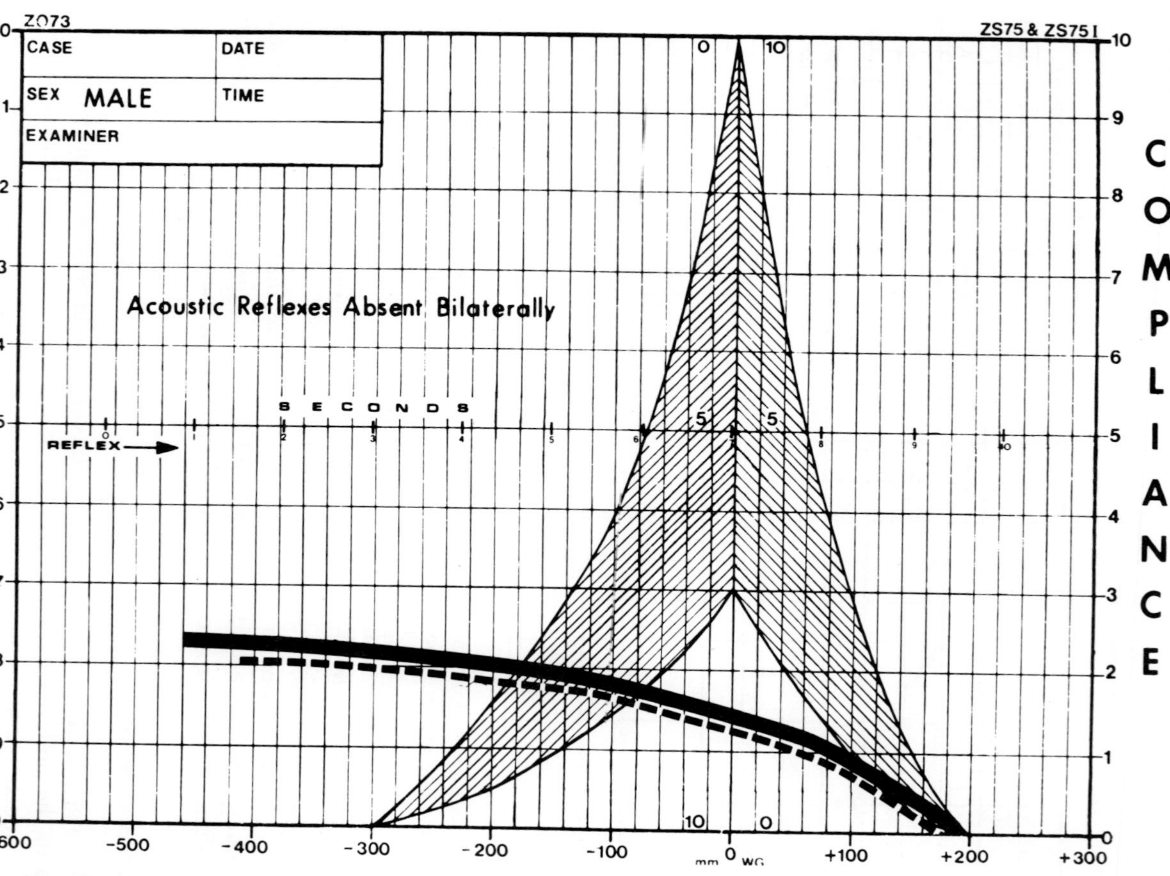

Fig. 7-2. Tympanogram of patient described in Figure 7-1. Note flat (type B) curves bilaterally seen commonly with effusion (○ = right, X = left ear).

reducing the swelling. The objective of antihistamine therapy is to counteract the effects of IgE-mediated histamine release, namely capillary membrane leakage. Table 7-2 lists the most common preparations and their adult and pediatric dosages and relative cost. Some authors believe that these drugs exert an additional direct effect on the middle-ear mucosa, leading to a decrease in effusion independent of tubal patency (Olson et al., 1978).

Politerization—Toynbee

As mentioned previously, reestablishment of eustachian tube function is a primary goal in treating serous effusion. In addition to medications that reduce allergic responses and vascular congestion, mechanical maneuvers are also helpful in promoting eustachian tube opening and reestablishing tubal patency (Fig. 7-3).

Politerization is performed through one nostril with a rapid blast of air from a 50- or 100-ml bulb syringe with the patient's other nostril and mouth held shut. This creates positive pressure in the nasopharynx and theoretically forces air up the eustachian tube and into the middle ear cavity. This maneuver is used on infants and young children and makes no use of physiologic swallowing or palate function in ventilating the middle ear.

The Toynbee maneuver, however, does employ functional opening of the eustachian tube via the tensor veli palatini function during swallowing. The patient is instructed to take a sip of water orally with the nose held shut and gently perform a mild Valsalva maneuver while swallowing the water. This not only generates positive pressure in the nasopharynx, but also employs tensor palatini function to open the eustachian tube while swallowing. This modified Toynbee maneuver is encouraged 8–12 times a day usually before meals and is an adjunct to conventional drug therapy.

Antibiotics

Serous effusions are not always sterile, and *Streptococcus pneumoniae, Hemophilus influenzae, Staphylococcus aureus,* and other bacteria can be cultured in varying percentages. In simple cases of serous effusion without bacterial pharyngitis, adenoiditis, or acute otitis, antibiotic therapy may be omitted. If, however, the patient's symptoms persist and the effusion has been present for some time with a change in constitutional symptoms such as nasal discharge, fever, or spontaneous otorrhea, broad-spectrum therapy such as ampicillin, amoxicillin, or other staphylococcus-active penicillins may be employed. Recent studies also support the efficacy of long-term prophylaxis of repeated bouts of acute otitis media sulfamethoxazole-trimethoprim (Bactrim, Septra) (Perrin et al., 1964).

Allergic Densensitization

Resistant serous otitis and signs of seasonal allergy warrant an allergic evaluation. Many "tough" cases of effusion, rhinitis, and sinusitis that are resistant to routine methods are successfully resolved following identification of specific allergies and subsequent desensitization therapy.

Whatever treatment regimen is used, follow-up examinations at frequent intervals with otoscopy, repeat tympanometry, and audiometric examination are necessary to evaluate the efficacy of medical therapy. Patients unresponsive to medical management should be referred for surgical treatment.

Table 7-2 *Commonly Used Antihistamine-Decongestant Combinations*

Product	Ingredients/Dose		Average Dose	Cost Ratio*
	Antihistamine	Decongestant		
ADULTS				
Sustained-release				
Chlor-Trimeton Decongestant Repetabs	Chlorpheniramine maleate 8 mg	Pseudoephedrine sulfate 120 mg	1 q12h	16
Novafed A Capsules	Chlorpheniramine maleate 8 mg	Pseudoephedrine sulfate 120 mg	1 q12h	15
Ornade Spansules	Chlorpheniramine maleate 12 mg	Phenylpropanol amine HCl 75 mg	1 q12h	18
Drixoral Tablets	Dexbrompheniramine maleate 6 mg	Pseudoephedrine sulfate 120 mg	1 q12h	20
Dimetapp Exentabs	Brompheniramine maleate 12 mg	Phenylpropanolamine HCl 15 mg	1 q12h	13
Naldecon Tablets	Chlorpheniramine maleate 5 mg Phenyltoloxamine citrate 15 mg	Phenylpropanolamine HCl 40 mg Phenylephrine HCl 10 mg	1 tid	24
Capsules, Tablets, and Liquid				
Chlor-Trimeton Decongestant Tablets	Chlorphemiramine maleate 4 mg	Pseudoephedrine HCl 60 mg	1 q4–6h	7
Actifed Tablets	Triprolidine HCl 2.5 mg	Pseudcephedrine HCl 60 mg	1 tid	7
Actifed Tablets	Triprolidine HCl 2.5 mg	Pseudoephedrine HCl 60 mg	1 tid	7

Actifed Syrup	Triprolidine HCl 1.25 mg	Pseudoephedrine HCl 30 mg	10 ml tid or qid (Children under 2 yr, 5 ml/24 hr; over 2 yr, 10 ml/24 hr given tid or qid)	6
Disophrol Tablets	Dexbrompheniramine maleate 2 mg	Pseudoephedrine sulfate 60 mg	1 qid	10
Naldecon Syrup	Chlorpheniramine maleate 2.5 mg Phenyltoloxamine citrate 7.5 mg	Phenylpropanolamine HCl 20 mg Phenylephrine HCl 5 mg	5 ml 3–4h	14
Dimetapp Elixir	Brompheniramine maleate 4 mg	Phenylpropanolamine HCl 5 mg Phenylephrine HCl 5 mg	5–10 ml tid or qid (Children—1 ml/2.25 kg q24h)	6
CHILDREN (ingredients are per 5-ml dose of syrups or 1-ml dose of drops)				
Rynatan Pediatric Suspension	Chlorpheniramine tannate 2 mg, pyrilamine tannate 12.5 mg	Phenylephrine tannate 5 mg	$\frac{1}{3}$ tsp (1.7 ml)/2 years of age up to 2 tsp (10 ml) q12h	16
Naldecon Pediatric Syrup	Chlorpheniramine maleate 0.5 mg Phenyltoloxamine citrate 2 mg	Phenylpropanolamine HCl 5 mg Phenylephrine HCl 1.25 mg	2.5 ml for a 6–12 month, 5 ml for 1–6 yr, 10 ml for 6–12 yr q3–4h†	13
Naldecon Pediatric Drops	Chlorpheniramine maleate 0.5 mg Phenyltoloxamine citrate 2 mg	Phenylpropanolamine HCl 5 mg Phenylephrine HCl 1.25 mg	0.25 ml/3 months of age ≤1 ml for up to 6 yr q3–4h†	30

(continued)

Table 7-2 *(continued)*

Product	Ingredients/Dose		Average Dose	Cost Ratio*
	Antihistamine	Decongestant		
CHILDREN (ingredients are per 5-ml dose of syrups or 1-ml dose of drops)				
Rondec Syrup	Carbinoxamine maleate 4 mg	Pseudoephedrine HCl 60 mg	5 ml qid (0.5 ml/kg q24h)	11
Rondec Drops	Carbinoxamine maleate 2 mg	Pseudoephedrine HCl 25 mg	0.25–1 ml qid (0.2 ml/kg q24h)	18
Triaminic Oral Infant Drops	Pyrilamine maleate 10 mg Pheniramine maleate 10 mg	Phenylpropanolamine HCl 20 mg	1 drop/2 lb qid	28

*Cost ratio is an approximate ratio between the products for a cost/dose (i.e., a cost ratio number of 2 is one-half the cost of 4 per dose).
†Not to exceed four doses in a 24-hour period.

Case History

A 6-year-old white male first presented with a 2-month history of decreased hearing reported by the parents. No recurrent acute infections were reported. His past medical history was remarkable only for *Hemophilus influenzae* meningitis at age 1 year (source unknown). There was no history of allergies.

Physical examination revealed bilateral tympanic membrane hypomobility with serous fluid, R > L (right to left). Marked tonsil and adenoid hypertrophy was noted on oral and nasopharyngeal examination. Typical "adenoidal facies" were also present. Tuning forks at 256 and 512 Hz revealed a bilateral conductive hearing loss. He was placed on Actifed and Triple Sulfa Syrup and scheduled for reevaluation in 3 weeks.

On return the patient had an acute left otitis media and persistence of serous effusion in his right ear. He was treated with Ampicillin and Dimetapp and instructed to return in 2 weeks. An audiogram showed a mild conductive loss bilaterally, worse on the right (10–15 dB airbone gap (ABG), 15 speech reception threshold (SRT). He returned 3 weeks later with bilateral actue otitis media and was placed on phenoxymethyl penicillin (PCN VK) and Actifed and was scheduled for adenoidectomy and bilateral placement of tympanostomy tubes on March 6, 1980. At operation, thick mucoid material was suctioned from both middle-ear cavities. Postoperatively he did well for about 18 months, at which time he developed a right acute otitis media with the tube in place and was treated with PCN VK for 10 days. His ears drained intermittently for 1 month thereafter, and he was placed on polymyxin-B-neomycin-hydrocortisone (Cortisporin) ear drops and sulfisoxazole (Gantrisin Syrup) and Actifed. Two months later, however, examination revealed extrusion of both tubes with dry intact mobile tympanic membranes. Repeat examinations and audiometric tests, including tympanometry, have since shown minimal conductive loss and reasonable aeration of the middle ear.

This case epitomizes the unpredictable course of eustachian tube dysfunction and the various complications and modes of therapy. In this case, repeated acute infections developed with persistence of serous effusion. This situation was effectively handled with timely placement of tympanostomy tubes and adenoidectomy after repeated attempts at antibiotic and decongestant therapy. Of particular importance is the necessity of close otologic follow-up with serial audiograms and tympanometry in assessing the long-term efficacy of the treatment plan used. When medical therapy fails to eliminate the effusion, chronic changes may occur (i.e., the "glue ear" seen at operation), and surgical intervention is needed to avoid further complications and chronic hearing loss.

Surgical Management

Tympanocentesis

Routine office myringotomy without placement of tympanostomy tubes is often insufficient in treating serous effusion of the middle ear cavity due to rapid healing of the tympanic membrane. The underlying ventilation problem is unaltered and spontaneous closure of the puncture wound and reaccumulation of fluid occur rapidly. Recently, tympanocentesis, along with a tapered dose of oral steroids, has produced a significant reduction in recurrence of effusion rather than myringotomy alone or with antihistamine therapy.

Myringotomy and Tympanostomy Tube Placement

The decision to place tympanostomy tubes follows failure of adequate medical treatment over a reasonable length of time (Figure 7-3). Some clinicians use a set period to evaluate their medical regimen while others opt for placement at an earlier

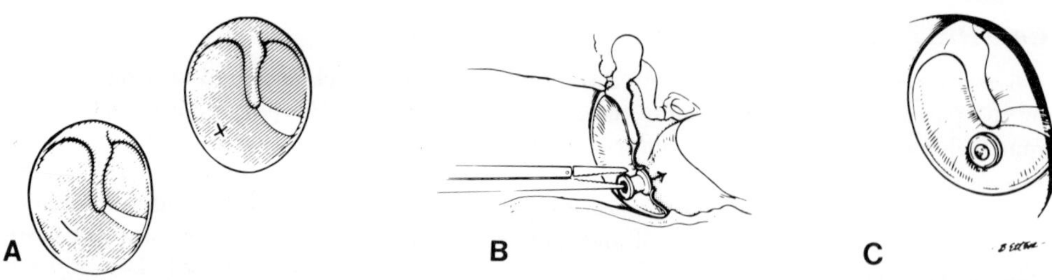

Fig. 7-3. Myringotomy and tube placement: (A) incision in anteroinferior quadrant of the tympanic membrane; (B) placement of tympanostomy tube under direct microscopic vision with alligator forceps; (C) appearance of eardrum and tube after placement. From Saunders, W. M., Paparella, M. M., & Miglets, A. W.: *Atlas of ear surgery* (ed. 3). St. Louis, Mosby, 1980, p. 171. With permission.

date based on personal clinical experience or the patient's symptomatology. In cases with persistent effusion, flat tympanograms or depressed air audiograms, a six-week regimen using decongestant therapy has been employed, with or without long term antibiotics, and politerization before myringotomy and tube placement. Complications of tympanostomy tubes include a persistent tympanic membrane perforation, early extrusion, and persistence of mucopurulent otorrhea secondary to external contamination. However, the morbidity of persistent serous middle ear effusion is overriding, and failure to treat this problem results in more serious complications. These include recurrent bouts of acute infectious otitis media (OM), chronic hearing loss with possible secondary speech developmental changes, and progression to chronic OM with tympanic membrane retraction, chronic mastoiditis, and even cholesteatoma formation. For this reason, patients who fail to respond to conventional medical management should be referred for re-evaluation and possible myringotomy and tube placement.

Adenoidectomy

The utilization of adenoidectomy in the management of serous otitis is controversial. The issue remains whether or not adenoidectomy is effective on the basis of removing a mechanical blockage to the eustachian tube orifice. Although controversial studies have not completely answered this question, clinical experience has shown that adenoidectomy may be of some value. The discovery that allergic etiologies for persistant serous fluid play a critical role in selected cases is important since adenoidectomy in these instances has proven less effective than proper desensitization and drug therapy.

Conclusion

Serous otitis media, a form of nonsuppurative middle-ear effusion, can be regarded as a continuum of events beginning with eustachian tube dysfunction and progressing to serous effusion. This then may develop into suppuration, chronic

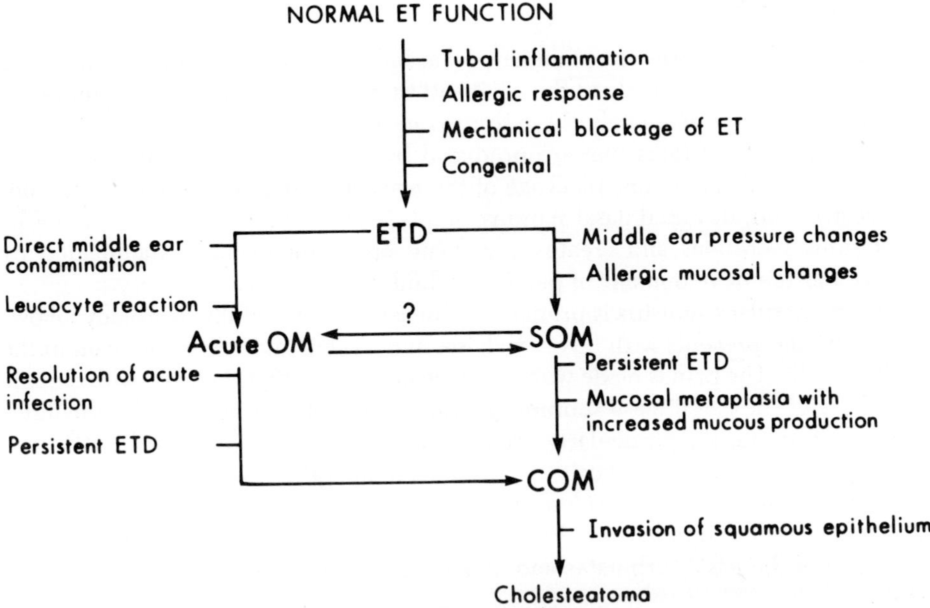

Fig. 7-4. Sequelae of persistent eustachian tube dysfunction (ET = eustachian tube; ETD = eustachian tube dysfunction; SOM = serous otitis media; COM = chronic otitis media).

mucus effusion, or resolution with restoration of eustachian tube function as shown in Figure 7-4.

To avoid the sequelae of chronic suppuration and cholesteatoma, the physician treating eustachian tube dysfunction must make an accurate assessment and begin early medical management. Antihistamine/decongestant therapy, allergic desensitization, eustachian tube aeration, and timely surgical intervention should avoid further complications of infection, chronic effusion, and permanent hearing loss.

ACUTE AND CHRONIC SINUSITIS

General Considerations

Acute and chronic sinus disease confront the practicing physician daily. The sinuses frequently become secondarily involved following URI and allergic rhinitis. This results in swelling of the mucosal lining, increased secretions, and obstruction of the ostia and produces headache, fever, facial pain, and nasal obstruction. Chronic sinus disease commonly presents as persistent "postnasal" drainage, chronic nonproductive cough, halitosis, and persistent nasal discharge. Recurrent or seasonal reactions may be an integral part of the patient's history. Acute and/or chronic bacterial infection may develop and, less frequently, viral and fungal illnesses.

Acute Maxillary Sinusitis

The maxillary sinuses are pneumatized at birth and reach a stable volume of 15 ml at age 18. They lie directly to the orbit and lateral to the nasal wall. The maxillary ostia are located approximately three-fourths up the medial wall and open into the middle meatus. Secretions that are produced by the sinuses are swept toward the nasal cavity by ciliary action. Blockage of the maxillary ostia by mucosal induration, nasal obstruction, deviated nasal septum, or foreign bodies prevents adequate clearing of sinus secretions and creates a stagnant environment for contamination by bacteria and the development of persistent fluid.

Acute maxillary sinusitis is primarily a disease of young adults. It usually follows a mild URI and presents with fever, malaise, and a vague dull throbbing pain in the cheek or teeth. The pain is made worse with change in position. Patients with chronic nasal allergies, deviated nasal septum, poor dentition, or maxillofacial abnormalities such as cleft palate are particularly prone to acute maxillary sinusitis.

Physical examination reveals an elevated temperature; tenderness in the infraorbital region; and mucopurulent drainage in the middle meatus, on the inferior turbinate, or in the oropharynx. Evidence of nasal allergies including polypoid degeneration of the nasal turbinates and hypertrophy of the nasal mucosa may also be seen.

Radiographically, there is mucoperiosteal thickening, air-fluid levels, or complete opacification of one or more sinuses. Nasal, antral, and choanal polyps may be evident.

Diagnosis depends on a combination of clinical, radiographic, and bacteriologic information. Acute infection is evident from the time course, presence of fever and recent onset of pain, radiographic evidence of fluid or mucosal thickening in the sinus, and identification of the offending pathogens. Unfortunately, nasal cultures are of little benefit in identifying the sinus organisms, and direct antral irrigation or sinus puncture may be necessary (Fig. 7-5). Such cultures may reveal pneumococcus, streptococcus, staphylococcus (including coagulase-positive), *Haemophilus influenzae*, anerobic gram-positive cocci, and gram-negative rods. More than one organism is frequently isolated and usually represents secondary bacterial contamination in the wake of a viral or allergic attack.

Of particular note is the role of allergic responses as a predisposing factor in acute sinusitis. Mucosal damage with loss of ciliary function and induration with impedance of sinus drainage have been implicated in the pathogenesis of acute and chronic sinus infections. Thorough airborne antigenic evaluation should be undertaken in those patients who manifest allergic tendencies or in cases refractory to medical management.

Treatment of acute maxillary sinusitis has two objectives—to eradicate the acute infection and to reestablish adequate drainage and aeration. Broad-spectrum antibiotics such as ampicillin, tetracycline, and the cephalosporins have been employed empirically in cases where sinus cultures were not performed.

Decongestants are employed to reduce mucosal congestion. Oral preparations of phenylpropanolamine or pseudoephedrine and topical nasal vasoconstricting sprays of phenylephrine (Neo-Synephrine) are employed (see Table 7-2). Hydration and humidity play key roles in mobilizing nasal and sinus secretions. An increase in oral fluids and use of a cool system vaporizer are helpful.

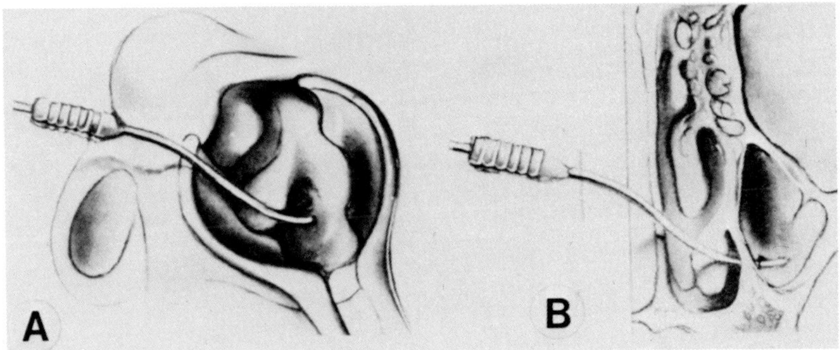

Fig. 7-5. Antral puncture and irrigation: (A) insertion of trocar transnasally in inferior meatus under local anesthesia; (B) position of trocar in maxillary sinus. From Saunders, W. M., Pararella, M. M., & Miglets, A. W.: *Atlas of ear surgery* (ed. 3). St. Louis, Mosby, 1980, p. 57. With permission.

Surgical therapy is indicated in severe infection or cases refractory to adequate antibiotic therapy. Patients should be referred to the ear, nose, and throat (ENT) specialist for surgery when there is evidence of sinus obstruction, chronic infection with marked mucosal thickening, or extension of the process beyond the involved sinus. Antral irrigation in the office has been used to clean mucus from the affected sinus under adequate topical anesthesia. Establishment of a larger nasoantral opening may be necessary to allow adequate drainage. This can be created transnasally under the inferior turbinate as seen in Figure 7-6. With severely thickened mucosa, mucocele, or retained mucopus, a Caldwell-Luc sublabial approach is performed to strip the sinus lining (Fig. 7-7). A nasal antrostomy is always performed in conjunction with this procedure. Adequate drainage and aeration is established, and normal nasal mucosa relines the sinus cavity.

Untreated or refractory maxillary sinusitis can lead to serious complications. Osteomyelitis of the maxilla with subsequent soft-tissue involvement may occur.

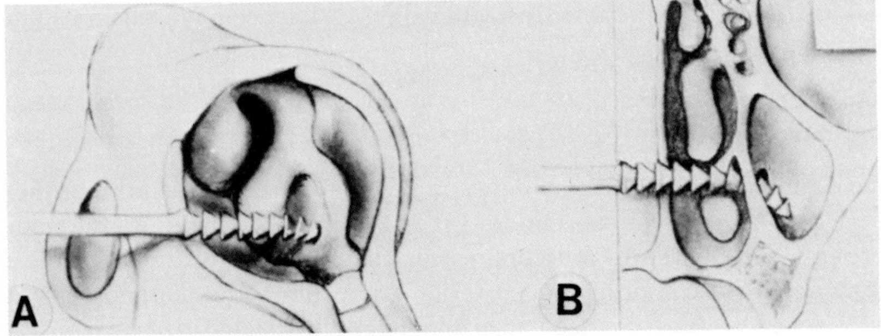

Fig. 7-6. Nasal antrostomy: (A) placement of ronguer in inferior meatus under local anesthesia; (B) entry into maxillary sinus and creation of nasoantral "window" that is larger and lower than the natural ostium. From Saunders, W. M., Paparella, M. M., & Miglets, A. W.: *Atlas of ear surgery* (ed. 3). St. Louis, Mosby, 1980, p. 59. With permission.

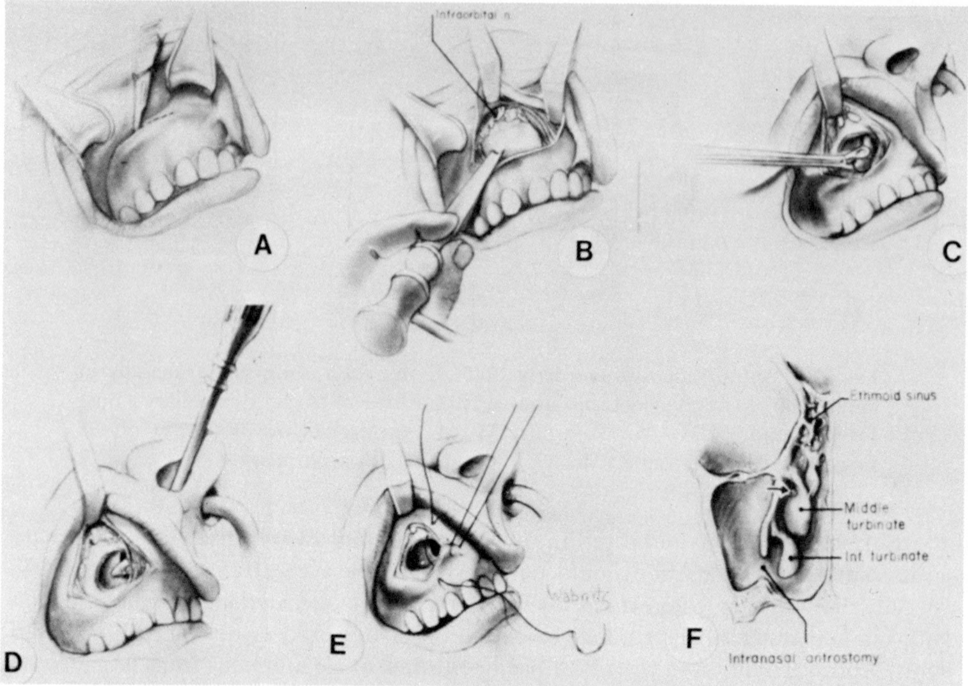

Fig. 7-7. Caldwell-Luc procedure: (A) sublabial incision above maxillary premolars; (B) elevation of mucoperiosteum and entry to sinus through anterior wall; (C) stripping of diseased mucosa and mucopus from sinus; (D) creation of nasal antrostomy; (E) closure of mucoperiosteum and oral mucosa; (F) position of surgical antrostomy in relation to inferior turbinate and natural ostium (arrow). Note ethmoid sinuses at root of middle turbinate. From Saunders, W. M., Paparella, M. M., & Miglets, A. W.: *Atlas of ear surgery* (ed. 3). St. Louis: Mosby, 1980, p. 61. With permission.

Orbital cellulitis secondary to extension of infection to the floor of orbit can lead to abscess formation and blindness. Intracranial extension occurs rarely in patients with maxillary sinusitis.

Ethmoid Sinusitis

The ethmoid sinuses develop between the medial wall of the orbit or the lamina papyracea and the roof of the middle turbinate and are anatomically divided into three groups. The anterior cells drain near the maxillary ostium into the middle meatus, whereas the middle and posterior group drain the superior meatus. The ethmoid sinuses are pneumatized at birth and reach a stable size by age 12.

Isolated acute ethmoid sinusitis is seen more commonly in childhood and presents as a swelling beside the nose or orbital cellulitis due to a dehiscence in the lamina papyracea. Adults suffer from this disease in combination with frontal or maxillary sinusitis on the basis of their common drainage point.

Symptoms include pain in the forehead, nasal bridge, and retroorbital area; nasal

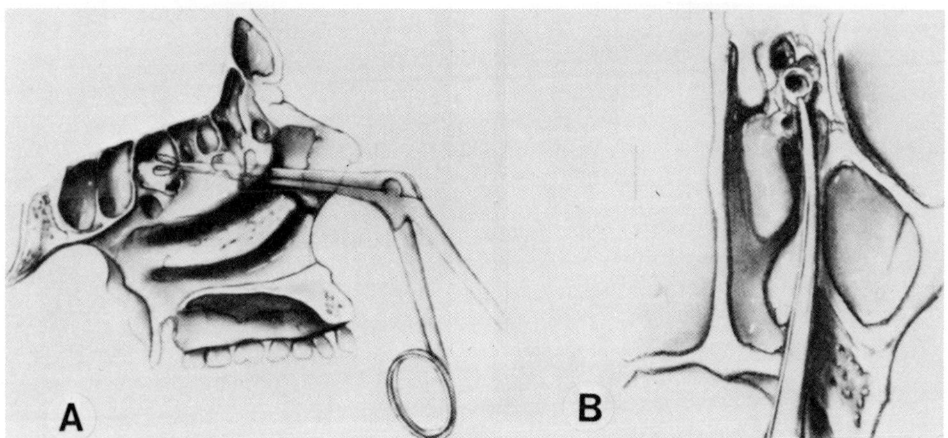

Fig. 7-8. Transnasal ethmoidectomy: (A) surgical access to ethmoid air cells through the middle meatus at the root of the middle turbinate; (B) coronal view of ethmoid cells and their relation to the middle turbinate, maxillary sinus, and medial wall of the orbit. From Saunders, W. M., Paparella, M. M., & Miglets, A. W.: *Atlas of ear surgery* (ed. 3). St. Louis: Mosby, 1980, p. 63. With permission.

congestion; fever; and malaise. Patients may describe a slowly or rapidly progressive swelling near the medial canthus.

Physical signs include nasal discharge, diffuse rhinitis, nasopharyngitis with fever, and pus in the middle or superior meatus. Pericanthal and periorbital swelling with tenderness and ectropion implicate the ethmoid complex. Radiographic evidence of ethmoid cloudiness is diagnostic.

The general measures of decongestants—hydration and humidity—are instituted. Intravenous antibiotic therapy is indicated in most cases as retroorbital abscess with proptosis and blindness can develop rapidly over 24–48 hours. Anatomic extension by hematogenous spread can lead to meningitis and brain abscess. Surgical intervention via an external approach with incision and drainage is indicated at the first signs of orbital involvement. For more chronic ethmoid disease, exenteration via a transversal or transantral approach is employed (Figure 7-8).

Frontal Sinusitis

The frontal sinuses develop late in fetal or even postnatal life and are not clinically significant before puberty. In fact, 15% of adults have only one sinus and 5% have no frontal sinus at all. Drainage occurs via the nasofrontal duct, which arises from the medial aspect of the sinus floor and runs through the ethmoid labyrinth before entering a groove near the anterior end of the middle meatus.

Clinically, frontal sinusitis is rare in children and is almost always associated with anterior ethmoiditis in adults as a result of their close anatomic relationship. Symptoms include fever, malaise, and a characteristic head pain that is located above the eyebrows. This pain is present on arising, worsens by midday, and then lessens toward evening. Clinical signs include tenderness and swelling or erythema over the

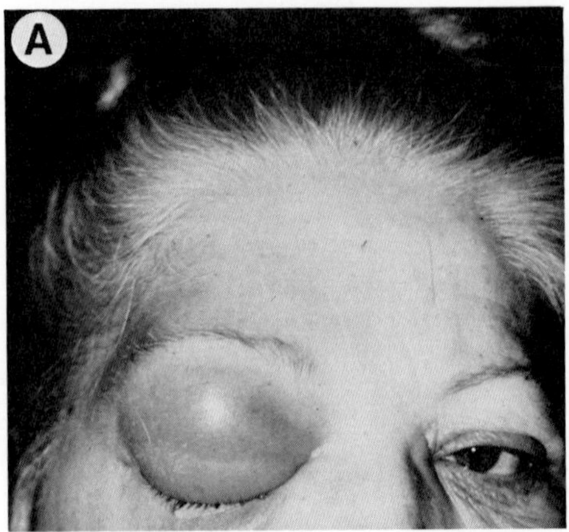

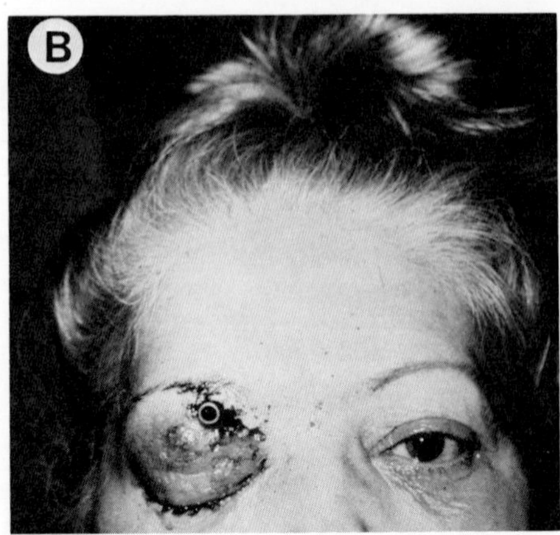

Fig. 7-9. Fifty-five-year-old white female with frontal sinus mucocele: (A) preoperatively—note periorbital swelling and displacement of orbital contents inferolaterally; (B) postoperative trephine procedure—note catheter in right frontal region for irrigation.

frontal sinuses. Occasionally an abscess or infected mucocele causes a mass effect pushing the globe inferiorly and laterally. Mucopus high in the nasopharynx on mirror examination may also be seen.

Radiographically, the frontal sinuses show mucoperiosteal changes, air-fluid levels, or an opacification that must be differentiated from aplastic frontal sinuses. In addition, ethmoidal cloudiness is usually seen in adults.

After frontal sinusitis is diagnosed, medical treatment is immediately instituted and includes oral broad-spectrum antibiotics, decongestants, hydration, humidity, warm compresses, and analgesics. Of particular concern in frontal sinusitis is the avoidance of intracranial complications secondary to osteomyelitis or venous spread and with resultant subdural abscess, empyema, acute meningitis, brain abscess, or cavernous sinus thrombosis. In addition, orbital cellulitis and abscess formation with blindness can occur. Trephination and catheter irrigation is necessary when there are impending complications or unsatisfactory progression on IV antibiotics (Figure 7-9).

Sphenoid Sinusitis

The sphenoid sinuses result as an ingrowth of nasal epithelium in fetal life into the body, greater and lesser wings of the sphenoid bone. Pneumatization occurs late in childhood and reaches full capacity by 15 years of age. Its close association to the cavernous sinus, superior orbital fissure, and pituitary gland make the sphenoid sinus a dangerous region for complications.

Fortunately, isolated sphenoid sinusitis and skull-base complications are rare. Sphenoid sinusitis may accompany maxillary, frontal, or ethmoid sinusitis (pansinusitis), and hence its symptoms, signs and treatment are interrelated. Specific symptoms include retroorbital pain and headache with referred pain to the vertex of the skull. Complications such as osteomyelitis of the sphenoid bone, superior orbital fissure syndrome, cavernous sinus thrombosis, and intracranial extension are usually avoided by early adequate treatment.

Chronic Sinusitis

The treatment of chronic sinusitis is often difficult. The identification of predisposing factors resulting in chronic sinus drainage are perplexing. Allergic states with chronic changes in the mucosa, impaired drainage secondary to anatomic obstruction, congenital abnormalities, and immunodeficient states all contribute to impaired sinus aeration and subsequent repeated infection.

The common denominator in the pathogenesis of chronic sinus disease is impaired mucosal function. Repeated insults to the nasal respiratory mucosa promote many changes. Increased mucous content and thickness of secretions and induration and hypertrophy of the mucosa occur early in the course. These changes lead to repeated infection and result in loss of ciliary function and impaired mobilization of drainage fluid. This, in turn, predisposes to chronic bacterial colonization of the sinus cavities and persistent infection. The treatment of chronic sinus disease, therefore, consists of reducing or eliminating the chronic irritative factors, controlling recurrent bacterial (or fungal) overgrowth, and reestablishing mechanical drainage. These factors contribute in varying proportions in each case and, therefore, complete otolaryngologic, allergic and general medical evaluation is necessary in treating this problem.

Symptoms of chronic disease are generally vague and nondiagnostic by themselves. Excluding exacerbations that mimic acute sinusitis, nasal congestion, chronic thick secretions in the throat, halitosis, chronic cough with mild pharyngitis or laryngitis, and a fullness in the head constitute the majority of symptoms. Patients may complain of symptoms secondary to airborne allergies or seasonal rhinitis, frequent winter colds, or epistaxis. A history of nasal polyps requiring removal is common. Symptoms may vary with climate. Profuse edematous sinus drainage occurs in moist climates, whereas obstructive or episodic variety is found in drier climates, and with wide temperature extremes both may occur.

Physical findings include nasal polyposis with mucosal thickening or atrophy, polypoid degeneration of the turbinates, thick mucoid drainage on the posterior oropharynx, deviated nasal septum, and mild injection of the laryngopharynx and vocal cords secondary to chronic cough. Unless an acute exacerbation is occurring, fever, severe pain, and throbbing headaches are absent.

Radiographically, evidence of mucoperiosteal thickening with partial or complete opacification of the involved sinuses is seen. Air-fluid levels seen on serial sinus films are consistent with chronic sinus blockage. Occasionally mucoceles, antrochoanal polyps, and nasopharyngeal obstruction by soft tissue are noticed.

Once the diagnosis of chronic sinus disease is made and the etiology is suspected, treatment consists of three modalities: removal of the underlying agent of the mucosal injury, control of acute exacerbations, and removal of diseased mucosa and reestablishment of drainage. Allergic desensitization and avoidance of particular antigens is of great benefit in susceptible individuals. Treatment of nasopharyngitis, adenoiditis, and viral syndromes is necessary. Acute therapy is initiated early at the first sign of infection. Chronic sinusitis is a disease of multiple bacterial organisms and is best treated with broad-spectrum antibiotics. Increased humidity and adequate hydration are important, as are trial courses of oral decongestants. Nasal steroid preparations are now available for use in cases of nasal polyposis and allergic rhinitis. Persistent mechanical causes and effects of chronic disease of the paranasal sinuses may eventually necessitate surgical treatment.

Case History

A 22-year-old white male was admitted to Barnes Hospital with a 2-day history of severe right frontal "headache." Several days previously he complained of nasal congestion, cough, and sore throat. He was seen 24 hours prior to admission by his private otolaryngologist where sinus films were "nonconclusive for sinusitis," and he was treated with PCN VK 250 mg qid and acetaminophen (Tylenol) No. 3 for pain. He presented to the emergency room that evening with increased right frontal pain, mild photophobia, and more localized tenderness above his right eye.

Physical examination revealed a temperature of 37.4°C. The tympanic membranes were normal and mobile. Nasal speculum exam revealed pus in the right middle meatus that reaccumulated after suctioning. There was marked tenderness over the right medial brow and some erythema but no fluctuance. Extraocular motion was grossly intact with minimal pain. There was no proptosis.

An ophthalmologic examination revealed no lid edema, chemosis, proptosis, or acuity changes. Neurologic examination was nonfocal with no evidence of intracranial or cavernous sinus complications.

Routine laboratory tests were normal except for a white blood count of 10.6 with a normal differential. Sinus films showed a right frontal air-fluid level with mucoperiosteal thickening. Similar changes were seen in the right maxillary sinus.

The patient was admitted, blood cultures were done, and high-dose antibiotics were begun IV. Warm compresses, nasal decongestants, and q4h vital signs with vision checks were also started. Repeat sinus films at 1 and 2 days after admission showed persistence of the air-fluid levels and interval clouding of the right ethmoid sinus. The patient spiked a temperature of 38.2°C orally on the second day and was taken to the operating room for right frontal sinus trephination and a right maxillary antrostomy. Gross mucopus was found in both sinuses. A drain was left in the frontal sinus for irrigation.

Postoperatively the patient did well on IV antibiotics and bid irrigations of the right frontal sinus. Methylene blue dye placed in the frontal sinus drain appeared in the nasal cavity, indicating frontonasal duct patency on the third postoperative day. The drain was removed, and the patient was discharged the following day on oral antibiotics, nasal saline, and decongestant drops. Follow-up office examination 2 weeks later showed no clinical evidence of persistent sinusitis. Repeat films revealed resolution of all air-fluid levels.

This is a good example of the progression of "undertreated" frontal sinusitis and the anatomic relationship between the anterior ethoids and the maxillary and frontal sinuses. This patient probably started with a viral URI or isolated rhinitis that then proceeded to block the common drainage point of the three involved sinuses in the middle meatus. This was followed by fluid collection in the blocked cavities and progression to a right-sided "pansinusitis." In this case, no intracranial or orbital complications developed, but failure of clinical improvement and persistence of the air-fluid levels after 48 hours of medical treatment warranted surgical intervention. This is, of course, an example of the extreme case of frontal disease that goes to surgery, and indeed the majority of instances of frontal sinusitis will resolve with antibiotic and decongestant therapy. The practitioner, however, must be aware of the indications for surgery when medical therapy fails as seen here. The presence of mucoperiosteal thickening probably represents chronic changes and may indicate the need for further evaluation after the acute episode is controlled.

REFERENCES

Dees, S. C., & Lefkowitz, D. *Am. J. Dis. Childh.*, 1972, *124*, 364.

Ishikawa, T., Bernstein, J., Reisman, R. E., et al. *J. Allergy Clin. Immunol.* 1972, *50*, 319.

Olson, A. L., Klein, S. W., Charney, E. *Pediatrics*, 1978, *61*, 679.

Oppenheimer, R. P. *Eye, Ear, Nose Throat Mon.*, 1976, *54*, 316.

Perrin, J. M., Charney, E., MacWhinney, J. B., McInerny, T. K., Mikker, R. L., Wazaeian, L. F. *New Engl. J. Med.*, 1964, *29*, 13.

Shambaugh, G. E., & Glasscock, M. E. *Surgery of the ear*. Philadelphia: Saunders, 1980.

SUGGESTED READINGS

Adams, G. L., Boies, L. R., & Paparella, M. M. *Fundamentals of Otolaryngology*, Philadelphia: Saunders, 1978.

English, G. N. *Otolaryngology, a textbook*. New York: Harper & Row, 1976, chap. 18.

Lierle, D. M., & Benstem, L. In G. M. English (Ed.), *Otolaryngology*, 1976, Vol. III, chap. II.

Paparella, M. M., & Shumrick, D. H. *Otolaryngology*. Philadelphia: Saunders, 1980, Vols. I, II.

Paradise, J. L. *Pediatrics*, 1977, *60*, 86.

Paradise, J. L. *S. Med. J.*, 1949, *69*, 9.

Patterson, R. *Allergic diseases, diagnosis and management*. Philadelphia: Lippincott, 1980.

Rynvel-Dagoo, B., Ahlbom, A., & Schiratzki, H. *Ann. Otol.*, 1978, *87*, 272.

QUESTIONS

1. A 7-year-old boy is seen for unilateral acute otitis media and treated for 10 days with amoxicillin and decongestants. On follow-up examination two weeks later, the patient has a serous effusion and a flat tympanogram. The following alternatives are reasonable *except:*

   a. Prolonged (6–12 wk) decongestants/antihistamine therapy
   b. Close follow-up
   c. Renew 7–10 day course amoxicillin +/− decongestants
   d. Suggest myringotomy and tube placement (M&T)
   e. Teach modified Valsalva minimum

2. A healthy 6-week-old infant develops an acute otitis media in the left ear while at home. Physical exam reveals a dull tympane membrane. There are no signs or symptoms of meningitis. The temperature is 101°. Which of the following measures is *not* warranted at this point:

   a. Hydration
   b. Decongestants
   c. Broad spectrum antibiotics covering *S. pneumoniae, H. influenzae,* and *S. viridans*

d. Spinal tap to r/o meningitis
e. Tympanocentesis and culture

3. A 6-year-old boy is referred for evaluation of rhinitis and nasal speech. Sinus films reveal increased adenoidal tissue in the nasopharynx and an "opacified frontal sinus". The most likely explanation is:

a. Blockage of the fronto-nasal duct by the adenoids
b. Tumor of the frontal sinus
c. Pus in the frontal sinus
d. Chronic allergic sinusitis
e. Misinterpretation of the films

4. A 30-year-old female is seen for chronic nasal stuffiness and hay fever. She admits to using over-the-counter nasal sprays for years, but has had little relief in recent months. On physical exam her nasal mucosa is boggy and congested with a thin clear rhinorrhea. The most appropriate therapy is to:

a. Prescribe stronger symptomatic nasal spray
b. Stop the nasal spray and start oral decongestants
c. Continue the nasal spray and add salt water nose drops
d. Stop the nasal spray and start topical steroid preparations
e. Suggest septal surgery to relieve obstruction

5. Treatment of chronic sinusitis in adults includes:

a. Adequate environment control and desensitization for allergic causes
b. Broad-spectrum antibiotics for acute exacerbations
c. Topical steroid and saline nasal preparations for airway congestion
d. Surgery for irreversible mucosal disease with pain or retained pus
e. Adequate hydration and humidity
f. All of the above

Answers can be found in Appendix B at the end of the book.

Lawrence Samuels

8

Cutaneous Allergy: Allergic Contact Dermatitis and Atopic Dermatitis

CUTANEOUS ALLERGY

"Cutaneous allergy" refers to a cutaneous hypersensitivity characterized by certain clinical and laboratory findings. Diseases of the skin characterized by a cutaneous hypersensitivity include two large categories with numerous etiologies: eczematous dermatitides and urticaria. Urticaria is reviewed in detail in Chapter 9, and our present discussion focuses on the clinical manifestations, pathophysiology, and treatment of eczematous dermatitides.

The term "dermatitis" indicates any cutaneous inflammation, whereas an eczematous dermatitis should indicate a cutaneous eruption consisting of erythema, pruritus, and skin lesions that range from papulovesicular to scaly in nature, depending on the stage of the eruption. An eczematous dermatitis can be further subdivided into acute, subacute, and chronic stages, depending on the clinical nature of the skin lesions. Four main divisions of eczematous dermatitis can be established: dermatitis resulting from exogenous agents such as allergic contact eczematous dermatitis (Table 8-1), endogenous agents such as autosensitization phenomenas, cases in which no clear etiology has been established such as in atopic eczematous dermatitis (Table 8-2), and diseases that have an eczematous dermatitis as part of their clinical picture (Table 8-3). Obviously, a discussion of cutaneous allergy encompasses many disease states, and the purpose of this chapter is to familiarize the reader with an eczematous dermatitis and to focus on two specific clinical conditions that are commonly encountered in clinical practice with regard to their clinical manifestations, pathophysiology, and treatment. These two clinical cutaneous diseases are allergic contact eczematous dermatitis and atopic eczematous dermatitis.

Eczematous dermatitis is worldwide, and etiologies vary slightly according to the locale. It is difficult to estimate the socioeconomic impact of severe eczema. Economically, this is manifest by poor work performance, lost work hours, school

ALLERGY: THEORY AND PRACTICE
ISBN 0-8089-1619-X

Table 8-1 *Eczematous Dermatitis Associated with Exogenous Agents*

Exogenous Agent	Clinical Disease
Plant resins	allergic contact eczematous dermatitis
Cosmetics and topical medications	allergic contact eczematous dermatitis
Metals	allergic contact eczematous dermatitis
Fabrics	allergic contact eczematous dermatitis
Ultraviolet light	polymorphous light eruptions, eczematous type

absenteeism, and the numerous medical care costs related to its treatment. Just as important are the marked psychological and social problems encountered by the patient with severe eczema. This is reflected in one's own self-image and relationship to family and friends. Estimates suggest that 25–30% of dermatologic patient visits are related to eczema; therefore, it is clear that this has an enormous impact on society. It is hoped that through a better understanding of the disease process, its treatment, and its implication on the patient's relationship to society, physicians can reduce both the economic as well as the psychological impact of this problem.

Pathophysiology

The underlying pathophysiology for many cases of eczematous dermatitis are unknown; thus the clinical and histologic patterns seen in any given case, depend on the clinical appearance of the lesions as described in the preceding section. Specific information regarding the pathophysiology of allergic contact eczematous dermatitis and atopic eczematous dermatitis is discussed in the appropriate sections of this chapter.

Clinical Manifestations

The clinical features of an acute eczematous dermatitis include areas of diffuse erythema and edema resulting in small, nonumbilicated, vesicular lesions that may exude serum, eventually leading to crust formation (Fig. 8-1). Histopathologically, there is significant intercellular edema in the epidermis (spongiosis), which can result in the development of intraepidermally located vesicles or bullae. The spongiotic portions of the epidermis may have an inflammatory infiltrate (exocytosis) composed predominately of mononuclear cells, but with some scattered neutrophils. Crusted lesions reveal a parakeratotic stratum corneum with areas of coagulated plasma. The dermis is edematous with vascular dilutation and a perivascular mononuclear cell infiltrate (Fig. 8-2). Clinical features characteristic of a chronic eczematous dermatitis include lesions that are reddish-brown in color with thickening of the skin noted by marked accentuation of the normal skin line (lichenification) and scaliness (Fig. 8-3). Histologic features include mild intercellular edema with epidermal hyperplasia

Table 8-2 *Eczematous Dermatitis of Unknown Etiology*

- Atopic eczematous dermatitis
- Dyshidrotic eczematous dermatitis
- Eczematous statis dermatitis
- Nummular eczematous dermatitis
- Idiopathic eczematous dermatitis

Table 8-3 *Immunodeficiency Disorders Associated with Eczematous Dermatitis*

Clinical Disease
• Wiskott-Aldrich Syndrome
• Hyper-IgE Syndrome
• DiGeorge Syndrome
• Nezelof Syndrome
• Selective IgA deficiency
• Louis-Bar Syndrome
• Acquired Agammaglobulinemia

Table 8-4 *Order of Potency of Topical Steroids in Descending Order*

Group Number	Topical Steroid
1	Halog Cream 0.1% Lidex Cream 0.5% Topicort Cream 0.25%
2	Valisone Ointment 0.1% Diprisone Cream 0.05% Aristocort Cream 0.5%
3	Kenalog Ointment 0.1% Synalar Ointment 0.025% Cordran Ointment 0.05%
4	Aristocort Cream 0.1% Valisone Cream 0.1% Westcort Cream 0.1% Locoid Cream 0.1% Synalar Cream 0.025%
5	Tridesilon Cream 0.05% Locorten Cream 0.03%
6	Hytone Cream 1.0% Nutracort Cream 1.0%

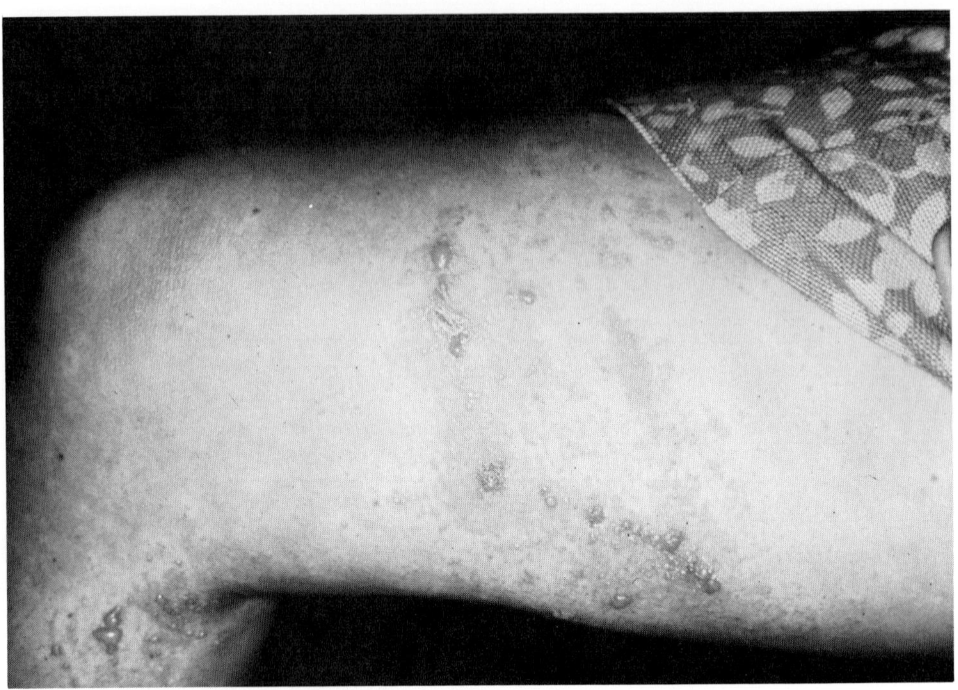

Fig. 8-1. Acute eczematous dermatitis demonstrated by linear erythematous vesicular bullous lesions.

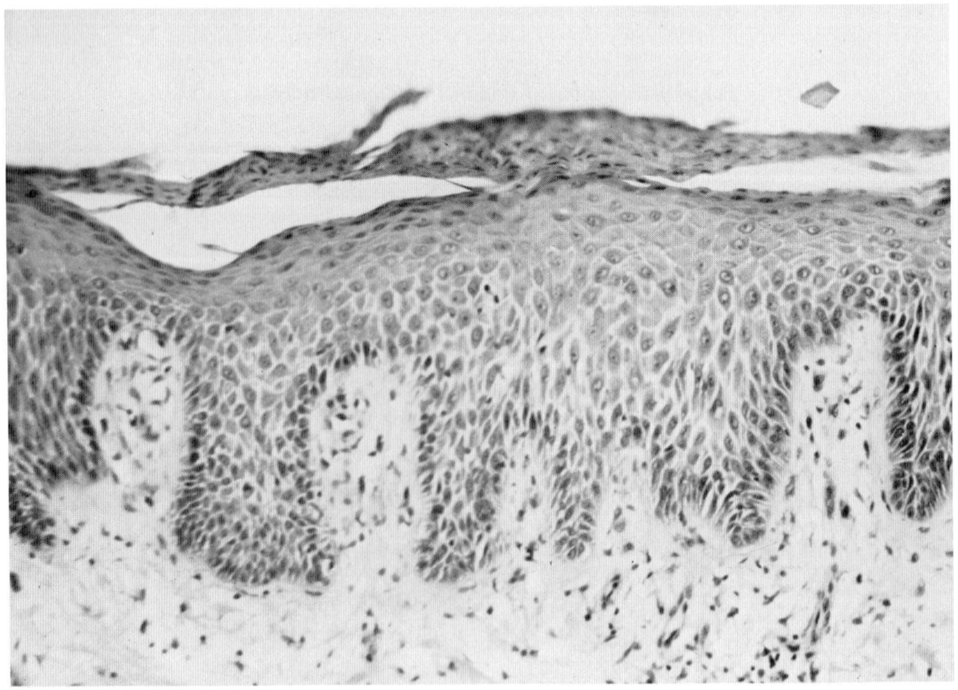

Fig. 8-2. Histologic features of an acute eczematous dermatitis demonstrated by intercellular edema with the formation of an intraepidermal vesicle. There is vaso dilutation in the papillary dermis with accompanying dermal edema.

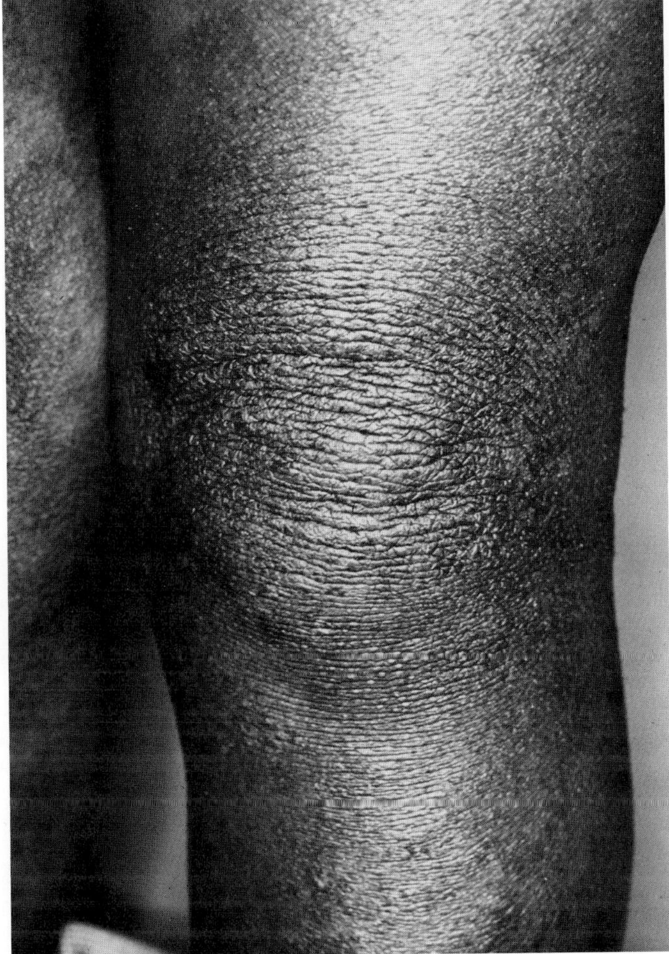

Fig. 8-3. Chronic eczematous dermatitis demonstrated by marked accentuation of the skin lines and skin thickening.

(acanthosis) and hyperkeratosis with areas of parakeratosis. The upper dermis has a mild perivascular mononuclear cell infiltrate (Fig. 8-4). Clinical features of a subacute eczematous dermatitis reveal lesions of both types; that is, lesions characteristically seen in acute eczematous dermatitis and chronic eczematous dermatitis. The histologic appearance depends on the type of lesion present.

Diagnostic Test

Routine laboratory testing in cases of eczematous dermatitis reveal no specific diagnostic abnormalities. As noted in Tables 8-1–8-3, there are specific diseases that have an eczematous dermatitis as a clinical component of the disease, and specific tests should be directed at the underlying disease process.

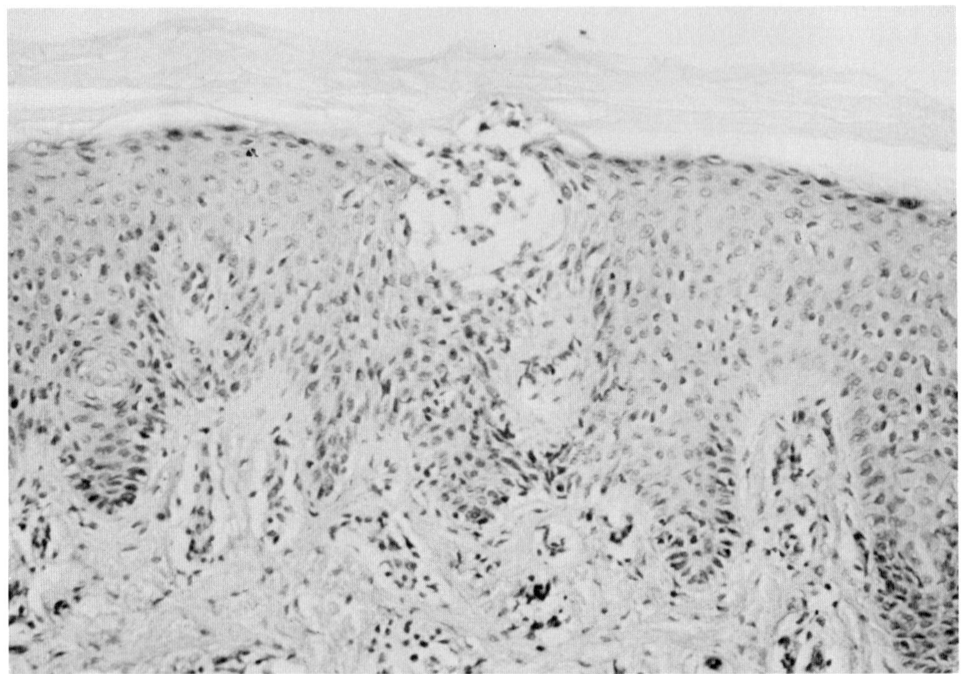

Fig. 8-4. Histologic features of a chronic eczematous dermatitis with intercellular edema in the epidermis with thickening of the epidermis and overlying parakeratosis. The vaso dilutation in the papillary dermis and dermal edema is less marked than that in an acute eczematous dermatitis.

TREATMENT

There are certain general measures regarding the treatment of any eczematous dermatitis depending on the stage of the clinical lesions. In acute eczematous dermatitis with marked erythema, edema, papulovesicular lesions, and/or bullous lesions, frequent tepid to cool, moist, soothing compresses are needed. Compresses can be tap water or normal saline and may have a mild desiccant added such as packets of aluminum acetate (Domeboro) to increase the drying effect of the soaks. They should be applied to the skin for 20–60 minutes, removed, patted dry, and the lesions then left to air-dry. The frequency of applications depends on the severity of the eruption and ranges from 2 to 6 times daily. Drying lotions such as calamine lotion or a corticosteroid spray are more effective during this stage than corticosteroid creams or lotions. Topical agents containing local anesthetics such as benzocaine should be avoided as they can cause secondary sensitization. Systemic antipruritics, such as diphenhydramine (Benadryl) 25–50 mg, hydroxyzine HCl (Atarax, Vistaril) 25–50 mg, or cyproheptadine (Periactin) 4 mg given every 6 hr can be used for symptomatic treatment. In selected cases when an acute eczematous dermatitis is widespread and involves areas such as the face or genitalia, a tapering course of oral corticosteroids should be used. Initial adult dosage should range from 40 to 60 mg of prednisone per day (1 mg/kg of prednisone daily for children) and tapered over a 7–14-day period. The patient should be encouraged to use topical care as the systemic corticosteroid is reduced. In cases of chronic eczematous dermatitis or resolving stages of an acute eczematous dermatitis when the lesions are marked by pruritus, erythema, and lichenification, moist compresses and drying agents should be specifically avoided. The patient should be instructed on the long-term treatment and maintenance of good local skin care, which is generally required to control or eradicate the eczematous dermatitis. Rather than trying to alter one's personal hygiene to extreme levels, it is generally more efficacious to encourage baths of shorter duration with tepid water and the use of soothing bath oils and mild soaps. There are many mild soaps, liquid cleansers, and lipid-free cleansers on the market, and since all brands are effective, the one most preferred by the patient should be used. This applies also to bath oils and moisturizers, as most are very effective and are more likely to be used if they are preferred by the patient. It is important to emphasize to the patient that treatment should be directed toward proper skin care and the use of topically applied cortisone creams and ointments. A list of commonly used corticosteroid preparations are presented in the table according to their strength (Table 8-5). Because of the side effects of topical steroids, it is advisable to use the lowest strength that will achieve the appropriate clinical results. In addition, general guidelines would indicate the use of mild corticosteroid preparations for the facial area including the ears, medium-strength topical steroids for the major portion of the body, and more potent corticosteroid preparations for the hands, feet, elbows, and knees. Once again, systemic antipruritics can be important, particularly at bedtime, to alleviate some of the nighttime scratching. It should be emphasized that these agents help only to reduce the symptomatology and that it is the purpose of the topical treatment to eradicate the cutaneous eruption. Although there is no role for long-term systemic steroid therapy in controlling a chronic eczematous dermatitis, a short tapering course in a setting of an acute exacerbation of a chronic eczematous dermatitis can sometimes be helpful in managing these patients while appropriate topical treatment is started. Although unusual, at times a generalized chronic eczematous dermatitis; an acute exacerbation of a chronic eczematous dermatitis; or a severe generalized acute eczematous dermatitis involving widespread areas of vesiculation, oozing, or encrusting may require hospitalization for initiation of treatment. In the hospital, skin care is reflective of treatment noted above; however, it can be provided on a much more intensive and extensive basis. There are also certain measures available during hospital care that are not routinely available for home patient care, that is, ultraviolet (UV) light phototherapy or larger doses of antipruritics that may produce significant sedation.

ALLERGIC CONTACT ECZEMATOUS DERMATITIS

Contact dermatitis is divided into two distinct groups. An allergic contact dermatitis due to a specific allergenic sensitization, which is elicited by contact with the skin and a primary irritant contact dermatitis, results in cutaneous injury due to a direct toxic effect. This chapter is concerned only with an allergic contact eczematous dermatitis.

Table 8-5 *Common Contact Allergens*

Medications, preservatives & fragrances	*AAD 1980, Allergen Test Tray Number**
Neomycin sulfate, 20%	7
Ammoniated mercury 1%	5
Ethylenediamine dihydrochloride, 1%	14
Parabens (methyl, ethyl, propyl, and butyl 3% each) 12%	6
Wool alcohols, 30%	3
Caine mixture, 8%	11
Lanolin, 100%	10
Benzyl alcohol, 5%	1
Quarternium 15, 2%	22
Imidazolidinyl urea 2%	16
Fragrance mix 16%	21
Metals	
Potassium dichromate, 0.5%	2
Nickel sulfate, 2.5% (optional)	23
Rubber chemicals	
Mercapto mix, 1%	13
MBT 1%	4
Thiuram mix, 1%	19
Black Rubber p-Phenyleneddiamine mix 0.6% (P.P.D., mix 0.6%)	17
Carba mix, 3%	8
Others	
Formaldehyde (in water), 2%	20
p-Phenylenediamine, 1%	9
Epoxy resin, 1%	12
p-tert-Butylphenol, 2%	18
PCMX, 1%	15

*Standard test tray (1980) recommended by the North American Contact Dermatitis Group.

Pathophysiology

The occurrence of an allergic contact eczematous dermatitis is based on the application of an allergenic substance applied to the skin, thus eliciting a clinical cutaneous eruption. This is a type IV or cell-mediated hypersensitivity (see Chapter 2). The antigen sensitizes the patient by binding to skin and/or other tissue proteins. Since preparation of the immunogen below the horny layer is essential for antigenic activity, breaking of the normal existing skin barrier by trauma also may favor sensitization. Certain clinical states are often associated with an increased incidence of allergic contact sensitization, presumably because they present unusually favorable opportunities for conjugation of the antigenic substance with the carrier proteins below the horny layer. Examples are eczematous eruptions over burned skin, eczematous eruptions associated with statis dermatitis, and secondary eczematous reactions associated with skin that is simultaneously undergoing nonspecific primary irritation. Sensitization of immunologically compotent cells to the contact antigen probably takes place both in the skin (peripheral sensitization) and centrally in the dermal lymphatics and draining lymph nodes. Current evidence suggests that contact antigens must be processed by Langerhans cells (a type of macrophage) before they can induce specific sensitization. Langerhans cells, apparently, pick up the contact antigen in the skin and carry them via dermal lymphatics to the draining lymph nodes. This completes the so-called phase of sensitization, which takes about 4 days following the contact of the antigen to the skin. On reexposure to the antigenic substance, there is transformation of sensitized lymphocytes and the release of a series of lymphokines. Lymphocytes are thus the principal mediators of allergic contact eczematous dermatitis.

Clinical Manifestations

The distribution of a cutaneous eruption can be of great aid in arriving at an appropriate clinical diagnosis. This is particularly important at the beginning of a cutaneous eruption. For example, eruptions restricted only to exposed areas of the body are quite characteristic of airborne allergens. These cutaneous eruptions are marked by very sharp cut-offs, as they are absent from areas where clothing covers the skin. Cutaneous eruptions may be restricted only to the head and neck, and this may indicate an allergic reaction to a hair dye or other cosmetic agent. Eruptions confined to sun-exposed areas may indicate a phototoxic or photoallergic dermatitis. Besides the distribution, the pattern and shape of an eczematous dermatitis may furnish clues to the nature of the causal agent. This is exemplified by the characteristic linear lesions associated with various contact sensitivities, particularly poison ivy. It should be emphasized that a very characteristic clinical feature of contact dermatitis is the artifactual, angulated lesions in a localized, but characteristic, distribution (Figs. 8-1 and 8-5). In addition to the obvious features mentioned above, it is noteworthy that the scalp, palms, and soles have a greater resistance to contact sensitization than do other areas of the skin. It is quite common with various hair dyes that the scalp is likely to be uninvolved, although there is a marked eczematous eruption of the face, ears, and neck area. There are also various nonspecific contributory factors that may influence the occurrence, severity, and site of involvement of an allergic contact eczematous dermatitis. They include friction, pressure, heat, and perspiration. Although contact eruptions usually extend to the mucous membranes of the mouth, clinical involvement of the oral mucosa is uncommon. The hypersensitivity in a contact allergy, as a rule, involves the entire cutaneous surface, but in exceptional cases, hypersensitivity restricted to particular areas has been reported (Figs. 8-6–8-8). Flare-ups limited to the original site of sensitization after systemic exposure to a contact allergen also indicates that there are pronounced local differences in the degree of hypersensitivity.

Diagnostic Tests

Establishing a diagnosis of an allergic contact skin sensitivity can be greatly aided by a thorough history, concentrating on recent exposures as well as by a thorough physical examination of the entire cutaneous surface, paying particular attention to

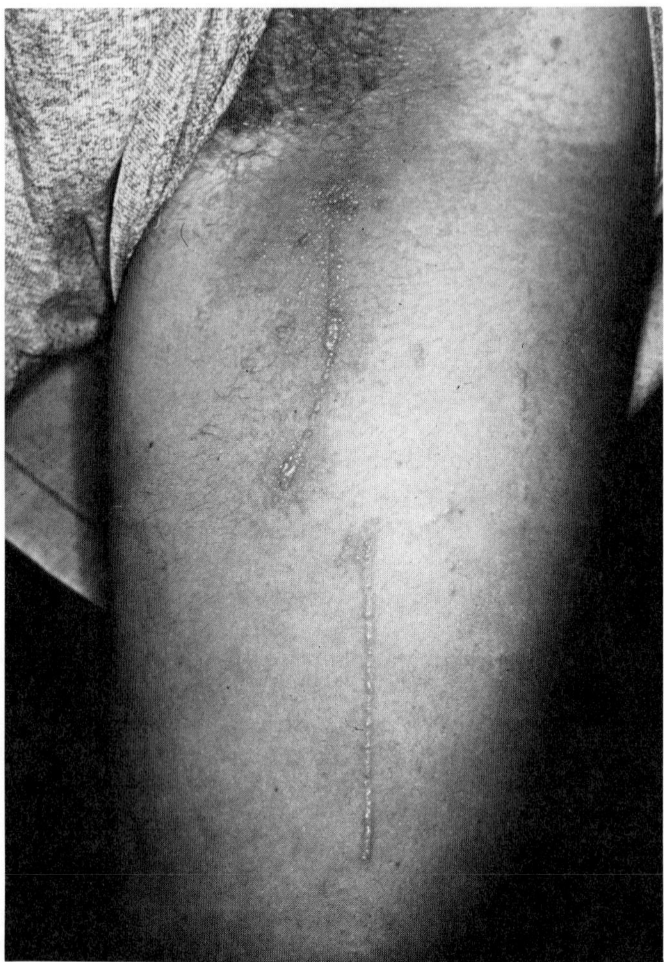

Fig. 8-5. Characteristics of poison ivy showing linear erythematous papular vesicular lesions.

the distribution and pattern of the lesions. There are usually no specific laboratory abnormalities noted, and there is, in general, no peripheral eosinophilia. Unfortunately, skin biopsies reveal very nonspecific changes. The most pronounced histologic findings are those noted in the various other forms of eczematous dermatitis that have been reviewed previously. Although the microscopic findings may be suggestive of an allergic contact hypersensitivity, microscopic findings are by no means diagnostic.

Patch tests, if properly used, are reliable and useful methods for diagnosing specific contact hypersensitivity. There are several manufactured patch test kits for various antigens. Table 8-5 demonstrates a list of common contact allergies and their appropriate test concentrations as recommended by the North American Contact Dermatitis Group. Specific patch testing trays are available for various types of contact dermatitis. These include fragrance materials, shoe materials, preservative materials, and others. Information regarding these test kits can be obtained from the North

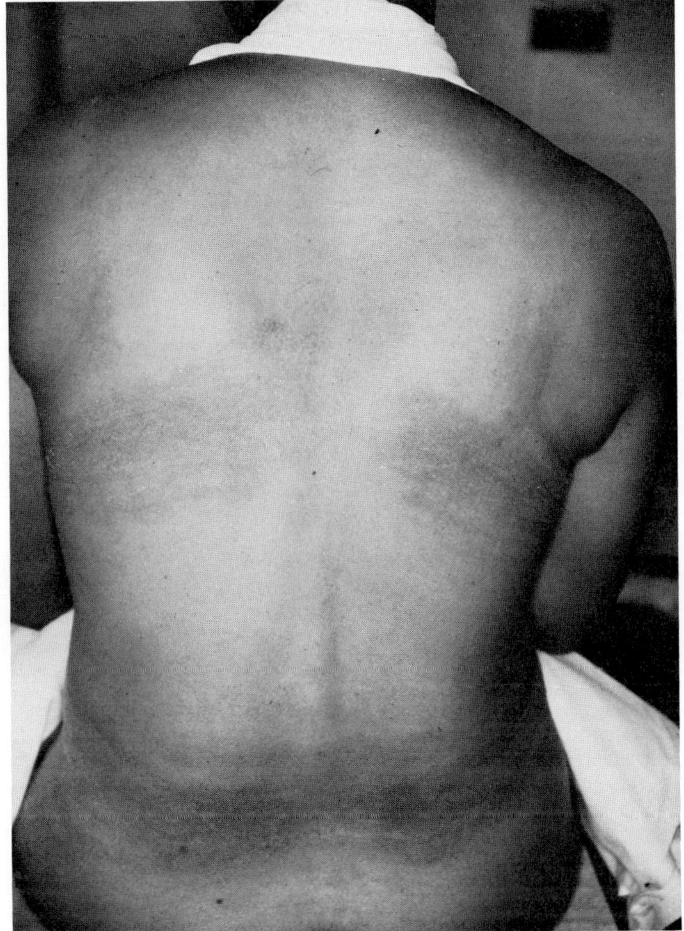

Fig. 8-6. Clinical characteristics of an acute allergic eczematous dermatitis due to a rubber accelerator.

American Contact Dermatitis Group. Regardless of the test tray utilized, the allergenic substances are applied to the skin, usually the back and the arms, under a small occlusive dressing. It is important to use recommended concentrations to avoid nonspecific primary irritant reactions. The patch test is left in place for 48 hours and the results recorded 30 minutes after removal of the patch test and again in 24–48 hours. A positive patch test with a 2+ reaction to nickel sulfate is noted in Figure

Table 8-6 *Interpretation Key For Patch Test Results*

−	Negative reaction
+	Weak positive reaction: erythema and possibly somewhat palpable
+ +	Strong positive reaction: erythema, papules, and vesicles
+ + +	Extreme positive reaction: bullous formation

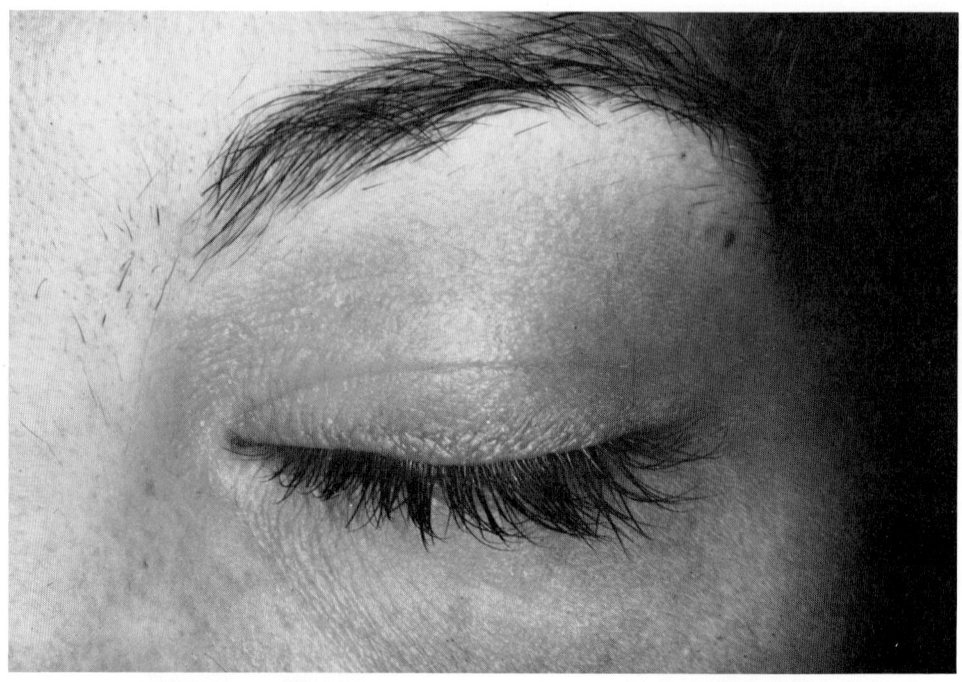

Fig. 8-7. Clinical characteristics of an allergic contact dermatitis due to nail polish.

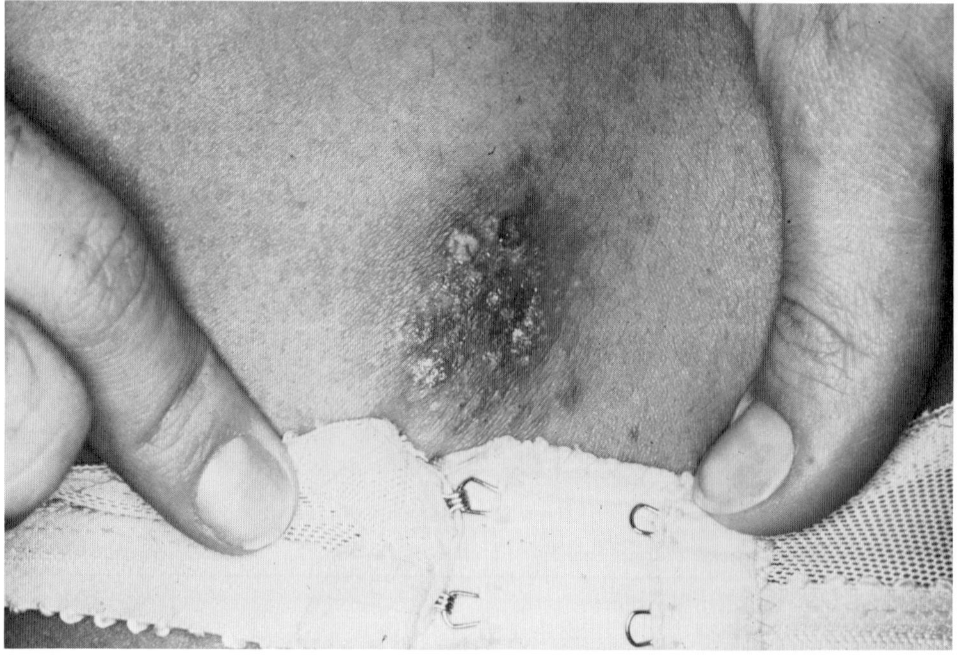

Fig. 8-8. An allergic contact dermatitis due to nickel in bra strap clasp.

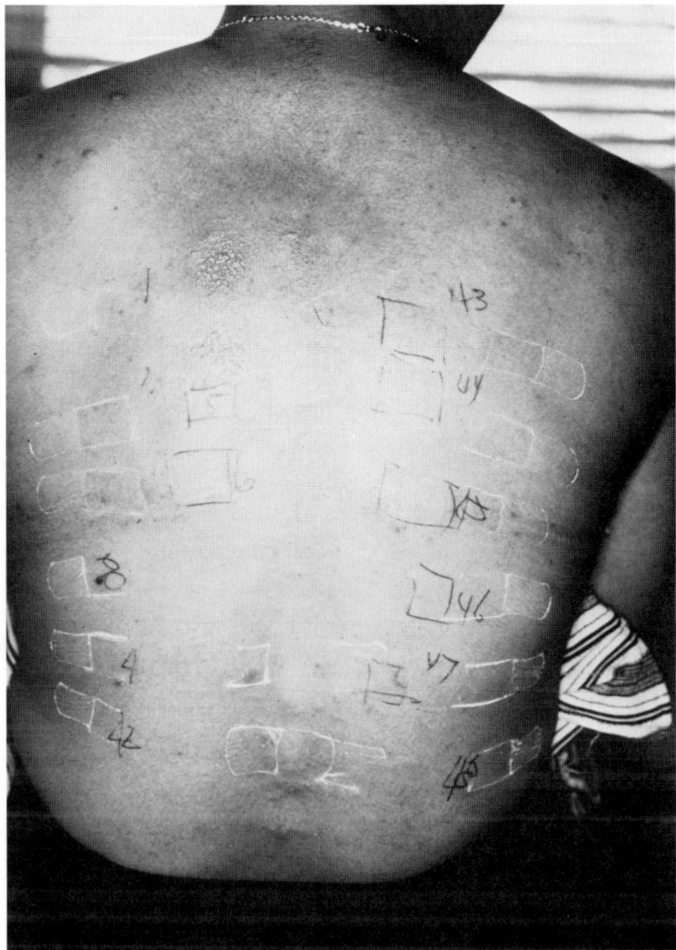

Fig. 8-9. Demonstration of a patch testing procedure with a positive test to nickel sulfate on the upper portion of the back.

8-9. Table 8-6 demonstrates the appropriate method for recording patch test results. Before substances that have elicited positive reactions can be accepted as causes of the presenting eruption, the results of the patch test should be correlated with the history of an allergenic exposure and the clinical findings.

Treatment

Treatment of an allergic contact eczematous dermatitis is similar to that of other forms of eczematous dermatitis (see above). Obviously, elimination and avoidance of the causal antigenic substance is the most effective preventive and therapeutic measure. Once a sensitizing agent has been identified, it is important to avoid inadvertent contact with chemically related substances that may produce a similar sensitization as well as to thoroughly investigate the wide range of materials that

Table 8-7 *Diagnostic Criteria for Atopic Dermatitis**

Absolute features—Must have each of the following:

- Pruritus
- Typical morphology and distribution:
  - Flexural lichenification in adults.
  - Facial and extensor involvements in infancy
- Tendency toward chronic or chronically-related dermatitis

PLUS

Two or More of the Following Features:

- Personal or family history of atopic disease (asthma, allergic rhinitis, atopic dermatitis).
- Immediate skin test reactivity.
- White dermographism and/or delayed blanch to cholinergic agents.
- Anterior subcapsular cataracts.

OR

Four or More of the Following Features:

- Xerosis/ichthyosis/hyperlinear palms
- Pityriasis alba
- Keratosis pilaris
- Facial pallor/infraorbital darkening
- Dennie-Morgan infraorbital fold
- Elevated serum-IgE
- Keratoconus
- Tendency toward nonspecific hand dermatitis
- Tendency toward repeated cutaneous infections

*Hanifin, J. M. and W. C. Lobitz, Jr., Arch. Dermatol. Vol. 113:663-670, 1977.

may contain the known sensitizing agent. In most cases, topical treatment alone is adequate for the treatment of most types of contact dermatitis; however, in selected cases when contact dermatitis is widespread or involving areas such as the face or genitalia, a tapering course of an oral corticosteroid should be used. Once again, the initial dosage should range from 40–60 mg of prednisone or its equivalent per day and tapered over a 7–14 day period.

There are several points worthy of mention that apply specifically to the treatment of plant contact allergic reaction. Generally, specific hyposensitization, particularly by the oral route, although effective, takes many months or several years to achieve adequate therapeutic results and thus is somewhat restricted clinically. At present, immunotherapy in acute plant allergic contact dermatitis is not recommended. In addition, it is not indicated in patients who are subject to occasional attacks of poison ivy contact dermatitis as conservative measures easily control most cases regardless of the severity. Consideration for a clinical trial with immunotherapy is reasonable in those individuals extremely sensitive to plant allergens whose professions require them to come into frequent contact with these substances. This would include farmers, telephone workers, lineworkers, highway workers, and others. If the above measures are unable to adequately control the patients allergic contact sensitivity, specific changes in work or locale are necessary.

Table 8-8 *Patients with Atopic Dermatitis**

	Percent
Patients with a personal history of allergic rhinitis or asthma	31
Patients with a family history of allergic rhinitis or asthma	62
Neither a personal nor a family history of allergic rhinitis, asthma, or other atopic diseases	21

Atopic dermatitis often occurs in association with a personal or family history of atopy, i.e., allergic rhinitis, asthma, or hay fever, however, a significant percentage of patients have neither a personal nor a familial history of respiratory allergic disease.

*150 patients

ATOPIC ECZEMATOUS DERMATITIS

Atopic eczematous dermatous dermatitis is a chronic, pruritic eruption of the skin with characteristic cutaneous morphology, often occurring in association with a personal or family history of atopy. Understanding the difference between atopic dermatitis and other forms of eczematous dermatitis is more difficult than understanding the distinction that exists between it and allergic contact eczematous dermatitis. As noted in Table 8-2, atopic eczematous dermatitis is an eruption of unknown etiology. It is both proper and necessary that certain criteria be met to establish the diagnosis of atopic eczematous dermatitis (Table 8-7). Atopic dermatitis was first well described by Coca and Cooke in 1923 as a chronic, pruritic eruption of the skin with characteristic cutaneous morphology, often occurring in association with a personal or family history of atopy. However, it is noteworthy that a significant percentage of patients have neither a personal or family history of respiratory allergic disease (Table 8-8). It is important to note that most patients have either a personal or a family history of atopy.

The incidence of atopic dermatitis varies depending on the diagnostic criteria used. A recently completed national screening survey estimated the prevalence to be 7–24/1000. The age of onset for atopic dermatitis is usually after the second month of life and 60% of the patients have onset in the first year of life (Table 8-9). Significantly, although 85% of the cases appear before age 5, there is still a small percentage

Table 8-9 *Onset of Atopic Dermatitis*

Age of Onset	Percent
2 months to 1 year	60
1 year to 5 years	30
6 years to 10 years	5
10 years to 20 years	4
over 20 years	1

The age of onset for atopic dermatitis is shown above and usually appears after the second month of life.

that occur later in life. The evolution of any individual case of atopic dermatitis is impossible to predict. However, if one takes all the patients with atopic dermatitis, 50% will at some point in time have respiratory allergic manifestations. The incidence of asthma is increased if the atopic dermatitis starts early in life and is extensive, or if there is a family history of allergic rhinitis or asthma. Follow-up studies generally agree that 40–50% of the patients have marked improvement between puberty and 20 years of age. Patients with the most severe atopic eczematous dermatitis and those associated with severe asthma or other allergic respiratory disease are twice as likely to have persistent disease.

Pathogenesis

The pathogenesis of atopic eczematous dermatitis is unknown and is probably multifactorial involving genetic factors, miscellaneous precipitating factors, abnormal humoral immunity, abnormal cellular immunity, altered physiologic activity, and altered pharmacologic reactivity. With regard to genetic factors, there have been increased frequencies of certain HLA antigens; however, its relation to pathogenesis is unknown. The role of precipitating factors, such as overbathing, irritation from various contactants, and adverse environmental conditions are probably just that, and that there is no relationship regarding pathogenesis. Many patients with atopic dermatitis have been found to have increased IgE levels. There is great controversy as to whether increased IgE levels are correlated with the severity of the atopic dermatitis, and about 20% of the patients with atopic dermatitis have normal IgE levels. To confuse the issue further, there are increased IgE levels in other types of dermatitis, clinically dissimilar to that of atopic eczema. Patients with atopic dermatitis have an increased incidence of positive skin test reactions to common environmental allergens; however, its clinical significance is unknown. Although increased IgE levels are a feature of atopic dermatitis, it has neither diagnostic or prognostic significance at present. In addition to abnormal humoral immunity, patients with atopic eczematous dermatitis have abnormal cellular immunity. This is exemplified by an increased incidence of various cutaneous infections, particularly with herpes virus, vaccina, verruca, molluscum contagiosum, and superficial fungal infections. They also have a decreased tendency to develop allergic contact dermatitis. A defect in chemotaxis of polymorphonuclear cells and monocytes has been observed, but its relationship to the pathogenesis is unknown. With respect to specific allergens, it is felt that common aeroallergens are inconsequential as causative agents in most patients with atopic eczema. Although controversy exists regarding food allergens and atopic dermatitis, there is increasing evidence that a clinical trial with an elimination diet may be worthwhile.

Patients with atopic dermatitis have several altered physiologic processes. They have increased sweat production to acetylcholine. However, sweat secretion itself is normal. Sweat delivery in some patients may be severely impaired; thus patients occasionally experience a sweat retention syndrome. Transepidermal water loss is increased in both involved and normal skin of atopic patients. Patients with atopic dermatitis appear to have a low threshold for induced pruritus. Abnormal cutaneous vasoreactivity is demonstrated by decreased digital temperature, white dermatographism consisting of linear pallor where the skin is stroked as opposed to the normal red response, and delayed blanche response to cholinergic agents consisting of paradoxic white dermatographic reaction to intradermal injection in contrast to the normal response of erythema. The altered physiologic responses can be explained by an altered sensitivity to pharmacologic activity in atopic dermatitis. Altered reactivity is revealed by an increased sensitivity to histamine, cholinergic agents, and alpha-adrenergic agents. Information regarding histamine in atopic dermatitis is abundant. Basophils and mast cells have a lower threshold for histamine release. Once again this pharmacologic abnormality is demonstrated by white dermatographism, delayed blanche response to cholinergic agents, and abnormal cutaneous basoreactivity. The role of kinins and prostaglandins in atopic dermatitis remains investigational. Pharmacologic activity reveals an increased sensitivity of vascular and pilomotor smooth muscles to alpha-adrenergic stimulation and the increased sensitivity of sweat glands to acetylcholine. There is also a decreased pruritus threshold and abnormal cell proliferation (lichenification). Lymphocytes, mast cells, and polymorphonuclear cells, including basophils from patients with atopic dermatitis, show a decreased physiologic response to beta-adrenergic stimulation, suggesting adrenergic blockage. It must be remembered that the underlying cellular and biochemical defects have not been established, and it is likely that the mechanism will be revised until a pathogenesis is finally established. At present it appears that various precipitating factors, immunologic abnormalities, altered physiologic activity, and altered pharmacologic activity are interrelated and dictate the clinical expression and prognosis for each patient with atopic eczematous dermatitis.

Clinical Manifestations

The clinical presentation of eczematous dermatitis varies depending on the age of the patient. Regardless of the age, the dermatitis is usually marked by periodic exacerbations. In infants (up to 2 years of age) the eruption usually begins by the sixth to eighth weeks of life. The lesions tend to be pruritic, erythematous, papulovesicular lesions with oozing and crusting. Most often, the eruption involves the face, scalp, ears, and extensor surfaces of the extremities (Figs. 8-10 and 8-11) and less often the buttocks, thighs, trunk, and anogenital region. Clinical features of atopic eczematous dermatitis in the infantile phase are pictured in Figures 8-12 and 8-13. Atopic eczematous dermatitis may begin in childhood (2–12 years of age) or be a continuum from infancy. The lesions become characterized by erythematous papules and lichenification, particularly in the flexoral folds (antecubital and popliteal fossa), flexor and extensor aspects of the wrists, and sides and nape of the neck. Clinical features of atopic eczematous dermatitis in the childhood phase are demonstrated in Figures 8-14 and 8-15. During the adolescent or adult phase, the lesions are characterized by hyperpigmentation with scaliness and lichenification. Again, the flexural areas and neck are the most commonly involved sites. Clinical features characteristic of atopic eczematous dermatitis in the adult phase are demonstrated in Figures 8-16 and 8-17. On rare occasions a patient with atopic eczematous dermatitis may present with a exfoliative erythroderma. There are other associated skin findings in patients with atopic eczematous dermatitis. These include xerosis, ichthyotic-like skin changes, Dennie-Morgan infraorbital fold (crease just beneath the margin of the lower eyelid), and Hertoghe's sign (thinning or absence of the lateral

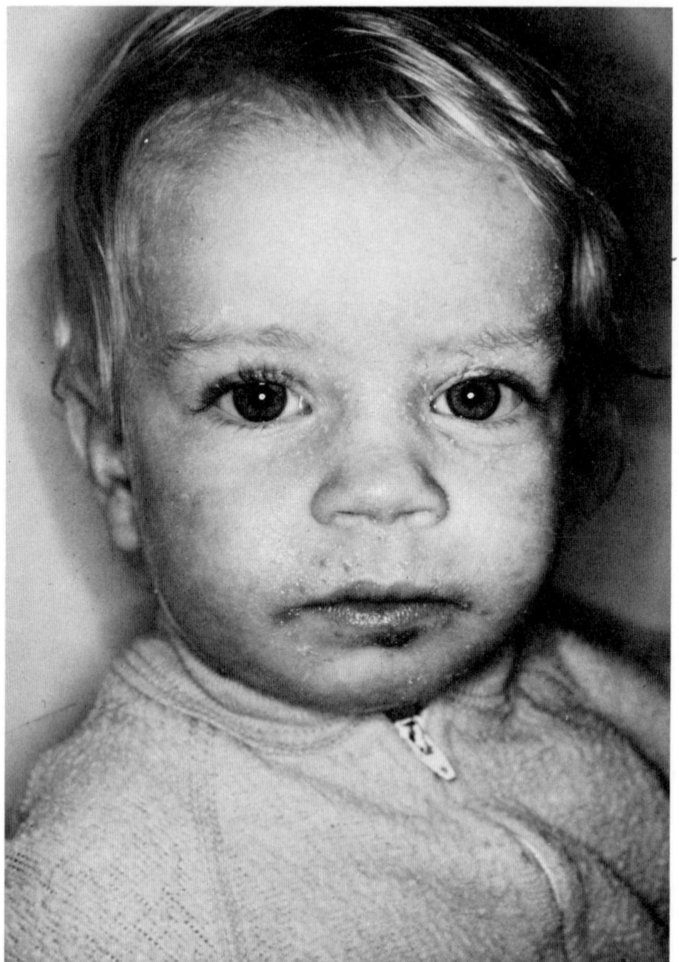

Fig. 8-10. Characteristic eruption on the face of a child with atopic dermatitis.

eyebrows). As noted in the table on diagnostic criteria (Table 8-7), patients with atopic dermatitis have an increased incidence of other noncutaneous clinical findings. These include ocular abnormalities such as the early formation of cataracts, which may develop in approximately 10–15% of patients with a peak incidence in the second decade of life. It is usually bilateral, develops rapidly, is capsular, and involves the posterior or anterior superficial cortex, or both. Keratoconus and retinal detachments are rare. Skin lesions always precede the ocular abnormalities by several years. Several complications have been noted with atopic eczematous dermatitis. The most significant involves pyogenic infections, primarily due to *Staphylococcal aureus* with the development of furunculosis, cellulitis, erysipelas, and external otitis. Results from one such study, culturing areas from both involved and uninvolved skin, is noted in Table 8-10 along with antibiotic sensitivities (Table 8-11). Patients with

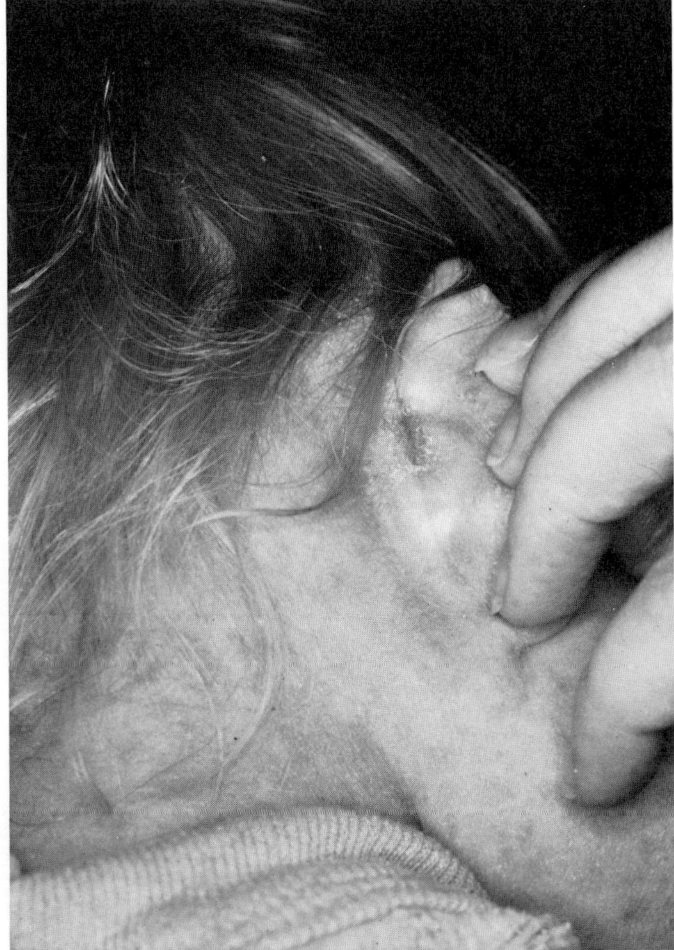

Fig. 8-11. Characteristic erythematous scaly lesions around the neck and ear in a patient with atopic eczematous dermatitis.

atopic dermatitis also seem to be particularly susceptible to infections with certain viruses, especially herpes simplex and vaccina, but also molluscum contagiosum and verruca vulgaris, but not varicella or zoster virus. Eczema vaccinatum and eczema herpeticum, formally Kaposi's disease and varicelliform eruption, can be seen in patients with atopic dermatitis vaccinated with vaccinia or patients who have developed herpes simplex infections, respectively.

Diagnostic Tests

Although other types of eczematous dermatitis can be similar to atopic dermatitis, its age of onset, clinical presentation, and associated findings usually aid in distinguishing it from any other skin diseases. Systemic diseases whose skin eruptions

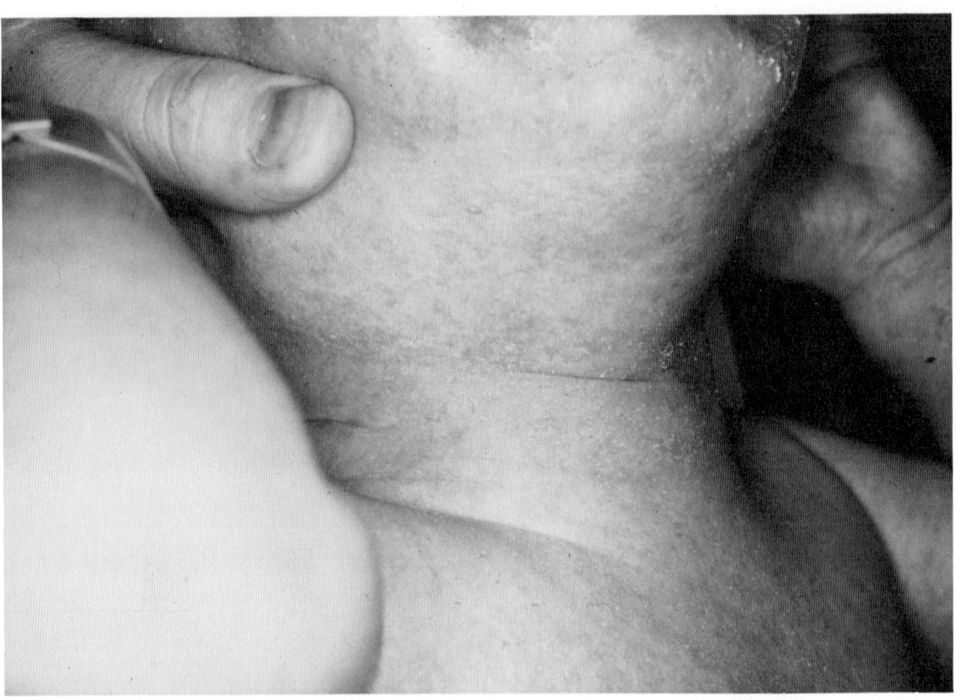

Fig. 8-12. Characteristic cutaneous lesions in the neck area of a child with atopic eczematous dermatitis.

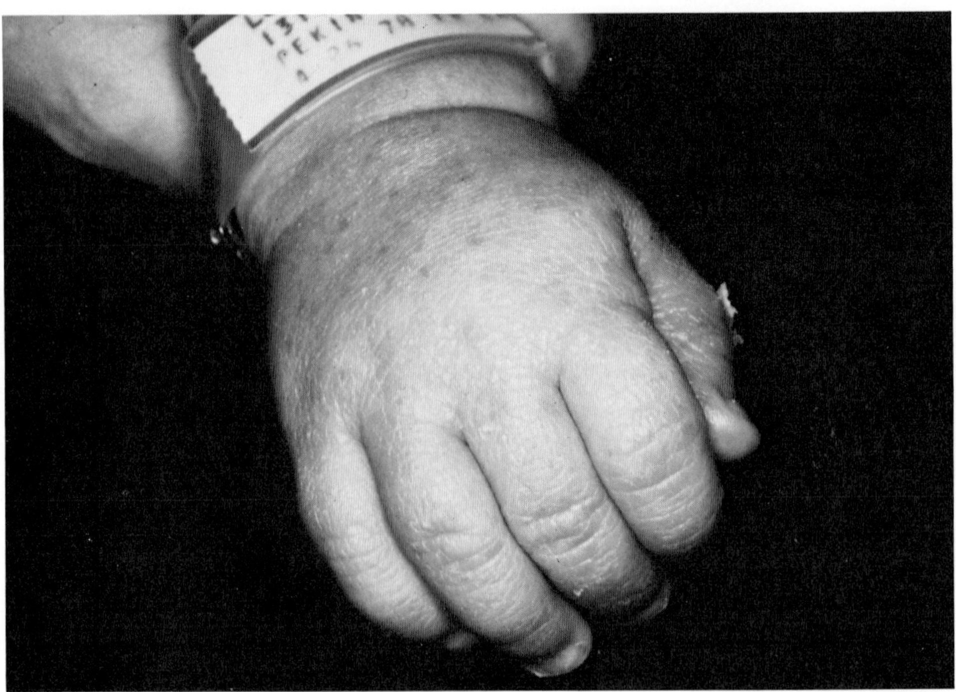

Fig. 8-13. Erythematous scaly pruritic skin lesions on the dorsal surface of the hand in a child with atopic eczematous dermatitis.

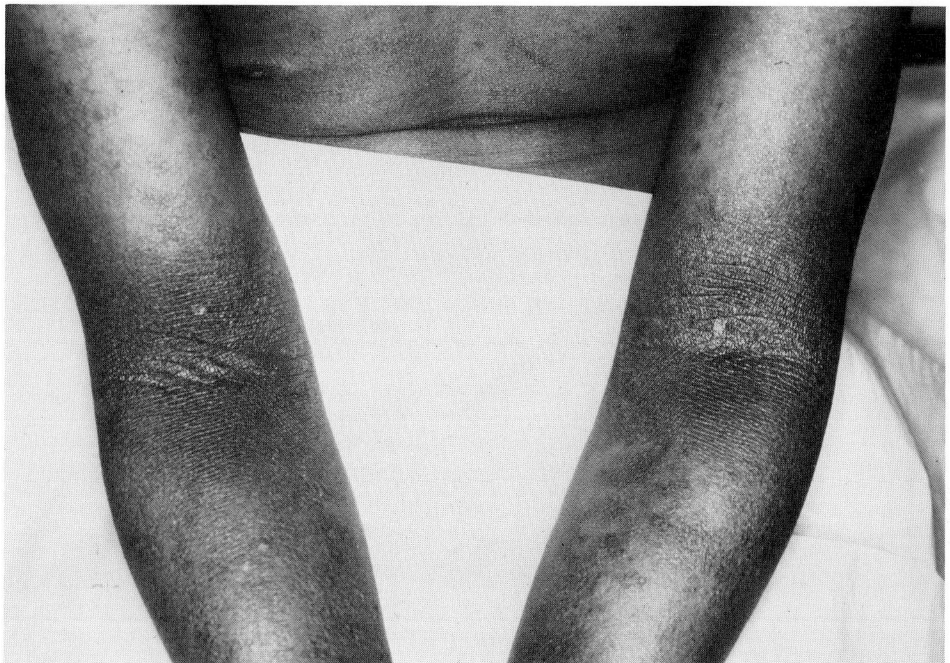

Fig. 8-14. Characteristic skin eruption involving the antecubital fossa in a patient in the childhood phase of atopic eczematous dermatitis.

may simulate those of atopic eczematous dermatitis can be divided into two groups: the metabolic diseases and the immunologic disturbances. Once again, from a diagnostic standpoint, histology on skin biopsy is very nonspecific. Although many immunologic and pharmacologic abnormalities have been discussed under the section on pathogenesis, no specific abnormalities is diagnostic in atopic eczematous dermatitis but can be suggestive of the diagnosis in the evaluation of difficult cases. It is noteworthy that many of the systemic conditions that can mimic atopic eczematous dermatitis have specific laboratory tests that can be performed to differentiate the disease processes. The primary skin diseases that may mimic atopic eczematous dermatitis are few in number. They include seborrheic dermatitis, Leiner's disease, and contact dermatitis. Once again, differential diagnosis depends on clinical examination, personal and family history of atopic disease, and available laboratory data. Attempts to skin-test atopic dermatitis individuals are usually unsuccessful from a diagnostic and therapeutic standpoint because of the increased incidence of positive cutaneous reactions in these patients, making positive test results difficult to interpret.

Treatment

Treatment of routine cases of atopic eczematous dermatitis does not differ significantly from that outlined previously for other forms of acute, subacute, and chronic forms of eczematous dermatitis. Obviously, if agents that produce exacerbations can

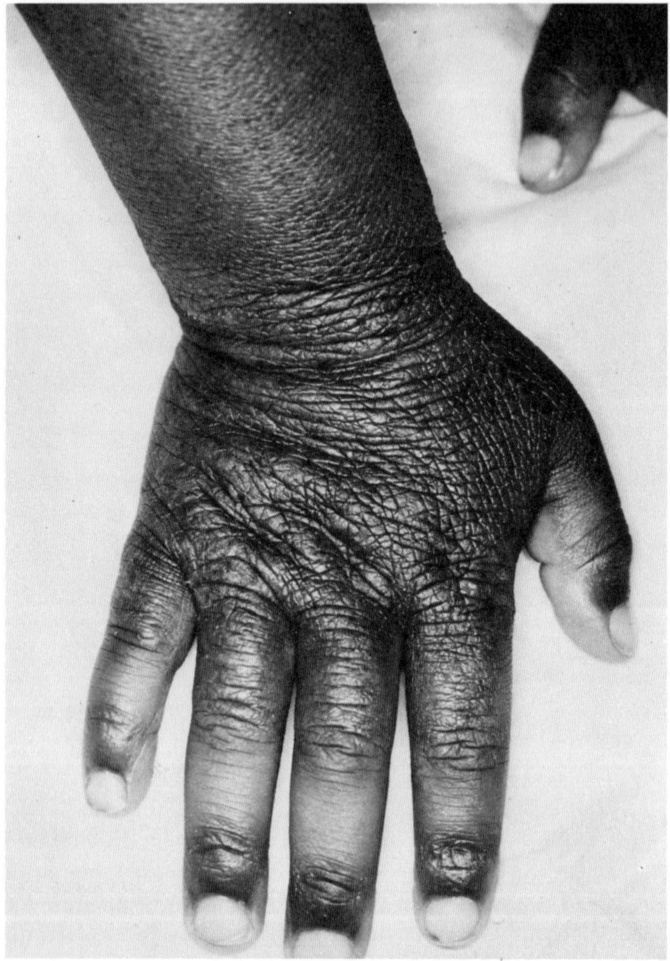

Fig. 8-15. Characteristic hyperpigmented, lichenified skin on the dorsal surface of the hand in the childhood phase of a child with an atopic eczematous dermatitis.

be identified, such as foods and inhalants, they should be avoided and improvement will almost always be noted. In the treatment of any case of atopic eczematous dermatitis, certain general considerations are important because of the chronicity of the disease. Most important, is communication between the physician, patient, and family so that all parties concerned understand the natural history of the disease process, the goals desired through treatment, and the working relationship that is necessary to maintain adequate control. Most eczematous eruptions, including atopic eczematous dermatitis, are worsened during cold winter months with cold temperatures and warm household heat with low humidity. Adequate environmental conditions at home with proper humidification and avoidance of dust laden areas can thus be important. Loose-fitting, nonwoolen clothing is recommended. The patient

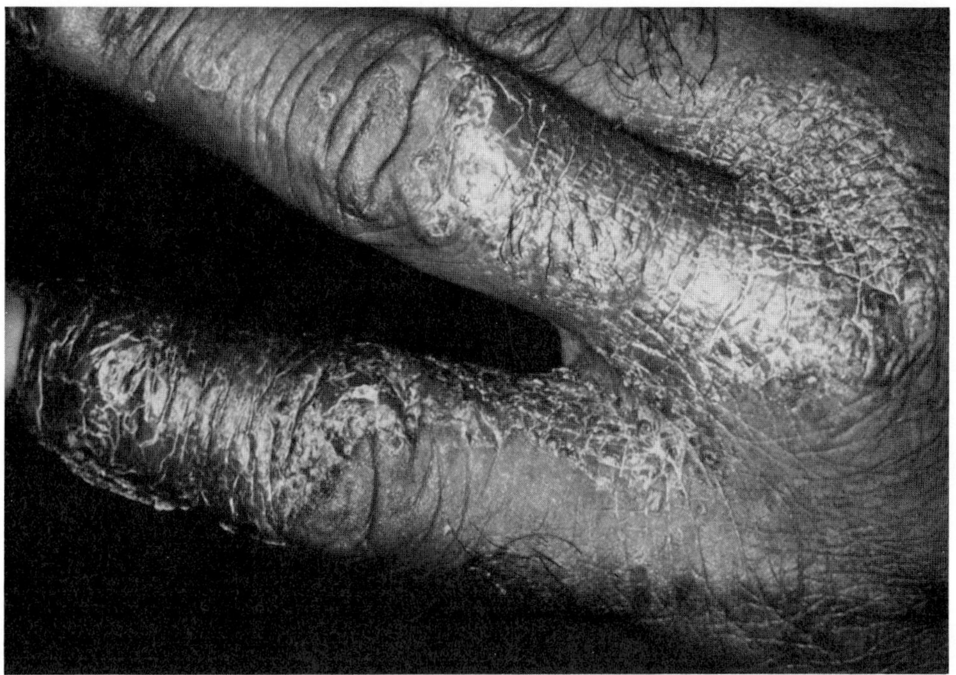

Fig. 8-16. Closer view of the characteristic hyperkeratotic, lichenified skin in a patient with atopic eczematous dermatitis.

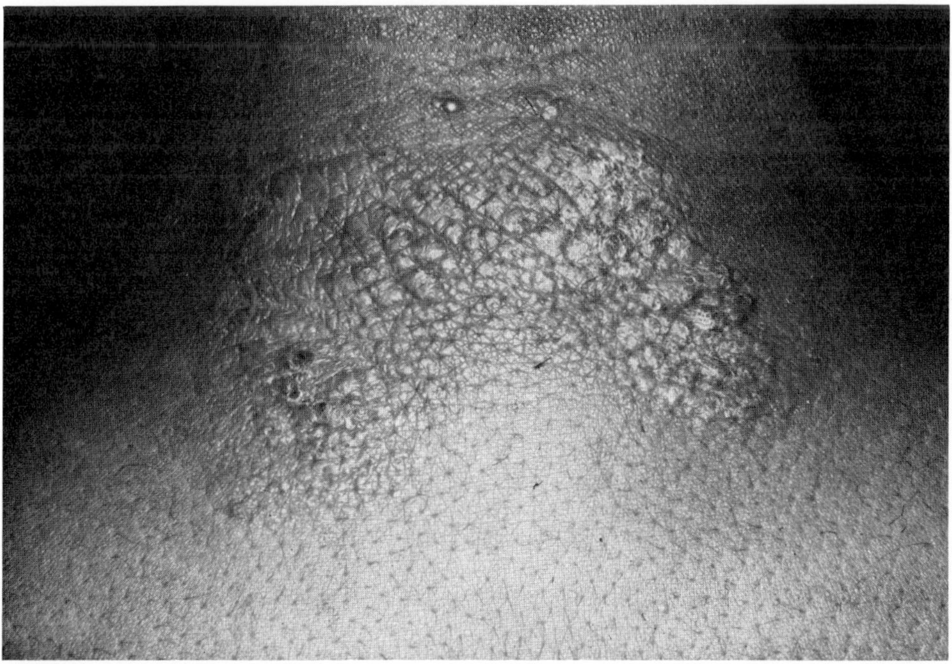

Fig. 8-17. Characteristic phase of the hyperkeratotic lichenified skin lesions in a patient with chronic atopic eczematous dermatitis.

Table 8-10 *Percent Incidence of Microorganism in 39 Patients with Atopic Eczema*

Microorganism	Lesions (%)	Normal Skin (%)
Staphylococcus aureus	93	76
Coagulase-negative staphylococci	79	82
Micrococci	13	25
Streptococci	0	2
Nonlipophilic diphtheroids	15	18
Lipophilic diphtheroids	0	2
Bacillus species	15	20
Gram-negative rods	5	5
Yeasts	0	2

should be instructed not to overbathe and to avoid irritating detergents and solvents that may aggravate the eczematous process. Although some authorities recommend water avoidance in patients with atopic dermatitis, this author from a practical standpoint prefers the judicious use of water and mild cleansing agents. If a patient expresses skin exacerbation related to a specific food ingestion, that food should be avoided. Because of the chronic nature of atopic eczematous dermatitis with the hyperpigmented, scaly, lichenified lesions, topical steroid ointments are preferrable to steroid creams or oral corticosteroids because of their therapeutic efficacy and lubricating effect. During chronic phases, nonsteroidal lubricants and antipruritic lotions may be adequate to control symptoms. As with other forms of eczematous dermatitis, secondary infections must be cultured and treated with an appropriate systemic antibiotic as well as adequate local skin care. Acute exacerbations of atopic eczematous dermatitis may require a short course of oral corticosteroids while topical

Table 8-11 *Antibiotic Resistance in 140 Patients with Atopic Dermatitis*

Antibiotic	Resistance (%)
Penicillin (2 units)	63
Penicillin (10 units)	58
Cephalothin (30 μg)	0
Tetracycline (5 μg)	14
Erythromycin (2 μg)	20
Oxacillin (1 μg)	8
Novobiocin (5 μg)	2
Neomycin (5 μg)	1

treatment is maintained in order to control some patients. In severe generalized cases, hospitalization may be required for more intensive topical therapy. Phototherapy is an additional treatment regimen that may be used in these severe cases unresponsive to more conservative methods of treatment. Immunotherapy is not indicated for atopic eczematous dermatitis.

REFERENCES

Coca, A. F. and Cooke, R. A. On the classification of the phenomena of hypersensitiveness. *J. Immunol.*, 1923, *8*, 163.

SUGGESTED READINGS

Fisher, A. A. *Contact Dermatitis* (Second Ed.). Lea & Febiger, 1975.

Fitzpatrick, T. B. et al. *Dermatology in general medicine* (Second Ed.) 1979, 507–531.

Hanifin, J. M. Atopic Dermatitis. *Jnl. Am. Acad. Dermatol.* 1982, 1–13.

Lever, W. F. et al. *Histopathology of the skin* (Fifth Ed.), 1975.

Raza, A. et al. Microbial Flora of Atopic Dermatitis. *Arch. Dermatol.* 1977, *113*, 780–782.

QUESTIONS

1. True or False—Most patients with atopic eczematous dermatitis have a personal or family history of atopy.
2. True or False—A skin biopsy is the most definitive diagnostic procedure in the evaluation of an allergic eczematous contact dermatitis.
3. True or False—Allergy shots are the most effective treatment for allergic eczematous contact dermatitis because they have been shown effective for other Type I immune reactions.
4. Atopic eczematous dermatitis has been associated with the following disorders and/or complications.
   a. A likelihood to develop generalized infections with herpes simplex or vaccinia virus (Kaposi's varicelliform eruption).
   b. An increased susceptibility to the wart virus and molluscum contagiosum.
   c. The skin of atopic eczematous dermatitis patients tend to harbor more staphylococcal bacteria even without any clinical evidence of infection.
   d. Patients with atopic eczematous dermatitis have an increased incidence of certain abnormal ocular problems.
   e. All of the above.

5. A true statement regarding allergic eczematous contact dermatitis is:
   a. It only occurs in individuals with personal or family history of other atopic disorders.
   b. The pattern and distribution of the cutaneous lesions can aid in making a proper diagnosis which can further be confirmed by patch testing.
   c. It should always be treated with systemic steroids.
   d. Topical anesthetics are the most effective preparations currently available for the topical treatment of this condition.
   e. Once a person has developed an allergic eczematous contact dermatitis due to poison ivy, he or she is immune to further reactions with re-exposure to the poison ivy resin.

Answers can be found in Appendix B at the end of the book.

Susan Bromberg Schneider
John P. Atkinson

9

Urticaria and Angioedema

Urticaria and angioedema are readily recognized, common medical problems that approximately 20% of the population experience at least once in their lifetime (Kaplan, 1978; Mathews, 1974; Mathews, 1980; Schneider & Atkinson, 1981; Warin & Champion, 1974; Yecies & Kaplan, 1980). Both lesions may occur simultaneously, or one—usually urticaria—may predominate. Urticaria presents as variably distributed, erythematous, pruritic wheals with serpiginous borders and central pallor. Angioedema is smaller in size, has less erythema and itching, evolves more slowly, and has a deeper location. Its common distribution includes the face and extremities, but the trunk, genitals, and mucosal surfaces such as the larynx and gastrointestinal (GI) tract may be affected. In some patients lesions known as "giant hives" have features of both urticaria and angioedema in that they are pruritic and erythematous but involve the deeper dermis.

MORBIDITY AND MORTALITY

Laryngeal edema is certainly the most serious and only life-threatening feature of urticaria and angioedema. Fortunately, airway involvement is uncommon in acute urticaria and angioedema and rare in all forms of chronic angioedema except hereditary angioedema. In any other location urticaria and angioedema resolve completely without residua. Patients primarily complain of itching, cosmetic effects, and the unpredictable timing of the eruptions.

PATHOPHYSIOLOGY

The histologic picture of urticaria and angioedema is that of interstitial edema, dilated lymphatics and vessels, and a paucity of inflammatory cells. Immunofluorescence is routinely negative for IgG, IgM, C3, or C4, and biopsy reports such as "no pathologic diagnosis" are common. Vasoactive mediators released from tissue mast cells are thought to produce this pathologic picture (Kaplan, 1981; Soter &

ALLERGY: THEORY AND PRACTICE
ISBN 0-8089-1619-X

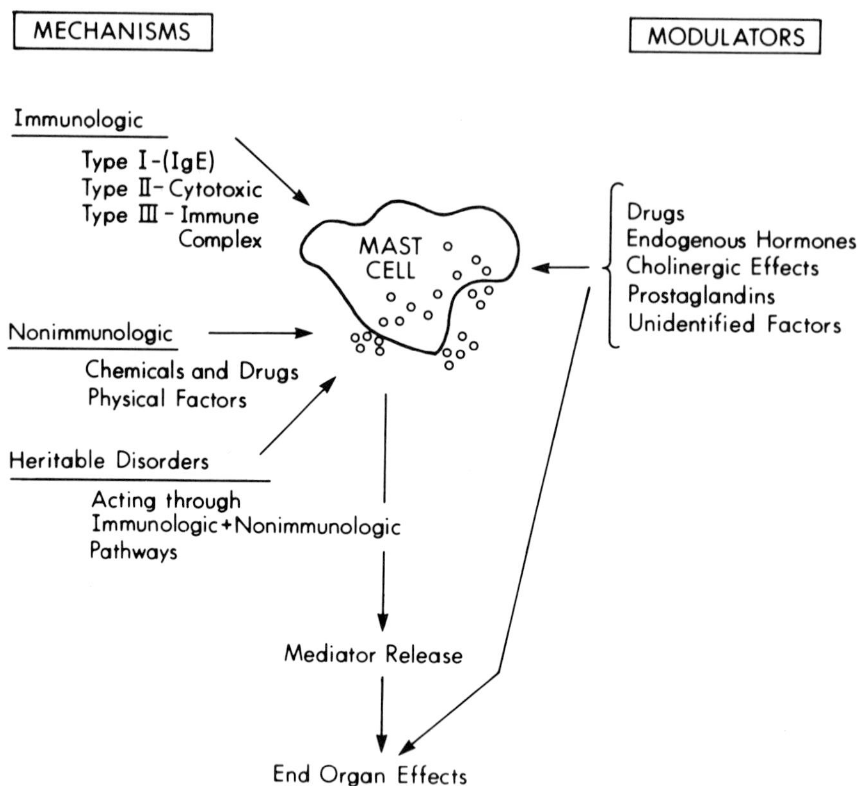

Fig. 9-1. Scheme of pathophysiologic events. From Schneider, S. B. & Atkinson, J. P. Urticaria and angioedema. In T. B. Fitzpatrick, et al., *Update: Dermatology in General Medicine* New York: McGraw-Hill, 1983, p. 65.
Adapted from Mathews, K. P. *Med. Clin. N. Amer.*, 1974, p. 188. With permission.

Wasserman, 1979). Since there is no necrosis and sparse inflammation, mediators with reversible actions, such as histamine, are considered by most students of this disease to be largely responsible for the urticaria and angioedema. Injection of histamine, in fact, produces a typical urticarial lesion. Other mediators, including serotonin, acetylcholine, kinins, arachidonic acid metabolites, and undoubtedly other factors (schematically presented in Fig. 9-1) also may mediate or modulate these lesions. Alcohol, stress, emotion, exercise, and hormonal milieus do not appear in most cases to initiate the lesions but may enhance or decrease mediator release, thereby modulating the condition.

DIFFERENTIAL DIAGNOSIS

The diagnosis of angioedema and urticaria is rarely a problem. Lesions that do not fit the criteria listed in Table 9-1 often indicate a need for a biopsy. For example, "urticaria-like" lesions that do not resolve within 24 hours suggest that a vasculitic process such as erythema multiforme or a form of urticarial vasculitis may be present.

Table 9-1 *A Comparison of Urticaria and Angioedema*

	Urticaria	Angioedema
Onset	Acute as lesions appear within minutes	Subacute as lesions evolve over hours
Symptoms	Pruritis Erythema prominent	Stinging or burning, or tingling sensation at eventual site of swelling; erythema usually not prominent
Duration	Hours	Hours to days
Histopathology	Dilatation of blood vessels Tissue edema ± Perivascular infiltrate	Dilatation of blood vessels Tissue edema ± Perivascular infiltrate
Location	Dermis	Deep dermis and subcutaneous tissue, especially common about face
Number of Lesions	Usually multiple	Usually single

Modified from Schneider S. B. & Atkinson J. P. "Urticaria and Angioedema." In *Update Dermatology in General Medicine*. New York: McGraw Hill, 1983, p. 62.

Insect bites ("papular urticaria") can look very similar to true urticaria, but the lesions tend to have a more nodular quality or indurated "feel" and usually persist for longer than 24 hours.

ETIOLOGIC CONSIDERATIONS

Drugs

A thorough history in relationship to possible drug exposure is essential in all cases of urticaria and angioedema. Drugs are the most commonly identified cause of nonidiopathic disease. In cases of multiple drug exposure, one can only statistically rank medicines as more or less likely to produce urticaria, realizing that potentially any drug can cause such reaction. Reliable skin tests exist only for the assessment of immediate hypersensitivity and not for any of the other mechanisms by which drugs can cause reactions, such as immune complex formation, nonspecific histamine release, complement activation, or effects on arachidonic acid metabolism. Moreover, such skin tests are available only to high-molecular-weight substances such as insulin or adrenocorticotropic hormone and to penicillin with which extensive work in defining major and minor immunologic determinants has been performed. Skin tests for other compounds are not a reliable method for determining if sensitivity exists.

In clinical practice, drugs most commonly causing urticaria and angioedema are as follows: the penicillins; the sulfonamides; animal protein derivatives such as insulin, adrenocorticotrophic hormone, thyroid extract, parathormone, and specific antisera; diuretics; aspirin and other nonsteroidal anti-inflammatory agents; opiate analgesics such as codeine, demerol, and morphine; and radiocontrast materials. Reintroduction of drugs may be accompanied by a more severe reaction than with initial use and should be avoided if at all possible. One should also avoid use of structurally similar drugs.

Blood Products

Acute urticaria and angioedema observed in association with the administration of blood products may occur by a number of mechanisms such as complement activation in the classic "*ABO* incompatibility" or by IgE or antibody and complement reactions to fresh frozen plasma, Factor 8, and cryoprecipitate. Reactions may also be directed to antigens "extrinsic" to blood, such as "contaminant" trace proteins or haptenic substances (food antigen, drugs, or drug metabolite) present in blood. Specific IgE antibody of donor origin may elicit urticaria and angioedema in blood recipients. The etiology of the urticaria occurring in this clinical setting seldom is found.

Food

Urticaria and angioedema can occur within minutes to hours after exposure to a responsible food. The normal route of exposure is via ingestion, although touch or inhalation of more potent antigens may precipitate local or systemic reactions in exquisitely sensitive individuals. Immediate IgE mediated "allergic" reactions are seen most commonly with nuts, fish, seafood, eggs, berries, and aliphatic aldehydes (present in odorous food such as garlic, or as a combustion product of broiling or frying). Late allergic reactions, occurring within hours of exposure, are less common, but have been observed with cereals, milk, eggs, potatoes, beef, pork, legumes, and oranges. In delayed reactions, documentation of the precipitant is more difficult because of interim ingestion of other foods and the lack of obvious temporal "cause and effect." "Dose-related" urticaria may occur with ingestion of large quantities of nonspecific histamine releasors, such as strawberries, lobster, and crayfish. Natural or synthetic additives, including salicylates, benzoates, metabisulfites, azo dyes, and yeast, have been implicated as occult etiologies in a limited number of cases of urticaria and angioedema.

Aeroallergens and Contactants

A history of seasonal exacerbations of urticaria, with associated rhinitis, conjunctivitis, and/or asthma, is helpful for the diagnosis of pollen-induced urticaria and angioedema. A seasonal pattern is, of course, not seen with sensitivity to antigens such as house dust, feathers, perennial molds, and animal epithelium. Contact urticaria and angioedema can be seen to a large number of ubiquitous items, such as toothpaste, mouthwash, shampoo, fabrics, detergents, and perfumes.

It is unnecessary and expensive to skin-test all patients with chronic urticaria for immediate hypersensitivity (for aeroallergens) or delayed hypersensitivity (for contactants). Only when clinical suspicion and observed patterns warrant should such testing be performed.

Primary therapy of aeroallergen or contact-induced urticaria and angioedema is avoidance. The efficacy of desensitization has not been established.

Infection and Infestation

Case reports of the association of urticaria and angioedema with almost any type of infection are found in the literature. Approximately 25% of patients with viral hepatitis and 6% of patients with infectious mononucleosis suffer urticaria in their prodrome or acute illness. Some authors quote as high as a 20% incidence of yeast sensitivity in their chronic urticaria population, although we have been unable to substantiate such a high number. Parasitic infections, uncommon in the United States, have been associated with urticaria. Acute urticaria may be associated with new onset of pyogenic infections; however, so-called hidden infections (dental abscess, sinusitis or gallstones) are rarely the cause of chronic urticaria and angioedema.

Bites and Stings

Systemic urticaria may occur with local envenomization by spiders, snakes, and insects. Therapy of such urticaria is, of course, avoidance. In certain patients with reactions to hymenoptera stings, hyposensitization is indicated. Patient instruction with regard to the use of self-administered epinephrine in the acute situation may be life-saving.

Physical Urticarias

The pathognomonic feature shared by the physical urticarias is their consistent reproducibility by their respective physical stimuli (cold, cholinergic, pressure, solar; see Table 9-2). From recent studies of experimentally induced lesions (Kaplan, 1978; Kaplan, 1981; Soter & Wasserman, 1979) we know that histamine and other mediators are released temporally in association with lesion development.

Cold Urticaria

Cold urticaria is precipitated by temperature change rather than absolute temperatures and typically manifests itself with the rewarming of a cold-exposed part. It may occur as a primary disease entity or may be associated with illnesses such as cryoglobulinemia, cryofibrinogenemia, cold-agglutinin disease, or paroxysmal hemoglobinuria of the Donath-Landsteiner type. A familial form of the disease, with immediate and delayed variants, also exists. Most cases are idiopathic. The provocative test for cold urticaria is performed by placing an ice cube on the volar surface of the patient's forearm for 4 minutes and then observing for 10 minutes.

Cholinergic Urticaria

Cholinergic urticaria is mediated by the release of acetylcholine. Liberation of acetylcholine may be precipitated by heat, exercise, sweating, and possibly strong emotions. Cholinergic urticaria appears as "punctate" lesions of around 1–2 mm in diameter occurring locally or scattered over the upper trunk and limbs. Provocative tests for cholinergic urticaria include (a) the intradermal injection of 100 μg of methacholine (Mecholyl), with a resultant wheal and flare surrounded by smaller satellite lesions; (b) the application of warm water locally with the development of focal

Table 9-2 *Etiologic Considerations in Urticaria and Angioedema*

Drugs	Systemic diseases
Blood Products	Serum sickness
Foods	Connective tissue disease
Aeroallergens and contactants	Malignancy
Infections and infestations	Endocrinopathies
Bites and stings	Urticaria pigmentosa
Physical agents	Systemic mastocytosis
Cold	Genetic diseases
Cholinergic or heat	Hereditary angioedema
Pressure	C3b inactivator deficiency
Dermatographism	Serum carboxypeptidase B deficiency
Solar	Amyloidosis with nerve deafness and limb pain
Vibratory	Type VI solar urticaria (erythropoietic protoporphyria)
Aquagenic	Hereditary cold urticaria and angioedema
	Hereditary vibratory angioedema
	Idiopathic

From Schneider, S. B., & Atkinson, J. P. Urticaria and angioedema. In T. B. Fitzpatrick et al (Eds.). *Update: Dermatology in general medicine*. New York: McGraw-Hill, 1983, p. 65. With permission.

urticaria, and (c) a 10-minute run in the doctor's office with the production of a generalized urticaria.

Pressure Urticaria and Angioedema

Patients with pressure-induced disease typically complain of involvement of the buttocks and back after a long trip or of the soles of the feet after a long walk. Other common sites of lesions are beneath bra straps, belts, or other tight garments. After a stimulus of sustained pressure, onset may be immediate (i.e., within minutes of the stimulus) or delayed (i.e., within several hours). Systemic symptoms such as fevers, chills, and nausea may be associated with the delayed variant. There are no standardized, reliable provocative tests for the diagnosis of pressure urticaria. A suggestive history and repeated examination of a patient's lesions are helpful in arriving at the correct diagnosis.

Dermatographism

In dermatographism, the "ability to write on skin," stroking the skin, results first in a white line of vasoconstriction, followed by pruritus, erythema, and swelling. This wheal and flare classically occurs immediately and resolves within 30 minutes. A rare delayed variant, occurring within 3–6 hours of stimulus and resolving in 24–48 hours, has been described. In approximately 50% of the population with dermatographism, the wheal and flare is mediated by IgE. Dermatographism is seen in 5%

of the "normal" population and can be elicited in some patients with chronic idiopathic urticaria. In most individuals, dermatographism is a curiosity only and rarely requires therapeutic intervention.

Solar Urticaria

This uncommon form of urticaria is characterized by the development of lesions in light-exposed areas. These lesions usually develop within minutes of exposure and resolve within hours. A delayed form, occurring 18–72 hours after solar exposure, has also been described. The provocative test for solar urticaria is performed by exposing the patient to a broad-spectrum fluorescent tube to which individual filters have been appended for transmission of desired wavelengths. A dermatologist's assistance in evaluating these patients is usually necessary.

Vibratory Angioedema

This rare physical angioedema occurs within minutes of a vibratory stimulus and may be provoked by placement of a laboratory vortex to a patient's forearm for 4 minutes.

Aquagenic Urticaria

A rare disorder with lesions similar to cholinergic urticaria, aquagenic urticaria is produced by water exposure. A provocative test consists of a water compress applied to the forearm.

Heritable Disorders

Hereditary angioedema is a rare cause of recurrent angioedema but a not uncommon diagnostic consideration (Atkinson, 1979; Gelfand et al., 1976; Schneider & Atkinson, 1981). This disease is associated with considerable morbidity and a relatively high mortality. Now that effective therapy is available, correct diagnosis is most important. In hereditary angioedema, the swelling is *not* accompanied by urticaria. Lesions are characteristically nonpainful, nonerythematous, nonpruritic, and nonpitting. Swelling evolves over several hours and lasts for 24–72 hours. A nondescript, transient, serpiginous, erythematous rash precedes or accompanies the angioedema in about one-fourths of patients. The attacks usually begin in childhood, but the frequency of episodes increases during adolescence and into the third and fourth decades. For most episodes there are no apparent initiating factors, although minor trauma is a clear precipitant in many patients. Since hereditary angioedema is inherited in a dominant fashion, family history is usually positive.

The description of the lesions by the patient, especially their association with hives, readily discriminates this entity from acquired angioedema. In patients with a compatible clinical picture for hereditary angioedema, the screening test of choice is a determination of C4. This widely available assay is low in over 80% of patients at all times and is always low in association with an acute attack. A normal or high C4, especially during an episode, rules this entity out. If the C4 level is low, a specific antigenic or functional C1 inhibitor determination needs to be performed to confirm the diagnosis. This confirmation is necessary since immune-complex-mediated diseases can occasionally present with a combination of angioedema and low C4.

Other rare forms of heritable urticaria and angioedema have been reported. They include C3b inactivator deficiency, in which serum C3 and properdin factor B are low and C3b inactivator is absent; serum carboxypeptidase deficiency (Mathews et al., 1980), in which the protein inactivating complement-derived anaphylatoxins is reduced; amyloidosis with nerve deafness and limb pain, an autosomal dominant disorder; erythropoeitic protoporphyria, type VI solar urticaria; and rare forms of cold and vibratory urticaria and angioedema.

Systemic Diseases

Although the association of urticaria and angioedema with various systemic illnesses has been widely reported, the actual incidence of systemic disease as a causative factor to chronic urticaria, and angioedema is probably very low.

Serum sickness is often accompanied by urticaria and angioedema. Transient serum-sickness-like reactions probably occur frequently in association with many infectious diseases, especially viral illnesses, as during the prodrome stage (antigen excess) of serum hepatitis. The drugs most frequently implicated in serum sickness are the penicillins, cephalosporins, sulfonamides, streptomycin, and heterologous antiserum.

Connective tissue disorders may be associated with urticaria and angioedema. At some time in their course, 5–20 percent of patients with systemic lupus erythematosus (SLE) will manifest urticarial lesions. Patients with acute rheumatic fever and juvenile rheumatoid arthritis may exhibit nonpruritic urticaria-like lesions. There are now numerous reports of hypocomplementemic vasculitic syndromes in which chronic urticaria is a major clinical manifestation (Mathison et al., 1977; Phanuphak et al., 1980). These syndromes vary in severity from a very benign form, in which skin involvement is the principal manifestation, to a severe form resembling lupus, in which systemic disease is present. The benign form is distinguished from chronic idiopathic urticaria by the presence in the former of longer-lived lesions and the biopsy appearance of an inflammatory infiltrate invading the vessel wall. The more severe type is seen predominantly in women, is characterized by persistent urticaria, occasionally life-threatening angioedema, arthralgias and arthritis, abdominal pain, neurological abnormalities such as seizures, mononeuritis, and noninfectious meningitis, and, rarely, glomerulonephritis. Skin biopsies in these patients reveal leukocytoclastic angiitis. Immunofluorescence demonstrates immunoglobulin deposition. Laboratory tests may disclose diminished C1q, C4, C2, and C3 and elevated erythrocyte sedimentation rate. Although these patients clinically resemble SLE cases, the antinuclear antibody test is negative. In practice, the systemic complaints and elevated sedimentation rate usually readily separate this group from patients with chronic idiopathic urticaria and angioedema.

There are case reports of urticaria and angioedema in association with carcinomas and lymphoreticular neoplasms. The more commonly reported ones are dysproteinemias; polycythemia vera; Hodgkin's disease; chronic lymphocytic leukemia; reticulum cell sarcoma; and cancer of the colon, rectum, and lung. Immune complex formation involving tumor antigens may be responsible for the urticaria and angioedema. An acquired C1 esterase inhibitor deficiency has also been described in patients with lymphoma. This group of patients clinically resembles those with hereditary angioedema, and laboratory analysis reveals both low C1 esterase inhibitor and C4. The associated malignancy and low C1 titers (in hereditary angioedema the C1 titer is normal) help to separate this group from hereditary angioedema.

Uncommonly, certain endocrine disorders have been associated with urticaria and angioedema. These include reports of urticaria with thyrotoxicosis that resolves with therapy of hyperthyroidism and of cycling of the severity of chronic urticaria with the menstrual cycle.

Idiopathic

The majority of patients with chronic urticaria and angioedema must be classified in the idiopathic group. In this patient population, despite a thorough initial evaluation and several year follow-up, no etiology to their disease state is evident. Although occasional series claim a greater than 50% success in identifying a cause, most investigators attain a 5–20 percent success. In many instances, even when other diseases are discovered, a causal relationship is not conclusively demonstrated, as therapy or removal of the presumed "underlying etiology" does not result in resolution of urticaria and angioedema. There is no increased incidence of atopy in these patients. Typically, they manifest no systemic symptoms such as fevers, arthralgias, or malaise, and the sedimentation rate is normal. Although a frustrating problem to its sufferers, the natural history of the chronic idiopathic state is a benign one. To our knowledge there have been no reported deaths from laryngeal obstruction. Furthermore, the spontaneous remission rate is such that approximately 50% of patients are symptom-free by 6 months, 70% by 1 year, and 90% by 5 years.

CLINICAL EVALUATION

There is *no substitute* for a detailed history (see Chapter 4). A physical examination to rule out underlying or associated diseases is mandatory. During this examination, light stroking of the skin should be performed to assess for dermatographism. The number, size, character, and position of all skin lesions should be noted and recorded. If symptoms are suggestive of a physical urticaria, provocative testing with the appropriate stimulus should be performed.

DIAGNOSTIC TESTS

Screening laboratory tests for most patients include a complete blood count, urinalysis, chemistry profile, sedimentation rate, and chest x-ray. An elevated sedimentation rate is not found in most patients with urticaria and angioedema and should signal the physician to carefully consider an underlying systemic illness. Other laboratory procedures are reserved for appropriate indications, as revealed through the history, physical examination, and likely etiologic factors (Table 9-3). The history, physical examination, screening laboratory tests, and judicious use of these additional tests and procedures allow for a sensible and accurate evaluation (Jacobson et al.,

Table 9-3 *Evaluation of Patient with Urticaria and Angioedema*

HISTORY

- Description of present illness
- Past medical history
- Drugs
- Occupation
- Travel
- Family history

Physical examination

Provocative physical tests, if indicated

Screening laboratory

- Complete blood count with differential
- Chemistry profile
- Sedimentation rate
- Chest x-ray
- Urinalysis

Selective laboratory, if indicated

- To rule out allergy: skin tests to aeroallergens patch tests to contactants, IgE, RASTs for specific antigens, eosinophil count
- To evaluate cold-induced disease: cryofibrinogens, cryoglobulins, cold agglutinins, VDRL, immune complexes
- To rule out connective tissue disease: antinuclear antibody, rheumatoid factor, immune complexes, total hemolytic complement, C3, C4, cryoglobulins, skin biopsy
- To rule out hepatitis: hepatitis antibody and antigen
- To evaluate infections: stool for ova and parasites; appropriate radiographic studies
- To rule out neoplasm: protein electrophoresis; appropriate radiographic and other studies
- To evaluate food sensitivities: diary; RASTs to foods; elimination diet
- For hereditary angioedema: C4, C1 inhibitor

From Schneider, S. B., & Atkinson, J. P. Urticaria and angioedema. In T. B. Fitzpatrick et al (Eds.). *Update: Dermatology in general medicine,* New York: McGraw-Hill, 1983, p. 76. With permission.

1980; Schneider & Atkinson, 1983). A thorough reevaluation is indicated in patients with persistent disease if atypical features or new signs and symptoms develop.

THERAPY

For patients in whom an etiology for the urticaria and angioedema is found, avoidance of the causative agent or therapy for the underlying disease is obviously the treatment of choice. Then, if this is ineffective, or in cases of idiopathic disease where no etiology is recognized, the physician can usually provide adequate symptomatic relief through medications. For idiopathic disease, patient education is a vital therapeutic adjunct to allay anxiety and lessen frustration. Patients are naturally concerned about the prognosis of their disease and the possibility of an underlying systemic illness. After the evaluation, most patients may be informed that (a) although the cause of their disease is unknown, no underlying disease has been detected; (b) although attacks may be aggravating, they are not life-threatening; (c) the natural course of the disease is such that spontaneous remissions occur in most patients; and (d) until a remission ensues, the lesions can usually be adequately controlled with medication.

For purposes of determining the best therapeutic approach to idiopathic disease, we prefer to divide our patients into two groups—those with infrequent episodes and those with frequent episodes.

For those patients with "infrequent" episodes—that is, less often than approximately one attack per month, our philosophy is to observe and treat attacks as they occur. These are patients with seldom occurrences of a non-life-threatening disease and for whom prophylactic medication rarely is justified. In an effort to assess frequency and severity of episodes, patients are instructed to keep a diary. If lesions are not present on initial evaluation, the patient is asked to return when fresh lesions occur so that the diagnosis of urticaria may be confirmed. Patients are also advised to take hydroxyzine or cyproheptadine when episodes occur.

For patients with frequent episodes—that is, at least one or more per week—our approach is to prevent rather than "chase" attacks with medications. The drug armamentarium includes antihistamines, phosphodiesterase inhibitors, sympathomimetics, and corticosteroids.

Antihistamines

The H_1 blockers, the mainstay of therapy, are available in several forms. Hydroxyzine and cyproheptadine seem to have less soporific effects and possess the additional advantage of anticholinergic and antiserotinin properties. In addition, cyproheptidine is often more effective in patients with cold urticaria.

Once lesions are present, antihistamines reduce itching but do not hasten resolution of urticaria. When given prophylactically, they may decrease the frequency and severity of attacks.

Recent evidence suggests that an H_1 blocker plus an H_2 blocker, cimetidine (Tagament) may be effective in some patients for treating disease where H_1 blockers alone do not work (Harvey et al., 1981). About 50% of patients do not improve with either H_1 or H_1 plus H_2 blocker therapy. The tricyclic antidepressant sinequan, which has both H_1 and H_2 blocking activity, has been shown to be effective in some cases of urticaria at low doses (i.e., 5 to 10 mg qid).

Phosphodiesterase Inhibitors

Various theophylline preparations are commercially available, including the easier-to-take sustained-release forms. They act, presumably, by elevating intracellular cyclic AMP (cAMP), an inhibitor of mast cell and basophil histamine release. Lower therapeutic levels than are necessary to treat asthma (8–15 μg/ml) are usually adequate. Theophylline preparations are often effective in the relatively recalcitrant pressure urticaria and angioedema. If antihistamines and phosphodiesterase inhibitors are both ineffective alone, a trial of both together is worthwhile.

Sympathomimetics

Agents such as terbutaline, albuterol, and ephedrine are generally ineffective as single agents, but in combination with antihistamines or phosphodiesterase inhibitors may act in concert to decrease disease activity. They should be used with caution in elderly patients or in those with organic heart disease, hypertension, and hyperthyroidism.

Corticosteroids

Steroids are rarely, if ever, indicated for long-term therapy of chronic and relatively benign disease but are useful agents in unusual patients not responding to the previously mentioned drugs (see below).

An example of a sequential drug trial is outlined for patients with frequent disease of greater than 6 weeks' duration who have had appropriate evaluation. Each drug is used continuously for at least 48 hours. Patients are instructed to proceed to the next step in their therapeutic trials if one or two episodes of urticaria and angioedema occur after 48 hours of therapy:

1. Cyproheptadine, 4 mg 3–4 times a day.
2. Hydroxyzine, 20–50 mg 3–4 times a day.
3. Hydroxyzine, 20–50 mg 4 times a day and cimetidine, 300 mg 4 times a day.
4. Hydroxyzine, 20–50 mg 4 times a day and a long-acting theophylline preparation twice a day.
5. Theophylline preparation plus terbutaline, 2.5–5 mg 3 times a day.
6. Hydroxyzine 20–50 mg 4 times a day, long-acting theophylline preparation twice a day, and terbutaline 2.5–5 mg 3 times a day.
7. For the unusual patient with severe disease and poorly tolerated morbidity who does not respond to the above therapy, prednisone is administered. A starting dose of ~1 mg/kg (40–80 mg in a single A.M. dose) for one week is used, with subsequent rapid tapering over 4–6 weeks. If lesions recur, steroid dose is reduced more slowly on a daily or an alternate-day schedule. The goal is to find the lowest dose that will control the lesions. Further, every 1–3 months attempts must be made to withdraw this medication. Antihistamines and theophylline preparations are often used in conjunction with the prednisone. These should be continued following discontinuation of the steroids.

Case 1

A 29-year-old sales manager was referred to our division for evaluation of chronic urticaria and angioedema refractory to therapy. The patient offered a 10-month history of almost daily angioedema involving predominantly the lips and eyelids. This swelling was often associated with hives of the trunk and extremities. A thorough evaluation by his referring physician had revealed a normal physical examination and unremarkable complete blood count, erythrocyte sedimentation rate (ESR), blood chemistries, chest x-ray, and urinanalysis. The patient denied any obvious physical precipitants to his disease. He denied history of inhaled, contact-induced, food or drug allergies. His general health was excellent. Other than the antihistamines he took for relief of itching, his only other medications were occasional acetaminophen for headaches and rare smoking of marijuana. In addition, he smoked one pack of cigarettes per day and drank one martini each night.

He was frustrated by the fact that he had tried "every antihistamine" (diphenhydramine, hydroxyzine, cyproheptadine, and chlorpheniramine) without effective control of his disease. Episodes were frequent, and because of cosmetic reasons, he had missed "too many" work days. He had seen many physicians for the same problem to no avail. Describing himself as an anxious person, he said he was "at the end of his rope."

During the initial consultation with the patient, a thorough history was obtained, and the physical examination was normal except for the presence of urticaria. Several hives were scattered over the anterior thorax, arms, and legs. It was learned that the patient had taken his many antihistaminic medications only when lesions appeared, and never on a prophylactic basis. It was also elicited that the patient suspected that his urticaria and angioedema were representative of a serious underlying illness.

On the basis of our evaluation, the patient was diagnosed as having chronic idiopathic disease. He was educated regarding his illness, especially its benign nature and natural course. His questions were answered, and he was instructed to keep a diary of the frequency, location, and severity of lesions while off all medications. On follow-up, it was determined that episodes occurred almost daily. A sequential drug trial was initiated as outlined in the "Therapy" section of this chapter. The patient achieved complete remission of his disease with hydroxyzine 25 mg 4 times a day. After a 3-month disease-free period, the patient was successfully tapered off hydroxyzine with no further episodes. Episodes recurred approximately 3 months and 15 months later, both times in association with upper respiratory tract infections. The process again responded to hydroxyzine.

This case illustrates several points in the management of patients with chronic urticaria and angioedema. First, the disease is both frustrating to the patient and vexing to the physician. It is not unusual for a patient to seek help from many physicians when the lesions do not resolve. Furthermore, patients commonly worry about their mysterious "affliction"—what it means, whether it will get worse, and whether they can die from it? Thorough patient understanding is a vital adjunct to effective therapy and patient compliance to the drug trial. Finally, in patients with frequent episodes of chronic disease, therapy administered after lesions occur does not decrease the frequency or severity of disease. Only medicine administered prophylactically will result in prevention of disease. Hence alleged "therapeutic failures" often achieve disease remission with simple type I antihistamine therapy administered prophylactically.

REFERENCES*

Atkinson, J. P. *Ann. Allergy*, 1979, *42*, 348–352.

Gelfand, J., Atkinson, J. P., & Frank, M. M. *Ann. Intern. Med.*, 1976, *84*, 580–593.

Harvey, R. P., Wegs, J., & Schocket, A. L. *J. Allergy Clin. Immunol.*, 1981, *68*, 262–266.

Jacobson, K. W., Branch, L. B., & Nelson, H. S. *JAMA*, 1980, *243*, 1644–1646.

Kaplan, A. P. In E. Middleton, E. Ellis, & C. Reed (Eds.), *Allergy: Principles and practice*. St. Louis: Mosby, 1978, pp. 1080–1099.

Kaplan, A. P. *Am. J. Med.*, 1981, *70*, 755–758.

Mathews, K. P. *Med. Clinics N. Am.*, 1974, *58*, 185–205.

*These references were selected because the majority are recent reviews and pertinent to this chapter, and thereby serve as entry to the literature. In addition, the authors of this chapter have published a similar, but more detailed review. Schneider, S. B. and Atkinson, J. P. *Update: Dermatology in General Medicine* Eds: Fitzpatrick, T. B., et al, New York: McGraw-Hill 1983, pp. 61–79.

Mathews, K. P. *J. Allergy Clin. Immunol.*, 1980, *66*, 347–357.

Mathews, K. P., Pan, P. M., Gardner, N. J., & Hugli, T. E. *Ann. Intern. Med.*, 1980, *93*, 443–445.

Mathison, D. A., Arroyave, C. M., Bhat, K. N., Hurewitz, D. S., & Marnell, D. J. *Ann. Intern. Med.*, 1977, *86*, 534–538.

Phanuphak, P., Kohler, P. F., Stanford, R. E., Schocket, A. L., Carr, R. I., & Claman, H. N. *J. Allergy Clin. Immunol.*, 1980, *65*, 436–444.

Schneider, S. B., & Atkinson, J. P. "Urticaria and Angioedema." In T. B. Fitzpatrick, Eisen, A. Z., Wolff, K., Freedberg, I. M., Austen, K. F. *Update: Dermatology in General Medicine*. New York: McGraw-Hill, 1983, pp. 61–79.

Soter, N. A., & Wasserman, S. I. *Int. J. Dermatol.*, 1979, *18*, 517–532.

Warin, R. P., & Champion, R. H. In *Major problems in dermatology*. Philadelphia: Saunders, 1974, Vol. I, pp. 1–164.

Yecies, L. D., & Kaplan, A. P. In C. W. Parker (Ed.), *Clinical immunology*. Philadelphia: Saunders, 1980, pp. 1283–1315.

QUESTIONS

1. Chronic urticaria and angioedema are frequently associated with which of the following:

   a. "Hidden" infections.
   b. Unsuspected foods and food additives.
   c. Seasonal inhalant allergens.
   d. Chronic fungal infections.
   e. Unknown factors.

2. Which of the following statements in regard to the association of underlying systemic illnesses and chronic urticaria and angioedema is *false*?

   a. A thorough history, physical examination, and laboratory evaluation will in most cases readily uncover an underlying illness.
   b. Chronic viral hepatitis, rheumatic diseases, and malignancies are underlying illnesses occasionally associated with urticaria and angioedema.
   c. If the urticaria and angioedema have been present for 6 months and no systemic disease has been discovered, it is unlikely that one will be found.
   d. Patients are not concerned about the possibility of an underlying illness but only want the hives to disappear.

3. Which of the following statements in regard to the management of acute urticaria and angioedema is *false*?

   a. Severe symptoms (massive swelling, laryngeal edema, decreased blood pressure) should be treated with antihistamines and corticosteroids.
   b. Itching can partially be ameliorated by antihistamines.
   c. This illness is usually an isolated, nonrecurrent event or that of a self-limited series of many events.
   d. The patient is often aware of or has a good idea of the cause of the lesions.

4. Regarding the role of histamine and antihistamines in this illness, which one of the following statements is *false*?

a. Histamine is thought to be the most important mediator of urticaria and angioedema.
b. Antihistamines are effective in many patients but not in others. This may be because other mediators are sometimes involved or because local concentrations of antihistamines are inadequate.
c. In chronic urticaria and angioedema antihistamines are most effective if given as soon as the lesions first appear.
d. If one type of antihistamine does not work, one should try a different class.

5. Which of the following statements is *true* in regard to the etiology of acute and chronic urticaria and angioedema?

a. Emotions are important inciting agents and may be the most common cause of both acute and chronic urticaria.
b. Large doses of various vitamins often will prevent urticaria and angioedema.
c. "Allergic" individuals have the same incidence of chronic urticaria as patients without an allergic background.
d. Skin testing for foods and aeroallergens often reveals a likely cause for acute and chronic urticaria.

Answers can be found in Appendix B at the end of the book.

Gerald S. Shatz

10

Anaphylaxis

The term "anaphylaxis" has several meanings, most of which refer to a rapidly developing usually systemic reaction that is potentially fatal in outcome. On a practical level, however, it is very important for the practicing physician to realize that anaphylaxis is a continuum of systemic allergic reactions ranging from the very mild to the life-threatening. Such seemingly trivial problems as itching of the hands and feet while eating a crab meat appetizer, rhinorrhea noted soon after taking an antibiotic, and cramping abdominal pain following a yellow jacket sting thus are all in a very real sense anaphylactic reactions and may be the harbingers of more serious problems that may emerge in the future. Fortunately, most anaphylactic reactions are not life-threatening, but all have the capacity to rapidly become so. Early therapeutic intervention with epinephrine may halt progression. Some reactions, however, are so sudden and unexpected or may involve critical areas such as the laryngopharynx that even optimal treatment in an emergency room setting will not readily reverse the process.

The release of chemical mediators from tissue mast cells and/or circulating basophilic leukocytes is felt to be responsible for the multiple and often varied clinical manifestations of this syndrome. The mechanisms of mediator release can be divided into immunologic (or "anaphylactic") and nonimmunologic (or "anaphylactoid") (see Fig. 10-1). Of the immunologically mediated variety, the most common in humans is the cytotropic (type I) anaphylactic reaction. Here release is triggered by the interaction between foreign antigenic substances and mast-cell-bound IgE antibody or possibly IgG_4 antibody specific to the foreign substance. Cytotoxic (type II) and aggregate (type III) anaphylactic reactions occur as a result of soluble or insoluble immune complex activation of the compliment system with production of the anaphylatoxins C3a and C5a. The interaction of these macromolecules with receptors on basophil and mast cell membranes also leads to extrusion of the chemical mediators of anaphylaxis. Although purely speculative at this time, certain types of anaphylactic

ALLERGY: THEORY AND PRACTICE
ISBN 0-8089-1619-X

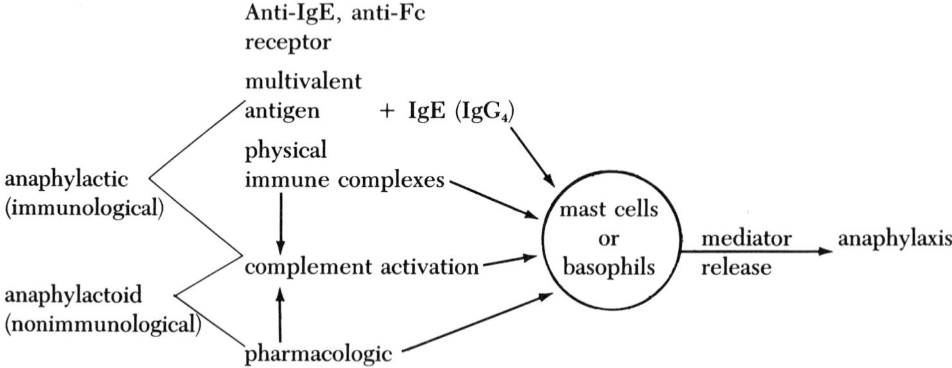

Figure 10-1. Depicted here is the final common pathway in anaphylaxis, namely mast cell (basophil) mediator release. Immunological and non-immunological mechanisms are shown.

reaction may occur as a result of autoimmune phenomena. Postulated autoantigens include the Fab fragments of cell-bound IgE antibody and vacant F_c receptors for IgE antibody.

Anaphylactoid reactions are dealt with separately in Chapter 11, and the remainder of this section is devoted to true anaphylaxis only.

EPIDEMIOLOGY

Although it seems obvious that patients with personal or family history of allergic problems would be at greater risk of developing anaphylaxis, no consistent correlation has been made. It appears, however, that asthma may be a predisposing factor for fatal penicillin–anaphylactic reactions. Also, it is clear that the more invasive the route of antigen administration, such as parenteral versus oral, the more likely it is for systemic reactions to occur. Otherwise, there are no constitutional factors that might indicate to the physician those individuals at risk for severe or fatal reactions.

CLINICAL MANIFESTATIONS

Skin

Of the shock organs under attack during systemic anaphylaxis, the skin is most commonly involved. This involvement may result in urticaria, angioedema, flushing, pruritus, or just a burning or stinging sensation. These symptoms may occur singly or in any combination. Skin reactions are not usually considered dangerous, although massive histamine release leading to hypotension has been well documented in cold-induced urticaria patients when swimming in cold water.

Upper Airway

Sneezing, rhinorrhea, and nasal obstruction are legitimate signs and symptoms of the anaphylactic syndrome that in and of themselves are not serious but may precede more serious problems. The upper airway can become obstructed by edema of the tongue, soft palate, oropharynx and hypopharynx, epiglottis, larynx, and even the trachea. These patients may initially complain of a lump or pain in the throat or dysphagia or develop hoarseness of the voice. If swelling continues, stridor, cyanosis, and respiratory arrest can ensue.

Lower Airway

Asthmatic symptoms of tightness in the chest, cough, shortness of breath, and wheezing indicate bronchial involvement. In some patients, pulmonary capillary permeability is markedly increased and florid pulmonary edema may ensue. Auscultatory findings, including moist rales, would then be present. Fortunately this seems to be a short-lived problem and does not change the basic treatment strategy of lower respiratory symptoms in anaphylaxis (see section on treatment).

Gastrointestinal Tract

Although not widely appreciated, the GI tract is a relatively common shock organ in anaphylaxis. Signs and symptoms include nausea, vomiting, cramping, abdominal pain, and diarrhea and may occur, especially if the route of antigenic administration is oral.

Cardiovascular System

Marked increase in vascular permeability at the capillary and post capillary venular level can rapidly produce a picture of hypovolemic shock with orthostatic hypotension and syncope. The ability of histamine to exert this effect on the vascular system is well known and most certainly is operative in vascular collapse of allergic etiology. However, vascular collapse due to primary cardiac dysfunction, hypoxemia, and acidemia may also be operative in anaphylaxis. Indeed, it has been speculated that a chemical factor released during anaphylaxis may have a cardiodepressant action. Cardiac tissue has recently been shown to possess histamine receptors of both the H_1 and H_2 varieties, and thus histamine may be the cardiodepressant factor. Obviously, severe antecedent respiratory obstruction producing hypoxemia and acidemia can result in metabolic cardiovascular collapse and this picture is the one most commonly seen in fatal anaphylactic shock.

Other Clinical Manifestations

Clinical manifestations of anaphylaxis include pelvic cramping pains due to uterine contraction. This symptom is easy to understand since the uterus has an abundance of mast cells. Epiphora and conjunctivitis may also occur due to conjunctival involvement.

ETIOLOGY

The feature shared in all forms of immediate hypersensitivity is host responsiveness to extrinsically derived antigens. The sources of antigenic exposure capable of inducing the anaphylactic syndrome include injectant, ingestant, inhalant, and contactant. Certainly, some antigens can be introduced by more than one route, but only the most common are emphasized (Table 10-1).

Injectants

Whereas intravenous (IV) and intramuscular (IM) injection of allergens are most effective in inducing anaphylaxis, the sub-Q, ID, and intradiscal routes also have this potential. During the first four decades of this century, prevention and treatment of many infectious disease processes were carried out by the use of hyperimmune antisera of heterologous, usually equine, origin. Most of the early fatalities from anaphylaxis have been attributed to this form of therapy. With the advent of the antibiotic era, ability to obtain antisera of human origin, and widespread sophisticated immunization programs, serum therapy is now an uncommon cause of anaphylaxis. Immunosuppressants employing horse antihuman lymphocyte sera currently has a place, albeit limited, in the prevention of renal allograph rejection. Antisera directed against tumor-specific antigens has been and continues to be scrutinized for efficacy.

Unfortunately, the replacement of serum therapy by antibiotics did not bring anaphylaxis to an end. In fact, penicillin alone is thought to be responsible for up to 500 deaths per year in the United States. This capacity to induce anaphylaxis is best explained in the ability of penicillin's *in vivo* metabolites to readily form covalent bonds with endogenous proteins. This high degree of protein reactivity facilitates the production of high density, multivalent antigen complexes able to reach sensitized tissue mast cells and circulating basophils with relative ease. This facility for protein reactivity seems to be shared by other B-lactam antibiotics and certainly is a major reason why patients with penicillin allergy are at risk for subsequent anaphylaxis if given semisynthetic penicillins or cephalosporins (see Chapter 28).

Stinging insect hypersensitivity accounts for at least 40 deaths per year in the United States. The insects of other *Hymenoptera* are involved and include the honeybees, wasp, hornets, yellow jacket, and imported fire ant. Some authorities feel that up to 0.4% of the general population are sensitized to one or more venom antigens and if stung, have a 5–10% chance of developing systemic reactions (see Chapter 27).

Most insulins currently in use are of porcine and bovine origin and are a rare cause of life-threatening anaphylaxis. Local reactions are common, and most allergic phenomena can be avoided by using a "pure" preparation. For some patients, purity means using a single-species insulin such as pork instead of mixed beef and pork. Other patients become sensitized to high-molecular-weight noninsulin proteins present in trace amounts in all commercially available insulins. This type of impurity problem can usually be bypassed by using the even more highly purified single component or monocomponent preparations. More recently human insulin, produced in bacteria by recombinant DNA techniques has become available. However patients sensitive to pure-pack insulin are also sensitive to human insulin.

Allergen extracts used for diagnosis and treatment of allergic disease always pose the threat of inducing severe anaphylactic reactions. Fortunately, if testing is per-

Table 10-1 *Causes of Anaphylaxis**

Route of Antigen Administration†
Injection
• *heterologous antisera*
snake venom, rabies, diptheria, anti-lymphocyte serum, anti-tumor antibody, clostridia
• *heterologous culture media for vaccines*
flu, measles
• *antibiotics*
beta lactum—penicillin, semi-synthetic, penicillins, cephalosporins
others and tetracyclines, aminoglycosides, chloramphenicol, amphotericin B, vancomycin, polymixin, bactracin
• *venoms*
hymenoptera
other—deer fly, kissing bug, snake, other insects
• *blood products*
red blood cells
plasma factors—IgA, gammaglobulin, clotting factors
• *hormones*
insulins, ACTH, methylprednisilone‡
enzymes‡, chymotrypsin, chymopapain, trypsin, penicillinase, l-asparigenase
• *allergen extracts*
diagnostic
therapeutic
• *miscellaneous*
dextrand
Ingestant
• *foods*
nuts, berries, beans, legumes, many others
• *drugs*
• *others*
bee pollen tablets
Inhalant
• penicillin, cromolyn, fish
Topical
• *skin*—antibiotics, certain physical stimuli
• *intravaginal*—sperm and seminal products
• *ophthalmic*—fluorescein dye
Unknown
• exercise induced anaphylaxis, idiopathic anaphylaxis, systemic mastocytosis
Miscellaneous
• echinoccus cyst

*Incomplete list.
†Certain antigens that have more than one route of administration.
‡Immunological mechanism possible but not proven.

formed with antigens of certain quality, concentration, and by the proper route of administration in appropriately selected patients, such reactions are rare. Much the same can be said about immunotherapy. Extra care in insuring correct dosage and subcutaneous route of antigen administration as well as avoiding large time gaps between allergy shorts can limit the possibility of anaphylaxis to immunotherapy.

Local anesthetic agents or "caine" drugs can cause many types of untoward reaction, most of which are nonallergic and include toxic central nervous system and cardiovascular reactions, vasovagal syncope, hyperventilation, and other anxiety-related symptoms. Some problems can be attributed to the sympathomimetic effects of epinephrine that is commonly given with the anesthetic during dental procedures. However, a small number of patients exhibit symptoms consistent with anaphylaxis, which seems to be nonimmunologically mediated in all but a few case reports (Chapter 11). It is estimated that more than 95% of patients labeled as sensitive to local anesthetics will be able to tolerate one or another of these drugs if appropriate dose testing is carried out.

Radiocontrast material and many drugs such as those used during induction of anesthesia are capable of inducing anaphylaxis. But since no convincing evidence suggests an immunologic basis for these reactions, they are discussed in the chapter concerned with anaphylactoid reactions.

Ingestants

Many foods contain antigens capable of eliciting severe anaphylactic reactions especially seafoods, nuts, berries, and legumes. Usually symptoms occur within minutes to several hours after ingestion, and patients learn to recognize the causative food(s). Some, however, are delayed for up to 12 hours and identification by history becomes more difficult. The problem is further compounded by our relatively primitive knowledge regarding the physiochemical nature of most food antigens. For the most part, therefore, reliable diagnostic reagents for skin testing, passive transfer, RAST testing, and provocative challenge are lacking. With the exception of RAST tests, the aforementioned methods of diagnosing are potentially dangerous and if undertaken should be performed under strictly controlled conditions. Food antigens recently described in the literature capable of inducing anaphylaxis include Wink soft drink, sesame seeds, and millet seeds. Only reactions to foods mediated by IgE antibody or of uncertain etiology are listed in Table 10-1. Of course, many other foods can induce severe anaphylactoid reactions.

Anaphylactic reactions to drugs taken by mouth are certainly less common than those that occur following parenteral administration. A good example of this is the experience with penicillin, where only six to eight deaths have been attributed to anaphylaxis after oral ingestion of the drug. The usual type of systemic reaction following drug ingestion is limited to the cutaneous and gastrointestinal systems. As in the case with certain foods, many drugs are capable of producing anaphylactoid as well as anaphylactic reactions, and some may possess both capabilities.

Several recent reports have documented oral ingestion of bee pollen, which is practiced by some health food enthusiasts, as yet another potential cause of anaphylaxis. Since much of the pollen contained in these tablets may come from composite weeds such as ragweed, it is not difficult to understand this phenomenon. At least one laboratory is now investigating the allergenic potential of honey produced by bees inhabiting hives in close proximity to large fields of ragweed.

Inhalant, topical, ophthalmic, rectal, and even the intravaginal routes have all been documented as portals of antigenic entry capable of inducing anaphylaxis in exquisitely sensitive individuals. One possible mechanism of sensitization in human seminal fluid allergy may involve cross-reactivity between Rho(D) immune globulin (RhoGAM), given to Rh-negative mothers after childbirth, and seminal proteins.

In a number of anaphylactic syndromes, the inciting antigens and the manner in which they are made available for interaction with IgE antibody have yet to be defined. Included in this category is the recently recognized syndrome of exercise induced anaphylaxis. Here the stimulus seems to be generated by rigorous exercise and shares certain qualities with the physical urticarias and exercise-induced asthma. However, it seems to be a distinct disease process and at times must be distinguished from cardiac dysfunction since a number of patients with this exercise-induced syndrome will experience collapse with or without syncope. One possible clue as to the origin of this problem is the observation in several patients that exercise-induced symptoms can be produced only following the ingestion of certain foods.

As the term implies, idiopathic anaphylaxis is used to connote patients experiencing episodic anaphylactic reactions whose diagnostic evaluation fails to reveal even a hint as to what the cause may be. Certainly as new data are accumulated, many of these patients will have an explanation for their problem. Indeed recent studies have suggested that a proportion of these patients have a form of systemic mast cell disease. This syndrome is important to identify since the symptoms can be controlled by a combination of H_1 and H_2 antihistaminics and aspirin.

At times a patient may be allergic to the only therapeutic agent available to them for treatment. Such could be the case in a penicillin-, insulin-, or horse-serum-sensitive patient. Rapid desensitization is then necessary, and since this procedure involves administering antigens to known sensitive individuals, anaphylaxis can and often will occur. For this reason desensitization is considered an example of "controlled" anaphylaxis and thus should be carried out only by physicians experienced with this procedure. In 22 reported cases of penicillin desensitization in history-positive and skin-test-positive patients, 5 experienced life-threatening anaphylaxis, one of which died. Work with monovalent haptens in penicillin allergic patients suggests desensitization may be attained safely by saturation of cell-fixed IgE antibody by antigens not capable of firing the mediator cells. Recently "oral desensitization" has been shown to be safe and effective in patients with beta-lactam antibiotic allergy.

DIAGNOSIS

Certainly the diagnosis of anaphylaxis must be entertained in any patient in shock, coma, and/or respiratory distress. Information gained from the history, if available, and physical exam usually suffice in confirming this diagnosis. The usual problem is to determine the etiologic agent(s) involved. Skin testing and provocative challenge are helpful in some situations but have the potential of inducing a recurrence. Thus these and other in vivo tests for anaphylaxis should be approached with extreme caution and only under controlled conditions. Passively transferring patient's serum (containing IgE antibody) into the skin of experimental animals whose mast cells are capable of fixing human IgE is a safer, although not generally available, way of skin testing with suspected and potentially dangerous antigens. *In vitro* testing such as RAST tests (Chapter 5) circumvent dangers inherent in *in vivo* tests but are not as sensitive and require precise knowledge of the biologically active antigenic determinants for accuracy. With the exception of penicillin, certain foods, and hormones, the identity and structure of the antigenic components are not known and thus only crude extracts are utilized in most RAST tests. Obviously, unless a minimum concentration of bioactive antigen is available in the crude extract, false-negative RAST scores may ensue. On the other hand, many borderline or obviously false-positive scores are often obtained, which may reflect one of the many inherent standardization and specificity problems in any radioimmunoassay. Thus in 1984, RAST testing and other *in vitro* assays such as leukocyte histamine release should be viewed as safe but only possibly helpful tools to use in establishing the cause(s) of anaphylaxis in an individual patient.

As mentioned above, any condition presenting with respiratory obstruction, cardiovascular collapse, or coma enters into the differential diagnosis of anaphylaxis. In vasovagal reactions, reflex bradycardia occurs which accounts for the orthostatic lightheadedness and/or syncope seen in the presence of normal or slightly lower blood pressure. Nausea, diaphoresis, and pallor are common. Patients improve by assuming the suppine position but at times may require atropine. Vasovagal syncope often follows an injection and thus must be differentiated from anaphylaxis as soon as possible. Upper-airway obstruction from trauma, foreign bodies, hereditary angioedema, acute epiglottis, and tumor should be ruled out. A case of acute non-traumatic laryngeal hemorrhage initially confused with anaphylactic laryngeal obstruction has been described in a patient on anticoagulant therapy. Similarly, nonallergic laryngeal edema was observed in a patient with sickle beta-thalasemia. Systemic anaphylactoid reactions are clinically identical to anaphylactic reactions and hence deserve similar, prompt treatment. Pseudo and factitious anaphylaxis are rare conditions but should be kept in mind in patients not responding to conventional treatment.

TREATMENT

Regardless of the cause of severity, once the diagnosis of anaphylaxis is made, immediate treatment with subcutaneous epinephrine is indicated. Since rapidity of onset and duration of symptoms seems to be correlated with mortality, it is only logical to intervene as soon as possible with the drug of choice, epinephrine. The precise dosage, concentration, and route of administration of this drug is open to some debate and of course depends on the clinical situation at hand. Suffice it to say that epinephrine should first be given by the subcutaneous route in a dosage of 0.01 ml/kg (1 : 1000 w/v aqueous) up to a maximum of 0.3 ml. This may be repeated every 15–20 minutes. If the reaction progresses or is obviously life-threatening from the start, intramuscular (IM) injection is preferred and dosage may be increased up to 0.5 ml in an adult without underlying cardiac irritability. If the causative antigen was injected such as in the case of an allergy injection, bee sting, or injection of penicillin, local infiltration with adrenalin (0.1–0.3 ml or 1 : 1000), along with tourniquet placement proximal to the site of injection may help by impeding systemic absorption. Some authorities feel that in anaphylactic shock with hypotension and poor peripheral perfusion, subcutaneous and IM adrenalin will not be readily absorbed systemically to exert beneficial effects. In general this is not true and should not preclude the use of subcutaneous (SC) and/or IM injection. In general intravenous (IV) epinephrine is not indicated for anaphylaxis therapy.

As is true with any resuscitation effort, immediate attention must be given to the airway that may be obstructed by laryngeal edema or bronchospasm. Oxygen, IV aminophylline, aerosolized bronchodilators, and IV antihistamines may help, but cricothyroidotomy and/or tracheotomy may be required if the upper airway is severely obstructed. The loading dose for aminophylline is 5 mg/kg over 10–20 minutes followed by continuous infusion at the rate of 0.6–0.9 mg/kg/hr (see Chapter 15). Diphenhydramine 1–2 mg/kg IV up to 50 mg is given by slow IV push.

Hypotension should be treated by adequate amounts of IV fluid and may require central venous pressure monitoring and vasopressors if normal blood pressure is not readily restored. No single antihypotensive agent is the drug of choice, but most experience has been with continuous IV infusion of metaraminінol (Aramine) 100 mg in 500-ml normal saline, epinephrine 1 mg in 50-ml saline, or levarterenol (Levofed) 8 mg in 500-ml normal saline. These agents work primarily by increasing peripheral vascular tone. Isoproterenol 1–2 mg in 500-ml normal saline or dopamine 100–200 mg in 500-ml normal saline may help by enhancing cardiac output. All the above drugs should be infused at rates necessary to maintain adequate blood pressure. In the clinical setting of peripheral edema, high hematocrit, and hypotension refractory to volume replacement with conventional crystalloid solutions (normal saline, Ringer's lactate), and vasopressors, use of colloidal fluid such as stable plasma protein solution and dextran may help. The oncotic properties of these substances may limit egress from and even promote return of extravasated fluid back into the vascular system. It should be obvious from the above discussion that the only appropriate setting for treatment of anaphylaxis is an intensive care unit.

Protracted anaphylaxis refractory to the usual forms of therapy is being recognized in patients taking beta-adrenergic blocking agents. These patients may benefit from more aggressive beta-agonist therapy.

Conventional H_1 blocking antihistamines may help to reduce airway edema and certainly will be helpful for pruritus and urticaria. There are data to support the use of the H_2 antagonist cimetidine (Tagamet) in combination with an H_1 blocking agent in the treatment of anaphylactic shock and may be used in a clinical situation such as a patient on beta-blocking agents. There is in addition evidence in animals that in this instance glucagon may lessen the $beta_1$ blockade and facilitate response to the beta agonist.

Steroids should be routinely given to any patient with a serious anaphylactic reaction not for an immediate effect, but rather to prevent recurrent, protracted, or late-phase anaphylaxis.

PREVENTION

As is true in all allergic diseases, avoidance of the allergen is the prophylactic measure of choice. This is a realistic possibility in many instances such as in food and drug reactions, but not in others like *Hymenoptera* sensitivity and idiopathic anaphylaxis. Medic alert cards or jewelery may expedite life-saving treatment in the unconscious patient and serve as a ready reference source enabling the patient to relay allergic information to any physician.

Although the true incidence of cross reactivity between penicillin and cephalosporin antibiotics is not known, all of these drugs should be avoided in the penicillin-allergic patient. A conscientious effort should be made to abandon the practice of IM injections of penicillin for outpatients since the oral route is much less hazardous.

Human versus heterologous antisera or hormones are preferred when available. Desensitization may have to be attempted when only equine, porcine, bovine, or fowl reagents are readily accessible. Tetanus immunizations should be kept up to date.

Patients with a convincing history for egg allergy should not receive flu vaccines because the viruses are grown in duck embryo. Rubella vaccine, which is prepared in embryo cells, has been reported to cause allergic reactions in egg-sensitive individuals. These patients should be skin tested with the vaccine prior to its administration.

Systemic reactions induced by *Hymenoptera* venom is an indication for specific venom immunotherapy, which may be necessary throughout the patient's entire life. Measures helpful in decreasing the likelihood of exposure should be stressed, especially in months of high insect activity (see Chapter 27).

Any person with a history of immunodeficiency or prior injection of gamma globulin should be screened for IgA deficiency before receiving a blood transfusion. If blood is required, IgA-deficient donors are preferred, but appropriately types and multiple-washed packed red cells are acceptable.

As already discussed, allergy immunotherapy should be performed only in appropriately selected patients utilizing antigens of proper quality and concentration. An observation period of 15–20 minutes following the injection is mandatory. If currently being given to patient taking beta-sympathic blocking agents, reevaluation of indications for immunotherapy is in order. Future use of allergoids—that is, substances that are highly immunogenic but less allergenic than traditional aqueous extracts—may be much safer to use in immunotherapy if efficacy is demonstrated.

Even though extreme caution has been painstakingly observed by the patient, inadvertent exposure to an allergen can and often does take place. Certain batches of milk may contain significant amounts of penicillin if this antibiotic is given to the dairy cow during milk production. Potatoes fried in the same oil used to prepare fish (as is often the case in fast food restaurants) can harbor enough antigen to provoke a severe anaphylactic reaction in the unwary fish-sensitive person. These points underscore the importance of educating the patient in the self administration of SC epinephrine. Several types of epinephrine kits are commercially available, and an adequate number should be purchased by these highly allergic individuals so they can have ready access to and initiate emergency treatment.

Prophylaxis with antihistamines, sympathomimetics, and steroids have helped individual patients with exercise-induced anaphylaxis and idiopathic anaphylaxis, but no consistent beneficial effects have been observed.

As the mysteries of the immune response continue to unravel largely through the efforts of research, better ways of identifying, protecting, and treating the anaphylactically sensitized patient will no doubt be found. Induction of tolerance to specific antigens by modulation of helper and suppressor T-lymphocyte function as well as by directly paralyzing IgE producing plasma cells and/or their precursors, IgE B lymphocytes, may one day be a reality.

Case History

A 24-year-old white female presented to an emergency room with a chief complaint of "I reacted to some food."

The patient was at a garden party and ingested a small meal consisting of Chinese hors d'oeuvres and drank a small quantity of beer. Within 5 minutes she noted the onset of swelling of her lips and tongue, intense pruritus over her entire body that was greatest in her hands and feet, a feeling of a lump in her throat, and lightheadedness. She was promptly transported to the emergency room, arriving approximately 10 minutes after she had eaten.

On arrival at the emergency room examination revealed an aggitated female in acute distress, with blood pressure 60 systolic (palpable). She was wheezing audibly and had mild stridor. There were numerous urticarial lesions over the entire body. Her face was markedly swollen, most pronounced in the perioral area, and the tongue was approximately twice the normal size. Examination of the chest revealed inspiratory and expiratory wheezes in all fields. The heart sounds were distant. There were no murmurs or gallops. The remainder of the examination was unremarkable.

The patient was immediately treated with 0.3 ml of aqueous epinephrine SC (1 : 1000) and a rapid infusion of 5% dextrose in one-half normal saline and because of difficulty in breathing was intubated. On this regimen her blood pressure rose to 80/40, and her wheezing decreased. Over the next 40 minutes she received two more injections of aqueous epinephrine SC and 2.5 liters of IV fluid and was also given 100 mg of diphenhydramine IM and 100 mg of methyl prednisolone (Solu-medrol) IV following her arrival in the emergency room. Her blood pressure had stabilized at 110/50, her facial and tongue swelling and urticaria had decreased dramatically, and she had only mild expiratory wheezing.

The patient was extubated without difficulty and was held in an observation unit for 24 hours. Because of continued wheezing she was begun on IV aminophylline 5.6 mg/kg initially and then 0.9 mg/kg hr^{-1}. She was given 75 mg of diphenhydramine q6h and 50 mg of methylprednisolone IV q6h. She did extremely well, and 24 hr following the incident her blood pressure was 120/84. Her urticaria and facial swelling had resolved entirely and she was wheeze-free. She was discharged on a rapidly decreasing dose of methylprednisolone and long-active theophylline.

Subsequent investigation revealed a 3+ positive RAST test to sesame. The chef who prepared the meal indicated that sesame oil had been used as a flavoring in several of the dishes. The patient was advised to avoid any food that might contain sesame oil and to carry injectable epinephrine with her when she ate out.

SUGGESTED READINGS

Lamson, R. W. Fatal anaphylaxis and sudden death associated with the injection of foreign substances, *JAMA*, 1924, *82*, 1091.

Richet, C. *Anaphylaxis* (translated by J. M. Bligh). Liverpool: The University Press, 1913.

Sobotka, A. K., Valentine, M. D., Benton, A. W., and Lichtenstein, L. M. Allergy to insect stings. I. Diagnosis of IgE-mediated hymenoptera sensitivity by venom-induced histamine release, *J. Allergy Clin. Immunol.*, 1974, *53*, 170.

Vaughan, W. T. and Pipes, D. M. On the probable frequency of allergic shock, *Am. J. Dig. Dis.*, 1936, *3*, 558.

Wasserman, S. I. Anaphylaxis. In E. Middleton, C. E. Reed, and E. F. Ellis, (Eds.) *Allergy: Principles and Practice*, St. Louis. C. V. Mosby Co, 1983.

QUESTIONS

1. The initial drug of choice for the treatment of anaphylaxis is:
   a. subcutaneous epinephrine
   b. intramuscular antihistamine
   c. intravenous steroid
   d. intravenous vasopressor
2. Which of the following examples of anaphylaxis is not immunologically mediated?
   a. hypotension and urticaria during a blood transfusion
   b. wheezing soon after peanut butter ingestion
   c. angioedema and urticaria during an IV pyelogram (IVP)
   d. generalized pruritus noted 10 minutes after IM muscular injection of penicillin
3. Reliable skin-testing antigens are available for detection of all but which one of the following?
   a. horse serum
   b. penicillin allergy
   c. insulin allergy
   d. sulfa allergy
4. Definition of the agent responsible for anaphylaxis should include all except
   a. a thorough history
   b. skin testing if available
   c. complete physical examination
   d. oral challenge
   e. diet diary
5. The most important measure needed to be taken to prevent anaphylaxis is:
   a. using oral rather than parenteral route for drug administration
   b. instruction in avoidance of known allergens
   c. obtaining a thorough drug and food allergy history
   d. all of the above

Answers can be found in Appendix B at the end of the book.

Susan Bromberg Schneider

11

Anaphylactoid Reactions

The term "anaphylactoid" translates literally into "like anaphylaxis." Anaphylactoid reactions (ARs) are acute reactions involving the target organs—skin, respiratory tract, cardiovascular system, and gastrointestinal (GI) tract. The symptoms and signs of ARs are secondary to the release of mediators by mast cells and basophilic leukocytes. Whereas in anaphylaxis the trigger to mast cell mediator release is a reaginic (IgE) antibody–antigen interaction (Austen, 1974), in Ars liberation of mediators results from nonimmunologic mechanisms.

By definition, in Ars no previous sensitizing exposure to the precipitating agent is necessary, no IgE specific for antigen is found, and the ability to transfer "sensitivity" to the agent by the Prausnitz-Kustner method is absent. It is of importance to emphasize that the clinical presentation of anaphylactic and anaphylactoid reactions are indistinguishable. Both are medical emergencies requiring immediate physician intervention and therapy.

MORBIDITY AND MORTALITY

The incidence of morbidity and death varies with the individual agent responsible for ARs. Reaction severity can range from a mild discomforting pruritus to hypotension, laryngeal edema, and death.

CLINICAL MANIFESTATIONS

The target organ manifestations of ARs occur within seconds to minutes of exposure to an oral, intravenous (IV), intramuscular (IM), inhaled, or topical inciting agent. They include the following:

SKIN. Urticaria, angioedema, flushing, or acrocyanosis.
RESPIRATORY TRACT. Wheezing secondary to bronchoconstriction and stridor secondary to laryngeal, hypopharyngeal, or tracheal edema.

ALLERGY: THEORY AND PRACTICE
ISBN 0-8089-1619-X

GASTROINTESTINAL TRACT. Nausea, vomiting, diarrhea, or colicky abdominal pain.
UTERUS. Uterine cramping.
CARDIOVASCULAR SYSTEM. Arrhythmias, ischemia, hypotension, or frank cardiovascular collapse.

CLASSIFICATION OF "INCITING AGENTS"

Agents triggering ARs act through direct mast cell action or complement pathway activation. It is also postulated that some may operate through their effects on arachidonic acid metabolism and SRS-A production.

The systematic classification of these agents is difficult because of their diverse properties. In general, they are either "selective" or noncytotoxic in their actions on mast cells, or "nonselective" or cytotoxic in effecting histamine release (Kazimierczak, 1978). Physical agents, such as high temperatures, freezing, thawing, ultraviolet (UV) light, roentgen rays, and other ionizing radiation, release histamine by chemical or osmotic injury. Nonselective chemical histamine releasors, such as detergents, acids, bases, and organic solvents, induce histamine release by irreversible changes in the membrane continuity and cellular function of the mast cell. The more clinically relevent agents causing ARs act selectively—that is, they do not damage the mast cell or other tissues. They include polymeric amines (e.g., compound 48/80), polysaccharides (e.g., dextrans), polybasic compounds (e.g., morphine), antibiotics (e.g., polymyxin B), leukocyte-derived cationic proteins, radiographic contrast materials, venoms (from cobras and bees), enzymes (e.g., chymotrypsin), aggregated proteins, complement-dependent IgG, and nonsteroidal anti-inflammatory agents (presumably acting via prostaglandin synthetase inhibition).

INDIVIDUAL ETIOLOGIC AGENTS CAUSING ARS

Some of the more common causes of ARs are reviewed below (see also Table 11-1).

Radiographic Contrast Material

Radiographic contrast material (RCM) is a water-soluble iodinated aromatic compound for intravascular administration. Approximately 5 million radiographic studies using this hypertonic substance are performed yearly. Adverse reactions with its use include (a) most commonly, nausea, vomiting, and flushing, probably secondary to vasovagal response or to anxiety; (b) cardiopulmonary failure and convulsions, attributable to the hemodynamic effects of intravascularly administered hypertonic solution, and most pronounced in patients with pulmonary hypertension; (c) acute renal failure, seen more frequently in patients with preexisting renal disease and characterized by osmotic diuresis, vasoconstriction, increased blood viscosity in small vessels, and diminished glomerular filtration; and (d) anaphylactoid reactions, occurring almost immediately after the administration of RCM, with urticaria, pruritus, rhinitis, angioedema, conjunctivitis, wheezing, and/or hypotension. Anaphylactoid

Table 11-1 *Major Etiologies: Anaphylactoid Reactions*

Radiographic contrast material
Albumin and plasma protein fractions
Synthetic volume expanders
Anesthetic agents
Protamine
Aspirin and other prostaglandin inhibitors
Chemotherapeutic agents
Miscellaneous
Additives, chelating agents, dyes
IgG anti-IgA reactions
Physical agents

radiographic contrast media reactions are seen in 1–2% of all contrast procedures (Greenberger et al., 1981). Patients with a history of previous reaction have a 17–35% risk of subsequent reaction on repeat exposure to radiographic contrast (Greenberger et al., 1981). Fatal events are seen in 1 in 10–50 thousand studies.

The mechanism of AR to RCM is a subject of much controversy. Reports of anticontrast medium IgM or IgE antibodies are infrequent, and in such cases a cause-and-effect relationship of antibody to reaction has not been established. For the majority of RCM reactions, an antibody-mediated mechanism is not implicated; the pathophysiology is either nonspecific activation of complement or direct release of mast cell contents.

Premedication with steroids and diphenhydramine will in most cases diminish the frequency and severity of ARs to RCM in patients with previous reactions (see Table 11-2 for protocol). In a recent prospective study examining the efficacy of

Table 11-2 *Premedication for Prevention of Anaphylactoid Reactions to Radiographic Contrast Material**

Time Prior to Procedure (Hours)	Medication Administered
13	Prednisone, 50 mg orally
7	Prednisone, 50 mg orally
1	Prednisone, 50 mg orally plus diphenhydramine (Benadryl) 50 mg IM

*For emergency procedures, in which a 13-hour premedication period is not possible, no data are available regarding results of any pretreatment program. One suggested regime is diphenhydramine 50 mg IM 1 hour before the procedure, plus hydrocortisone 200 mg IV immediately q 4h until the procedure is completed. (*Note:* The efficacy of this emergency approach has not been documented) (Greenberger et al., 1981).

premedication (prednisone 50 mg orally every 6 hours for three doses prior to the procedure with the last dose 1 hour before the procedure; and diphenhydramine, 50 mg IM one hour prior to the procedure), the incidence of recurrent reactions was only 7.5%. Recurrent reactions were milder than the initial ones, but for one serious event (0.3% or 1 out of 318 procedures). This was characterized by transient hypotension, wheezing, and urticaria that responded to therapy (Greenberger et al., 1981).

Albumin and Plasma Protein Fractions

Albumin is the most commonly used intravascular volume expander in the United States. It is also used as an additive to parenteral preparations so as to prevent adherence of medication to syringes, containers, or tubing. As radiolabeled microspheres, it is utilized diagnostically for nuclear medicine perfusion studies (Littenberg, 1975). Purified plasma protein fraction, another human blood derivative, is employed clinically as a source of coagulation factor, hyperimmune globulin, simple gamma globulin, and C_1 esterase inhibitor.

The best known side effect of albumin or plasma protein administration is the transmission of hepatitis. A more dramatic untoward reaction is anaphylactoid, ranging in severity from mild to fatal. It is distinct from anti-IgA reactions to blood products seen in IgA-deficient patients. It characteristically is a single event occurrence in patients without history of previous blood product exposure. It is treatable with epinephrine therapy and other supportive measures as indicated.

As for the mechanism of ARs to albumin and purified protein fractions, bacterial, endotoxin, or pyrogen contamination of administered fluid and IgA-deficiency in the patient have been ruled out repeatedly in many case reports. Notably, Prausnitz-Kustner sensitivity to albumin and plasma protein is not transferrable. The most likely cause of histamine release to albumin and plasma protein is activation of complement by aggregated protein through both classic and alternate pathways (Ring et al, 1979). Notably, 5–15% of the total protein content of commercially produced albumin and purified protein fraction is aggregated.

Synthetic Volume Expanders

The synthetic volume expanders include the dextrans, used in the United States, as well as the gelatins and starches, approved for use in Europe. Dextran, to which we shall devote this discussion, is a product of the Leuconostic mesenteroides B512 bacterial conversion of sucrose. It occurs in nature as a contaminant of beet and cane sugar. Dextrans have been available for clinical use since 1945, for purposes of intentional hemodilution, volume substitution, facilitation of the microcirculation, and antithrombogenesis. They are also used as vehicles complexed to iron (Imferon) for parenteral replenishment of iron deficiency. The marketed forms of the dextrans include Dextran 40, Rheomacrodex, Dextran 60/75, and Macrodex.

The advantages of synthetic colloid therapy over albumin are its easy availability, its lower costs, and its longer shelf life. The disadvantages are its relatively rapid disappearance from the intravascular space, the fact that only a limited amount of volume can be safely replenished with it, and its toxicities such as impaired platelet function, renal damage and altered coagulation. Finally, untoward anaphylactoid reactions may occur with dextran use (Collins, 1979). Histamine release induced by dextran is probably nonspecific. The incidence of ARs to dextrans is lower with the low-molecular-weight forms (e.g., Dextran 40) than with the heavier, generously side-branched forms (e.g., Dextran 60/75). Several published series reveal that the incidence of Ars to Dextran 40 is approximately 0.007% and to Dextran 60/75 is 0.69% (Ring & Messmer, 1977).

Anesthetic Agents

The rate of complications to general anesthesia in the United States is approximately 1%. Untoward reactions to induction agents and muscle relaxants include hepatic toxicity, aspiration, arrhythmias, myocardial depression, cardiovascular collapse, and anaphylaxis or anaphylactoid reactions. The New Zealand Adverse Drug Committee reported, in their 1966–1974 series, that approximately 2% of their anesthesia complications were severe histamine-related and that of these, 10% were fatal (Fisher, 1975). The incidence is much higher with the induction agents.

Among the drugs used in general anesthesia are several dibasic and polybasic compounds that can potentially act not only as immunogens, but also as direct histamine liberators. They include amphetamines, atropine, codeine, decamethonium (Syncurine), D-tubocurarine (Tubarine), gallamine (Flaxedil), hydralazine (Apresoline), meperidine (Demerol), methohexital (Brevital), morphine, papaverine (Pavabid), propanidid (Epontol), succinylcholine (Anectine), thiopental (Pentothal), tolazoline (Priscoline), and trimetaphan (Arfonad).

There are, at present, no reliable diagnostic tests to distinguish whether reactions occur by anaphylactoid versus anaphylactic mechanisms. A history of previous anesthesia or previous sensitizing dose is not at all diagnostic of IgE hypersensitivity. Furthermore, the use of multiple drugs concomitantly makes pinpointing of a single etiologic agent most difficult. False-positive skin tests occur with histamine releasors, as well as with improper storage, administration, and preparation of the antigen. False-negative tests occur, with improper preparation and storage of antigen, use of the whole drug rather than the antigenic determinant responsible for an IgE reaction, or application of skin tests during the refractory postanaphylaxis period.

Protamine

Protamine is a polycationic polypeptide used for heparin neutralization in cardiopulmonary bypass, blood component donation, and cell separation techniques. Adverse reactions to protamine are anaphylaxis-like and include urticaria, wheezing, acrocyanosis, and hypotension. The mechanism of such reactions is probably nonimmunologic. Protamine degranulates mast cells *in vitro* and is anticomplimentary. A protamine-specific IgG antibody may be responsible for a limited number of anaphylaxis-like reactions.

Aspirin and Derivatives

Untoward reactions to aspirin [acetylsalicylic acid or (ASA)] are often misdesignated as aspirin "allergy" rather than aspirin "idiosyncrasy" or "sensitivity." Notably, such adverse reactions—to include urticaria, angioedema, and bronchospasm—are seldom IgE-mediated (see Chapter 29).

Chemotherapeutic (Cytotoxic) Agents

The usual side effects ascribed to chemotherapeutic agents include nausea, vomiting, diarrhea, myelosuppression, dermatitis, alopecia, ulcerative stomatitis, defective oogenesis and spermatogenesis, teratogenesis, liver and renal toxicities, hemorrhagic enteritis, hemorrhagic cystitis, and the syndrome of inappropriate antidiuretic hormone. More unusual untoward reactions to IV or topical chemotherapy are immediate systemic ones, characterized by urticaria, angioedema, chest tightness, and cardiovascular collapse (Weiss & Bruno, 1981). The mechanism of these systemic events varies with the cytotoxic agent.

L-Asparaginase, a parenterally administered polypeptide derived from *Escherichia coli,* is used in the therapy of acute lymphocytic leukemia and T-cell lymphoblastic lymphoma. Systemic reactions to L-asparaginase usually occur weeks into the course of twice- or thrice-weekly therapy. Specific IgE and IgG antibody have been isolated in such patients, and anaphylactic deaths have been reported.

Use of cisplatinum in genitourinary neoplasms has been associated with reactions such as pruritus, bronchospasm, urticaria, angioedema, and hypotension. Such systemic reactions occur more frequently when cisplatinum is used in combination with other chemotherapeutic drugs. Reactions are not dose-related. Pretreatment with antihistamines and steroids seems to decrease the frequency and severity of such events in patients with a previous history. Specific IgE has not been isolated in any case. Such reactions are probably anaphylactoid.

Urticaria, angioedema, and hypotension have been reported with use of the cytotoxic antibiotics daunorubicin and doxorubicin in therapy of acute leukemia. Doxorubicin administration in dogs increases serum histamine levels, with resultant hypotension. The mechanism of systemic reactions to cytotoxic antibiotics is believed to be anaphylactoid, via direct mast cell degranulation or complement activation.

"Pseudoanaphylactic" reactions, characterized by fever, confusion, wheezing, and hypotension, have been reported with first-time use of bleomycin. Circulating pyrogens have been implicated as the cause in animal studies.

Systemic reactions have been reported with oral and parenteral methotrexate by unknown mechanisms. An anaphylactic reaction in which specific antibody was isolated and successful desensitization was performed has been reported to cytarabine, another antimetabolite.

Anaphylactoid reactions to first-dose VP-16-213 (etoposide) or VM-26 (teniposide), the epidophyllotoxins, has been seen.

Systemic reactions of unknown mechanism have been reported with the alkylating agents topical nitrogen mustard and intravesicle topical thiopeta. Cyclophosphamide therapy has been associated with systemic reactions, with IgE homocytotropic antibody isolated in one case.

Miscellaneous

Additives, Chelating Agents, and Dyes

A variety of anaphylaxis-like reactions have been reported with the use of additives, chelating agents, and dyes. Their mechanisms have either been unstudied or undetermined. These are (a) methylparabens, commonly used preservatives in drugs and topicals; (b) sodium bisulfite, an antioxidant used as an antifermentative preservative; (c) desferroxamine, a chelating agent used in hemochromatosis; and (d) indocyanin green, a cardiac dye solution used to measure cardiac output, ophthalmic blood flow, liver function, and (e) fluorescein. These agents have been used in retinal angiography and have all been associated with the development of urticaria, hypotension, wheezing, and laryngeal edema.

IgG Antibody Reactions

Any IgG reaction in which complement is activated may mimic IgE reactions. The classic example is in IgA-deficient patients receiving blood products, in whom IgG mounted against IgA can cause anaphylaxis-like reactions, with hypotension and death (Pineda & Taswelly, 1975; Vyas et al., 1969).

Physical Agents

Physical agents, such as light, pressure, vibration, heat, cold, and exercise, may cause histamine release and anaphylaxis-like reactions. The most dramatic example is with cold urticaria, in which submersion into cold water, as with diving into a swimming pool, can result in massive histamine release with hypotension and even death. Although a subgroup of patients with cold urticaria have IgE-mediated disease, reaginic antibody has not been isolated in the remainder of the idiopathic group.

The syndrome of exercise-induced anaphylaxis is characterized by warmth, pruritus, and generalized urticaria to exercise, with or without associated respiratory distress, abdominal colic, or syncope (Sheffer & Austen, 1980). Although exercise-induced anaphylaxis does not occur with every exercise experience, no consistent relation to an environmental antigen has been determined. It is distinct from cholinergic urticaria by the appearance of its lesions and its associated syncope.

DIFFERENTIAL DIAGNOSIS

The differential diagnosis of AR includes any reaction that causes acute onset and rampent course of true (or factitious) vascular collapse. Diseases that should be considered are:

ANAPHYLAXIS. This has already been discussed in detail in Chapter 10.

PHARMACOLOGIC, TOXICOLOGIC, OR IDIOSYNCRATIC REACTIONS. Many drugs, via pharmacologic, toxic, or idiosyncratic effects, cause hypotension with bradycardia, tachycardia, or other arrhythmias. Such reactions are primarily cardiac and are distinct from ARs by the absence of histamine release.

DRUG-UNRELATED REACTIONS. These include psychomotor reactions, such as hyperventilation with dyspnea, paresthesia, dizziness, and loss of consciousness; vasovagal reactions with loss of consciousness and bradycardia; and sympathetic stimulation with production of endogenous epinephrine.

SYNCOPE. Myocardial infarction, insulin reaction, intracranial bleeds, and vasovagal events may present with syncope. Laboratory and physical findings distinguish these from histamine-related events.

FACTITIOUS DISEASE. This includes malingering and hysterical conversion (Patterson & Schatz, 1975).

SYSTEMIC MASTOCYTOSIS. Systemic Mastocytosis has recently come to the forefront as a cause of anaphylactoid reactions. It is characterized by repeated episodes of intense flushing followed by profound hypotension, sometimes in association with other symptoms as outlined above, and usually resulting in collapse. When the patient is brought to the emergency room, the most frequent finding is low or absent blood pressure. Treatment consists of epinephrine and fluids; the patient generally responds promptly. When a patient is evaluated by conventional techniques, little is found and the patient generally carries a diagnosis of ideopathic anaphylaxis. If the attacks are bizarre, the patient is felt to have some undefined psychological illness, as has been the case with several patients that have been diagnosed at Washington University.

Pathology is greater than normal numbers of mast cells in the skin and, in some patients, other organs such as the bone marrow. These patients have a general overproduction of the mediators of anaphylaxis as evidenced by an increase in the serum or urinary concentration of PGD_2 (measured in the urine as a metabolite of PGD_2). In some patients an increase in the 24 hr urine histamine concentration can be measured and a recent report suggests that an increase in histamine metabolites is seen in all patients with this disease. Skin biopsy should also be performed. It is important, however, that proper technique be utilized. Rather than produce a bleb with local anesthetic and biopsying in the middle of the bleb, which is the usual procedure, the area *around* the biopsy site should be infiltrated. This avoids the problem of the local anesthetic inducing mediator release. We prefer to stain the biopsy with the Leader stain that is highly specific for mast cell granules, although the metachromatic stain toluidin blue or Giemsa stain can also be used. The number of mast cells in several high power fields are counted and, if the number is greater than 9, this is presumptive evidence of systemic mastocytosis.

Since symptoms of mastocytosis are the result of aberrant release of mediators, probably because mast cells in this disease are inherently unstable, therapy is directed against the production, release, or effect of the mediators. The currently recommended protocol is a combination of H_1 and H_2 antihistaminics to prevent the end organ effects of histamine, and aspirin to prevent the synthesis of PGD_2. Since the cyclooxygenase of the mast cell is relatively resistant to inhibition by aspirin, it must be used in large quantities. We generally start with 12 aspirin (60 grains, 3.9 grams) of aspirin per day. This will generally give a blood level approaching 20 μG/ml which is sufficient to block PGD_2 production. On this regimen we have found that it is possible to completely block the symptoms of mastocytosis.

Table 11-3 *Therapy for Anaphylactoid Reactions*

Administer subcutaneous epinephrine 1:1000 aqueous dilution immediately for acute reversal of histamine effect; this may be repeated at a 5–30-minute interval if necessary
- Children's dosage 0.01 mg/kg
- Adult's dosage 0.3–0.5 ml

Stabilize vital signs: evaluate airway patency, respiratory status, blood pressure, and pulse; if indicated, establish airway by endotracheal intubation or tracheostomy; establish IV line for fluids and medications

Administer appropriate drugs

- For ongoing histamine release
  - *Antihistamines:* diphenhydramine (Benadryl) 50 mg IV, IM, or orally may be administered at the onset of anaphylactoid reaction and repeated every 6 hours as necessary
  - *Steroids:* to prevent late or prolonged effects of anaphylactoid reactions, an initial IV bolus of 7–10 mg/kg hydrocortisone or a hydrocortisone equivalent can be administered; this may be followed by a dose of 5 mg/kg q6h for 48–72 hours, with subsequent rapid tapering over 3–5 days
- For hypotension, if present
  - Fluids (preferably normal saline) should be administered rapidly through a large bore peripheral or central line
  - If fluids alone are ineffective in restoring blood pressure, one of the following basopressors should be added:
    - Metaraminol bitartrate (Aramine), an alpha and beta agonist that can be administered by slow bolus or constant infusion with cardiac monitor in place; as a bolus dose.
      - For slow IV push, adults 2–5 mg; children 0.01 mg/kg
      - As a constant infusion, titrated to a rate to maintain systolic pressure of 100: adults 25–200 mg/500 ml; children 0.01 mg/kg
    - Levarterenol bitartrate (Levophed), an alpha and beta agonist more potent than Aramine; dose: As constant infusion, adults 4–8 g/1000 ml, titrated to maximum of 2 ml/min; children 1 mg/250 ml, titrated to maximum of 0.5 ml/min
  - Dopamine (Intropin), a beta agonist; dose: As constant infusion, 200 mg/500 ml, at a rate of 0.3–1.2 mg/kg hr
- For bronchospasm, if present
  - Intravenous aminophilline, at a loading dose of 3–6 mg/kg in 250–400 ml of fluid over 15–30 min; then constant infusion of 0.4–0.9 mg/kg hr by infusion pump

THERAPY

The therapy for anaphylactoid reactions is the same as that described for anaphylaxis in Chapter 10. An outline of a suggested approach can be seen in Table 11-3.

It should be emphasized that, by the nature of the disease, therapy for ARs *must* be immediate. The therapeutic mainstays include *epinephrine,* to counteract peripheral histamine effect, *antihistamines* for ongoing histamine release, and *steroids,* to suppress the occurrence of late events. Supportive measures, including central line, intubation or tracheostomy, bronchodilators, and pressor agents may be necessary.

FOLLOW-UP AND PROGRESS

Patients with a previous history of a reaction should wear "Medic Alert" necklaces or bracelets and should be educated regarding the use of self-administered epinephrine. Commercial epinephrine kits include the Anakit and the Epipen.

Case History

A 59-year-old white male was admitted to the hospital for evaluation of nocturia and hesitancy. His past history was remarkable for degenerative joint disease. His only medication was aspirin as needed for knee pain. He had no history of drug or inhalant allergies. A physical examination revealed a uniformly enlarged prostate without nodules. The patient was scheduled for a cystoscopy and intravenous pyelogram (IVP). Within seconds of receiving radiographic contrast medium, he complained of generalized warmth and peripheral tingling. His skin began to itch, and diffuse hives developed. His eyes were tearing, he sneezed repeatedly, and he complained of throat thickening. The patient began to cough, and then (approximately 2 minutes after receiving contrast) his speech became slurred and he lost consciousness. His blood pressure was 60 palpable, and his pulse 150.

Therapy for this anaphylactoid reaction was begun immediately. Subcutaneous epinephrine, 0.3 ml of 1 : 1000 dilution and IM Benadryl 50 mg were administered at the onset of pruritus. With the development of laryngeal edema, airway patency was secured by an endotracheal tube. The existing IV line with normal saline was opened wide, but still blood pressure remained palpable only. A second central line was started, and a solution containing Levophed was begun, titrating it to a systolic pressure of 100. Aminophylline at a loading dose of 5.6 mg/kg over 20 minutes was administered for bronchospasm, after which a maintenance dose of 0.6 mg/kg hr^{-1} was given by continuous infusion. A gram of hydrocortisone was also administered intravenously. Supportive therapy was continued for 2.5 hours, until the patient's vital signs stabilized. He was uneventfully extubated. An electrocardiogram during the hypotensive period that demonstrated diffuse T-wave inversions reverted to normal with resolution of the hypotension. Follow-up sequential myocardial enzymes were negative. The patient's speech and state of consciousness returned entirely to normal.

There are several points that should be made regarding this episode and other anaphylactoid events: (a) there is no dependable predictor of who might develop anaphylactoid reactions to agents such as radiographic contrast; (b) medical personnel and equipment necessary for emergency care must be on standby for any radiographic contrast procedure; (c) corticosteroids are administered early during an anaphylactic or anaphylactoid reaction, not for acute therapy, but to prevent prolonged or late reactions; (d) although most fatalities occur within the first 30 minutes of an acute reaction, patients may require supportive care for hours to days after the reaction; and (e) sequellae of hypotension to be considered and looked for after anaphylactoid reactions include myocardial infarction, renal failure, shock liver, shock lung, and stroke.

REFERENCES

Austen, K. F. *New Engl. J. Med.*, 1974, *291*, 661–664.
Collins, J. A. *Vox Sag*, 1979, *36*, 39–49.
Fisher, M. *Anesth. Intens. Care*, 1975, *3*, 180–197.
Greenberger, P. A., Patterson, R., Simon, R., Lieberman, P., & Wallace, W. *J. Allergy Clin. Immunol.*, 1981, *67*, 185–186.
Kazimierczak, W., & Bertil, D. *Progr. Allergy*, 1978, *24*, 295–365.
Littenberg, R. L. *J. Nucl. Med.*, 1975, *16*, 236–237.
Patterson, R., & Schatz, M. *J. Allergy Clin. Immunol.*, 1975, *56*, 152–159.
Pineda, A. A., & Taswell, H. F. *Transfusion*, 1975, *15*, 10–15.
Ring, J. & Messmer, K. *Lancet*, 1977, *1*, 466–469.
Ring, J., Stephan, W., & Brendel, W. *J. Allergy*, 1979, *9*, 89–97.
Samter, M., & Beers, R. F., Jr. *J. Allergy*, 1967, *40;* 281–293.
Sheffer, A. L. & Austen, K. F. *J. Allergy Clin. Immunol.*, 1980, *66*, 106–111.
Vyas, G. N., Perkins, H. A., Fudenberg, H. H. *Lancet*, 1968, *2;* 312–315.
Weiss, R. B., & Bruno, S. *Ann. Int. Med.*, 1981, *94*, 66–72.

SUGGESTED READINGS

Harnett, J. C., Spector, S. L., & Farr, R. S. In *Allergy: Principles and practice*. E. Middleton, E. Ellis, & C. Reed (Eds.), St. Louis: Mosby, 1978, pp. 1002–1022.
Lakin, J. D., Blocker, J. J., Strong, D. M., & Yoam, M. W. *J. Allergy Clin. Immunol.*, 1978, *61*, 102–107.

QUESTIONS

1. A patient enters the emergency room with diffuse hives, throat thickening, and mild bronchospasm 1 hour after ingestion of a cephalosporin tablet and an empirin with codeine. The drug that should be administered first to treat this anaphylactic or anaphylactoid reaction is:
   a. Diphenhydramine
   b. Steroids
   c. Epinephrine
   d. Aminophylline
   e. Levophed
2. A 69-year-old male with diabetes mellitus controlled by diet and insulin loses consciousness while shopping in a grocery store. A witness describes that he became acutely short of breath, agitated, and sweaty prior to losing consciousness. The only pertinent past medical history is that of a previous heart attack 4 years ago, degenerative joint disease, and a long history of aspirin sensitivity. His medications include digoxin, hydrochlorthiazide, potassium, and insulin. He also takes occasional over-the-counter remedies for the knee pain from his degenerative joint disease. He allegedly took a new over-the-counter remedy just prior to shopping. The most likely diagnosis for his acute event is:

a. Uncomplicated insulin reaction
b. Vasovagal reaction
c. Cardiopulmonary event such as myocardial infarction, pulmonary embolus, or arrhythmia.
d. Anaphylactoid reaction to over-the-counter medicine or other unknown agent.
e. Either c or d.

3. Which of the following can distinguish anaphylactic from anaphylactoid reactions?

   a. Prausnitz-Kustner transfer testing
   b. Radioallergosorbent (RAST) testing
   c. Provocative challenge testing
   d. a, b, and c
   e. a and b

4. A 31-year-old stewardess was admitted to the hospital for evaluation of recurrent renal stones. As part of her workup, an IVP was ordered. Before injecting contrast, the radiologist asked her if she had had any previous untoward reaction to radiographic contrast. She reported a mild pruritus and two hives with a previous IVP. She described it as "transient and insignificant," requiring no therapy. With this information, the appropriate course taken by the radiologist should be:

   a. Proceed with the study. Her previous reaction was insignificant, and repeat reactions in such cases are never more severe than the initial episode.
   b. Cancel the IVP. Then consult with her primary physician regarding the necessity of the study. Only if the study is vital to her workup should he proceed with the steroid and diphenhydramine premedication protocol. During the IVP, medications and personnel to treat a possible anaphylactoid reaction should be present.
   c. Cancel the IVP and reschedule after premedication by steroid and diphenhydramine protocol. Consultation with her primary physician and reconsideration of the necessity of the study is unnecessary since the prophylaxis protocol prevents untoward reactions.
   d. Cancel the IVP. Even if the study is vital to her workup, it cannot be done in light of her history of previous reaction.
   e. Cancel the IVP. Place varying concentrations of skin test reagent to radiographic contrast material on patient. If the skin tests are negative, the radiologist may safely proceed with the study.

5. In the event blood transfusion is required in a patient with IgA deficiency, blood may be received by all but *which one* of the following ways?

   a. Washed red cells
   b. Autotransfusion
   c. IgA-deficient blood
   d. Packed red cells

Answers can be found in Appendix B at the end of the book.

PART 4

Treatment of Allergic Diseases

Anthony Kulczycki, Jr.

12

Environmental Control

Avoidance of the antigen responsible for allergic disease is the treatment of choice. In some cases the offending antigen can be removed from a patient's environment and the disease is cured. If the responsible antigens cannot be *completely* avoided then minimizing exposure to them is still important and useful in treating allergic problems.

The majority of asthmatic patients have allergens implicated in the causation of their disease (reviewed by Kulczycki, 1981). It is essential that the physician accurately identify by history and laboratory evaluation (usually skin testing) which antigens are significant in the etiology of the patient's allergic problem (see Chapters 4 & 5). He must ask when (seasons, days of week, hours of day) and where (parts of country, home or place of work, room) allergic symptoms occur. He must determine which environmental factors initiate symptoms (dusting, cutting grass, playing with pet, going into damp moldy areas, sleeping on feather pillow) and which factors relieve symptoms (leaving job, entering air-conditioned building). The physician must have a thorough knowledge and understanding of the patient's environmental history in order to effectively counsel the patient.

Every allergic patient should have recorded in a separate section a history entitled "Environmental History." The physician must include (see Table 12-1) where the patient lives, the type of heating and air conditioning (if any), whether pets or other animals are in the home, whether cockroaches are present, and whether smokers are in the home. The physician must also record whether feather antigens are present and if conditions are favorable for the growth of mites and molds (humidity, temperature, and substrate) and the accumulation of antigens (rugs, etc.). Are dehumidifiers or humidifiers, air cleaners, or electrostatic precipitators used? How often is the furnace filter changed? How and how often is housecleaning done? Are there any leaks in basement, pipes, or roof? Are fabric softeners used in the dryer? Also, the patient's past responses to environmental changes must be evaluated and recorded.

ALLERGY: THEORY AND PRACTICE
ISBN 0-8089-1619-X

Table 12-1 *Environmental History*

Home
- Location: urban, suburb, rural
- Rented or owned
- Age of home; length of time in home
- Surroundings: drainage, trees, plants

Construction
- Frame, brick, other
- Number of floors, rooms
- Basement: finished, unfinished, none
- Crawl space

Heating and cooling
- Forced-air heat, radiator, electric baseboard; thermostat setting, start of heating season
- Filter system: fiberglass, permanent, electrostatic, HEPA, none, and frequency of changing and cleaning
- Cooling: central air, window units, swamp cooler, fan use

Pets
- Type, age, sex, fertility, degree of family attachment
- Location: outdoor only, patient's bedroom
- Unwanted animals (rats, mice, roaches)

Feathers
- Pillows, dusters, down jackets, sleeping bags, and birds

House dust and mite antigen
- Use of air-conditioning and dehumidification in summer
- Age and encasement of mattresses, box springs, and pillows
- Upholstery: leather, vinyl, cloth
- Housecleaning: carried out by person other than patient or by patient (? with mask), frequency
- Type of vacuum: canister, upright, water-filtered
- Techniques: damp dusting, damp mopping, dry mopping

Mold and moisture
- Leaks: basement walls, sewer, pipes, roof, none
- Condensation, mildew: basement, pipes, windows, walls, bathrooms, none
- Dehumidifier: basement, none; cleaning frequency
- Humidifier: furnace, cold or hot mist; frequency of use and cleaning

Clothes dryer
- Type of fabric softener: quarternary ammonium compound for dryer, liquid for washer
- Dryer location and venting

Wool
- Does all wool cause itching? (If so, what wool items are used, blankets, rugs, clothes?)

Patient's bedroom
- Location, size, number of occupants, pieces of furniture
- Flooring: wood, tile, linoleum; wall-to-wall carpet, area or throw rug
- Rug: wool, cotton, synthetic
- Pad: felt, rubber, synthetic
- Windows: shades, blinds, drapes, curtains
- Heating vent: near bed, across room
- Beds: mattress—innerspring, foam, covered, enclosed; springs—box, coil, covered, enclosed
- Blankets and spread: synthetic, wool, cotton
- Pillows: Dacron, polyester, foam, feather
- Pieces of furniture, shelves, books, toys, plants, boxes, clutter

Other rooms
  Floors, rugs, pads, furniture composition, plants, pillow composition
Smoking
  By whom: patient, parent, other
  Location and amount of smoking
Irritants encountered
  Smog, hair spray, other aerosolized sprays, fumes, smoke, paint

---

The physician, having assessed the patient's allergic problem and environmental history, should initiate appropriate measures for environmental control. If the patient is allergic to multiple allergens, the physician should use reasonable judgment in providing practical choices for the initial environmental control measures and in describing potential benefits realistically. Sometimes patients need to see for themselves whether relatively simple measures (e.g., discarding feather pillows, fabric softeners and old rugs; wearing masks during housecleaning) are effective before they invest in more expensive measures (central air conditioning, air filtration systems). Patients may be more receptive to extermination of vermin (cockroaches, mice) than to elimination of pets or habits (smoking). The physician must evaluate in the follow-up whether (and which) environmental control measures were undertaken and their efficacy just as he asks whether drugs were taken properly and whether they were effective. Of course, initial environmental control measures of limited scope often will be insufficient to significantly lower antigen exposure, and additional measures will be required. Patients must be educated about potential antigens in their environment and must be alerted to and reminded of possible environmental effects on their symptoms. In many cases, patient education can prevent acquisition of new sources of antigens in the home.

HOUSE DUST

The most common antigen implicated as a cause of asthma* is house dust, and the bulk of the antigen in house dust is derived from fecal pellets of house mites of the *Dermatophagoides* species (Tovey et al., 1981). *Dermatophagoides*, "skin-eaters," thrive on shed epidermal cells (i.e., dander, dandruff) of humans or animals. They require warmth (at least 27°C) and humidity for growth (a relative humidity of 80% is ideal for mites) (Murray & Zuk, 1979). Mites die if relative humidity is under 50%. Mattresses, pillows, and stuffed furniture have the highest mite populations in homes. The extent of environmental control recommended should be proportional to the severity of allergic disease.

Mite Populations

The primary concern for dust-allergic patients should be to minimize the mite populations in their homes, particularly in their bedrooms. In most parts of the United States it is quite helpful to reduce the indoor temperature and humidity

---

*It is suggested that much of "intrinsic" asthmatic may be secondary to mite and mold antigens, which may be clinically significant because of their high concentrations in spite of relatively low specific IgE antibody concentrations (Kulczycki, 1981).

during the summer by air conditioning (especially central air conditioning) and dehumidification (especially in basements). One should urge the patient to reduce the dander (human as well as animal dander) available to mites: (a) by not having pets,† (b) by encasing mattresses and box springs completely in plastic or allergenproof material, (c) by replacing pillows with Dacron (or other polyester) pillows, which are encased in "allergenproof" material and/or are washed regularly and dried thoroughly, (d) by using vinyl or leather couches and chairs, and (e) by thorough housecleaning, as discussed below. (Plastic enclosures to completely encase mattresses and box springs are often available at department stores, but usually for only standard-sized beds.)‡

It should not be surprising that pediatricians repeatedly make the clinical observation that asthma often starts when a child is transferred from the crib with its plastic encased mattress to a bed with an old unprotected mattress and an old pillow. If patients are unwilling or unable to properly encase bedding material, the physician should insist on weekly vacuuming of the mattress and a suitable mattress cover. Obviously, food should be eaten only in dining areas to minimize dispersal of food remnants that nourish house mites.

Fecal Particles

The dust-sensitive patient should not be exposed to dispersal of the antigenic mite fecal particles. Proper housecleaning is essential to the management of dust allergy not only because it removes much of the substrate for mite growth (dander, food remnants, etc.), but also because it removes much of the house mite's antigenic fecal particles that would otherwise be dispersed later. Often the crux of the problem with housecleaning is that the dust-sensitive patient, who is often the individual best educated and motivated regarding housecleaning procedures, should *not* be exposed to the antigenic mite fecal particles during dusting and vacuuming.

The ideal solution particularly for dust-sensitive patients is to have housecleaning carried out, at least once a week, and *only* when the patient is out of the home. The patient should not return until 1 hour after cleaning has been completed. If this is possible, the patient does not need a mask and the housecleaner(s) need not be concerned as much about antigen dispersal as about thorough cleaning. For example, if multiple nonwashable rugs are unavoidable, it would be wise to recommend a good quality vacuum cleaner with a "rug-beating" attachment.

The less desirable alternative is to have the patient involved in housecleaning. For this alternative the patient must use a mask when cleaning. (Masks, such as 3M pollen masks, are often available at pharmacies and masks can be ordered from Allergen-Proof Encasings, Inc.) After cleaning, the patient must leave areas, particularly bedrooms, where dust has been dispersed. Housecleaning done by the patient

---

†It is important that dust-allergic asthmatics *not* have indoor pets, even if the asthmatics are not allergic to the pets. Animal dander can only increase the amount of mite antigen present. If pets cannot be avoided, they must be banned from the patient's bedroom and bathed frequently (see section on animal dander).

‡Alternative enclosures can be ordered from Allergen-Proof Encasings, Inc., 1450 East 363rd St., Eastlake, Ohio 44094.

should minimize dispersal of mite antigens. Dusting should be carried out with gentle containing motions using a damp cloth (water-dampened cloths are suitable for painted surfaces) or silicone-type pick-ups (e.g., Endust). Damp mopping of floors is preferable to using dust mops or brooms. Dust should be removed from bedspreads, throw rugs, pillows, and cushions out of doors. Since mite antigens are widely dispersed during vacuuming, the amount of vacuuming done by the patient should be kept to a minimum (i.e., by using washable cotton throw rugs instead of wall-to-wall carpeting) or the patient should use a vacuum cleaner that blows exhaust through water (i.e., Rainbow cleaner). (Before recommending the latter option one must consider whether the expense and weight of the vacuum are appropriate for the patient.)

Other Dispersals of Antigenic Mite Fecal Particles

The dust-sensitive patient must consider other dispersals of antigenic mite fecal particles and means of minimizing them. Constant air circulation by forced-air heat is particularly inadvisable for dust-sensitive patients; in fact, many asthmatics report annual exacerbations at the onset of the heating season. This is probably due to the shower of antigenic mite fecal particles and mold spores that had accumulated in the heating ducts. One should point out to patients that radiator heat and electric baseboard heat are preferable to forced air heat. If dust-allergic patients must live with forced air heat, they should stay away from the home the first heating day of the winter and filter the circulating air as much as is feasible. An electrostatic air cleaner for the entire home (Honeywell, Emerson Electric, Carrier, etc.) is particularly useful if the patient's problems are worse during the heating season or if the same air circulation system is used for heating and cooling. Patients unable to purchase electrostatic filters installed (current cost approximately $600–$800) must be counseled to replace their less efficient fiberglass filters regularly (at least monthly during periods of use). Shutting vents or placing muslin cloth over vents to the patient's bedroom (which may necessitate multiple nonallergenic blankets or an electric blanket) may be of some benefit if electrostatic filters cannot be obtained.

High-efficiency particulate air (HEPA) filters can be used as an alternative to electrostatic filters. The HEPA filtration units are now available both for central installation and for individual rooms.§ The expenses of central installation and periodic filter replacement and the very high blower pressure required are to be taken into account if a central unit is considered. The individual HEPA portable units (Cleanaire, ATI; Space-Gard, Research Products Corp.) are best used in bedrooms with doors shut (current cost approximately $250). Individual room units are often available for rental. Portable unit filters may become clogged in particularly dusty homes, and it may be wise to use them in conjunction with an electrostatic filter system for the entire home. The more effective the filter system is the less difficult (and antigenic) the housecleaning will be.

---

§Air Techniques, Inc., 1717 Whitehead Rd., Baltimore, MD 21207 or Research Products Corp., Madison, WI 53701.

Control of Dust

Regardless of the measures above, it is still necessary to minimize the "dust-catchers and dustbins" of a home. Otherwise, patients may still be exposed to localized accumulations of house mite antigen, certain filter systems may become overloaded, the housecleaning tasks may be insurmountable, and so on. Elimination of clutter and inappropriate storage (boxes of useless items) is important. The use of encasing pillows, mattresses, and box springs was stressed above. Similarly, upholstered furniture should be discouraged. Bare wood, tile, or linoleum floors are to be encouraged. Stuffed animal toys, animal skins, and hides must be eliminated. Shag rugs, wall-to-wall carpets, fuzzy blankets, and heavy drapery should be eliminated as much as possible in favor of washable synthetic area rugs, washable synthetic or cotton blankets, and light washable curtains. (Shag and long pile rugs are less desirable than short pile rugs.)

Special attention is directed toward the patient's bedroom. In fact, the bedroom should have simple easy to clean surfaces without dust-catching items, that is, no shelves, pennants, pictures, mirrors, and toys. Necessary items are to be kept in closed drawers. Bookcases should have enclosed shelves. Only clothing in current use should be kept in bedroom closet and the closet door must be kept closed. Venetian blinds should be replaced by window shades.

POLLENS

The principal allergens involved in allergic rhinitis throughout much of the United States are derived from pollen grains. The physician must assess the severity of the patient's problem, the length of the pollen season(s), and often the patient's tolerance for medication and general life-style before attempting drastic modifications of the patient's environment. However, pollen-allergic patients should be acquainted with the pollens to which they are particularly sensitive and with local pollination seasons. Patients should learn that moderate rainfall will clear the outside air of pollen and that indoor pollen counts are minimal (unless windows are open or air conditioners are set to bring in "fresh air"). They should also be aware that highest pollen counts are present in the early morning (at least near pollination sources).

Since tree pollens are the heaviest of the allergenic pollens they travel relatively short distances. Thus urban areas with relatively few trees have less tree pollen. For long-range planning, patients allergic to elm pollen, for example, should not move into a neighborhood full of elm trees nor plant them. For short-range planning, camping or picnicking in the woods may not be particularly appropriate during the middle of the tree-pollination season. It may be wise to encourage extremely sensitive individuals (particularly those with short seasons of involvement) to tend to remain indoors with windows closed and to go outdoors mainly during or after rainfalls or with masks. Air filtration systems that work only with the heating or air-conditioning system turned on will be ineffective for tree allergic individuals since tree pollination normally occurs when such systems would be idle. However, most filtration systems are operational with only the blower fan.

Grass and weed pollens are relatively light and travel great distances. The particular location of the sensitive patient may not be as important as for tree-sensitive individuals. Extremely sensitive individuals should consider weather conditions because warm sunny days favor pollen dissemination, whereas cool cloudy days do not. Cutting and raking grass are not recommended, especially for grass-allergic individuals. (Many grass-allergic patients will experience pruritus on prolonged contact with grass when sitting or lying on lawns.) The 24-hour ragweed count outdoors is about 3 times higher than the pollen count inside with windows open. Indoor pollen is practically zero in centrally air-conditioned homes. In many parts of the United States grass and weed pollination occurs during the air-conditioning season; thus patients with moderate to severe problems should be encouraged to install central air-conditioning systems. The cost of installing central air conditioning minus the increase in the value of the home is considered as a legitimate medical expense for tax purposes depending on the severity of the patient's problems and the documentation (e.g., skin testing) by the physician as to its necessity.

A minority of patients may be able to avoid pollen entirely by vacationing on islands or on ocean cruises or in areas with lower pollen counts (not tax-deductible expenses). Most ragweed species are not present west of the Rocky Mountains; however, grass pollination is perennial in much of California. Most patients will not be able to escape the pollination seasons, in fact, some may work outdoors. Nevertheless, some environmental control can still be exercised at home and in transportation (car windows should be up when driving).

Ragweed-sensitive individuals should avoid pyrethrum in the environment. Pyrethrum is a powder derived from a plant botanically related to ragweed that is often found in insecticides. Honey often contains ragweed pollen and may cause allergic symptoms.

MOLD SPORES

Inhalation of airborne mold spores is known to cause both asthma and allergic rhinitis. Although an enormous number of species of fungi exists and fungal spore concentrations are in vast excess of pollen concentrations, our understanding of mold-induced allergic respiratory disease is limited (Salvaggio & Aukrust, 1981). In many parts of the United States mold spore concentrations may peak after the initial spring warming, persist throughout summer, and peak again during the fall. Mold-sensitive patients thus rarely have a brief well-defined seasonal allergy, and symptoms often may span much of the year or may be perennial. Patients experiencing amelioration of respiratory symptoms after the first winter snowfall are often found to be allergic to outdoor fungal spores. (This pattern is distinct from ragweed allergy since ragweed pollination ceases with the first frost.) Spores of some fungi are dispersed during damp or even rainy weather; alternatively, other fungal spores are blown into the atmosphere when humidity is low and wind speed high. Thus different mold-allergic patients may note that differing weather conditions exacerbate their symptoms.

Obviously, one aspect of environmental control for mold-sensitive patients is to stay indoors during periods when the concentrations of the outdoor mold spores (to which they are allergic) are high. Some patients may learn which weather pattern aggravates symptoms and, for example, will minimize their errands outdoors "when the weather changes" just before a rainfall. Mold-allergic individuals should neither cut grass nor rake leaves. Other aspects of outdoor environmental control are to have well-drained property; to eliminate vines and shrubs growing directly against the walls; to have dead leaves removed; and to avoid compost heaps, mulch, and barns.

Fungi can also propagate indoors, particularly in damp and dark areas, and may initiate perennial symptoms. The prime sites for domestic mold growth include damp basements, crawl spaces, shower curtains and stalls, bathrooms, window moldings, portable air-conditioning units, irregularly cleaned or improperly functioning dehumidifiers and humidifiers, vaporizers, refrigerator drip trays, and garbage containers. Mold growth can be curtailed by reducing basement moisture (sealing walls, repairing sewers, installing basement dehumidifiers) and repairing leaks in roof, pipes, etc. If crawl spaces contain water, drains should be installed; if damp, the ground should be covered with sturdy polyethylene sheets to provide a vapor lock, preventing moisture and mold access to the home. Mold growth may be substantial on walls, floors, and items in bathrooms because of moisture. Moldy areas must be cleaned regularly (e.g., with Lysol or Clorox solutions) and kept dry. Moldy shower curtains and wallpaper should be discarded. Vaporizers should be properly cleaned with soap and water daily; humidifiers, dehumidifiers, and air conditioners must be checked for mold growth and cleaned. Flow humidifiers (e.g., Aprilaire) do not have reservoirs and avoid problems with fungal growth. Vaporizer or humidifier use (restricted to only dry winter months) is deemed excessive if room walls, rugs, bedding, or other objects become damp. It is also important not to soak carpeting and carpet pads during do-it-yourself cleaning because prolonged dampness may foster mold growth. Clothes should be dried promptly. Dead leaves of house plants should not accumulate in pots to provide decaying substrate for fungi. Patients with severe mold allergy should have no plants (or only desert plants). Although fruit stored in basements may also be a substrate for mold growth, the more common problem is that nonessential mold-prone items are stored in most basements.

It is important to realize that pillows (especially foam), mattresses, and box springs can harbor mold growth as well as mite growth. This makes Dacron polyester pillows and encasement of bedding material especially important.

Apart from reducing the substrate (and humidity) to slow fungal growth, mold retardants could be considered. Roccal, Zephiran, and paraformaldehyde are among the useful fungicides. Removal of mold spores by electrostatic or HEPA air cleaners (discussed above) is also a useful environmental control measure. Quantitation of outdoor mold spores (Salvaggio & Aukrust, 1981) and indoor fungal spores (Kozak et al., 1980) may be difficult and time-consuming. Exposure of multiple culture plates of Sabouraud's agar throughout a patient's home is admittedly not a very quantitative procedure. Nevertheless, it dramatically alerts patients to the areas of greatest mold growth and has a certain impact which is lacking in discussions about microscopic mold spores. It thus often stimulates appropriate environmental control measures by patients and their families.

Occasionally patients with mold allergy will notice that mold-containing foods may exacerbate respiratory symptoms. Such patients should limit their consumption of beer, wine (especially red wine), canned tomatoes, aged cheeses, and mushrooms especially during periods when outdoor mold spore concentrations are high.

FEATHERS

Feathers are so commonly involved in causing allergic asthma and rhinitis that the initial advice often given to patients with allergic respiratory symptoms by internists and pediatricians is to discard their feather pillows. This is usually sound advice because old feather pillows may contain abundant house mite antigen in addition to feather and mold antigen. Such patients often have exacerbations of symptoms during sleep or on waking.

It is important that allergic individuals replace all pillows in the home with Dacron or other polyester pillows. The new pillows should be encased in an allergenproof material (to prevent dander from getting in) and/or should be washed regularly and dried thoroughly (to remove any accumulated substrates and antigens). (Few individuals enjoy airtight enclosures on pillows, and "featherproof" ticking is a totally ineffective barrier to the feather and mite antigens. Foam pillows may support mold growth.)

Feather-sensitive individuals must remove other sources of feather antigen from their homes. Feather beds, comforters, and dusters, down jackets and sleeping bags, and birds are often overlooked as sources of feather antigen.

The physician should also be careful that hospitalized asthmatic patients are not given feather pillows.

ANIMAL DANDER

Animal dander presents two separate problems to the physician caring for the allergic patient: the patient may be allergic to the dander (or secretions) of the pet, and/or the patient may be allergic to house dust, and the animal dander provides a rich substrate for the growth of mites that exacerbates the dust allergy.

In dealing with animal-sensitive and dust-sensitive patients the clinician usually encounters common pets. As a basis for communicating with patients, it is sometimes helpful for the physician to record details such as the age, sex, and fertility of pets as well as whether the pets are kept indoors and how attached family members are to the pets.

In cases with allergic asthma or rhinitis with (a) at least moderate severity and (b) evidence of IgE antibody to an appropriate dander *or* to house dust antigen, one usually recommends that families find another home for their pet. If this advice is given in a tactful, understanding manner, some families and children will accept and follow it. In some cases a trial separation from the pet is warranted. After a cat or dog has been removed from the home it is important to thoroughly clean the home of animal dander. One should remember that cat antigens may remain in the home for some time, even after extensive cleaning. One must anticipate that many families will be unwilling or unable to follow such advice and one should provide some alternatives: (a) agree that new pets (including pet offspring) will not be acquired, (b) keep pet(s) out of patient's bedroom and as far from the bedroom as possible (preferably out of doors), and (c) bathe animals regularly (this is practical with dogs, but not cats). Obviously, animals should be groomed out of the home and not by the allergic patient. Saliva of animals can also be antigenic, causing localized urticaria after contact.

Cats can be a problem because of their longevity and their aversion to water. One should also point out to cat owners that feline urinary proteins can be highly allergenic. Therefore, litter boxes should be cleaned frequently* and should not be near vents or areas regularly used by the patient.

The physician must also inquire about other pets such as rabbits, gerbils, and hamsters as well as horses and farm animals and must consider whether patients are exposed to rats or mice in basements or squirrels (or bats) in attics and air vents. A large proportion of urban asthma appears to result from exposure to rodent antigens. Veterinarians and some laboratory workers receive prolonged exposures to numerous epidermal antigens and a significant proportion (approximately 32% of exposed laboratory workers) may acquire job-related animal allergy (Schumacker et al., 1981).

Nonliving sources of animal dander antigen must also be considered. Furs, hides, and stuffed animals may have significant allergenic activity depending on their size and the tanning procedures used. Horse hair, cow hair, and hog hair may be found in furniture or rug pads and can produce allergic symptoms.

COCKROACHES

Cockroach antigen appears to be a major cause of asthma in exposed individuals. In a Chicago study 58% of 106 adult asthmatics and 69% of 48 asthmatic children had IgE antibodies to cockroach and presumably had asthmatic symptoms because of roaches (Kang & Sulit, 1978). In a Boston study 41% of 200 children with asthma and/or rhinitis had cockroach exposure, indicating the prevalence of home infestation for allergic individuals in an urban area (Twarog et al., 1977). Symptoms may be perennial or may be exacerbated during the heating season. It is not yet known whether the antigen is derived from the exoskeletons discarded by growing roaches or from roach excrement.

Since cockroaches are seldom seen during daylight hours infestations may be underestimated or even undetected. Roaches may enter homes through cracks in walls or doorways and through sewer systems. Sealing cracks and keeping water traps intact in the sewer system will minimize roach immigration. Cockroaches are often found in the food-producing industry warehouses and eggs may enter homes when cases, cartons, and boxes are brought indoors. Roaches have an affinity for kitchens (because of food particles), basements, and bathrooms (because of moisture).

Allergic individuals with history and skin tests consistent with cockroach allergy should have roaches eradicated (organophosphates and carbamates are most commonly used). Eradication requires at least two applications of chemicals (preferably by an exterminator) because eggs are not affected by the first application of chemicals. The second visit should be timed to eliminate the newly hatched roaches before they become fertile. After eradication, roach debris should be removed to avoid increasing the antigenic load.

---

*Cat-allergic patients should not clean litter boxes. Pregnant women should also avoid cat litter (because of the potential for toxoplasmosis).

WOOL

It is difficult to assess the importance of wool as an antigen in allergic individuals. Patients who do not itch wearing wool next to their skin need no environmental control measures regardless of skin test results. Patients who itch when wearing wool next to their skin may either have an irritation due to coarse wool fibers or may have wool allergy. If patients itch with all types of woolens and are skin-test-positive, they usually require environmental control. Such individuals may dismiss the problem by stating that they always have other clothes between their skin and their sweaters and coats (or sheets between themselves and woolen blankets). It is often necessary to point out that woolen particles from clothes and blankets can act as inhalant antigens. Woolen blankets should be replaced with cotton or electric ones. Woolen clothes, if not replaced, should be stored in plastic garment bags when not in use.

KAPOK

Kapok is the fibrous material derived from seed pods of the kapok tree. It is used in cushions for boats and pools and in sleeping bags because it is buoyant and impervious to water. Kapok can also be found in mattresses, furniture, and toys and can be allergenic.

FABRIC SOFTENERS

Sensitivity to the product "Bounce" has been described both in asthmatic patients and in previously normal individuals (Mauceri & Rosan, 1976; Oster, 1976). Reactions to Bounce, "Cling-Free," and other quarternary ammonium compound fabric softeners can be quite severe. Although the incidence of fabric softener-induced asthma is not known, it seems wise to instruct all allergic individuals to refrain from using Bounce or similar *cloth* fabric softeners designed for use in a dryer. The use of liquid fabric softeners in washing machines appears to be a safe alternative.

ACTIVE AND PASSIVE CIGARETTE SMOKING

Cigarette and other tobacco smoke appear to be irritants more often than allergens. Asthmatics have been warned for many years against active smoking. However, the effect of passive smoking on allergic diseases may have been badly underestimated. A study in East Boston (Weiss et al., 1980) revealed that 30 of 31 children with persistent wheezing were from households with at least one parent currently smoking. Deaths from asthma in nonsmoking women appeared to correlate with their husbands' smoking habits (Hirayama, 1981).

It seems reasonable to urge patients with allergic respiratory diseases *and* their families not to smoke. Family members who are unable to break smoking habits should not smoke in patient's presence, should minimize their smoking in the home and car, and should keep ashtrays clean. Electronic air filtration is also quite helpful in reducing passive smoking. In many cases it may be wise to have patients avoid public places that have concentrations of smokers without effective air cleaning.

POLLUTANTS AND METABISULFITES

Even mild asthmatics may have asthmatic attacks after inhalation of sulfur dioxide concentrations (1, 3, and 5 ppm) well below the federal limit for occupational exposure (Sheppard et al., 1980). Sulfur dioxide and other oxides of sulfur are produced mainly by combustion of bituminous coal.

Of course, such patients should not work in environments with high SO_2 concentrations. Asthmatics should be advised not to move to highly polluted locations (major highway intersections, industrial areas) and to remain indoors when media report "poor air quality" or smog alerts.

Certain patients with sensitivity to sulfur dioxide will have acute asthmatic attacks after ingestion of metabisulfites (Stevenson & Simon, 1981). Such patients should be identified and counseled to avoid foods containing metabisulfites. Metabisulfites are antioxidants commonly used in food processing as (a) sanitizing agents, (b) preservatives, and (c) antioxidants and inhibitors of discoloration of foods. Wine bottles or their corks, for example, are commonly exposed to metabisulfite solutions. Restaurant foods such as salads, fruit, vegetable dishes and dips (particularly potatoes and avocado dip), and shellfish may contain up to 100 mg of metabisulfite.

OTHER ENVIRONMENTAL FACTORS

Numerous substances have been identified that cause allergic reactions, nonallergic immunologic reactions, or irritation due to occupational exposure. Occupational asthma is reviewed in Chapter 22. One should consider that substances can be transported into a home from the work environment (e.g., on clothes) and cause symptoms in family members.

Patients with food allergy may have respiratory symptoms when exposed to dispersal of heat-stable food antigens during cooking (e.g., fish). Additives to foods can initiate asthma attacks either immediately after ingestion (e.g., tartrazine, metabisulfites) or many hours later (e.g., monosodium glutamate). Food allergy and adverse food reactions are detailed in Chapter 26.

Noxious irritants should also be eliminated from the environment, such as strong perfume, spray deodorant, hair spray, "air fresheners," furniture and floor waxes, cosmetics, paint, gasoline, cleaning fluid, and fumes and smoke from any source (including fumes from formaldehyde insulation).

MOVING TO NEW LOCATION

In some cases it is wise to recommend that the patient move from one dwelling to another. This is usually more feasible for renters than owners because they have more mobility and less control over their environment. A cockroach-allergic patient renting a unit in a large complex teeming with roaches, with a landlord unwilling to eradicate them, should move. Similarly, moving from an industrial zone producing air pollutants may be advisable.

However, physicians should be cautious in considering changes of *geographic* location for medical reasons. One must consider all current sensitivities (a ragweed-allergic individual will improve in California *unless* that individual is also grass-sensitive, since grass is perennial in much of California). A trial visit for a month to the new area is a good idea but does not guarantee that allergic problems will be reduced. After successful trial visits the physician must still be concerned that the patient may have seasonal problems at the new location or may eventually (2–4 years later) acquire sensitivity to new allergens in the new environment. The physician should be aware that patients may cite "allergic problems" to rationalize a move that may be unsound socially and economically. Most allergists advise against long-distance moves except in rare instances.

Case History

A 27-year-old waitress presented with wheezing; cough; shortness of breath; rhinorrhea; sneezing; nasal obstruction; maxillary sinus discomfort; and itching of her eyes, nose, and throat for 6 months. Two months prior to the onset of symptoms the patient acquired a baby Siamese cat. The patient's symptoms were worse at home, especially on her bed (the cat's favorite resting place) and when dusting. The patient stopped smoking and took antihistamines and theophylline but had little improvement in symptoms. Physical examination (in an air-conditioned clinic) revealed no wheezes. Skin testing was remarkable only for a 4+ reaction to prick test with cat epithelium extract.

Subsequently, the patient found a new home for her kitten. She cleaned her home thoroughly and took antihistamines, decongestants, and theophylline during the cleaning period. Thereafter, she became symptom-free without medication.

This illustrates a case of "cat asthma," the potency of cat antigen in the environment and in testing, and the benefit of allergen avoidance. Itching of eyes, nose, and throat is quite typical of respiratory allergy to inhalant antigens.

REFERENCES

Hirayama, T. *Br. Med. J.*, 1981, *282*, 183–185.

Kang, B., & Sulit, B. *Ann. Allergy*, 1978, *41*, 333–336.

Kozak, P. P., Gallup, J., Cummins, L. H., & Gillman, S. A. *Ann. Allergy*, 1980, *45*, 167–176.

Kulczycki, A. Jr. *J. Allergy Clin. Immunol.*, 1981, *68*, 5–14.

Mauceri, R. A., & Rosan, J. R. *New Engl. J. Med.*, 1976, *294*, 907.

Murray, A. B., & Zuk, P. *J. Allergy Clin. Immunol.*, 1979, *64*, 266–269.

Oster, M. W. *New Engl. J. Med.*, 1976, *294*, 1297.

Salvaggio, J., & Aukrust, L. J. *Allergy Clin. Immunol.*, 1981, *68*, 327–346.

Schumacher, M. J., Tait, B. D., & Holmes, M. C. *J. Allergy Clin. Immunol.*, 1981, *68*, 310–318.

Sheppard, D., Wong, W. S., Uehara, C. F., Nadel, J. A., & Boushey, H. A. *Am. Rev. Resp. Dis.*, 1980, *122*, 873–878.

Stevenson, D. D., & Simon, R. A. *J. Allergy Clin. Immunol.*, 1981, *68*, 26–32.

Tovey, E. R., Chapman, M. D., & Platts-Mills, T. A. E. *Nature* 1981, *289*, 592–593.

Twarog, F. J., Picone, F. J., Strunk, R. S., So, J., & Colten, H. R. *J. Allergy Clin. Immunol.*, 1977, *59*, 154–160.

Weiss, S. T., Tager, I. B., Speizer, F. E., & Rosner, B. *Am. Rev. Resp. Dis.*, 1980, *122*, 697–707.

SUGGESTED READINGS

Gutman, A. A. Allergens and other factors important in atopic disease. In R. Patterson (Ed.), *Allergic Diseases, Diagnosis and Management*. Philadelphia: Lippincott, 1980, pp. 100–147.

Mansmann, H. C., Jr. Environmental control. In E. Middleton, Jr., C. E. Reed, & E. F. Ellis (Eds.), *Allergy, principles and practice*. St. Louis: Mosby, 1978, pp. 957–964.

QUESTIONS

1. A 29-year-old blood bank technician has had perennial rhinitis, chronic sore throat, cough, fatigue, and nasal voice for 5 of the past 6 years. A psychiatrist believes she is suffering from depression. For the past year she has been renting an unfurnished apartment in a very old building. The apartment has unfiltered forced-air heat and window air conditioning. She has been using old furniture, rugs, and bedding obtained from her brother in this and previous apartments, including a feather pillow, soiled area rugs, and an unenclosed mattress and box spring. One year she had almost no symptoms while working in rural Nevada (without her brother's furnishings). She has no pets or plants. Her symptoms are improved at work. Physical examination reveals boggy, pale turbinates, an edematous uvula, episodic cough, nasal voice, but no wheezes. Skin tests demonstrate 4+ reactions to only house dust, house dust mite, and feather antigen. Antihistamine-decongestant combinations have given slight relief but troublesome side effects. Initially you should:

   a. Defer treatment until psychiatric therapy is completed
   b. Try different antihistamine-decongestant combinations while initiating immunotherapy
   c. Have patient discard feather pillow and rugs, enclose mattress and box spring, filter forced air (or turn down heat and use electric blanket and electric space heater), and clean regularly with a mask
   d. Culture patient's throat, and recommend house plants and humidifier to increase humidity

2. A 47-year-old salesman has an acute onset of shortness of breath and wheezing walking past his neighbor's basement window if the neighbor's clothes dryer is in use. He has similar symptoms when walking near the detergent and soap aisle in supermarkets. Several years ago he had severe wheezing when his wife tried a new fabric softener. This man has:

   a. mild asthma aggravated by irritants
   b. exercise-induced asthma
   c. sensitivity to quarternary ammonium compounds
   d. sensitivity to metabisulfites

3. A 6-year-old boy has had asthma since age 1. Despite therapeutic levels of theophylline and oral prednisone, he averages one admission monthly for asthma for the past several years. Because of prednisone his growth has slowed, dropping from 40th

percentile to 90th. He lives in an inner-city housing project. Skin tests to house dust, mold, weeds, feathers, and dog and cat epithelium are negative. No smokers are in the household. You recommend:

a. inhaled beclomethasone to decrease requirement for systemic steroid
b. skin testing with cockroach antigen, mouse and rat antigens, and appropriate control measures if positive
c. skin testing to cigarette and tobacco smoke and, if positive, appropriate control measures
d. breathing exercises and a beta$_2$-sympathomimetic drug

4. Which of the following substances can precipitate an asthma attack?

a. sodium metabisulfite
b. monosodium glutamate
c. cigarette smoke
d. cockroach antigen
e. all of the above

Answers can be found in Appendix B at the end of the book.

Scott R. Sale

13

Immunotherapy

The introduction into the body of a foreign substance that initiates immunologic events in order to reduce an allergic, IgE-mediated response is termed *immunotherapy* or *hyposensitization*. Immunotherapy (IT) was first described in 1911 by Noon and by Freeman in the same year (Freeman, 1911). They successfully treated 16 of 18 patients with grass pollen-sensitive allergic rhinitis by subcutaneously injecting extracts of grass pollen. Although these studies were not double-blind or placebo-controlled, they demonstrated the efficacy of allergen injection therapy.

EFFICACY OF IMMUNOTHERAPY

Since 1911, many studies have shown the usefulness of IT in controlling responses to inhaled antigens in persons with allergic rhinitis, asthma, or both. Adequate, controlled studies for some allergens have been difficult to achieve because of imprecise separation of symptoms due to overlapping allergic seasons, especially those for molds and ragweed, and concomitant viral infections that may mimic or exacerbate symptoms. Nevertheless, as shown in Table 13-1 and summarized in more detail by Zeiger (1981), extracts of trees, grass, ragweed, and mites, the major allergen in house dust, have been used effectively in double-blind, placebo-controlled studies to treat allergic rhinitis, whereas grass, dust, mites, animal dander and a mix of pollen, dust, and some mold extracts have been successful in lowering symptom scores in asthmatics. Although well-defined studies of trees, ragweed, and mold in asthma have not been performed, implications about the effectiveness of ragweed and mold therapy can be made from Johnstone & Dutton's study (1968), in which a mix of pollens, mold, and dust was used to treat asthmatic children. Children on higher dose treatment regimens responded better overall than those on small doses of antigen or placebo injections, especially during the ragweed and mold seasons.

Immunotherapy with cat pelt extract was shown to reduce bronchial reactivity

ALLERGY: THEORY AND PRACTICE
ISBN 0-8089-1619-X

Table 13-1 *Efficacy of Aqueous Immunotherapy*

Allergen	Allergic Rhinitis	Extrinsic Asthma	References*
Tree (mountain cedar)	Yes	NS†	Pence et al., 1976
Grass (timothy, rye, mix)	Yes	Yes	Frankland & Augustin, 1954
Ragweed (unpurified)	Yes	NS	Lichtenstein et al., 1971
Dust (unpurified)	NS	Yes	Aas, 1971; Bruun et al., 1949
Mites	Yes	Yes	Gabriel et al., 1977; Smith, 1971
Molds	NS	NS	—
Pollen, mold, dust mix	NS	Yes	Johnstone & Dutton, 1968
Animal dander	NS	Yes	Taylor et al., 1978; Wahn & Siraganian, 1980

*Double-blind, placebo-controlled studies.
†No significant data.

in 5 individuals with cat asthma (Taylor et al., 1978). Similarly, increases in IgG blocking antibody in laboratory workers with mouse, rat, and rabbit asthma correlated with an unquantitated reduction in symptoms compared to the results with placebo controls.

Other types of injections once considered to be immunotherapy have now been shown to have no proven benefit. Bacterial vaccines, once given to reduce an individual's sensitivity to colonizing and pathogenic bacteria that were thought to cause irritant asthma attacks, have no place as immunizing agents. It has been shown that viruses and mycoplasma were the precipitants of asthma attacks, and not bacteria. Injections of foods, urine, or automobile fumes are also dangerous, unproven, and unacceptable, whereas the treatment of migraine headaches, vasomotor rhinitis, urticaria, or atopic dermatitis with IT is no better than treatment with placebo.

IMMUNOLOGIC MECHANISMS OF IMMUNOTHERAPY

Although the ultimate explanation for the effectiveness of IT in allergic rhinitis or asthma is not precisely known, several immunologic events have been shown to occur in most patients receiving IT: not all mechanisms occur in all patients, but the success of IT in most cases probably could be explained by one or more of them.

1. Increased levels of blocking antibody, IgG
2. Decreased total and post seasonal rise in specific IgE
3. Decreased basophil reactivity and histamine release

4. Increased specific T suppressor activity for IgE antibody
5. Decreased lymphokine production in the presence of specific allergens
6. Increased production of secretory IgA and IgG

The first immunologic change described with IT was the markedly increased production of a specific IgG directed against the antigen injected. These antibodies were thought to prevent interaction between antigen and cell-bound IgE and are called *blocking antibodies*. Blocking antibody begins to appear in significant amounts after a treatment regimen has progressed approximately to the injection of 2500 protein nitrogen units (PNU) or 25 μg of protein (Table 13-2). (One PNU/ml is the equivalent of 1×10^{-5} mg of nitrogen precipitated by phosphotungstic acid from 1 ml of an allergenic extract.) Although IgG antibody is detectable in atopic and normal individuals before IT is initiated, the amount of additional IgG antibody produced is proportional to the amount of antigen injected. There is a limit, however, to the amount of blocking antibody produced and the maximum amount seems to correlate with a reduced risk of adverse reactions from pollen IT injections. The rate of production and maximum levels of IgG antibody may be determined by the amount of antigen given and the intervals between injections during the early weeks of immunization.

The exact function of blocking antibody is not known. It may prevent antigen from combining with IgE on mast cells and basophils, and may also combine with the antigen to form soluble immune complexes that are removed by the reticuloendothelial system and thus not deposited in tissues. It must be pointed out that the correlation between IgG levels and a decrease in allergic sensitivity is poor blocking at best, casting some doubt on the role of these antibodies.

The importance of IgE antibody levels is also not known. After adequate doses of IT the normal postseasonal rise in IgE antibody levels in allergic individuals is blunted (Levy & Osler, 1967). Total serum IgE, which initially rises for several months after immunotherapy is begun, will fall if adequate antigen doses are administered. These changes in total and specific IgE levels may take 1–2 years to occur. Like blocking antibody, however, the total IgE or specific IgE does not correlate well with symptom scores (Lichtenstein et al., 1973). Just as a perfect correlation does not exist between IgG or IgE antibody levels and symptom scores, decreases in basophil reactivity and subsequent histamine release with IT do not always occur or correlate with reduced symptoms (Lichtenstein et al., 1971).

Whereas increases in blocking antibody may account for the symptomatic improvement after IT has been initiated, changes in lymphocyte reactivity may be the key to prolonged improvement. The presence of increased specific T suppressor cells (Katz, 1978; Rocklin et al., 1980) with histamine receptors after adequate IT correlates with reduced IgE antibody production and decreased symptom scores. There is also a decrease in overall lymphocyte proliferation and lymphokine production (Evans et al., 1976; Gatien et al., 1975). These suppressor cell responses are specific for the allergen injected and presumably with multiple allergen IT, multiple IgE-specific T suppressor cells will be activated. The dose of allergen and the interval between injections may be the determinants of sustained production of suppressor cells and a decreased allergic response. Suppressor cell measurements, however, are not yet generally available to the practicing clinician.

Increased levels of specific nasal secretory IgA and IgG have been detected

Table 13-2 *Sample Schedule for Perennial Aqueous Immunotherapy*

Week	Concentration (w/v)*	Weekly Dosage (ml)	PNU	PNU (Total)	Micrograms of Protein	Total Micrograms of Protein
1	1 : 10,000	0.05	2.5	2.5	0.025	0.025
2		0.10	5.0	7.5	0.050	0.075
3		0.15	7.5	15	0.075	0.15
4		0.20	10	25	0.10	0.25
5		0.30	15	40	0.15	0.40
6		0.40	20	60	0.20	0.60
7		0.50	25	85	0.25	0.85
8	1 : 1000	0.05	25	110	0.25	1.10
9		0.10	50	160	0.50	1.60
10		0.15	75	235	0.75	2.35
11		0.20	100	335	1.00	3.35
12		0.25	125	460	1.25	4.60
13		0.30	150	610	1.50	6.10
14		0.35	175	785	1.75	7.85
15		0.40	200	985	2.00	9.85
16		0.45	225	1210	2.25	12.10
17		0.50	250	1460	2.50	14.60
18	1 : 100	0.05	250	1710	2.50	17.10
19		0.10	500	2210	5.00	22.10
20		0.15	750	2960	7.50	29.60
21		0.20	1000	3960	10.0	39.60
22		0.25	1250	5210	12.5	52.10
23		0.30	1500	6710	15.0	67.10
24		0.35	1750	8460	17.5	84.60
25		0.40	2000	10460	20.0	104.60
26		0.45	2250	12710	22.5	127.10
27	Maintenance	0.50	2500	15210	25.0	152.10

*Conversion of w/v to PNU is only an approximation and differs from antigen to antigen.

during IT while nasal secretory IgE may be diminished. Whether the IgA and IgG in respiratory and ocular secretions act as blocking antibody to bind the antigen and prevent attachment of the antigen to IgE on mast cells or impair diffusion across the mucosal barrier is unknown. No correlation can be made between symptom scores and either secretory antibody levels or changes in secretory antibody : serum antibody ratios.

In summary, although the exact mechanism and sequence of immunologic events that determine the success or failure of IT have not yet been fully delineated, IT continues to be used effectively when the proper antigens are selected and the IT is given in adequate doses.

INDICATIONS FOR IMMUNOTHERAPY

For the practicing clinician the decision to refer a patient to an allergist for IT is seldom an easy one. Before IT should be considered, the first two principles of allergy must be heeded. Avoidance of the allergen along with adequate and reasonable pharmacologic therapy must be attempted to control symptoms. If avoidance and noninjurious medications are ineffective, IT should be considered. The following groups of persons listed will be the ones with the best success rate: there are no data to show that IT will prevent persons with hay fever from developing asthma.

1. Persons with some seasonal variation in upper or lower respiratory tract symptoms and positive skin tests that confirm the history
2. Persons experiencing only one season with symptoms and in whom symptoms cannot be controlled with noninjurious medications and avoidance or result in persistent loss of sleep, work or school time, or ability to perform daily functions
4. Persons with positive skin tests who have perennial asthma or rhinitis that is refractory to conventional medications
5. Children with recurrent serous otitis media secondary to hyperplastic sinusitis and positive skin tests
6. Persons who desire a possible cure of their rhinitis or asthma

Not everyone with allergic symptoms needs IT. Many persons have only one season during which they have symptoms, in either the upper or lower respiratory tract. Usually their symptoms can be controlled with medication alone; even short courses of adequate topical or systemic corticosteroids may be given to palliate exacerbations. If the symptoms cannot be controlled with easily tolerated and noninjurious medications or result in the inability to attend school or function well at work, IT should be considered.

There are a number of individuals with perennial asthma or rhinitis whose symptoms persist despite avoidance and pharmacologic therapy. They may or may not have seasonal variations in their symptoms, but their skin tests are positive and correlate with their symptoms. Many of these persons may benefit from IT; their medication requirements might be reduced and steroids found not to be necessary.

Children with recurrent serous otitis media often have concomitant allergic rhinitis. They may develop severe nasal congestion with thickened turbinates, which is known as *hyperplastic sinusitis*. Middle-ear effusions often develop. If avoidance of known allergens (often dogs, cats, or dust) and pharmacologic therapy are not effective, and if appropriate positive skin tests are demonstrated, IT should be given a trial. Hearing losses are often reversed as a consequence.

Finally, there are those allergic individuals who wish to be cured of any symptoms that require medications for control. These individuals with only one or two seasons of IgE mediated allergic rhinitis, asthma, or both have a small chance for complete ablation of their symptoms. Although there is no way of predicting who will respond with a cure, however, most individuals appropriately given adequate IT do show significant improvement.

TYPES OF IMMUNOTHERAPY

There are three different techniques of pollen IT: perennial, preseasonal (also known as rush or cluster), and coseasonal. The well-established method is perennial IT, in which allergen injections of increasing dose and concentration are given weekly for approximately 6 months until maintenance concentrations have been reached. Maintenance doses vary among allergists, but generally about 2500 PNU per antigen per injection or its equivalent, 0.5 ml of a 1 : 100 w/v dilution, is needed. One of the keys to successful IT is that enough antigen be given to sustain an immunologic response since the maximum amount of antigen given with each injection is more important than the cumulative amount of antigen given. Table 13-2 gives one example of an allergen extract injection protocol.

Once the maintenance dose of antigen has been reached, different schedules of injections are used to reach a steady state of one injection every 4 weeks. Some allergists will gradually increase the interval between injections over a 2–3 year period; others will increase the interval more rapidly over 4–6 months. Both methods are accepted. There are a few individuals who require weekly or biweekly injections indefinitely to maintain their immunity and minimize large local or systemic reactions. Rarely does an individual have to be maintained on less than 2500 PNU per antigen because of large reactions. Immunotherapy is then stopped when there have been 1 or 2 allergic seasons with marked symptomatic improvement. If asthma is being treated with IT, injections may need to be continued longer.

In order to prepare some individuals for their allergic season rapidly, preseasonal (rush or cluster) IT is administered. Injections may be given daily over a 1-month period (Tipton & Nelson, 1982), 2–3 times per week over a 3–4-month period, or two to three injections may be given 1 day every 3 weeks (Van Metre et al., 1982), effecting a more rapid progression to maintenance concentrations. The injections may be discontinued or given less frequently at the onset of the allergic season and then continued in this manner during the nonallergic season. The procedure is repeated prior to each allergic season. Coseasonal immunization is the use of higher doses of extracts given during the allergic season with shorter intervals between injections. Both preseasonal and coseasonal methods may be associated with more local and systemic reactions than with the perennial method, although Tipton & Nelson (1982) reported no increased adverse reactions among patients given daily IT. The standard injection schedule of aqueous IT remains a gradual increase in amount and concentration of antigen attained by weekly injections.

The Rinkel technique of hyposensitization has received publicity from nonallergists since its inception (Rinkel, 1949). In a well-controlled, double-blind study by Van Metre et al. (1979), however, there was no significant difference between the results with placebo therapy and the results with Rinkel IT. Neither treatment compared favorably with standard IT, which produced a significant decrease in ragweed rhinitis symptoms, increase in blocking antibody levels, and decreases in postseasonal rises of IgE antibody. Similarly, an American Academy of Allergy–sponsored multicenter study comparing Rinkel IT with histamine placebo in 155 subjects with ragweed, grass, or mountain cedar rhinitis showed no significant differences between the Rinkel-treated group and the placebo group (Hirsch et al., 1981).

STANDARDIZATION OF ALLERGEN EXTRACTS

Since 1933 allergists have used PNU determinations to measure the concentrations of allergenic extracts. Phosphotungstic acid precipitates all proteins, and whereas skin-reactive protein allergenicity decreases with time, the protein nitrogen that precipitates does not change. Therefore, PNU determinations may be the same, but the allergenicity of different extracts will vary.

Currently the PNU method is used along with the weight/volume (w/v) index as concentration standards for manufacturers of allergenic extracts. According to the w/v method, there will be 1 g of crude allergen in 50 ml of extracting solution. A rough conversion factor is 0.5 ml of 1 : 100 w/v = 2500 PNU. Other equivalents that were formerly used are shown in Table 13-3.

Improved methods of allergen characterization and potency are being sought by the Bureau of Biologics. Better purification of crude extracts is being developed so that there will be more specific immunologic responses; decreased hazards of hyposensitization to contaminants, improved clinical efficacy, and higher levels of IgG antibody may result (Kjellmann & Lanner, 1980). A disadvantage of purified extracts may be the loss of some low- and high-molecular-weight allergens and haptens. Eventually international reference sera of common allergens will be available for standardization.

Tests for determination of the potency and consistency of allergenic extracts, namely RAST inhibition (Gleich et al., 1974), isoelectric focusing (Varga & Ceska, 1972), and crossed immunoelectrophoresis (Weeke et al., 1974), have been available for years but are only recently being utilized by manufacturers. Titration of skin test sensitivity in humans remains the best test available, but it is not easily accomplished.

Table 13-3 *Approximate Equivalent terms in 0.5 ml of a 1:100 (w/v) Extract*

Term	Equivalent
Protein nitrogen units (PNU)	= 2500*
Protein nitrogen (μm)	= 25
Total nitrogen (units)	= 8500†
Total nitrogen (micrograms)	= 85†
Pollen, Freeman-Noon units	= 5000†

*Conversion of w/v to PNU is only an approximation and differs from antigen to antigen.
†No longer used.

The exact selection of the antigens depends on which skin tests are positive and correlate with the clinical history. If IT is initiated for grass and ragweed symptoms but skin tests are also positive to other allergens, only those allergens to which the individual has symptoms should be included in the extract. (Some allergists may include the other allergens to which the skin was reactive on the chance that the individual might develop symptoms to those allergens at a later date and thus would already be protected.) Antigens to which the skin is not reactive should never be included because the patient might then become sensitized to those antigens (Turkeltaub et al., 1978).

The decision to give *only* dust IT should not be made casually as isolated IgE-mediated symptoms due to dust are uncommon. Perennial upper or lower respiratory tract symptoms may be somewhat attributable to dust especially if there is pruritus or wheezing associated with dusty conditions. Pure dust rhinitis or asthma is uncommon, however, and the indication for IT to dust alone would be rare. The use of pure mite extract, as the major antigenic component in house dust, has been shown to be effective in the treatment of individuals with IgE-mediated rhinitis, asthma, or both in relation to dust symptoms. Similarly, Kang et al. (1982) have shown in a study without patient controls that cockroach antigenic extract is effective in reducing symptoms and raising blocking antibody in cockroach-sensitive asthmatics whose symptoms occur similarly to those in patients with dust-related symptoms. The use of this cockroach extract is not yet widely accepted.

INDICATIONS OF SUCCESSFUL IMMUNOTHERAPY

Determining whether IT has been useful is not always easy. Often the patient will complain that IT has not helped and the physician will need to find subtle indicators of improvement. These may include fewer medications needed or a reduction in steroids from daily to low-dose alternate day. Emergency room visits and hospitalizations during an allergic season may be fewer than in previous years. Similarly, there may have been fewer work or school days missed or more days spent comfortably.

UNSUCCESSFUL IMMUNOTHERAPY

Although IT has not been perfected as of 1983, with appropriate indications in properly selected patients, IT is significantly more effective than placebo in about 80% of patients with seasonal symptoms (Table 13-1). It is well known from many studies that there is symptomatic improvement in 25% of patients receiving placebo.

When IT does not seem to be effective, several factors should be considered:

1. Inaccurate history and selection of antigens
2. Treatment of vasomotor rhinitis or intrinsic (nonallergic) asthma
3. Poor environmental control re: dust, feathers, mold
4. Animals still at home causing a "priming effect;"

5. New IgE-mediated sensitivities present
6. Inadequate immunotherapy doses
7. Irregular injection schedule
8. Results expected too early in treatment program
9. Expectation of a complete cure (not always realistic)

If an inaccurate history is obtained, IT may be given to someone with nonallergic disease despite positive skin tests. Patients with vasomotor or perennial nonallergic rhinitis will not be affected by IT. Asthmatics with negative skin tests, whose attacks may be precipitated by viruses at the same time as the ragweed or mold seasons, will also not respond to allergen IT.

If there is poor control of dust, mold, feathers, or animal dander while IT is being given to control sensitivity to one or more of those allergens, symptoms may not improve. Furthermore, animal danders of any type, including cat, dog, bird, gerbil, hamster, or guinea pig, may prime the upper or lower respiratory tract in persons with positive skin tests to the respective animal. There may not be immediate onset of sneezing, coughing, or wheezing when the patient is around the animal, but with an infection severe rhinorrhea or asthma may occur. In households shared by pets and individuals who are allergic to animal dander, IT against all inhalant allergens may thus be futile until the animal dander is cleared from the household. If an individual's symptoms change for the worse, the physician must suspect either that a new inhalant allergy has developed or that a new animal has been brought into the home.

Inadequate doses and concentrations of IT are often used. Although thorough studies have not been done to determine the exact amount of PNUs needed to achieve symptomatic improvement and effect significant immunologic responses, it is generally thought that at least a total of 2500 PNUs of each antigen needs to have been given in order for any symptomatic improvement to have occurred.

Some patients expect immediate improvement (within 3–6 months), but decreased symptoms seldom occur until at least 9–12 months unless a rush program of IT is instituted. Rarely, 2 years of *adequate* IT may be required before symptomatic improvement begins. Because some people expect a complete cure the realistic potential of IT needs to be explained to the patient—even though complete cures do occasionally occur.

RISKS OF IMMUNOTHERAPY

The proper administration of allergenic protein is often associated with some local pain, erythema, and swelling. Occasionally, however, large local reactions consisting of pain, erythema, and induration more than a walnut in size will occur because the following techniques were not followed or too high a dose for that particular time was administered:

1. Give injections in a physician's office or under the supervision of a qualified medical person.

2. Make sure that epinephrine and antihistamines are available.
3. Use a $\frac{3}{8}$-inch, disposable 26- or 27-gauge needle on 1.0mi syringe.
4. Give the injection subcutaneously in the outer arm between the shoulder and the elbow.
5. Wipe the needle before injecting.
6. Use oblique angle of insertion.
7. Check for absence of blood return by pulling back on the plunger.
8. *Do not* rub at the site of injection.
9. Wait 20 minutes before releasing the patient.

These local reactions may occur after every injection and may develop from minutes up to 24 hours afterward. Often, repeating the dose on the next injection date or dropping back to the previous dose will obviate further local reactions. If the local reactions continue, the allergen to which the patient was most sensitive by skin testing should be given separately in a more stepwise and dilute method.

Local reactions may not occur until stronger concentrations of extract are being given and if increasing doses are given on the next injection date after a large local reaction, there may be a systemic reaction. Local reactions may also occur when a fresh vial of the maintenance concentration is used; therefore, the initial dose from a new vial should be reduced by 25–50%, with a return to maintenance levels with the subsequent injections. Persistent large local reactions may lead to noncompliance. The management of local reactions is summarized in the following list:

1. Apply cold locally.
2. Give oral antihistamine as needed.
3. Call the allergist.
4. Review injection technique.
5. Review dosage schedule—repeat same dose next week or drop back to the previous dose.

Systemic reactions with urticaria, angioedema and flushing, light-headedness, bronchospasm, shock, or cardiac arrest, as well as vasovagal reactions, can occur with allergen injections. These systemic reactions should be managed as any other anaphylactic reaction outlined in Chapter 10 and in addition local aqueous epinephrine (1 : 1000 w/v; 0.1–0.3 ml) should be given subcutaneously at the site of the allergen injection to reduce the allergen's absorption. The allergen dose should be reduced by at least 50% for the next injection.

Immunotherapy has also been investigated for its long-term safety. Studies by Levinson et al. (1978), Yang et al. (1979), and Kemler et al. (1979) have shown no immune complex formation or other adverse immunologic effects. Phanuphak & Kohler (1980), however, claimed that there was an association between the initiation of IT and polyarteritis nodosa in 6 of 20 patients, although some of these 6 patients may have had polyarteritis nodosa before the start of IT. Also, the amount of protein used in the IT was too small to account for circulating immune complexes in humans

(Kohler, 1979; Stein et al., 1978). More conclusive evidence is needed to incriminate IT as a cause of polyarteritis nodosa.

The safety of continuing IT during pregnancy has been shown (Turner et al., 1980), as long as systemic reactions are avoided; however, starting IT during pregnancy is not recommended (see Chapter 19).

ALTERNATIVES TO STANDARD AQUEOUS IMMUNOTHERAPY

Because of the prolonged course and incidence of local and systemic reactions associated with allergen IT, other methods have been devised to reduce the allergic response yet maintain the immunologic response (Table 13-4).

Repository therapy is used successfully with delayed absorption of antigens allowing for larger doses of antigen administration (Norman et al., 1972; Norman & Lichtenstein, 1978). Purification of allergen extracts was attempted for a while to reduce local reactions and avoid injection of unnecessary proteins (Norman et al., 1968; Malley & Perlman, 1970). This method was found to be no more effective than the use of crude extracts, yet more expensive, and it carries the risk of deleting certain minor antigens during the purification.

The conjugation of allergens to polyethylene glycol (Lee & Sehon, 1978), D-glutamic acid, D-lysine (Butterfield et al., 1981; Liu et al., 1979; Tse et al., 1978) or isologous gamma globulin (Borel et al., 1976) has been effective in suppressing IgE production in animals, but not yet in humans.

The use of glutaraldehyde to polymerize large amount of antigen has allowed for fewer injections resulting in comparable immunologic responses to aqueous extracts and fewer local and systemic reactions (Hendrix et al., 1980; Johannson et al., 1974; Metzger et al., 1981). These allergen polymers are available in Europe, but not yet in the United States.

Efforts to modify allergens with pyridine (Allpyral) have resulted in losses of antigenicity with ragweed (Lichtenstein et al., 1968), but in Europe, Allpyral has been found effective in grass extracts (Brown, 1979), allowing for fewer injections with fewer adverse reactions. As of December 31, 1981, Allpyral extracts were no longer available in the United States. The use of formalin to alter allergens (Allergoids) has been shown by Norman et al. (1981) and Marsh et al. (1970, 1981) to be safe and effective, with longer stability, fewer local reactions, and fewer injections needed compared to aqueous extracts. Urea, through its denaturation and subsequent recombination of allergenic proteins (Norman et al., 1980) causes an increase of T suppressor cells; however, no clinical efficacy in humans has been shown.

The oral route of pollen hyposensitization has been successful in animals (David, 1977) but not in humans. Humans, however, have been orally desensitized to bovine serum albumin (Korenblat et al., 1968) and penicillin (Sullivan et al., 1981). Intranasal IT with polymerized ragweed or timothy has been useful preseasonally to reduce symptoms with few side effects in humans.

Allergen immunotherapy is useful when indicated and when the proper antigens are given in adequate amounts. Continued efforts are being made to reduce the number of injections as well as the local and systemic reactions while improving the immunogenic response.

Table 13-4 *Alternatives to Conventional Aqueous Immunotherapy*

Method	Types	Antigens Used	Mechanism	Comments	References
Repository	Antigen suspended in mineral oil	Ragweed	Delayed absorption of antigen	No longer used because of granuloma formation and plasma cell tumors in mice	Loveless, 1957
	Aluminum monostearate precipitation (Alum)	Ragweed	Same as above	Larger doses of antigen may be given safely; similar efficacy to aqueous extracts; commercially available	Norman & Lichtenstein, 1978; Norman et al., 1972
Allergen purification	Aqueous	Ragweed AgE; AgK; Timothy AgD	Same as with aqueous extracts	Purified extracts are no more effective than crude whole extracts; some antigens may be deleted; purification process is expensive	Malley & Perlman, 1970; Norman et al., 1968
Allergen conjugation	Polyethylene glycol	Ovalbumin; Ragweed	Suppression of specific IgE	No human studies, but effective in mice	Lee & Sehon, 1978
	D-Glutamic acid and D-lysine	Ragweed AgE ovalbumin; short ragweed fraction A	Induces T-cell tolerance with suppression of IgE response to the hapten or antigen	Animal studies are effective, but humans are not yet	Butterfield et al., 1981; Liu et al., 1979; Tse et al., 1978
	Isologous gamma globulin	Benzyl penicilloyl (BPO)	Tolerance induction	Effective in mice	Borel et al., 1976
Allergen polymerization	Glutaraldehyde	Ragweed, grass mixture, tree mixture, bee venom	Decreased allergenicity with increased immunogenicity	Fewer side effects, controlled study shows efficacy with ragweed; grass therapy was effective in 6 patients; not yet commercially available	Hendrix et al., 1980, 1981; Patterson et al., 1980, 1981
	Glutaraldehyde linked, tyrosine absorbed (Pollinex)	12-grass mixture; short ragweed	Decreased allergenicity with increased immunogenicity	Uncontrolled study showing similar efficacy and immune response as Allpyral but fewer local reactions; 5 injections of preseasonal short ragweed were effective in a double-blind placebo-controlled study; Available in Europe	Johansson et al., 1974; Metzger et al., 1981

	Pyridine extraction and aluminum monostearate precipitation (Allpyral)	Ragweed, birch, timothy, rye, or cocksfoot	Altered antigen with delayed absorption	Ragweed antigens may be destroyed by the pyridine; grass therapy effective in Europe; no longer available in the United States	Brown, 1979; Lichtenstein et al., 1968
Allergen modification	Tetrahydrofuran extraction and aluminum sulfate precipitation (TEAP)	Pollen mixtures, Mold mixtures, dust	Altered antigen with delayed absorption	Marked granuloma formation in a poorly controlled study; studied only in Europe	Rudolph et al., 1978
	Formalinized allergen combined with a lysine adjuvant (Allergoid)	Rye grass group I, ragweed	Decreased allergenicity with normal immunogenicity	Low doses may be effective, but clinical efficacy has yet to be shown	Marsh et al., 1970, 1981
	Urea denaturation	Ragweed AgE	Loss of allergenicity but T suppressors increased	Increased side effects and no clinical efficacy yet, but promising	Norman et al., 1980
Nonallergenic immunogen	Anti-idiotype antibodies	Anti-epsilon antibody	Prevent IgE responses	In animals effective before but not after thee has been antigen exposure	Geczy et al., 1978
Different route	Oral	Ragweed, horse serum, bovine serum albumin, penicillin	Local increased IgA; Reduced serum specific IgE and IgG	Desensitization to pollen was effective in mice and rats; Humans have been desensitized to BSA and penicillin but not pollens	David, 1977; Korenblat, 1968; Sullivan, 1981
	Nasal	Aqueous and polymerized ragweed and timothy	Local increased IgA and IgG in some studies	Aqueous and polymerized allergens are effective; Aqueous extract was locally irritating	Georgitis et al., 1982; Johansson et al., 1979; Nickelsen et al., 1981

REFERENCES

Aas, K. *Acta Pediatr. Scand.*, 1971, *60*, 264–268.

Borel, Y., Kilham, L., Hyslop, N., & Borel, H. *Nature*, 1976, *261*, 49–50.

Brown, E. *Acta Allergol.*, 1979, *2*, 122–128.

Bruun, H. M., Thantney, N., & Jackson, F. *Clin. Allergy*, 1949, *9*, 465–472.

Butterfield, J. H., Gleich, G. J., Yunginger, J. W., Zimmerman, E. M., & Reed, C. E. *J. Allergy Clin. Immunol.*, 1981, *67*, 272–278.

David, M. F. *J. Allergy Clin. Immunol.*, 1977, *60*, 180–187.

Evans, R., Pence, H., Kaplan, H., & Rocklin, R. *J. Clin. Invest.*, 1976, *57*, 1378–1385.

Frankland, A. W., & Augustin, R. *Lancet*, 1954, *1*, 1055–1057.

Freeman, J. *Lancet*, 1911, *2*, 814–817.

Gabriel, M., Ng, H. K., Allan, W. G. L., Hill, L., & Nunn, A. J. *Clin. Allergy*, 1977, *7*, 325–336.

Gatien, J. G., Merler, E., & Colten, H. R. *Clin. Immunol. Immunopathol.*, 1975, *4*, 32–37.

Geczy, A. F., deWeck, A. L., Geczy, C. L., & Toffler, O. *J. Allergy Clin. Immunol.*, 1978, *62*, 261–270.

Georgitis, J. W., Mueller, U. R., Clayton, W. F., Kane, J., Wypych, J. I., Reisman, R. E., & Arbesman, C. E. *J. Allergy Clin. Immunol.*, 1982, *69*, 100.

Gleich, G. J., Larson, J. B., Jones, R. T., & Baer, H. *J. Allergy Clin. Immunol.*, 1974, *53*, 158–169.

Hendrix, S. G., Patterson, R., Zeiss, C. R., Pruzansky, J. J., Suszko, I. M., McQueen, R. C., Slavin, R. G., Miller, H. M., Lieberman, P. L., & Sheffer, A. L. *J. Allergy Clin. Immunol.*, 1980, *66*, 486–494.

Hirsch, S. R., Kalbfleisch, J. H., Golbert, T. M., Josephson, B. M., McConnell, L. H., Scanlon, R., Kniker, W. T., Fink, J. N., Murphree, J. J., & Cohen, S. H. *J. Allergy Clin. Immunol.*, 1981, *68*, 133–155.

Johansson, S. G. O., Miller, A. C. M. L., Mullan, N., Overell, B. G., Tees, E. C., & Wheeler, A. *Clin. Allergy*, 1974, *4*, 255–263.

Johansson, S. G. O., Deuschl, H., & Zelterstroem, O. *Int. Arch. Allergy Appl. Immunol.*, 1979, *60*, 447–460.

Johnstone, D. E., & Dutton, A. *Pediatrics*, 1968, *42*, 793–802.

Kang, B., Johnson, J., & Chang, J. L. *J. Allergy Clin. Immunol.*, 1982, *69* (No. 1, suppl.), 132.

Katz, D. H. *J. Allergy Clin. Immunol.*, 1978, *62*, 44–55.

Kemler, B. J., Franklin, W. D., Alpert, E., & Bloch, K. J. *Clin. Allergy*, 1979, *9*, 473–478.

Kjellman, I. M., & Lanner, A. *Allergy*, 1980, *35*, 323–334.

Kohler, P. F. *J. Allergy Clin. Immunol.*, 1979, *63*, 297–299.

Korenblat, P. E., Rothberg, R. M., Minden, P., & Farr, R. S. *J. Allergy*, 1968, *41*, 226–235.

Lee, W. Y., & Sehon, A. H. *Int. Arch. Allergy Appl. Immunol.*, 1978, *56*, 193–206.

Levinson, A. I., Summers, R. J., Lawley, T. J., Evans, R., & Frank, M. M. *J. Allergy Clin. Immunol.*, 1978, *62*, 109–114.

Levy, D. A., & Osler, A. G. *J. Immunol.*, 1967, *99*, 1068–1077.

Lichtenstein, L. M., Norman, P. S., & Winkenwerder, W. L. *Ann. Int. Med.*, 1971, *75*, 663–671.

Lichtenstein, L. M., Norman, P. S., & Winkenwerder, W. L. *J. Allergy*, 1968, *41*, 49–57.

Lichtenstein, L. M., Ishizaka, K., & Norman, P. S. *J. Clin. Invest.*, 1973, *52*, 472–482.

Liu, F. T., Bogowitz, C. A., Borgatze, R. F., Zinnecker, M., Kat, L. R., & Katz, D. H. *J. Immunol.*, 1979, *123*, 2456–2465.

Loveless, M. H. *J. Immunol.*, 1957, *79*, 68–79.

Malley, A., & Perlman, F. *J. Allergy Clin. Immunol.*, 1970, *45*, 14–29.

Marsh, D. G., Lichtenstein, L. M., & Campbell, D. H. *Immunology*, 1970, *18*, 705–722.

Metzger, W. J., Dorminey, H. C., Richerson, M. B., Weiter, J. M., Donnelly, A., & Moran, D. *J. Allergy Clin. Immunol.*, 1981, *68*, 442–448.

Nickelsen, J. A., Goldstein, S., Mueller, V., Wypych, J., Reisman, R., & Arbesman, C. E. *J. Allergy Clin. Immunol.*, 1981, *68*, 33–40.

Norman, P. S., Lichtenstein, L. M., Kagney-Sobolka, A., & Marsh, D. G. *J. Allergy Clin. Immunol.*, 1982, *70*, 248–260.

Norman, P. S., Winkenwerder, W. L., & Lichtenstein, L. M. *J. Allergy Clin. Immunol.*, 1968, *42*, 93–108.

Norman, P. S., Winkenwerder, W. L., & Lichtenstein, L. M. *J. Allergy Clin. Immunol.*, 1972, *50*, 31–44.

Norman, P. S., Ishizaka, K., Lichtenstein, L. M., & Adkinson, N. F. *J. Allergy Clin. Immunol.*, 1980, *66*, 336–341.

Norman, P. S., & Lichtenstein, L. M. *J. Allergy Clin. Immunol.*, 1978, *61*, 384–389.

Patterson, R., Suszko, I. M., Hendrix, S., Zeiss, C. R., & Pruzansky, J. J. *J. Allergy Clin. Immunol.*, 1980, *66*, 495–499.

Patterson, R., Suszko, I. M., Hendrix, S. G., & Zeiss, C. R. *J. Allergy Clin. Immunol.*, 1981, *67*, 162–165.

Pence, H. L., Mitchell, D. Q., Creely, R. L., Updegraff, B. R., & Selfridge, M. A. *J. Allergy Clin. Immunol.*, 1976, *58*, 39–50.

Phanuphak, P., & Kohler, P. F. *Am. J. Med.*, 1980, *68*, 479–485.

Rinkel, H. J. *Ann. Allergy*, 1949, *7*, 631–639.

Rocklin, R. E., Sheffer, A. L., Greineder, D. K., & Melmon, K. L. *New Engl. J. Med.*, 1980, *302*, 1213–1219.

Rudolph, R., Stand, R. D., Baumgarten, C., & Kunkel, G. *Lung*, 1978, *155*, 297–308.

Smith, A. P. *Br. Med. J.*, 1971, *4*, 204–206.

Stein, M. R., Brown, G. L., Lima, J. E., Nelson, H. S., & Carr, R. I. *J. Allergy Clin. Immunol.*, 1978, *62*, 211–216.

Sullivan, T. J., Wedner, H. J., Shatz, G. S., Yecies, L. D., & Parker, C. W. *J. Allergy Clin. Immunol.*, 1981, *68*, 171–180.

Taylor, W. W., Ohman, J. L., & Lowell, F. C. *J. Allergy Clin. Immunol.*, 1978, *61*, 283–287.

Tipton, W. R., & Nelson, H. S. *J. Allergy Clin. Immunol.*, 1982, *69*, 194–199.

Tse, K. S., Kepron, W., & Sehon, A. *J. Allergy Clin. Immunol.*, 1978, *61*, 303–309.

Turkeltaub, P. C., Marsh, D. G., Lichtenstein, L. M., & Norman, P. S. *J. Allergy Clin. Immunol.*, 1978, *61*, 171 (abstract).

Turner, E. S., Greenberger, P. A., & Patterson, R. *Ann. Int. Med.*, 1980, *93*, 905–918.

Van Metre, T. E., Adkinson, N. F., Amodio, F. J., Lichtenstein, L. M., Mardiney, M. R., Norman, P. S., Rosenberg, G. L.,Sobotka, A. K., & Valentine, M. D. *J. Allergy Clin. Immunol.*, 1979, *66*, 500–513.

Van Metre, T. E., Adkinson, N. F., Amodio, F. J., Kagey-Sobotka, A., Lichtenstein, L. M., Mardiney, M. R., Norman, P. S., & Rosenberg, G. L. *J. Allergy Clin. Immunol.*, 1982, *69*, 181–193.

Varga, J. M., & Ceska, M. *J. Allergy Clin. Immunol.*, 1972, *49*, 274–284.

Wahn, U., & Siraganian, R. P. *J. Allergy Clin. Immunol.*, 1980, *65*, 413–421.

Weeke, B., Lowenstein, H., & Neilsen, L. *Acta Allergol.*, 1974, *29*, 402–417.

Yang, W. H., Dorval, G., Osterland, C. K., & Gilmore, N. J. *J. Allergy Clin. Immunol.*, 1979, *63*, 300–307.

Zeiger, R. S., & Schatz, M. *Med. Clinics N. Am.*, 1981, (September), 987–1012.

SUGGESTED READINGS

Johnstone, D. E. *Ann. Allergy*, 1981, *46*, 1–7 (pt. 1) and 59–65 (pt. 2).

Lichtenstein, L. M. *Am. Rev. Resp. Dis.*, 1978, *117*, 191–197.

Norman, P. S. *J. Allergy Clin. Immunol.*, 1980, *65*, 87–96.

Patterson, R., Lieberman, P., Irons, J. S., Pruzansky, J. J., Melam, H., Metzger, W. J., & Zeiss, C. R. Immunotherapy. *In* E. Middleton (Ed.), *Allergic principles and practice*, St. Louis: Mosby, 1978, Vol. 2, pp. 877–898.

Zeiger, R. S., & Schatz, M. *Med. Clinics N. Am.*, 1981 (September), 987–1012.

QUESTIONS

1. What is the safest and most effective form of immunotherapy for ragweed hay fever?
   a. DGL ragweed injections.
   b. Coseasonal injections of aqueous ragweed extract.
   c. Sublingual ragweed extract.
   d. Perennial injections every 2–4 weeks of aqueous ragweed extract.
   e. None of the above
2. Injections of mold spore extract should be given to:
   a. Individuals who notice hives after eating blue cheese.
   b. Persons with asthma mainly in winter.

c. Persons with asthma which is worse after cutting grass, raking leaves, or being in a damp basement.
d. Farmers with chills and fever several hours after working with damp hay in a silo.
e. None of the above.

3. Which one of the following immunologic criteria is associated with successful timothy grass immunotherapy?

a. High pretreatment antitimothy nasal IgA.
b. Low serum antitimothy IgG.
c. High serum total IgE.
d. Low postseasonal antitimothy IgE.
e. None of the above.

4. Large local reactions to an immunotherapy injection should be treated with:

a. 0.2 ml 1 : 1000 epinephrine locally.
b. Arm elevation and warm soaks.
c. Ice applied to the injection site.
d. Oral corticosteroids for 3 days.
e. None of the above.

5. Aqueous immunotherapy has been associated with:

a. Chronic active hepatitis.
b. Fibrosarcomas.
c. Serum sickness.
d. Muscle atrophy.
e. None of the above.

Answers can be found in Appendix B at the end of the book.

Rand Dankner

14

Antihistamines

Antihistamines are compounds that antagonize the physiologic actions of histamine by competitive inhibition at specific histamine receptor sites. They have been available for clinical use in the United States since the 1940s primarily for the treatment of allergic diseases. There are currently over 100 antihistaminic preparations to choose from, and many contain decongestants or other agents as additives. These so-called "classic" or H_1 antihistamines act by blocking the action of histamine at its H_1 receptor. Two H_2 histamine receptor antagonists, cimetidine and ranitidine, are approved for clinical use in the United States and are effective in the treatment of a variety of gastrointestinal disorders by inhibiting histamine-induced gastric acid secretion. Cimetidine has been shown to be of value in the treatment of certain allergic diseases as well; ranitidine has not yet been studied for use in allergic disorders and therefore its use will not be discussed in this chapter.

This chapter begins with a brief review of the physiology of histamine with emphasis on its role as a mediator of allergic disease and its possible role as a modulator of the immune response. There follows a discussion of the pharmacology of antihistamines and their therapeutic uses in the treatment of selected allergic diseases.

HISTAMINE

Physiology

Endogenous histamine is synthesized by decarboxylation of L-histadine, a reaction catalyzed by the enzyme L-histadine decarboxylase and that requires pyridoxal phosphate as a cofactor (Fig. 14-1) (Beaven, 1978). Histamine is metabolized by one of two enzymes: diamine oxidase (histaminase) or histamine-*N*-methyltransferase. Metabolism through the diamine oxidase pathway yields imidazole acetic acid and

ALLERGY: THEORY AND PRACTICE
ISBN 0-8089-1619-X

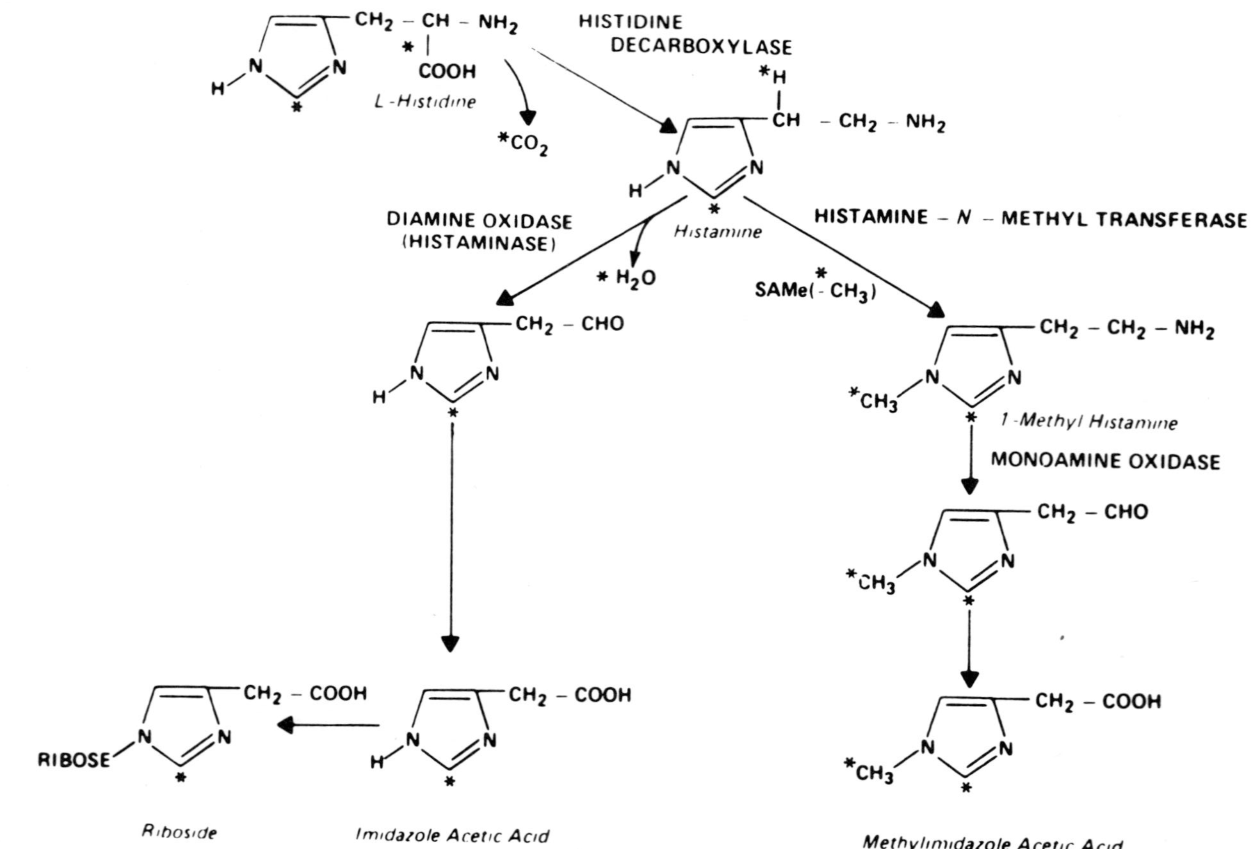

Fig. 14-1. Histamine synthesis and catabolis. M. A. *Monogr. Allergy*, 1978. *13*, 2. With permission.

then by ribosyl conjugation, ribosylimidazole acetic acid, an inactive metabolite. Beaven and colleagues (1978) have shown that the ribosylation of imidazole acetic acid is blocked by therapeutic doses of salicylates.

The predominant pathway of histamine catabolism in humans involves the ring methylation of histamine to form *N*-methylhistamine, a reaction catalyzed by histamine-*N*-methyltransferase. *N*-Methylhistamine is further metabolized to *N*-methylimidazole acetic acid. These metabolites are inactive and are excreted in the urine. The enzymes responsible for histamine metabolism are prevalent throughout body tissues. Degradative enzymes also circulate and excreted histamine is rapidly catabolized with a half-life of just a few minutes.

Storage and Release

The major storage site for histamine in humans is within the metachromatic granules of tissue mast cells and circulating basophils where preformed histamine is ionically bound to the proteoglycan-protein matrix of the granules (Wasserman, 1980). Histamine and other chemical mediators are released from mast cell and basophil stores by degranulation; this noncytolytic process involves the fusion of perigranular membranes with one another and with the external cell membrane, leading to extrusion of the granular contents from the cell. Degranulation can occur either as a result of immunologic or nonimmunologic mechanisms.

Actions

The actions of histamine at the cellular level occur through two receptors termed "H_1" and "H_2" (Ash & Schild, 1966; Black et al., 1972). The distribution of these receptors in any tissue determines the net action histamine will have on that tissue. Histamine-induced contraction of smooth muscle—whether in the lung, gastrointestinal (GI) tract, or elsewhere—is mediated through the H_1 receptor and is blocked by the "classic" antihistamines (H_1 antagonists). Histamine-mediated gastric acid secretion involves H_2 receptors and is blocked by the H_2 antagonists. Most other physiologic actions of histamine probably involve both receptors; for example, vascular effects of histamine including capillary dilatation, increased capillary permeability, cutaneous flushing, and perhaps local cutaneous (wheal and flair) as well as the systemic depressor response are best prevented by combined H_1 and H_2 receptor blockade (Plaut, 1979).

Histamine has many actions in hypersensitivity reactions in addition to its well-known effects on vascular permeability and smooth-muscle contraction. In humans, histamine has been shown to (1) suppress IgE-mediated histamine release from basophils, (b) suppress lysosomal enzyme release from neutrophils, (c) inhibit T-cell suppressor activity, (d) inhibit T cell proliferation and migration inhibitory factor production, and (e) inhibit granulocyte and eosinophil chemotaxis (Melmon et al., 1981; Plaut, 1979). These actions of histamine may be considered anti-inflammatory (Plaut, 1979) and appear to be mediated through the H_2 receptor. In addition, a subpopulation of suppressor T lymphocytes with surface H_2 histamine receptors has been identified in humans and appears to be decreased in atopic subjects but may increase in these subjects following specific immunotherapy (Beer et al., 1982; Rocklin et al., 1980). In view of the many actions histamine appears to have within the immune system, it seems likely that histamine functions as an important modulator of the immune response in addition to its role as a mediator of inflammation (Melmon et al., 1981). If histamine does indeed have an important role as an immunomodulator, its actions in this capacity would appear to be mediated through the H_2 receptor where stimulation results in increased concentrations of intracellular cyclic adenosine monophosphate.

The role of histamine as a mediator of immediate hypersensitivity reactions is well established. Histamine can reproduce various clinical manifestations of allergic disease such as rhinitis, urticaria, and anaphylaxis when administered by appropriate routes and is released by sensitized mast cells and basophils acutely in response to antigen challenge. The fact that histamine is not the sole mediator of many allergic diseases can be inferred from the limited efficacy of antihistamines in the treatment of a variety of allergic diseases. Antihistamines, nevertheless, are a very useful group of drugs in the management of certain allergic disorders.

ANTIHISTAMINES

Structure

Antihistamines are a group of compounds that bear a structural relationship to histamine. The H_1 antihistamines share the common core structure of a substituted ethylamine (Fig. 14-2). Substitution at either end of the molecule will alter specific properties of the drug and is the basis for the classification of H_1 antihistamines into six classes. Substitution at the *C*-terminal end of the ethylamine moiety generally involves a nitrogen, carbon, or ether linkage to two aromatic rings; a nitrogen linkage is present in the ethylenediamines, an ether linkage in the ethanolamines, and a carbon linkage in the alkylamines. The piperazines are characterized by a piperazine nucleus connected to the *N*-terminal end of the ethylamine side chain, whereas the phenothiazine and piperidine classes contain characteristic ringed substitutions, although their resemblance to native histamine is less striking. Cimetidine bears a structural similarity to histamine as well in that it contains an imidazole ring and a polar (although uncharged) side chain. Unlike the H_1 antihistamines, H_2 antagonists are polar, hydrophilic molecules; these properties contribute to their specificity of action at the H_2 receptor (Douglas, 1980).

Metabolism

The H_1 antihistamines are rapidly absorbed after oral administration with systemic effects developing 15–30 minutes later, with peak actions occurring at 1–2 hours (Douglas, 1980). Their duration of action varies from 3 to 12 hours depending on the preparation. The H_1 antihistamines also may be given parenterally with a more rapid onset of action, although rapid intravenous (IV) administration may result in hypotension (Pearlman, 1976). Hepatic metabolism is the primary mechanism of degradation of the H_1 antihistamines with very little of the unmetabolized drug appearing in the urine. The H_1 antihistamines have been shown to induce hepatic microsomal enzymes; consequently, their own metabolism as well as the metabolism of other hepatically inactivated drugs may be augmented after prolonged use. This theoretical possibility has not been shown to be of clinical relevance. The dose of

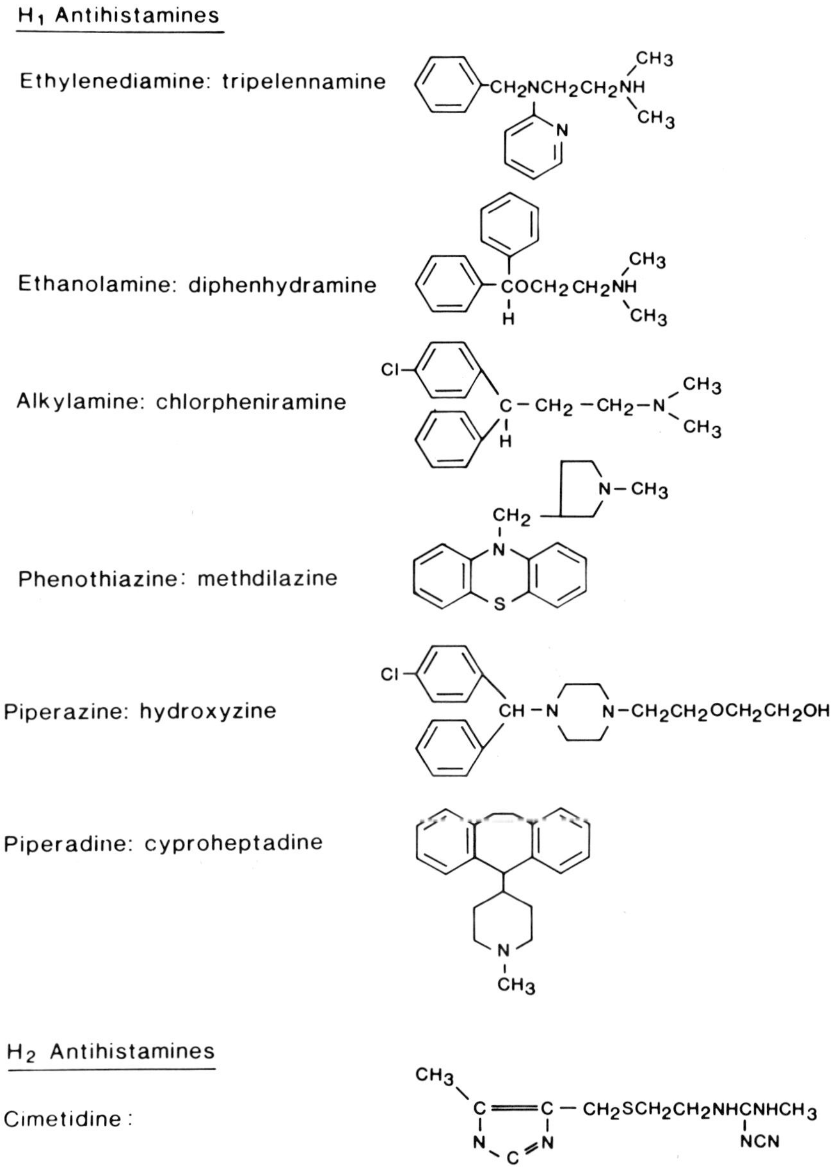

H_1 Antihistamines

Ethylenediamine: tripelennamine

$CH_2NCH_2CH_2NH(CH_3)_2$

Ethanolamine: diphenhydramine

$COCH_2CH_2NH(CH_3)_2$

Alkylamine: chlorpheniramine

Cl — $C - CH_2 - CH_2 - N(CH_3)_2$

Phenothiazine: methdilazine

CH_2 — N — CH_3

Piperazine: hydroxyzine

Cl — CH — N N — $CH_2CH_2OCH_2CH_2OH$

Piperadine: cyproheptadine

N — CH_3

H_2 Antihistamines

Cimetidine:

CH_3 — C = C — $CH_2SCH_2CH_2NHCNHCH_3$ (NCN)

Fig. 14-2. Representative structures of H_1 and H_2 antihistamines.

H_1 antihistamines should, nevertheless, be reduced in the presence of liver failure. Cimetidine is also rapidly absorbed from the gastrointestinal tract with peak blood levels occurring 60–90 minutes later (Finkelstein & Isselbacher, 1978); it may be safely administered by the IV route with rapid onset of action. Unlike the H_1 antihistamines, 50–70% of cimetidine is excreted unchanged in the urine 24 hours after administration; therefore, the dose or dose interval of cimetidine must be adjusted in patients with renal insufficiency.

Pharmacologic Properties and Side Effects

The H_1 antihistamines have a number of pharmacologic effects not related to their ability to competitively inhibit the action of histamine. These effects may be either clinically beneficial or deleterious (side effects) and can be divided into central nervous system (CNS) effects, anticholinergic effects, local anesthetic properties, and miscellaneous actions. The antihistamines readily cross the blood–brain barrier and can stimulate or depress the CNS resulting in symptoms such as agitation, restlessness, or (more commonly) drowsiness. The latter effect is the major side effect limiting the use of H_1 antihistamines in the treatment of allergic diseases. By virtue of a number of actions in the CNS, certain antihistamines are useful in the treatment of nausea, motion sickness, Parkinson's disease, and anxiety. Anticholinergic properties of antihistamines are responsible for a number of undesirable side effects such as dryness of the mouth and throat and urinary retention but may contribute to the therapeutic efficacy of H_1 antihistamines in the treatment of rhinitis and Parkinson's disease (Douglas, 1980). Less important properties of the H_1 antihistamines include local anesthetic effects, cardiac effects (increased ionotrophy and chronotropy), and effects on exocrine gland secretions (increased salivary, pancreatic and lacrimal gland secretions). The H_1 antihistamines also produce gastrointestinal side effects such as anorexia, nausea, vomiting, diarrhea, and epigastric distress. The classes of H_1 antihistamines differ from each other to some extent in the prominence of various pharmacologic actions and side effects (Table 14-1) and recommended dosages (Table 14-2); it should also be noted, however, that drugs within a given class may vary markedly with respect to the frequency and severity of specific side effects.

General Principles of Therapy

There are certain general principles that should guide the use of oral H_1 antihistamines in order to achieve the best therapeutic response. Since all antihistamines act by competitive inhibition at specific receptor sites and since histamine is rapidly released in excess in immediate hypersensitivity reactions, the drugs are most effective when given prophylactically before the stimulus to histamine release occurs. Thus H_1 antihistamines should be given on a continuous basis in the treatment of recurrent allergic symptoms during periods of antigen exposure. In addition to pro-

Table 14-1 *H_1 Antihistamine Properties: Group Comparisons*

	H_1 Blockade	Sedative Effects	Anticholinergic Effects	GI Effects
Ethylenediamines	+ + +	+ +	+	+ + +
Ethanolamines	+ + +	+ + +	+ + +	+
Alkylamines	+ + +	+	+	+
Piperazines	+ + +	+ +	+	+
Piperadines	+ + +	+ +	+	+
Phenothiazines	+ + +	+ + +	+ + +	+

Table 14-2 *Representative H_1 Antihistamines*

Generic Name	Brand Name	Oral Dosages (mg) Adult	Child (6–12 yr)	Dose Interval (Hours)
Ethylenediamines	PBZ	25–50	12.5	4–6
Tripelennamine	PBZ-SR	100	Not recommended	8–12
Ethanolamines				
Diphenhydramine	Benadryl	50	25	4–6
Carbinoxamine	Clistin	4–12	2	3–4
Doxylamine	Decapryn	12.5–25	6.25	4–6
Clemastine	Tavist	1.34–2.68	Not recommended	8–12
Alkylamines				
Brompheniramine	Dimetane	4	2	4–6
	Dimetane Extentabs	8–12	8	8–12
Chlorpheniramine	Chlor-Trimeton	4–12	4	4–6
	Teldrin	8–12	8	12
Triprolidine	Actidil	2.5	1.25	8–12
Dexchlorpheniramine	Polaramine	2	1	4–6
	Polaramine Repeatabs	4–6	2	8–10
Dimethindene	Forhistal	2.5	2.5	12
Phenothiazines				
Methdilazine	Tacaryl	4–8	4	6–12
Trimeprazine	Temaril tablets	2.5	2.5	6–8
	Temaril capsules	5	5	12/24*
Piperazines				
Hydroxyzine	Atarax, Vistaril	25–100	10–25	4–8
Piperidines				
Azatadine	Optimine	1–2	0.5–1	9–12
Cyproheptadine	Periactin	4	2–4	6–12

*Twelve hours in adults; 24 hours in children

ducing a more satisfactory therapeutic response, the uninterrupted use of antihistamines may lead to "tolerance" of undesirable CNS and other side effects of the drugs. There is no evidence that continuous prolonged use of antihistamines results in a decrease of their therapeutic effectiveness. As with most drugs, the dose of an antihistamine must be individualized; thus a low dose of a particular H_1 antihistamine may be ineffective, whereas a higher dose may be adequate to alleviate allergic symptoms. Conversely, a reduction in dose may allow continued therapeutic benefit without undue side effects. A final point is that if the desired therapeutic effect is not achieved with an antihistamine of one class or if undesirable side effects are a problem, switching to an H_1 antihistamine from another class may be beneficial. For this reason, the physician should become familiar with one or two drugs from each of the H_1 antihistamine classes.

Therapeutic Uses

Allergic Rhinitis and Conjunctivitis

Antihistamines are an integral part of the therapy of allergic rhinitis. They are estimated to be of some benefit to 70–95% of the patients with allergic rhinitis (Feinberg, 1947). The drugs are most effective in relieving the symptoms of sneezing, rhinorrhea, and itching of the eyes, nose, mouth and ears, although with oral administration they are generally less effective for allergic conjunctivitis than rhinitis. They are minimally effective in relieving nasal stuffiness as assessed subjectively or by measurements of nasal airflow (Connell, 1979). This may explain the clinical observation that H_1 antihistamines are generally more effective for seasonal allergic rhinitis than for perennial allergic rhinitis since patients with the latter entity seem to have more of a problem with nasal obstruction. Vasomotor rhinitis and other nonallergic causes of rhinitis, including the common cold, respond minimally to antihistamine therapy, although patients may derive some benefit from the anticholinergic properties of the drugs (Feller et al., 1950). Since the symptoms of allergic rhinitis are often most severe in the early morning, administration of a long-acting antihistamine at bedtime is an important part of therapy in patients with allergic rhinitis. This is particularly important for patients with seasonal allergic rhinitis and ragweed sensitivity since the ragweed pollen count is highest during the early morning hours. Again, the prophylactic use of antihistamines cannot be over-emphasized.

There is no advantage to combining two or more H_1 antihistamines, even from different classes; however, drugs that contain a combination of an H_1 antihistamine and a decongestant, usually pseudoephedrine, phenylephrine, or phenylpropanolamine, ameliorate nasal congestion in addition to other symptoms of allergic rhinitis. One study (Aschan, 1974) reported synergism between H_1 antihistamines (*N*-hydroxyethyl-promethazine or clemastine) and adrenergic agents (ephedrine or phenylpropanolamine) in relieving nasal congestion as measured by rhinomanometry in nonallergic patients with histamine-provoked nasal congestion or infectious rhinitis. Numerous studies have demonstrated the efficacy of these combination preparations in the treatment of allergic rhinitis (Aaronson et al., 1968; Empey et al., 1975). Patients taking such combination preparations complain less about drowsiness than do patients taking H_1 antihistamines alone. The overall incidence of adverse effects, however, is probably not different between the two groups (Empey et al., 1975). Patients taking sympathomimetic agents may experience the typical CNS or cardiovascular side effects of these drugs (Chapter 16).

Urticaria and Angioedema

Urticaria and angioedema are acute or chronic allergic reactions of diverse etiologies manifest as characteristic lesions in the skin (see Chapter 9). Antihistamines are an important part of therapy in the management of patients with urticaria or angioedema. The H_1 antihistamines are effective in reducing the pruritus of existing lesions and decreasing the frequency and severity of recurrent lesions. Antihistamines do not hasten the resolution of edema once urticaria or angioedema are present (Bromberg-Schneider & Atkinson, 1982).

Certain antihistamines may be more effective than others in the treatment of specific urticarial syndromes. Thus cold urticaria responds best to cyproheptadine, 12–16 mg/day in divided doses (Wanderer et al., 1977). Hydroxyzine is the drug of first choice in the treatment of cholinergic urticaria at doses of 100–200 mg/day in the adult divided into three or four doses daily (Moore-Robinson & Warin, 1968). Hydroxyzine is the initial H_1 antihistamine used by many physicians in the empiric treatment of urticaria of a variety of causes. In one recent study (Cook et al., 1973) comparing the effects of five oral H_1 antihistamines (Chlorpheniramine, tripelennamine, promethazine, diphenhydramine, and hydroxyzine) on the cutaneous response to allergen skin testing, hydroxyzine produced the greatest reduction in wheal size for the longest period of time following antigen challenge. In another study (Rhoades et al., 1975), hydroxyzine was the most effective of three antihistamines tested (cyproheptadine, chlorpheniramine, and hydroxyzine) in preventing the pruritus induced by intradermal injections of increasing doses of histamine. Hydroxyzine also has anxiolytic properties that may be useful in the treatment of urticaria and angioedema.

Combined H_1 and H_2 receptor blockade may be more effective than H_1 blockade alone in suppressing histamine-induced cutaneous wheal development (Harvey & Schocket, 1980), and cimetidine has been reported to be effective in combination with H_1 antihistamines in the treatment of urticaria and angioedema. In one study, the combination of cimetidine and cyproheptadine resulted in 90% improvement in 50% of patients with chronic urticaria previously unresponsive to conventional regimens that included H_1 antihistamines, ephedrine, and corticosteroids (Phanuphak et al., 1978). In a more recent study, the combination of hydroxyzine and cimetidine was found to be superior to the combination of hydroxyzine plus placebo, terbutaline, chlorpheniramine, or cyproheptadine in chronic idiopathic urticaria patients (Harvey et al., 1981). Cimetidine alone does not inhibit histamine-induced cutaneous wheal development (Nathan et al., 1981) and is not effective when used alone in the treatment of urticaria and angioedema.

Doxepin and other tricyclic antidepressent, are psychotherapeutic agents with H_1 antihistaminic properties although structurally dissimilar from drugs classified as H_1 antihistamines. These drugs also demonstrate some H_2 antagonist properties as well as antiserotonin and anticholinergic effects (Richelson, 1983). Sullivan et al.

(1982) showed that doxepin, on a molar basis, is a more potent H_1 antihistamine than any other available agent. Early clinical experience with this drug in urticaria patients has been encouraging with beneficial effects occurring at doses much lower than those usually used in the treatment of depression (Sullivan, 1981). The role of doxepin or other tricyclic antidepressants in the treatment of urticaria and other allergic diseases remains to be determined by clinical trials.

Anaphylaxis and Anaphylactoid Reactions

An antihistamine should never be the first drug used to treat serious systemic allergic reactions. Following epinephrine administration, however, most authors recommend that diphenhydramine be given IV or IM at a dose of 1.25 mg/kg up to 50 mg presumably to occupy any still available histamine receptors (Weiszer, 1980). Since antihistamines react relatively slowly and since massive histamine release has already occurred in anaphylaxis, the role of antihistamines in the management of this life-threatening condition must be considered secondary. The H_1 antihistamines have been shown to be effective as part of a regimen for the *prophylaxis* of radiocontrast material-induced anaphylactoid reactions in high risk patients (Greenberger et al., 1981). The current recommendation is that these patients receive 50 mg of diphenhydramine IM 1 hour prior to the procedure. These patients also receive prednisone, 50 mg orally every 6 hours for three doses, with the third dose given 1 hour before the procedure. This protocol reduces the incidence of recurrent allergic reactions by more than tenfold in high risk patients.

A role for H_2 antagonists in the prophylaxis of severe systemic allergic reactions had not been established, although their potential usefulness in combination with an H_1 antihistamine in this setting is suggested by the observation that combined H_1 and H_2 blockade can prevent morphine-induced hypotension (attributed to non-immunologic histamine release), whereas H_1 or H_2 blockade alone is ineffective (Philbin et al., 1981). It has been suggested that combined H_1 and H_2 antihistamine administration is appropriate for both prophylaxis and treatment of anaphylaxis since the vascular effects of histamine are mediated through both receptors (Plaut, 1979).

Asthma

Even recent literature has warned against the use of antihistamines in asthmatic patients primarily because of the possibility that H_1 antihistamines may interfere with the clearance of respiratory tract secretions secondary to their inherent anticholinergic properties. Subsequently, careful studies have demonstrated that the use of oral H_1 antihistamines in usual therapeutic doses does not produce worsening of bronchospasm (Grater, 1972; Karlin, 1972; Leopold et al., 1979). Therefore, asthmatics who have other allergic diseases likely to benefit from treatment with antihistamines should not be denied appropriate therapy with these agents, unless there is a clear history of respiratory symptoms provoked by antihistamine administration (Schuller, 1982). There is controversy as to whether H_2-receptor blockade with cimetidine increases bronchial reactivity to inhaled histamine in asthmatics (Nogrady & Beran, 1981; Schachter et al., 1982); further studies are required to clarify this issue.

The possible usefulness of H_1 antihistamines as therapy for asthma is currently a controversial subject; certainly other agents, including beta-adrenergic agents, theophylline, and corticosteroids, are more useful drugs in the treatment of asthma.

That H_1 antihistamines may have a role in the therapy of asthma is suggested by experimental data demonstrating that (a) histamine is released during IgE-mediated immediate hypersensitivity reactions in the lung; (b) histamine causes bronchial constriction in asthmatics at lower doses than in normals; (c) bronchial smooth-muscle contraction that occurs in response to antigen challenge in sensitized tissue is significantly reduced by the presence of an H_1 antihistamine; and (d) oral, inhaled, or intravenous (IV) H_1 antihistamine administration to asthmatics has been shown to improve baseline pulmonary flows and to decrease bronchial constriction in response to increasing concentrations of inhaled histamine (Casterline & Evans, 1977; Nathan et al., 1979; Pova, 1977). The bronchodilator effect of H_1 antihistamines is not a consequence of their anticholinergic properties (Nogrady & Bevan, 1978). Nevertheless, H_1 antihistamines have not been shown to be reliably efficacious in the therapy of asthma, perhaps because tissue concentrations are not adequate at specific receptor sites in the lung or more likely because other mediators such as leukotrienes are more important in the pathogenesis of asthma.

Two H_1 antihistamines, cinnarizine and ketotifen, may be efficacious in the treatment of asthma. Cinnarizine, a piperazine derivative, is also an inhibitor of calcium ion transport (Emanuel et al., 1979). Calcium ion transport across cell membranes is known to be important in smooth-muscle contraction, mast cell degranulation and goblet cell secretion, events implicated in the pathogenesis of asthma. Ketotifen, a tricyclic benzocycloheptathiophine derivative with H_1 antihistaminic properties, is an oral agent that in addition to its antihistaminic properties acts similarly to cromolyn sodium on mast cell membranes (Gobel, 1978). Both of these agents have shown promise in clinical trials in asthmatics, although their salutory effects are likely the result of pharmacologic properties not related to H_1 receptor blockade. Neither cinnarizine nor ketotifen are available for clinical use in the United States at this time.

In summary, antihistamines are not contraindicated in asthmatic patients, but neither are they indicated as therapy for this disease.

Topical Use

Topical H_1 antihistamines are effective in the treatment of pruritic dermatosis primarily because of their local anesthetic properties. Unfortunately, antihistamines are highly sensitizing when applied topically and thus may cause dermatitis following topical or oral readministration of the drug. Members from each of the six classes of H_1 antihistamines have been demonstrated to have sensitizing properties; in addition, phenothiazines may produce a photoallergic contact dermatitis. Committees from the American Medical Association and the American Academy of Pediatrics have urged strongly against the use of topical antihistamines (Yaffe et al., 1973). Topical ocular application of H_1 antihistamines alone or in combination with a decongestant are effective in the treatment of allergic conjunctivitis; however, antihistamines may be sensitizing by this route of administration as well.

Use in Pregnancy

The use of all medications during pregnancy (see Chapter 19) should be kept to a minimum. Information regarding the safety of antihistamines during pregnancy is limited. Diphenhydramine, tripelennamine, pheniramine, and chlorpheniramine are considered to be generally safe in pregnancy (Greenberger & Patterson, 1978). An epidemiologic study found brompheniramine to be associated with a statistically significant increase in teratogenic effects. Antihistamines of the piperazine class have been shown to have teratogenic effects in animals; antihistamines from this class, including hydroxyzine, should not be used during pregnancy. Data on newer H_1 antihistamines in pregnancy are unavailable; therefore, these drugs are best avoided in pregnant patients. There are also no data available on the safety of cimetidine during pregnancy, although cimetidine is known to cross the placenta and may interfere with fetal hepatic metabolism; therefore, at this time cimetidine should be avoided in pregnant patients.

Contraindications and Drug Interactions

There are few absolute contraindications in the use of H_1 antihistamines, although there are a number of relative contraindications; the therapeutic risk to benefit ratio must be kept in mind when using these drugs. Antihistamines are contraindicated in patients with a history of allergy to these drugs. A history of ethylenediamine sensitivity is a contraindication to the use of H_1 antihistamines from the ethylenediamine class; these patients should also avoid the use of piperazines including hydroxyzine because their metabolites may include ethylenediamine (Fisher, 1980). Other contraindications to the use of H_1 antihistamines relate to their anticholinergic properties; thus patients with glaucoma or urinary retention should avoid H_1 antihistamines. The use of antihistamines in pregnancy has already been discussed, and because H_1 and H_2 antihistamines do appear in breast milk, they are best avoided in nursing mothers. Since H_1 antihistamines are metabolized hepatically, they are contraindicated in the presence of significant liver dysfunction. Cimetidine, as already mentioned, is renally excreted and must be used with caution in patients with renal insufficiency.

In general, the CNS depressant effects of antihistamines will be additive with those of other CNS depressing drugs including ethanol; patients should be advised about the potential for increased sedation from the concomitant use of antihistamines and alcohol. The anticholinergic effects of H_1 antihistamines will be exacerbated by concomitant use of other drugs with anticholinergic properties; consequently, caution is advised when using H_1 antihistamines in patients maintained on tricyclic antidepressents, monoamine oxidase (MAO) inhibitors or other anticholinergic drugs. The theoretical possibility that H_1 antihistamines will alter the metabolism of other hepatically metabolized drugs by virtue of liver microsomal enzyme induction has not been demonstrated to be clinically important.

Cimetidine has been shown to decrease the clearance of a number of drugs including antipyrine, diazepam, warfarin, propranolol, phenytoin, and *theophylline*. Cimetidine produces a reduction in theophylline clearance by decreasing the rate of theophylline elimination (Campbell et al., 1981; Jackson et al., 1981; Reitberg et al., 1981). The effect of cimetidine on theophylline elimination is immediate and progresses over several days. Although specific guidelines have not yet been established, it has been recommended that serum theophylline concentrations be measured 1–2 days after the initiation of cimetidine therapy and 2–4 days after the discontinuation of cimetidine therapy in patients maintained on theophylline. It would seem prudent to decrease the theophylline dose by 25% in patients with adequate theophylline blood levels at the time of initiating cimetidine therapy. Though its usefulness in allergic diseases has not yet been investigated, ranitidine, an H_2 antagonist containing an aminoalkyl furan ring rather than an imidazole ring, does not interfere with the hepatic metabolism of theophylline and therefore may be preferable for patients requiring both theophylline and H_2 antagonist therapy (Medical Letter, 1982, 24: 111–113.)

SUMMARY

In summary, histamine, long recognized as an important mediator of allergic disease, exerts its actions at the cellular level through specific receptors. In addition to its role as a mediator of immediate hypersensitivity, histamine may be involved in immunoregulation. Since the beneficial effects of antihistamines in the treatment of allergic diseases result from competitive inhibition at histamine receptor sites, these drugs are most effective when given prophylactically. The use of H_1 antihistamines is limited by their side effects, particularly drowsiness; nevertheless, many patients derive substantial relief from allergic symptoms with these drugs, and the side effects may be minimized by appropriate dosing, choice of antihistamine and by continuous administration. The use of an H_2 antihistamine, often in combination with an H_1 antihistamine is effective for the treatment of certain allergic diseases.

REFERENCES

Aaronson, A. L., Ehrlich, N. J., Frankel, D. B., Gutman, A. A., & Aaronson, D. W. *Ann. Allergy*, 1968, *26*, 145–150.

Aschan, G. *Acta Otolaryngol.*, 1974, *77*, 433–438.

Ash, A. S. F., & Schild, H. O. *Br. J. Pharm. Chemother.*, 1966, *27*, 427–439.

Baraf, C. S. *Curr. Ther. Res.*, 1976, *19*, 32–38.

Beaven, M. A. *Monogr. Allergy*, 1978, *13*, 1–113.

Beer, D. J., Osband, M. E., McCaffrey, R. P., Soter, N. A., & Rocklin, R. E. *New Engl. J. Med.*, 1982, *306*, 454–458.

Black, J. W., Duncan, W. A. M., Durant, C. J., Ganellin, C. R., & Parsons, E. M. *Nature*, 1972, *236*, 385–395.

Bromberg -Schneider, S., & Atkinson, J. P. In T. P. Fitzpatrick, (Ed.), *Update: Dermatology in general medicine*. New York: McGraw-Hill, 1982.

Campbell, M. A., Plachetka, J. R., Jackson, J. E., Moon, J. F., & Finley, P. R. *Ann. Intern. Med.*, 1981, *95*, 68–69.

Casterline, C. L., & Evans, R. *J. Allergy Clin. Immunol.*, 1977, *59*, 420–424.

Connell, J. T. *Ann. Allergy*, 1979, *42*, 278–285.

Cook, T. J., MacQAueen, D. M., Whittig, H. J., Thornby, J. I., Lantos, R. L., & Virtue, C. M. *J. Allergy Clin. Immunol.*, 1973, *51*, 71–77.

Douglas, W. M. Histamine and 5-hydroxytryptamine (serotonin) and their antagonists. In Goodman, L. S., & Gillman, A., *The pharmacologic basis of therapeutics*. New York: MacMillan, 1980, pp. 607–646.

Emanuel, M. B., Chamberlin, J. A., Whiting, S., & Rigden, B. G. *Br. J. Clin. Pharmacol.*, 1979, *7*, 189–195.

Empey, D. W., Bye, C., Hodder, M., & Hughes, B. M. *Ann. Allergy*, 1975, *34*, 41–46.

Feinberg, S. M. *Am. J. Med.*, 1947, *3*, 560–570.

Feller, A. E., Badger, G. F., Hodges, R. G., Jordan, W. S., Rammelkamp, C. H., & Dingle, J. H. *New Engl. J. Med.*, 1950, *242*, 737–744.

Finkelstein, W., & Isselbacher, K. J. *New Engl. J. Med.*, 1978, *299*, 992–996.

Fisher, A. A. *Am. Acad. Dermatol.*, 1980, *3*, 303–306.

Gobel, P. *J. Int. Med. Res.*, 1978, *6*, 79–85.

Grater, W. C., Casebolt, J., Howard, L. A., Miller, J., Lanoff, G., & Rohr, J. H. *Ann. Allergy*, 1972, *30*, 95–97.

Greenberger, P. A., & Patterson, R. *Ann. Int. Med.*, 1978, *89*, 234–237.

Greenberger, P. A., Patterson, R., Simon, R., Lieberman, P., & Wallace, W. *J. Allergy Clin. Immunol.*, 1981, *67*, 185–187.

Harvey, R. P., & Schocket, A. L. *J. Allergy Clin. Immunol.*, 1980, *65*, 136–139.

Harvey, R. P., Wegs, J., & Schocket, A. L. *J. Allergy Clin. Immunol.*, 1981, *68*, 262–266.

Jackson, J. E., Powell, J. R., Wandell, M., Bentley, J., & Dorr, R. *Am. Rev. Resp. Dis.*, 1981, *123*, 615–619.

Karlin, J. M. *Ann. Allergy*, 1972, *30*, 342–347.

Leopold, J. D., Hartley, J. P. R., & Smith, A. P. *Br. J. Clin. Pharmacol.*, 1979, *8*, 249–251.

Melmon, K. L., Rocklin, R. E., & Rosenkranz, R. P. *Am. J. Med.*, 1981, *71*, 100–106.

Moore-Robinson, M., & Warin, K. P. *Br. J. Dermatol.*, 1968, *80*, 794–799.

Nathan, R. A., Segall, N., Glover, G. C., & Schocket, A. L. *Am. Rev. Resp. Dis.*, 1979, *120*, 1251–1258.

Nathan, R. A., Segall, N., & Schocket, A. L. *J. Allergy Clin. Immunol.*, 1981, *67*, 171–177.

Nogrady, S.G., & Bevan, C. *Thorax*, 1978, *33*, 700–704.

Pearlman, D. S. *Drugs*, 1976, *12*, 258–273.

Phanuphak, P., Schocket, A., & Kohler, P. F. *New Engl. J. Med.*, 1978, *299*, 992–996.

Philbin, D. M., Moss, J., Akins, C. W., Rosow, C. E., Kono, K., Schneider, R. C., Verlee, T. R., and Savarese, J. J. *Anesthesiology*, 1981, *55*, 292–296.

Plaut, M. *J. Allergy Clin. Immunol.*, 1979, *63*, 371–375.

Pova, V. T. *J. Allergy Clin. Immunol.*, 1977, *59*, 54–63.

Reitberg, D. P., Bernhard, H., & Schentag, J. J. *Ann. Intern. Med.*, 1981, *95*, 582–585.

Rhoades, R. B., Leifer, K. N., Cohan, R., & Whittig, H. J. *J. Allergy Clin. Immunol.*, 1975, *55*, 180–183.

Richelson, E. *Mayo Clin. Proc.*, 1983, *58*, 40–46.

Rocklin, R. E., Sheffer, A. L., Greineder, D. K., & Melmon, K .L. *New Engl. J. Med.*, 1980, *302*, 1213–1219.

Schachter, E. N., Brown, S., Lach, E., & Gerstenhaber *Chest*, 1982, *2*, 143–147.

Schuller, D. *J. Allergy Clin. Immunol.*, 1982, *69*, Suppl., 131.

Sullivan, T. J. *J. Allergy Clin. Immunol.*, 1982, *69*, 260–267.

Wanderer, A. A., Pierce, J. P., & Ellis, E. F. *Arch. Dermatol.*, 1977, *113*, 1375–1577.

Wasserman, S. I. *Int. J. Dermatol.*, 1980, *19*, 7–17.

Weiszer, I. In R. Patterson (Ed.), *Allergic diseases*. 1980, pp. 374–394.

Yaffe, J. S., Bierman, C. W., Cann, H. M., Gold, A. P., Kenny, F. M., Riley, H. D., Jr., Schafer, I., & Stern, L. *Pediatrics*, 1973, *51*, 229–302.

QUESTIONS

1. A 34-year-old woman has "chronic idiopathic urticaria" unresponsive to therapy including hydroxyzine, terbutaline, cyproheptadine, and corticosteroids. She is most likely to benefit from a trial of:

   a. A combination of several H_1 antihistamines, each from a different class.
   b. Cimetidine
   c. A combination of hydroxyzine plus cimetidine
   d. A long-acting H_1 antihistamine-sympathomimetic combination.

2. A 42-year-old woman with perennial allergic rhinitis reports decreased sneezing, rhinorrhea, and nasal pruritus since beginning therapy with brompheniramine 8 mg orally every 12 hours. She now complains of drowsiness and continued chronic nasal stuffiness. Appropriate modification of therapy would include:

   a. Increasing the dose of brompheniramine to 12 mg orally every 12 hours.
   b. Decreasing the dose of brompheniramine to 4 mg orally every 12 hours.

c. Switching from brompheniramine to a long-acting H_1 antihistamine-sympathomimetic combination.
d. Switching from brompheniramine to triprolidine 2.5 mg orally every 12 hours.

3. A 24-year-old man with allergic rhinitis and asthma has a history of urticaria following aminophylline administration. He is requesting therapy for rhinitis. You advise the patient that:

   a. Antihistamines are dangerous in asthmatics and should be avoided.
   b. His rhinitis may be a manifestation of continued theophylline administration.
   c. He may have ethylenediamine sensitivity and should not take antihistamines.
   d. He may have ethylenediamine sensitivity and should avoid antihistamines of the ethylenediamine and piperazine classes.

4. A 22-year-old woman with allergic rhinitis has excellent control of otherwise debilitating symptoms while taking brompheniramine 12 mg orally bid. She has just become pregnant. You recommend that she:

   a. Continue current therapy.
   b. Discontinue brompheniramine and begin chlorpheniramine 12 mg orally bid.
   c. Discontinue all antihistamines.
   d. Discontinue brompheniramine and begin hydroxyzine 50 mg orally tid.

5. Which of the following statements are true concerning the use of antihistamines in the treatment of anaphylaxis and anaphylactoid reactions?

   a. They should be avoided if bronchospasm is a feature of anaphylaxis.
   b. They are effective as part of a regimen for prophylaxis of certain anaphylactoid reactions, particularly radiocontrast sensitivity.
   c. They should be given rapidly and intravenously if hypotension is a component of anaphylaxis.
   d. They should be given only if urticaria are a component of anaphylaxis.

Answers can be found in Appendix B at the end of the book.

H. James Wedner

15

Theophylline

Theophylline (1,3-dimethylxathine) has been utilized for the treatment of asthma since 1937, when it was first described as being effective in reducing bronchospasm. Originally this drug was generally used in combination with ephedrine (4 : 1 or 5 : 1 ratios) and a variety of other agents including phenobarbital, mucolytic agents, and antihistamines. More recently a growing body of literature has demonstrated that theophylline (or its more water soluble salts such as aminophylline) alone is an effective therapeutic agent in the treatment of asthma. Indeed, most recent evidence indicates that fixed combinations of theophylline or its derivatives and other agents offer no advantages over theophylline itself (Weinberger & Bronsky, 1974). Fixed-ratio combinations do not allow individual drug dosing and may be detrimental since ephedrine may increase the toxicity of theophylline without augmenting the therapeutic benefit. For these reasons we do not recommend the use of these fixed dose combinations. In this chapter we shall not deal with these combinations but will concentrate on theophylline as a single modality for the treatment of asthma.

Theophylline belongs to the class of methylated xanthine derivatives and is chemically 1,3-dimethylxanthine (Fig. 15-1). It is related to other methylxanthines such as caffeine (1,3,7-trimethylxanthine) and theobromine (3,7-dimethylxanthine). The latter two although not therapeutically effective in asthma, are important since they interfere with some of the assays used to determine plasma theophylline levels.

Theophylline has limited solubility in water, and hence many preparations of theophylline salts have been made available for clinical use in asthma. Some of these are listed in Table 15-1. It is important to note that the salt in some cases makes up a significant portion of the weight of the drug, and this must be considered when prescribing these drugs. The salt does not alter the structure of the base compound; thus the circulating drug is in all cases theophylline. In recent years numerous studies have demonstrated that theophylline base is readily absorbed from the gastrointes-

ALLERGY: THEORY AND PRACTICE
ISBN 0-8089-1619-X

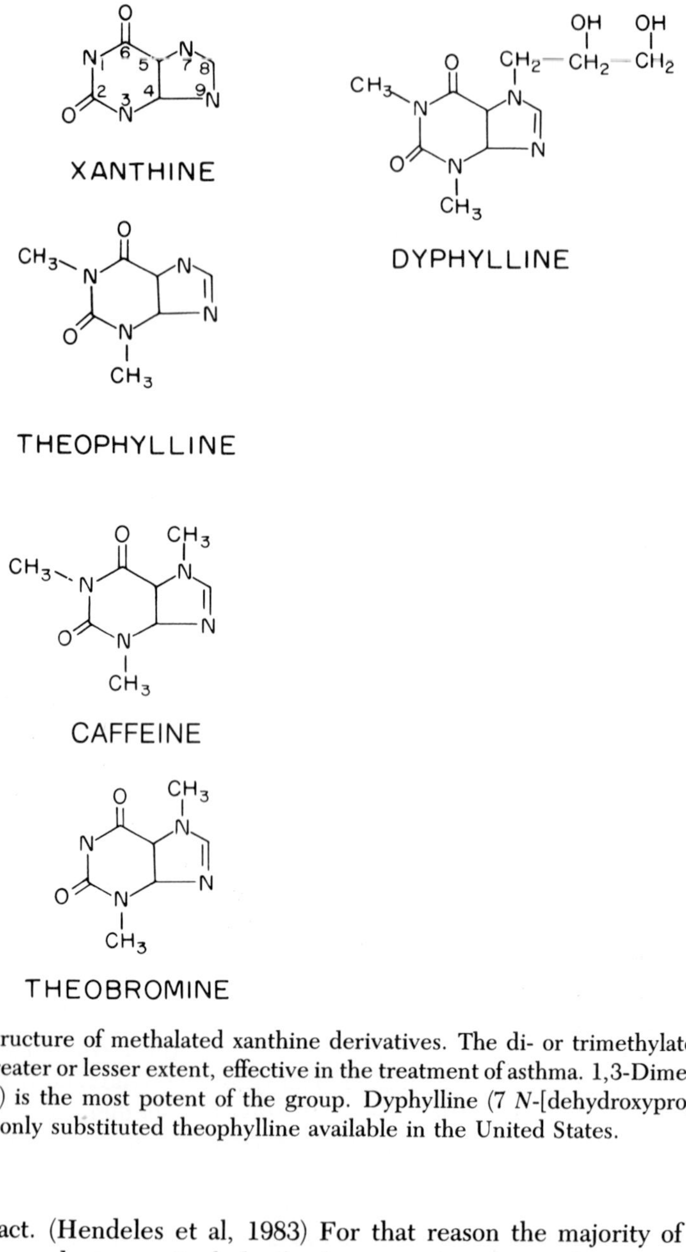

XANTHINE

DYPHYLLINE

THEOPHYLLINE

CAFFEINE

THEOBROMINE

Fig. 15-1. Structure of methalated xanthine derivatives. The di- or trimethylated xanthines are all, to a greater or lesser extent, effective in the treatment of asthma. 1,3-Dimethylxanthine (theophylline) is the most potent of the group. Dyphylline (7 *N*-[dehydroxypropyl]-theophylline) is the only substituted theophylline available in the United States.

tinal (GI) tract. (Hendeles et al, 1983) For that reason the majority of the newer theophylline products, particularly the longer-acting dosage forms, are pure theophylline base.

A number of substituted analogs of theophylline have also been produced. The majority of these are not available in the United States. The 7-*N*-dihydroxypropyl derivative is available in the United States as dyphylline (Lufyllin). It is important to note that, in contrast to the salts of theophylline, dyphylline is not accurately measured by the standard theophylline assays, and this must be taken into account when utilizing this drug. Dyphylline does have the advantage that it has neutral pH in solution and is the only preparation available for intramuscular (IM) use.

Table 15-1 *Theophylline Salts Used in Asthma*

Drug Preparation	Percent of Theophylline by Weight
Theophylline (anhydrous)	100
Theophylline monohydrate	91
Theophylline–ethylene diamine (Aminophylline Anhydrous)	85
Aminophylline hydrate	80
Theophylline ethanolamine	74
Theophylline sodium acetate	64
Theophylline calcium salicylate	49
Theophylline sodium glycinate	46
Choline theophylline	65
Dyphylline	70

Mechanism of Action

The role of the cyclic nucleotide cyclic adenosine monophosphate (cAMP) as a mediator and/or modulator of the allergic response is beyond the scope of this chapter. Although the sequence of events leading to the production and destruction of cAMP or cGMP is well known (Fig. 15-2), the exact role that these agents play in the biochemical machinery of cells involved in the allergic or asthmatic response is not clear. However, certain generalities can be made; namely, agents that tend to increase intracellular cAMP, either by increasing production or decreasing breakdown, inhibit the allergic response and agents that lower cAMP levels tend to augment the response.

Theophylline falls into the category of those agents that decrease the breakdown of cAMP, since it is a potent inhibitor of cyclic nucleotide phosphodiesterase, the enzyme that destroys cAMP. As a phosphodiesterase inhibitor, theophylline increases not only the basal levels of cAMP in cells, but also potentiates greatly the effects of other agents that increase cAMP levels such as β adrenergic agents. Theophylline would thus be expected to act synergistically with these agents, and as is discussed below, this is indeed the case.

Although the ability of theophylline to inhibit phosphodiesterase is well documented and is widely held to be the mechanism of theophylline action, it should be pointed out that this drug has other actions that may contribute to its antiasthmatic effects. Theophylline is much more active (on a molar basis) in certain tissues, such as lung, than in others, such as the isolated mast cell. Moreover, it is much more active *in vivo* than *in vitro*. Indeed, the K_i (the molarity for one-half maximal inhibition of phosphodiesterase) in broken cells is greater than 3×10^{-3} *M*, a concentration that can never be achieved by oral or parenteral administration of the drug.

For this reason investigators have looked for other actions of this drug. One of these is worth mentioning. Adenosine binds to receptors on many cells, including mast cells, and in the mast cell augments the release of histamine and other mediators.

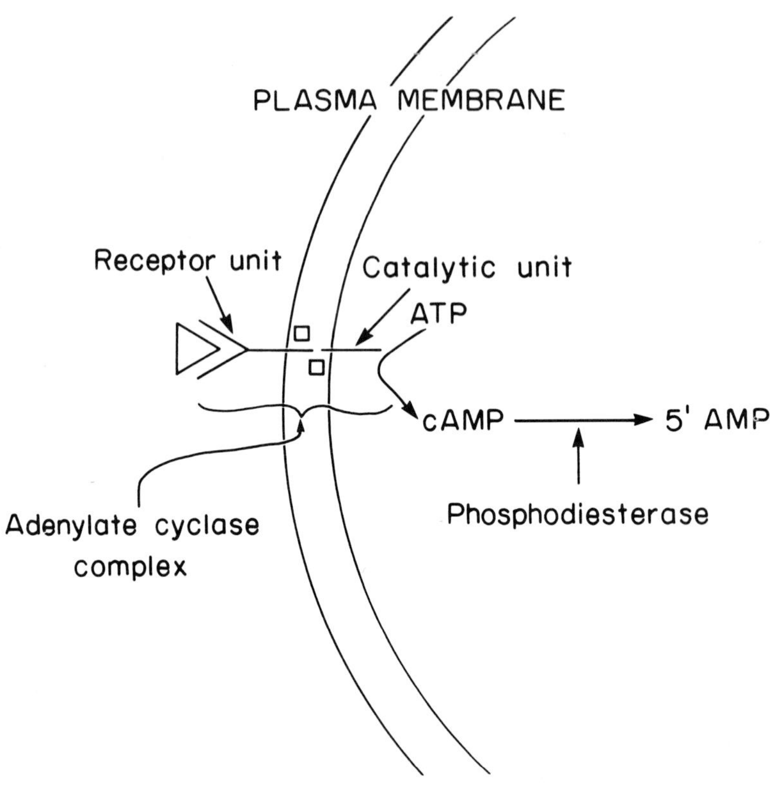

Fig. 15-2. Schematic representation of the adenylate cyclase complex. Adenylate cyclase is made up of a receptor subunit, a catalytic subunit, and one or two connecting proteins. The signal generated by the binding of a ligand to a receptor subunit activates the catalytic unit through the connecting proteins.

Since adenosine is released in areas of hypoxia, one might anticipate that this agent would be present in the asthmatic lung and might contribute to the asthmatic response. Sullivan and his coworkers (Marquard et al., 1978) have demonstrated that theophylline inhibits adenosine binding to mast cells and prevents the concomitant increase in histamine release. The concentrations at which theophylline is effective are very close to the therapeutic levels of theophylline, suggesting that this as an effect of theophylline. Whether this action of theophylline plays a major or minor role in the antiasthmatic potency of theophylline is not known.

ABSORPTIONS, BIOTRANSFORMATION, AND EXCRETION

As mentioned above, because of the limited aqueous solubility of anhydrous theophylline, a number of salts of theophylline have been produced (Table 15-1). Evidence has demonstrated however that the relative aqueous solubility of theophylline or its salts has little effect on the absorption of these preparations and within the limits of the dosage forms (short- or long-acting) all preparations should have identical absorptive characteristics (Weinberger et al, 1981). This does not mean that all preparations are identical. Other factors such as powder versus microcrystaline, hardness or compressions of the tablet, dissolution characteristics of the tablet, and overall bioavailability of the form utilized greatly affect the absorption characteristics. Weinberger et al (1981) has compared the rates of absorption and peak levels of a number of products, and the reader is referred to this article for a more general discussion.

Theoretically, liquid forms of theophylline are more rapidly absorbed than capsules or tablets. However, newer microcrystaline forms may approach the speed of aqueous or ethanolic solutions of theophylline. As shown in Table 15-2, liquids achieve reasonable levels within 15–30 minutes and peak levels are achieved in 30–60 minutes. It should be noted that there is little difference in the absorption of aqueous and alcoholic solutions of theophylline, and the latter should be avoided, particularly in children. Tablets are slightly delayed with peak levels seen in 60–90 minutes. Theophylline preparations are also available in the form of rectal suppositories or enemas. The absorption of theophylline from the rectum is good with peak levels seen in 60 minutes. This is particularly true where solutions are used. The absorption of theophylline from rectal suppositories can, however, be very erratic, probably as a result of incomplete or irregular dissolution of the suppository. In the unusual situation where rectal theophylline is deemed necessary, we recommend that the liquid form be used.

In the past 5 years a number of long-acting theophylline preparations have been introduced and the list of these preparations is growing almost daily. In theory, this dosage form provides an excellent means of achieving relatively stable blood levels with little peak to trough variability and a convenient twice-daily (bid), or more recently once-daily, dose schedule. There seems to be a great deal of variability in the bioavailability and absorptions of these forms, however, which makes a discussion of this group difficult. In general, the choice of a long-acting theophylline preparation should be based on the greatest percentage of bioavailability and lowest peak to trough variability (Weinberger et al., 1981).

After absorption of oral or rectal forms or intravenous (IV) injection, theophylline is distributed in the total body water. This is followed by elimination of the drug via biotransformation and excretion. The actual kinetic model for the decline of plasma theophylline is beyond the scope of this review. However, it is important to note that the decline in plasma theophylline concentration is linear when the log of plasma theophylline concentration is plotted against time. This analysis allows one to calculate the time for the plasma theophylline level to decrease by one-half ($T_{1/2}$). For any given patient, in the absence of other physiological factors the $T_{1/2}$ is a constant.

Theophylline is both excreted unchanged and oxidized by the liver microsomal oxidase system. Approximately 10% is excreted unchanged in the urine, and the

Table 15-2 *Short-Acting Theophylline Preparations*

Form	Onset (Minutes)	Peak (Minutes)
Liquid	15–30	30–60
Tablet	30–60	60–120
Rectal (liquid)	15–30	30–60

major metabolic products are 3-methyl xanthine, 1,3-dimethyluric acid, and 1-methyluric acid. Since the liver oxidase system is extremely variable from individual to individual in the normal state, the metabolic rates ($T_{1/2}$) vary greatly. For this reason it is impossible to predict the actual dose of theophylline necessary to maintain the patients plasma levels within the usual therapeutic range; and, as discussed below, it is imperative that the plasma levels be monitored. There are a number of factors that do predictably alter the plasma $T_{1/2}$, and these are discussed below.

PHARMACOLOGIC EFFECTS OF THEOPHYLLINE

The major pharmacologic effect of theophylline is related to its bronchodilating effect. In normal patients or patients with a history of asthma but who are symptom-free and off all drugs, theophylline has little or no effect on pulmonary function. In patients who have observable bronchospasm as evidenced by decreased FEV_1, MMEF, or peak flow theophylline in adequate doses does decrease bronchospasm when compared to placebo. The plasma level at which theophylline is effective has been examined by a large number of groups using both single-dose and steady-state techniques, and although the results vary from study to study, a plasma level of 10 μg/ml or greater should usually be obtained. Since the toxic level for theophylline is generally considered to be over 20 μg/ml, the therapeutic range is considered to be 10–20 μg/ml. This is not to mean that levels less than 10 μg/ml are ineffective in all patients. There are patients in whom levels of 5–10 μg/ml have proven significant benefit. In the majority of patients, however, levels of at least 10 μg/ml must be achieved. It is also important to note that the bronchodilatory effect of theophylline

Table 15-3 *Pharmacologic Effects of Theophylline*

System	Action
Respiratory	Decrease bronchospasm, increase response to hypoxia, stimulate respiration, increase diaphramatic muscle activity
Cardiac	Ionotrophic; chronotrophic—tachycardia; may decrease right atrial pressure
Vascular	Dilates pulmonary vessels and coronary vessels—decreases pulmonary hypertension and increases coronary flow; constricts cerebral vessels
Involuntary muscle	Relaxation
Kidney	Increases renal plasma flow, and GFR* may have a prominent diuretic effect; may cause hypokalemia
Adrenal	Releases catecholamines
Stomach	Irritates gastric epithelium—related to blood level *not* direct effect
Nervous	Stimulates—may cause convulsions at high blood levels

*Glomerular filtration rate.

increases within the therapeutic range. Thus adjusting the dosage to increase serum theophylline from 12 μg/ml to 18 μg/ml will induce a significant increase in bronchodilation and in some cases may produce therapeutic benefit where one was not seen before. Theophylline should not be abandoned as ineffective or a second agent added until the upper end of the therapeutic range has been explored.

A complete discussion of the pharmacology of theophylline is beyond the scope of this chapter. The major pharmacologic effects are shown in Table 15-3. Like the bronchodilatory effects, most of the actions shown in Table 15-3 are dose-related. In general, the nonpulmonary effects of theophylline are of little consequence when the plasma levels are kept within the therapeutic dose range. Some, such as the diuretic effects, however, may cause patients some concern. It is often possible to decrease the side effects without altering the therapeutic benefits by minor adjustment of the dosage.

ADVERSE REACTIONS

The major adverse reactions seen with theophylline are shown in Table 15-4. It is important to note that these are not idiosyncratic but are related to the blood level of theophylline. As pointed out by Ellis, (1983) the reason for toxicity differs between the adult and pediatric age groups. In children the major cause of toxicity is overdosage, with the majority of toxic reactions seen in patients receiving rectal forms. When analyzed, it was found that in the majority of cases the dose given was far in excess of what is considered adequate on a mg/kg basis. In adults the major causes of toxicity are disease states that decrease the clearance of theophylline by the liver. These include cardiac disease associated with congestive heart failure and hepatic failure. In these cases the dose of theophylline was not decreased to compensate for the increased $T_{1/2}$.

The most common adverse effect is gastrointestinal (Table 15-4). Early symptoms include nausea or anorxea and represent one of the earliest signs of theophylline overdosage, although CNS symptoms may predominate, particularly in adults. These are followed by vomiting, and occasionally hematemesis secondary to vomiting may occur. In the vast majority of cases the GI toxicity is related to the blood level of theophylline and is a central effect, it is *not* due to local irritation of the gastric mucosa. There are patients who experience an immediate feeling of nausea and will

Table 15-4 *Major Adverse Reactions Observed with Theophylline*

System	Action
Gastrointestinal	Anorexia, nausea, vomiting, occasional abdominal pain and diarrhea
Cardiovascular	Tachycardia, other arrythmias; palpitations; hypotension with shock; hypertension
Nervous	Anxiety, agitation, irritability; tremulousness, frank convulsions; insomnia
Other	Diaphoresis; hypokalemia with or without alkalosis

respond to an alteration of the dosage form. This is particularly true of long acting preparations in which little theophylline is released in the stomach, but these occasions are rare. One exception to this rule occurs in the use of elixirs of theophylline where there may be direct gastric mucosal irritation due to ethanol. Since the absorption of theophylline from aqueous solutions (<5% ethanol) is as rapid as that from ethanol solutions, the use of elixirs of theophylline is not warranted.

Central nervous system toxicity is also related to blood levels. The initial signs are irritability and restlessness. These may be followed by agitation and ultimately seizures. The latter symptoms are generally seen at very high blood levels (>35 μg/ml), and at Barnes Hospital all patients who experienced theophylline related seizures had blood levels in excess of 50 μg/ml. Increased respiratory rate and central hyperthermia may also occur, again usually where blood levels are extremely high. In most cases the onset of GI symptoms are a harbinger of more profound side effects; however, seizures in the absence of GI symptoms have been reported.

Cardiovascular toxicity is generally seen in adults, and in the majority of cases these symptoms are seen in patients receiving IV aminophylline therapy, usually in those patients receiving rapid IV infusions. There may be cardiac arrhythmias of the supraventricular or ventricular form, and these probably relate to transient very high levels of theophylline. Hypotension may also be associated with rapid infusions of theophylline.

It must be emphasized that all the toxic effects of theophylline are related to the blood levels of theophylline, and in general these are seen at plasma levels of 20 μg/ml or greater. Since the therapeutic effects are seen at levels of 10 μg/ml or greater, it is possible in the majority of cases to select a dose of theophylline that provides therapeutic benefits without toxicity. Since the therapeutics range is relatively narrow, however, this can be done only with the use of frequent blood theophylline levels, particularly when beginning therapy.

DRUG INTERACTIONS

Interactions between theophylline and other commonly utilized therapeutic agents, although not extensive, are important and should be considered. The majority of these interactions are shown in Table 15-5. In most cases these interactions result in an increase or decrease in the clearance of theophylline, that is, alterations in the $T_{1/2}$. For example, the macrolide antibiotics decrease the clearance of theophylline, and thus the $T_{1/2}$ is prolonged. Patients receiving these agents require a decrease in the theophylline dosage. Metoprolol, in contrast, increases the clearance of theophylline, and thus an increase in the dosage is often necessary to maintain adequate blood levels. The interactions shown in Table 15-5 should be kept in mind when adjusting theophylline levels.

USE OF THEOPHYLLINE

Theophylline serves as a first-line drug in the treatment of asthma. As such, proper use of the drug is critical to achieve maximum benefit. Frequent assessment of plasma theophylline levels cannot be overemphasized, particularly in light of the

Table 15-5 *Factors That Effect Theophylline Elimination*

Factor	Effect on Half-Life
Youth	Decreased
Smoking	Decreased
Obesity	Decreased
Congestive heart failure (acute pulmonary edema)	Increased
Hepatic failure	Increased
Severe COPD	Increased
Viral illness or viral immunization	Increased
Drugs	
Macrolide antibiotics (erythromycin, troleandomycin)	Increased
Cimetidine	Increased
Propranolol	Decreased
Metoprolol	Decreased
Phenobarbital	Decreased
Phenytoin	Decreased
High-protein diet	Decreased

marked differences at which normal individuals metabolize this drug. It is also very important to keep in mind those factors that influence theophylline clearance (see Table 15-5). Most of these factors are easily compensated for as long as they are considered. In general, the most important factors to be considered are age and smoking. The clearance of theophylline decreases with age. Children will require more theophylline than adults and often more frequent dosing. Smoking increases clearance, and thus smokers will require more theophylline than nonsmokers.

Intravenous Theophylline

Patients who present to the hospital in an acute asthmatic attack and who do not respond to inhaled or parenteral beta-adrenergic agents will require the use of IV aminophylline. The standard preparation is aqueous aminophylline (theophylline ethylenediamine). Recently an aqueous solution of theophylline has been introduced for IV infusion. We anticipate that it can be used in a fashion identical to aminophylline except that the dosage will have to be decreased by approximately 15%. In patients who are not receiving theophylline, a loading dose of theophylline is generally warranted. The standard dose is 5.6 mg/kg (6.0 mg/kg in children) given over about 20 minutes. This will generally achieve a blood level within the therapeutic range. In patients who are already receiving theophylline orally we do not recommend that a loading dose be utilized; however, some authors suggest using a loading dose of 2.5–3.0 mg/kg in this situation, and in most cases this provides an adequate level with little risk. In addition, there are tables published on the use of a loading dose of theophylline in patients on oral theophylline based on the blood levels. However, these require the availability of "stat" theophylline plasma levels that are not generally obtainable. In patients where theophylline biotransformation may be severely impaired such as congestive heart failure or hepatic disease, the loading dose should be omitted.

Following the loading dose a constant infusion of aminophylline is begun. In nonsmoking adults an infusion rate of 0.5–0.9 mg/kg/hr will usually provide adequate blood levels. Smokers and children may require greater infusion rates, up to 1.5 mg/kg hr^{-1} to achieve adequate blood levels. In calculating either loading dose or constant infusion rates, the lean body mass should be utilized. Obesity tends to increase theophylline clearance, however, and such patients may require slightly higher infusion rates when the dose is calculated using mean body mass. In all cases the factors that effect theophylline $T_{1/2}$ (Table 15-5) must be kept in mind and the dosages adjusted accordingly. A reduction of $\frac{1}{4}$–$\frac{1}{3}$ may be necessary, and when cardiac and/or hepatic disease is present, even greater reductions should be anticipated. Again, it is important that frequent theophylline blood levels be obtained to assure that a therapeutic level is achieved. This is particularly important where the factors that affect theophylline elimination come into play (Table 15-5). The constant infusion is generally maintained until the patient has stabilized and symptoms of asthma have remitted (see Chapter 21) at which time the patient can be switched to an oral theophylline preparation.

Oral Theophylline

Although there are multiple dosage forms of oral theophylline, these fall into three general classes: liquid, short-acting tablets or capsules and long-acting tablets or capsules. The two former require dosage on a q6h basis, whereas the latter is generally given on a q12h or q8h basis. In any case the total theophylline per 24 hours will be approximately the same, with the exception that patients on longer-acting preparations may require less medication in 24 hours. In the majority of our patients receiving oral theophylline we utilize the long-acting preparations (see below) because they tend to give more stable theophylline blood levels and are significantly more convenient for the patient and increase patient compliance.

Patients receiving IV theophylline may be switched directly to a long-acting

Table 15-6 *Maintenance Doses of Oral Theophylline*

Age	Daily Dose (mg/kg)	Average Daily Dose (mg)
<9 yr	24	—
9–12	20	900
12–16	18	900
>16	10–13	800
>16 smoker	18	1200
>16 heart failure	8	500
>16 hepatic insufficiency	5	350
>16 heart and liver failure	2	150

Table 15-7 *Oral Theophylline Dosage Based on Plasma Drug Levels*

Theophylline Blood Level	Alteration in Dose Necessary
<5*	Increase 100%
5–7.5	Increase 50%
8–10	Increase 20%
11–20	No change necessary unless symptoms persist
21–25	Decrease 20%
26–30	Decrease 33%
31–35	Decrease 50%
>35	Decrease 100%

*Blood levels less than 5 suggest poor patient compliance, and this should be checked before adjusting the dose. For levels greater than 25, omit one or two doses before continuing at a lower level.

theophylline preparation, or one may start with one of the shorter-acting preparations and then switch to a long-acting dose form. In patients who are started directly on an oral preparation we generally start with long-acting preparations, having found no advantage to beginning with short-acting dosage forms.

The recommended dose of theophylline for various age groups is shown in Table 15-6. Again, the various factors that influence the clearance of theophylline must be kept in mind when beginning theophylline, and one should obtain plasma drug levels. The manipulation of the oral dose based on plasma levels is shown in Table 15-7.

Once the patient has been stabilized at a dose within the therapeutic range (10–20 μg/ml), their drug needs should remain constant unless they develop complications such as influenza or other viral infections or receive drugs that alter the theophylline $T_{1/2}$. It is important to note that the plasma level that achieves maximum therapeutic benefit differs from patient to patient. Thus one patient may respond at a plasma level of 8 μg/ml, whereas another may require 17–18 μg/ml. If a patient has a theophylline level in the low therapeutic range and has not responded adequately, therefore, we recommend that the dose of theophylline be increased to reach the plasma levels of over 15 μg/ml before the patient is considered a theophylline failure.

Rectal Suppositories

There are innumerable liquid, short-acting, and long-acting preparations of theophylline or theophylline salts. As discussed above, there is no reason to believe that the actual form of theophylline is of any real benefit, although we discourage the use of alcoholic forms. The major factors are bioavailability, peak to trough variation, and cost. There have been a number of excellent review articles that compare the various forms of this drug in these terms, and the reader is referred to these (Weinberger et al., 1981). Rectal administration of theophylline deserves special comment. In the past rectal suppositories containing aminophylline have been utilized extensively in children. Absorption from this preparation is extremely erratic and has lead to frequent under or over dosing. We do not recommend the use of aminophylline suppositories. When rectal administration is desired, several enema preparations are available. These are well absorbed and should be used instead of suppositories.

CONCLUSION

Theophylline, or its salts, has been in clinical use for approximately 45 years. Recent experience with this drug indicates that it is an extremely valuable agent for the treatment of asthma. We generally use it as the first-line drug in our patients. Although it is not a difficult agent to use, it cannot be overemphasized that plasma levels must be monitored to assure that over- or underdosage does not occur. This combined with an accurate knowledge of drug interactions and disease states that alter the clearance of theophylline should allow one to utilize theophylline and achieve maximum benefit in the treatment of asthma.

Case History

A 24-year-old white male presented with a chief complaint of cough, dyspnea, and wheezing of 3 months' duration. He recently moved into a new home. The patient had a long history of allergic rhinitis and was skin-test-positive to a number of aeroallergens including house dust and mites for which he was receiving appropriate immunotherapy. His asthmatic symptoms were present during the entire day but tended to worsen at night. He had used several over-the-counter preparations for his asthma without any success. Physical examination revealed a boggy nasal mucosa, the chest was hyperresonant to percussion, and there were diffuse inspiratory and expiratory wheezes in all lung fields. Pulmonary function testing (PFT) reveals a forced expiratory volume (FEV_1) that was 60% of predicted and a maximum mid-expiratory flow (MMEF) that was 40% of predicted. Chest x-ray showed only modest hyperaeration.

A diagnosis of chronic moderate asthma was made and the patient was started on a long-acting theophylline preparation 300 mg every 12 hours and inhaled albuterol, 2 puffs every 8 hours. He was advised on the appropriate environmental control and was told to return in 1 week. On return the patient reported that he was considerably improved. He now had only episodic wheezing, generally at night. Physical examination revealed occasional expiratory wheezes in all lung fields. Pulmonary function was considerably improved; however, the MMEF was still less than 75% of predicted. A blood theophylline level was 7.5 μg/ml. The patient's theophylline dose was increased to 450 mg every 12 hours, and he was advised to continue his albuterol.

When seen 2 weeks later, the patient reported that he was symptom-free. Chest examination was entirely normal, and PFTs were greater than 80% of his predicted value. Blood theophylline level was 13 μg/ml. The patient was advised to continue theophylline and discontinue albuterol on a chronic basis. He was told that he could use the albuterol as needed.

One month later the patient developed abdominal pain and was seen by his internist. He was begun on antacids and cimetidine. Several days later he reported nausea and vomiting. Examination at that time revealed no wheezing. A blood theophylline level was 23.0 μg/ml. The patient was advised to decrease theophylline dosage to 300 mg bid and was told that this was necessary because of the cimetidine. He was advised to continue on the lower doses as long as he was taking the cimetidine but return to his former dose if this drug was discontinued.

This case illustrates the efficacy of long-acting theophylline in the treatment of chronic asthma. The need for frequent monitoring of the blood level of this drug is also evident. There are a number of instances where the dose of theophylline will have to be adjusted (Table 15-5), and the patient should be advised of these.

REFERENCES

Ellis, E. F. Theophylline and its derivatives. In Middleton, E., Reed, C. E., and Ellis, E. F. (Eds.) *Allergy Principles and Practice*, St. Louis: The C. V. Mosby Co., 1983.

Hendeles, L., Weinberger, M. Theophylline. In Middleton, E., Reed, C. E., and Ellis, E. F. (Eds.) *Allergy Principles and Practice*, St. Louis: The C. V. Mosby Co., 1983.

Marquardt, D. L., Parker, C. W., Sullivan, T. J. Potentiation of mast cell mediation release by adenosine. *J. Immunol*, 1978, *120*:871.

Weinberger, M. M., Bronsky, E. A. Evaluation of oral bronchodilator therapy in asthmatic children. *I. Ped*, 1974, *84*:421.

Weinberger, M., Hendeles, L., Wong, L. Relationship of formulation and dosing interval to fluctuation of serum theophylline concentration in children with chronic asthma. *J. Ped*, 1981, *99*:145.

SUGGESTED READINGS

Deutsch, R. I., Tashkin, D. P., Simmons, M., Calvarese, B., Wagner, J., & Lee, Y. E. *Ann. Allergy*, 1980 *45*, 137–143.

Fixley, M., Shen, D. D., & Azarnoff, D. L. *Am. Rev. Resp. Dis.*, 1977, *115*, 955–962.

Green, E. R., Green, A. W., Lanc, R., Slaughter, R., Middleton, F., Jr. *J. Pediatr.*, 1981, *98*, 832–834.

Lietman, P. S. *J. Pediatr.*, 1981, *99*, 145–152.

Reitberg, D. P. *Ann. Int. Med.*, 1981, *95*, 582–585.

Renton, K. W., Gray, J. D., & Hall, R. I. *CMA J.* 1980, *23*, 288–290.

Talseth, T., Boye, N. P., Bredesen, J. E., & Kornstad, S. *Ann. Allergy*, 1981, *46*, 279–280.

Westerfield, B. T. (1981) *Am. Rev. Resp. Dis.*, 1981, *124*, 17–20.

QUESTIONS

1. Each of the following is a normal pharmacologic action of theophylline except:
   a. Smooth-muscle relaxation
   b. Chronotropic action on the heart
   c. Ionotropic action on the heart
   d. Cerebral vasodilation
   e. Diuresis

2. A 6-year-old asthmatic child presents with nausea and vomiting. He has regurgitated all his oral medications, including theophylline. In this case the following is true:
   a. Theophylline should be discontinued since it will make the vomiting worse.
   b. The patient should be admitted to the hospital and placed on IV aminophylline to prevent an acute asthmatic episode.
   c. Aminophylline suppositories should be used as an alternative to oral theophylline.

d. Theophylline enemas may be used since the absorption of this form is highly predictable.
e. An elixir of theophylline should be used instead of the tablet form.

3. With the exception of elixir of theophylline, the GI symptoms associated with theophylline are:

   a. Related to the blood level
   b. Highly dependent on the salt of theophylline used
   c. Significantly reduced by the use of an aqueous solution of theophylline
   d. Seen in much greater frequency with the long-acting form of theophylline
   e. Greatly reduced if the drug is taken only with meals

4. A 44-year-old male presents to the emergency room with a 5-hour history of severe wheezing and shortness of breath. His blood gas reveals a PaO_2 of 58, a $PaCO_2$ of 30, and a pH of 7.45. There is significant depression of the FEV_1 and the MMEF. There is no history of smoking. He is not taking oral theophylline. In addition to other measures, the best procedure would be to:

   a. Start the patient on a long-acting theophylline preparation.
   b. Give the patient a loading dose of IV aminophylline 5.6 mm/kg over 20 minutes and then start IV aminophylline at 0.7 mg/kg hr^{-1}.
   c. Start the patient on IV aminophylline at 1.5 mg/kg hr^{-1}.
   d. Give a loading dose of 2.5 mg/kg over 20 minutes and then start IV aminophylline at 0.9 mg/kg hr^{-1}.
   e. Do not use aminophylline since it is not indicated in the acute situation.

5. For each of the following, indicate whether the dose of oral theophylline should be adjusted up, down, or no adjustment needed.

   a. A 44-year-old asthmatic has just been placed on cimetidine.
   b. A 23-year-old asthmatic has just developed an acute viral syndrome.
   c. The asthmatic in case b (above) develops a bacterial bronchitis and is started on erythromycin.
   d. A 37-year-old female with chronic renal failure secondary to pyelonephritis has been started on ampicillin.
   e. A 67-year-old male has just presented with the onset of congestive heart failure.

Answers can be found in Appendix B at the end of the book.

John Alvin Wood

16

Beta-Adrenergic Therapy for Asthma

Beta-adrenergic agonists are an important class of compounds used in treatment of asthma. The actions of these agents are the result of their sympathomimetic effects on the lung. These effects include relaxation of bronchial smooth muscle, inhibition of the release of chemical mediators from mast cells, pulmonary vasodilation, and increased ciliary motility in bronchial epithelium. The oldest of these drugs, epinephrine, is still being used; however, newer synthetic agents are currently available that have the advantage of greater specificity, longer duration of action, and efficacy by the oral route. This chapter deals with the physiology and pharmacology of these drugs and includes a review of the autonomic nervous system and its possible role in asthma.

ANATOMY AND PHYSIOLOGY OF THE AUTONOMIC NERVOUS SYSTEM

The autonomic nervous system controls the involuntary or visceral functions of the body. Some of these include arterial blood pressure, sweating, body temperature, and gastrointestinal (GI) function (Table 16-1). Many of these functions are controlled entirely by the autonomic nervous system, and some only partially.

The autonomic nervous system is controlled centrally in the brain and its outflow is transmitted through the body by two major subdivisions, the sympathetic and the parasympathetic systems (Figs. 16-1 and 16-2). In general, these two systems oppose each other in their actions, although not all organs have innervation by both. For instance, arterioles have almost sole sympathetic innervation. Some organs are innervated by both, although one may be more dominant in strength.

A summary of the sympathetic and parasympathetic functions (Table 16-1) shows that sympathetic stimulation causes excitatory effects in some organs but inhibitory effects in others, and the same is true of the parasympathetic system. Pertinent to this discussion are the effects on the heart and lungs. Sympathetic stimulation to the

ALLERGY: THEORY AND PRACTICE
ISBN 0-8089-1619-X

Table 16-1 *Autonomic Effects on Various Organs of the Body*

Organ	Effect of Sympathetic Stimulation	Effect of Parasympathetic Stimulation
Eye:		
Pupil	Dilated	Contracted
Ciliary muscle	None	Excited
Glands:		
Nasal	Vasoconstriction	Stimulation of thin, copious secretion containing many enzymes
Lacrimal		
Parotid		
Submaxillary		
Gastric		
Pancreatic		
Sweat glands	Copious sweating (cholinergic)	None
Apocrine glands	Thick, odoriferous secretion	None
Heart:		
Muscle	Increased rate Increased force of contraction	Slowed rate Decreased force of atrial contraction
Coronaries	Vasodilated	Constricted
Lungs:		
Bronchi	Dilated	Constricted
Blood vessels	Mildly constricted	None
Gut: Lumen	Decreased peristalsis and tone	Increased peristalsis and tone
Sphincter	Increased tone	Decreased tone
Liver	Glucose released	None
Gallbladder/bile ducts	Inhibited	Excited
Kidney	Decreased output	None
Ureter	Inhibited	Excited
Bladder:		
Detrusor	Inhibited	Excited
Trigone	Excited	Inhibited
Penis	Ejaculation	Erection
Systemic blood vessels		
Abdominal	Constricted	None
Muscle	Cosntricted (adrenergic) Dilated (cholinergic)	None
Skin	Constricted (adrenergic) Dilated (cholinergic)	Dilated
Blood		
Coagulation	Increased	None
Glucose	Increased	None

Table 16-1 *(continued)*

Organ	Effect of Sympathetic Stimulation	Effect of Parasympathetic Stimulation
Basal metabolism	Increased up to 100%	None
Adrenal cortical secretion	Increased	None
Mental activity	Increased	None
Piloerector muscles	Excited	None
Skeletal muscle	Increased glycogenolysis Increased strength	None

From Guyton, A. *Textbook of medical physiology*. Philadelphia: W.B. Saunders, 1981. With permission.

heart increases the rate and force of contractility, whereas parasympathetic stimulation decreases both rate and contractility. Sympathetic and parasympathetic nerves follow the major bronchi and blood vessels in the lung and penetrate into the acina and pleura. These nerves influence smooth muscle tone in the bronchi and blood vessels as well as partly control the secretory function of bronchial glands and type

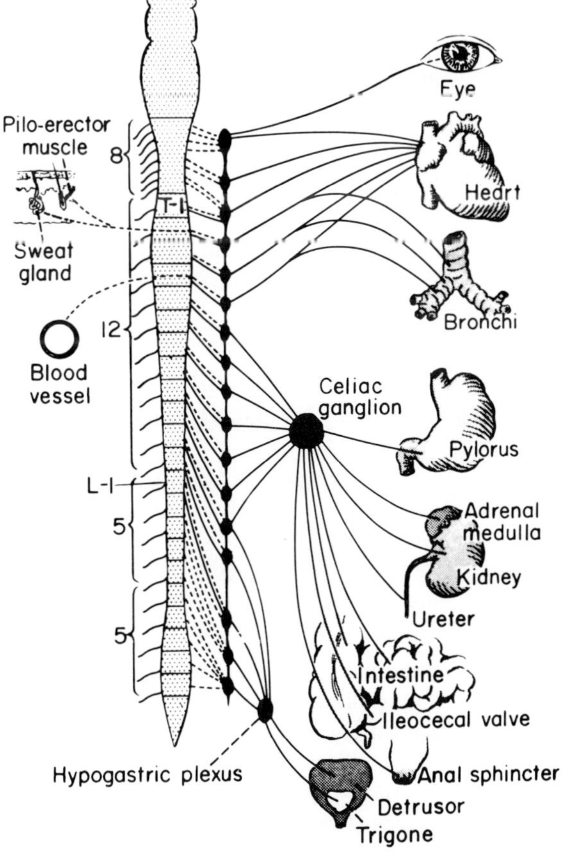

Fig. 16-1. The sympathetic nervous system. From Guyton, A. *Textbook of medical physiology*. Philadelphia: W.B. Saunders, 1981. With permission.

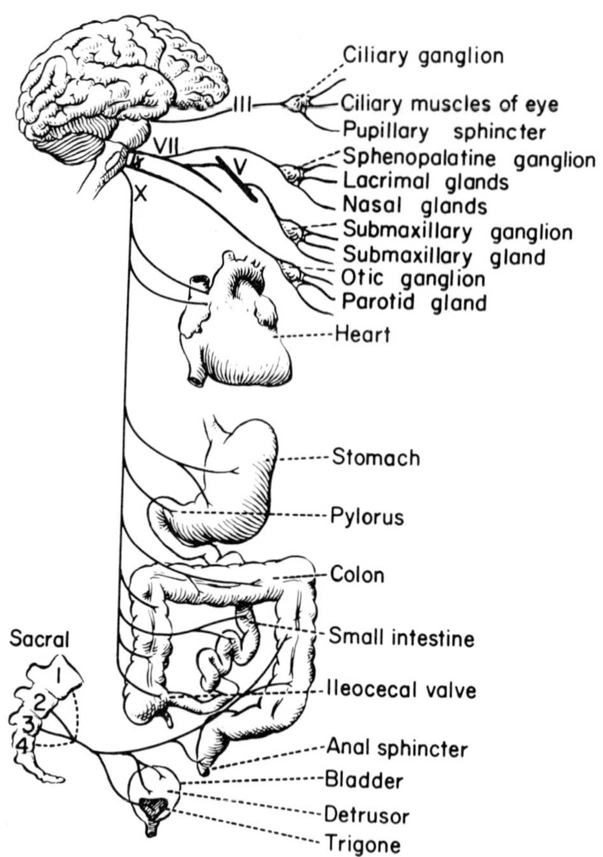

Fig. 16-2. The parasympathetic nervous system. From Guyton, A. *Textbook of medical physiology*. Philadelphia: W.B. Saunders, 1981. With permission.

II alveolar epithelial cells. Sympathetic stimulation causes relaxation of bronchial smooth muscle with resultant bronchodilatation, and parasympathetic stimulation causes increased bronchospasm and bronchial gland secretion (Table 16-2).

Parasympathetic nerves secrete acetylcholine at their nerve endings as their transmittor and for this reason are referred to as cholinergic. Sympathetic nerves secrete norepinephrine and are referred to as adrenergic nerves (Fig. 16-3). Epinephrine is not secreted by sympathetic nerves.

Another source of sympathetic stimulation is the production of norepinephrine and epinephrine by the adrenal glands. The adrenal glands converts norepinephrine into epinephrine. Circulating epinephrine and norepinephrine have almost the same action as sympathetic nerve stimulation, except the former lasts about 10 times longer since they are removed more slowly from the blood (10–30 sec). Norepinephrine has strong actions on the heart and smooth muscle in blood vessels. Epinephrine is almost the same as norepinephrine in its action except for (a) greater cardiac effects, (b) weaker vasoconstrictor activity, (c) greater metabolic effects, and (d) bronchial smooth-muscle relaxation. Norepinephrine has little bronchodiatory effect and may even cause bronchial constriction.

The structure of epinephrine and norepinephrine (Fig. 16-4) consists of a benzene ring with two hydroxyl groups at positions three and four. This part of the

Table 16-2 *Autonomic Innervation of the Lung*

	Sympathetic	Parasympathetic	
Structure	Innervation	Innervation	Role in Asthma
Airway smooth muscle	Causes bronchodilation	Involved in bronchospasm	Bronchospasm as a result of parasympathetic predominance
Goblet cells	No control	No control	Secretion occurs as a direct result of irritant stimulation
Bronchial glands	No control	Stimulation causes secretion	Secretions are more viscous during asthma attack
Mucosal blood vessels	Causes vasodilation	Effect is uncertain	Vasodilation is common in asthma attack: results in mucosal congestion
Lymphatics	No control	No control	Uncertain
Mast cells	Indirectly inhibits	Indirectly stimulates	Stimulation results in release of mediators that cause asthmatic response

From Zimet, I. *Respiratory pharmacology and therapeutics*. Philadelphia: W.B. Saunders, 1978. With permission.

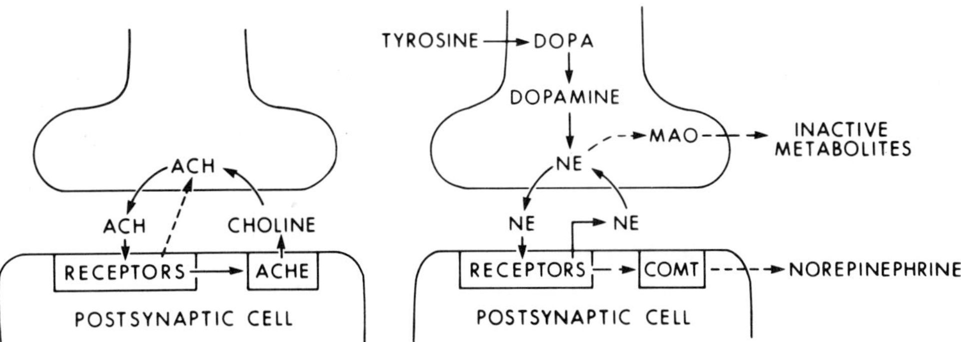

Fig. 16-3. Comparison of neutrotransmitter inactivation in cholinergic (A) and adrenergic (B) neurons. ACH = acetylcholine; ACHE = acetycholineterase; DOPA = dihydroxphenylalanine; MAO = monoamine oxidase; NE = norepinephrine; COMT = catechol-O-methyltransferase. The principal mechanisms for inactivation are indicated by heavy lines, the minor mechanisms by light dashed lines. Acetycholine inactivation by metabolic transformation is an exceptional case, and most neurotransmitters are inactivated by uptake into the presynaptic terminals following their release. ACHE may be localized within the postsynaptic membrane as shown, or within the synaptic clift (myoneural junctions). From Jenson, D. *The principles of physiology*. New York: Appleton Century Crofts, 1980. With permission.

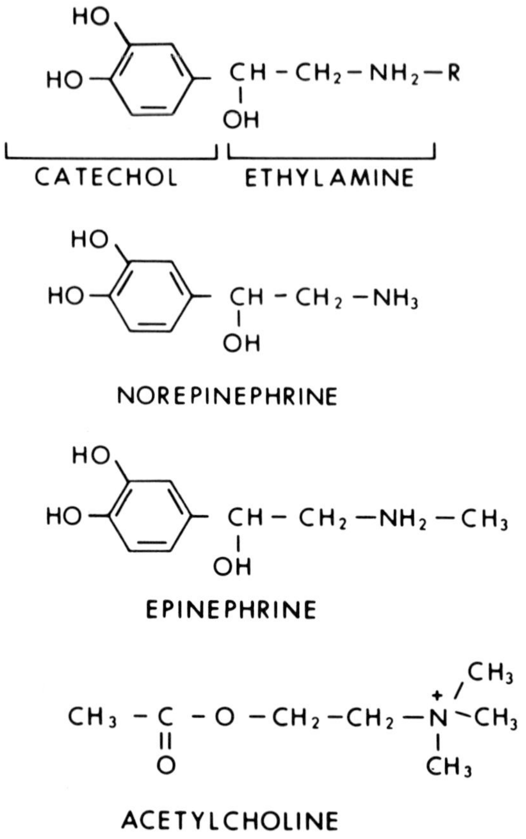

HO
HO — [benzene ring] — CH – CH_2 – NH_2 – R
| OH

CATECHOL ETHYLAMINE

HO
HO — [benzene ring] — CH – CH_2 – NH_3
| OH

NOREPINEPHRINE

HO
HO — [benzene ring] — CH – CH_2 – NH_2 – CH_3
| OH

EPINEPHRINE

CH_3 – C(=O) – O – CH_2 – CH_2 – N^+(CH_3)(CH_3)(CH_3)

ACETYLCHOLINE

Fig. 16-4. Comparison of the structure of catechol-amines and acetylcholine.

structure is referred to as a *catechol*. The catechol then has a side chain of two carbon atoms with a terminal amino group (ethylamine chain). Thus these structures are referred to as catecholamines. Epinephrine differs from norepinephrine by having a methyl (CH_3) group on the terminal amine.

The neurotransmittors acetylcholine and norepinephrine may be inactivated by two mechanisms: (a) metabolically by enzymatic conversion into an inactive compound and (b) reuptake into the presynaptic terminals following its release and interaction with postsynaptic receptors (Fig. 16-3). Acetylcholine is rapidly inactivated by the enzyme acetylcholinesterase. Norepinephrine and epinephrine may be inactivated by the enzymes monoamine oxidase (MAO) and catechol-*o*-methyltransferase (COMT).

In 1948 Ahlquist compared the relative potencies of a number of sympathomimetics and found the order of potency for smooth-muscle contraction to be epinephrine, norepinephrine, and isoproterenol. The order of relaxation of smooth muscle was isoproterenol, epinephrine, and norepinephrine. Cardiac stimulation was similar to those that caused relaxation of smooth muscle. To explain these responses, he theorized tissues had two types of adrenergic receptors—alpha and beta receptors. Epinephrine strongly stimulates both alpha and beta receptors, norepinephrine is more active on alpha, and isoproterenol is more active on beta. A summary of the

Table 16-3 *Response to Stimulation of Adrenoceptors*

Tissue or Process	Alpha Adrenoceptor	Beta Adrenoceptor
Smooth muscle		
Respiratory tract	Contraction (?)	Relaxation
Arteries in skin and viscera	Contraction	Little direct effect
Pulmonary circulation	Contraction	Relaxation
Bronchi	Contraction	Little effect (?)
Skeletal muscle	Contraction	Relaxation
Coronary circulation	Contraction	Relaxation
Intestinal tract	Relaxation	Relaxation
Uterus	Variable	Relaxation
Urinary bladder, trigone, and sphincter	Contraction	No effect
Heart muscle	Minor increase in rate and force of contraction	Increased rate and force of contraction
Skeletal muscle	No effect or facilitation of muscle twitch	Decrease in duration of muscle twitch due to increased rate of recovery
Mast cells sensitized with IgE or IgG antibody	Increased release of histamine and SRS-A after antigenic challenge	Decreased release of histamine and SRS-A after antigenic challenge
Gastric acid secretion	No direct effect	Decreased
Glycogenolysis	Stimulated (?)	Stimulated
Glycolysis	No direct effect	Stimulated
Lipolysis	Inhibited	Stimulated
Insulin secretion	Inhibited	Stimulated

From Middleton, C., Reed, C., & Ellis, E. *Allergy, principles and practice*. St. Louis: C.B. Mosby, 1978. With permission.

effects of stimulation of the alpha and beta receptors is seen in Table 16-3. It can be seen that both excitatory and inhibitory effects are seen in both receptors depending on the tissue or organ that is stimulated.

As an example, isoproterenol differs from epinephrine in that an isopropyl rather than a methyl group is substituted on the terminal amine. This change results in loss of most of the alpha effects of the parent catecholamine. Although isoproterenol is a potent stimulator of beta receptors and is used in the treatment of bronchospasm, it has significant cardiac side effects.

A further division of the beta system of receptors was devised by Lands et al. in 1967. They found other analogs of catecholamines with larger *N*-alkyl substitutes or certain other alkyl substitutes in the side chain were significantly more active in stimulating certain beta receptors than others (Figs. 16-5 and 16-6). The receptors that mediate these effects became known as subtypes $beta_1$ and $beta_2$. $Beta_1$ adrenoreceptors mediate their beta-adrenergic effects on the heart, intestine, and lipolysis. $Beta_2$, adrenoreceptors mediate their effects on smooth muscle in bronchi, uterus, and blood vessels, and glycolosis (Table 16-4).

Selective beta-adrenergic agents would allow one to use a higher dosage of beta

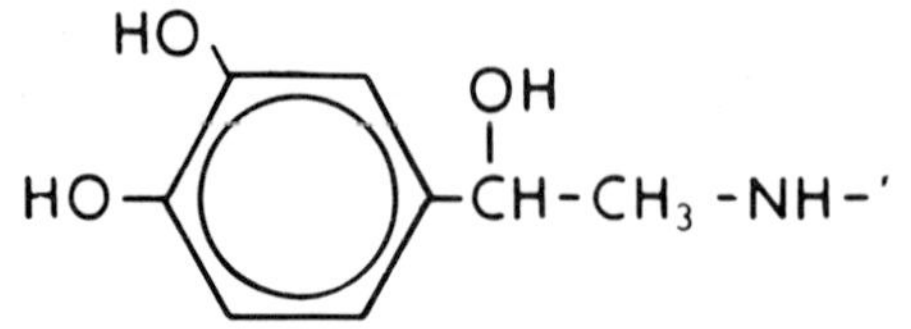

HO, HO (ring), OH

$HO-C_6H_3(OH)-CH(OH)-CH_3-NH-$'

R	Alpha Effects	Beta Effects	
		Beta$_1$	Beta$_2$
H-NOREPINEPHRINE	++	±	
CH_3-EPINEPHRINE	++	++	
$CH(CH_3)_2$ -ISOPROTERENOL	±	++	++
$C(CH_3)_3$ TER-BUTYL	0	+	++

Fig. 16-5. Effect of varying N-alkyl substituent on relative α and β effects in sympathominetic drugs.

stimulators without increasing cardiac toxicity. Thus a beta$_2$ agent would cause bronchodilatation with fewer cardiac effects. The selective beta$_2$ agents now available in the United States are isoethrine, terbutaline, albuterol, and metaproterenol. Other selective beta$_2$ agents, fenoterol and hexoprenaline, are not approved at this time for use in the United States (Fig. 16-6).

It has been shown that the effect of beta-adrenergic stimulation is mediated by the production of cAMP. In the asthmatic 3′5′-cAMP reduces bronchospasm by smooth-muscle relaxation. It also inhibits the release of mediators of inflammation and bronchoconstriction from leukocytes and mast cells respectively. Theophylline also exerts its effect through cAMP. Theophylline and beta-adrenergic products thus increase cyclic AMP by different mechanisms, and the two are additive in their effects.

PHARMACOLOGY OF BETA-ADRENERGIC AGENTS

Beta-adrenergic agents may be administered by aerosolization, parenterally [intravenously (IV) or subcutaneously (SC)], and orally. Some agents are better suited for administration by one route than another, and few are available in the United States in all three forms. Different agents may also be administered by different routes to the same patient. The choice of preparations and route of administration will vary according to the clinical situation. In general the aerosolized and parenteral preparations have a more rapid onset of action and shorter duration of action than

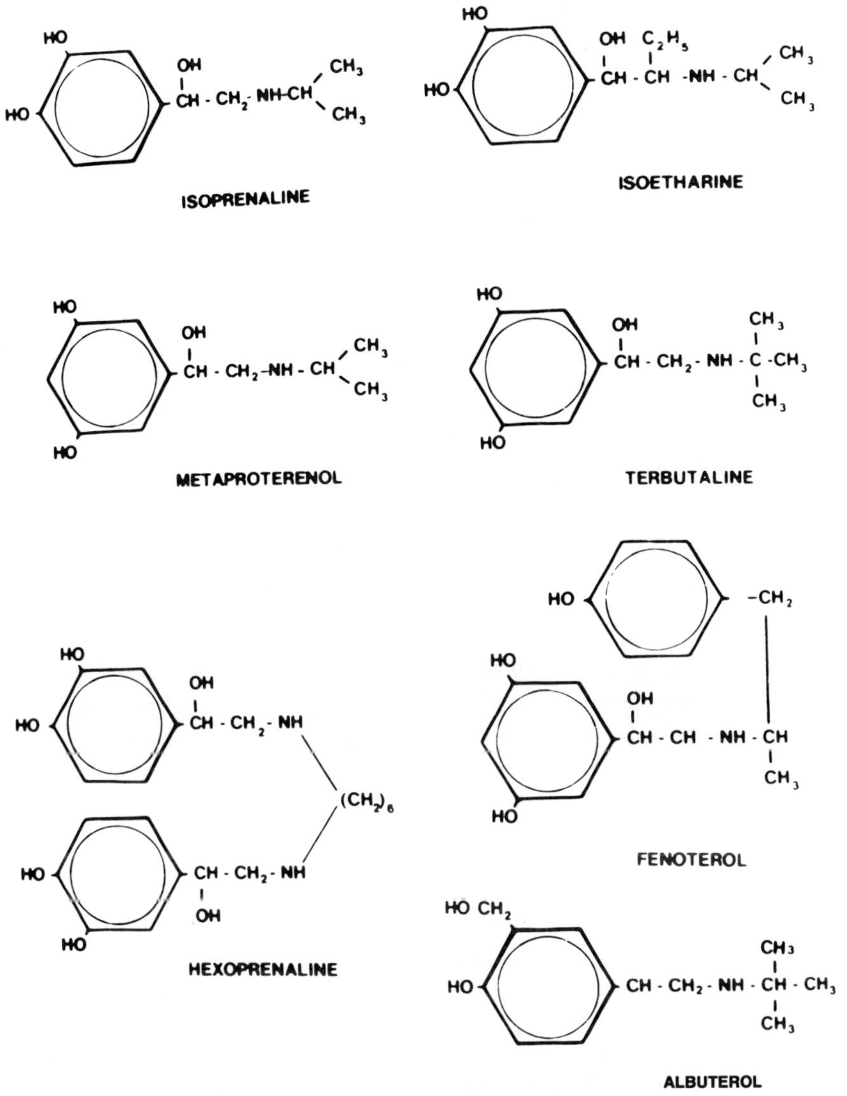

Fig. 16-6. Structure of beta$_2$-specific agonists. From Stein, M. *New directions in asthma*. Park Ridge, Ill: American College of Chest physicians, 1975. With permission.

the oral forms and are most helpful for acute or subacute flares in bronchospasm. Regardless of the mode of administration the desired effect is decreased bronchospasm with resultant decrease in airway resistance, decreased work of breathing, and improved blood gases and alveolar ventilation.

Aerosol

Administration of beta-adrenergic drugs by aerosolization for inhalation has the advantage of rapid onset of action, potent bronchodilatation, and good patient acceptance (Table 16-5). Unfortunately, some preparations are available without prescription and may be used with little patient understanding or direction and are

Table 16-4

Response Involving Beta$_1$ Adrenoceptors	Responses Involving Beta$_2$ Adrenoceptors
Cardiac chronotropy (rate) and inotropy (force of contraction)	Relaxation of smooth muscle in bronchi, uterus, and arteries in skeletal muscle beds
Dilation of coronary blood vessels	
Relaxation of smooth muscle of intestinal tract	Decreased duration of skeletal muscle twitch
Lipolysis but may be beta response in humans	Glycolysis
	Glycogenolysis
	Insulin secretion

From: Middleton, C., Reed, C., & Ellis, E. *Allergy, principles and practice*. St. Louis: C.V. Mosby, 1978. With permission.

potentially dangerous. An epidemic of asthma-associated deaths in Europe in the late 1960s was thought by some to be linked to abuse of aerosolized bronchodilators, although this association has not been seen in this country. Patients using aerosolized bronchodilators should be carefully instructed as to their proper use and cautioned to their potential abuse. Patients with acute bronchospasm may improve transiently with the use of an aerosolized bronchodilator but flare again in a short period of time. These patients should have their bronchodilator program reviewed by their physician if they require frequent use of their aerosolized bronchodilator.

Aerosolized beta-adrenergic drugs may be administered by several methods: hand bulb nebulizers, metered hand-pressurized inhalers, intermittent positive pressure breathing (IPPB), or compressed air-driven nebulizers. Hand-bulb nebulizers have been replaced by metered pressure-driven hand nebulizers because the latter is easier to use and delivers a more uniform dosage. A pressure-driven nebulizer (compressed air or oxygen) is frequently used in a hospital setting, although home pumps can be used in the same manner. Since most patients with bronchoconstriction are hyperinflated, delivery by IPPB is not rational and may potentially lead to increase in hyperinflation and resultant barotrauma (pneumothorax and/or pneumomediastinum).

In general, hand-pressurized nebulizers are intended for those patients who have only occasional wheezing or those taking chronic oral bronchodilators who need additional medication. Some patients are unable to tolerate the side effects of oral beta$_2$, preparations (see below) and aerosolized bronchodilators are often better tolerated. This is because a much smaller dose is needed to give the desired effect, and the drug is applied directly to receptors in the lung. In the hospital setting, aerosolized bronchodilators are an adjuvant to the patient's other bronchodilators and may even be administered by nebulization through a ventilator if the patient is in respiratory failure and intubated. Finally, one can use an aerosolized bronchodilator to determine the response to therapy by measuring pulmonary functions prior to and following administration of the drug. There has recently been an interest in the use of spacers between the patient and the nebulizer in an attempt to improve

Table 16-5 *Aerosol Bronchodilators*

Generic Name	Trade Name	Contents	Recommended Dose	Onset (Minutes)	Peak (Minutes)	Duration (Hours)	Comments
Epinephrine	Medihaler-Epi	0.3 mg/puff	1–2 puffs	1–5 (transient early peak)	<5 mg	2–3	Potent bronchodilator Alpha$_1$, beta$_1$, beta$_2$ effects; better selective beta agents available
	Primatene, Bronkaid	0.2 mg/puff	1–2 puffs, may repeat in 4 hr		90–120		
Isoproterenol	Isuprel, Mistometer	0.125 mg/puff	1–2 puffs up to 5 times/day	2–5	5–30	1–3	Short-acting; significant cardiac side effects; better selective beta agents available
	Solutions	1 : 200	5–15 inhalations q6h				
		1 : 100	3–7 inhalations q6h				
	Medihaler-Iso	0.075 mg/puff	1–2 puffs 4–6 times/day				
Metaproterenol	Alupent aerosol, Metaprel aerosol	0.65 mg/puff	1–3 puffs every q4–6	2–10	30–90	1–15	Longer-acting; more beta$_2$ selectivity
	Alupent solution	0.3 ml in 2 ml NS* every 6 hr				4–6	
Isoetharine	Bronkometer aerosol	0.34 mg/puff	1–2 puffs q4h	5	15–60	1–3	Shorter duration; beta$_2$-selective; No longer with phenylephrine
	Bronkosol	1% solution	0.5 ml in 2-ml NS				
Albuterol	Ventolin, Proventil	0.01 mg/puff	1–2 puffs q6–8h	5	30–60	4–6	Very beta$_2$-selective

*Normal saline.

delivery of the aerosol. The exact shape, length, and degree of added effectiveness of these spacers has yet to be determined.

Metered-hand nebulizers are available, containing isoproterenol, isoetharine, metaproterenol, albuterol, and epinephrine. Because of greater $beta_2$, specificity isoetharine, metaproterenol, and albuterol are usually preferred. Isoproterenol is a very potent bronchodilator and is used in some pulmonary function laboratories to determine the patient's response to bronchodilators. Unfortunately, it has the problem of significant cardiac effects and is of shorter duration of action than the other, more selective agents. The selective $beta_2$ agents may also be used in the same manner in the pulmonary function laboratory.

Solutions of isoproterenol, isoetharine and metaproterenol are available for mixture with saline and administration by a pressure-driven nebulizer with compressed air or oxygen. The advantage of this form of administration is that one can take longer to administer the medication and thus be sure that a full dose is delivered. The disadvantage is that trained personnel and special equipment are required to deliver the medication, and this adds to the expense of this form of therapy.

Oral Administration

Orally administered beta-adrenergic drugs (Table 16-6) can be given alone or in conjunction with other bronchodilators. In general, they are used as an adjuvant to theophylline but are often limited in their dosage by their side effects. Wolfe et al. (1978) have shown the degree of bronchodilatation in asthmatics by terbutaline and theophylline to be additive when used together (Fig. 16-7).

The oral selective beta-adrenergic drugs available are terbutaline, metaproterenol, and albuterol. Ephedrine has been used for years but is not a selective $beta_2$ agent. Tachyphylaxis may be seen when ephedrine is used for long periods of time.

Terbutaline, metaproterenol, and albuterol are administered every 6–8 hours, and the dosage is 2.5–5 mg, 10–20 mg, and 2–4 mg, respectively. It is best to start with the lower dosage because of better patient tolerance and then increase as clinically warranted. The dosage should be adjusted according to patient response and the degree of tolerance by the patient. The disadvantage of oral therapy is that the therapeutic blood level required for bronchodilatation is usually sufficient to produce stimulation of other $beta_2$ and often $beta_1$ receptors at other sites. Oral preparations therefore often have a higher incidence of side effects than administration by aerosolization. The main side effects of these drugs are cardiac (tachycardia, palpitations, arrhythmias) and neuromuscular (nervousness, tremor) and are often dose-related. These side effects are seen early in their use and will often decrease over time. There is also considerable patient variation in these side effects. In general, younger patients tolerate oral beta agonists better than do older patients.

The oral preparations are relatively slow and inefficient for achieving a rapid therapeutic effect. The oral preparations have a peak of action at 2 hours and a duration of action of 4–6 hours and thus are of less benefit in the acute situation. They do, however, have the advantage of ease of administration and consistency of dose delivered.

Parenteral Administration

The parenteral route of administration is usually limited to the acute situation. Both epinephrine and terbutaline can be given subcutaneously (Table 16-7). They have a rapid onset of action (10–15 minutes) and are of short duration of action (1–4

Table 16-6 *Oral Beta Agents*

Generic Name	Trade Name	Content	Recommended Dose	Onset (Minutes)	Peak (Hours)	Duration (Hours)	Comment
Ephedrine	Many available	Varies according to preparation	15–50 mg 4–6 times/day			4–6	Not a $beta_2$ agonist; has $alpha_1$, $beta_1$, $beta_2$ actions; tachyphylaxis occurs; to be avoided for more selective agents
Ephedrine–theophylline combinations	Marax	Ephedrine 25 mg, theophylline 135 mg, Atarax 10 mg	1 tablet 2–4 times/day				Fixed combination of agents makes individual drug adjustments difficult
	Tedral	Theophylline 130 mg, ephedrine 24 mg, phenobarbital 8 mg					Low dose of theophylline per tablet Individual dosages preferred rather than fixed combinations
Metaproterenol	Alupent, Metaprel	20 mg	10–20 mg q6–8h	30	2–2.5		Selective $beta_2$ actions, 17% adverse effects
Terbutaline	Brethine, Bricanyl	2.5, 5 mg	2.5–5 mg q6–8h	30	2–4	4–6	Selective $beta_2$ actions, 20–33% rate of tremor (5-mg dose)
Albuterol	Ventolin, Proventil	2, 4 mg	2–4 mg q6h	30	1–3	4–6	

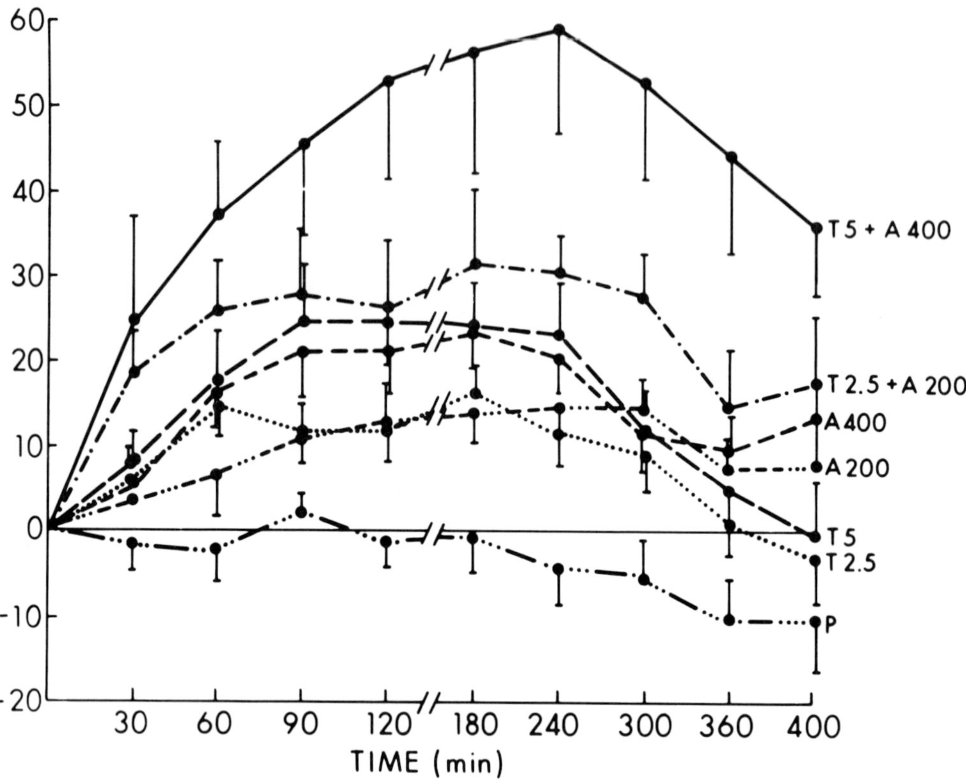

Fig. 16-7. Mean percentage changes in forced expired volume in one second with time after oral administration of drug or placebo. A denotes aminophylline; P denotes placebo; T denotes terbutaline; and the numbers after those letters show the dose in milligrams. From Wolfe, J., Tashkin, D., Calvarese, B., & Simmons, B. *New England Journal of Medicine*, 1978, *298*, 363. With permission.

hours). Repeated epinephrine doses can be given every 20–30 minutes. A total dose of 1–1.5 mg is commonly accepted; however, the exact total dose is not clearly established. Care must be taken to ensure that the correct dose is given since a larger dose could be dangerous because of its potent stimulation of other receptors. The solution should be clear in color, as a brown color represents harmful breakdown of products. Terbutaline 0.25 mg may be administered subcutaneously and if needed may be repeated in 30 minutes. A total of 0.5 mg of terbutaline should not be exceeded within a 4-hour period. Epinephrine is not a selective $beta_2$ agent and activates alpha and beta receptors. Terbutaline when given parenterally loses most of its selective $beta_2$ actions and thus is similar to epinephrine in its action.

Intravenous isoproterenol and terbutaline have been used in the treatment of status asthmaticus. Although this form of therapy may be effective in relieving severe bronchospasm, its hazards are potentially serious and even fatal. Intravenous beta-adrenergic therapy should be reserved for those *very experienced in the use and complications of parenteral sympathomimetics and should be limited for use in an intensive-care setting*.

Table 16-7 *Parenteral Beta Agents*

Generic Name	Trade Name	Content	Recommended Dose	Onset	Peak (Hours)	Duration (Hours)	Comment
Epinephrine	Adrenalin (various preparations)	1 : 1000 solution	0.2–3 ml SC every 20–30 min up to 1.5 mg (1 mg/ml)	10–15 ml	1	1–4	Both alpha and beta actions; caution in patient with cardiac disease
	Sus-Phrine (aqueous plus crystalline solution)	1 : 200	0.05–0.03 ml every q4–6h			8–10	Longer duration of effect
Terbutaline	Bricanyl, Brethine	1 mg in 1 ml	0.25 mg SC; may be repeated in 15–30 min and q4–6h ≤0.5 mg q4–6h	5–15 min	0.5–1	1.5–4	Little $beta_2$ specificity when given parenterally

TOXICITY

Patient intolerance to $beta_2$-adrenergic drugs often results from stimulation of $beta_2$ receptors other than those in the lung. Since $beta_2$ agonists are not totally selective, they may also stimulate $beta_1$ receptors. Finally, side effects may occur that are nonspecific and are unrelated to either $beta_1$ or $beta_2$ receptor stimulation. (See Table 16-8 for a list of relative and absolute contraindications to the use of these drugs.)

$Beta_1$ Effects

It is common with the use of $beta_2$ agonists to see tachycardia or palpitations that, although minor, are often annoying to the patient. Premature artial or ventricular beats may be exaggerated by beta agonists. These drugs may exacerbate abnormal rhythms in patients who have a prior history or arrhythmias. The physician will need to determine whether these effects are minor or of a more serious nature and make necessary dosage adjustments.

$Beta_2$ agonists should be used with caution in patients who have a history of serious arrhythmias or underlying cardiac disease (coronary artery disease, congestive heart failure, congenital heart disease, and valvular heart disease). In those patients use of these agents requires careful observation and monitoring. If there is concern about arrhythmias, 24-hour monitoring will give a more accurate assessment over a longer period of time. Since $beta_1$ stimulation increase rate and force of contraction, angina may be worsened in those with coronary artery disease. Cardiac output may be a problem in those with valvular heart disease, particularly if arrhythmias are precipitated. The effect of beta stimulation may be variable in hypertensive patients. If cardiac output is increased, blood pressure may increase, whereas if peripheral vascular resistance is decreased due to smooth muscle relaxation, blood pressure may fall. Beta agents should be used with caution in patients with thyrotoxicosis.

$Beta_2$ Effects

Since the central nervous system (CNS) and skeletal muscle have $beta_2$ receptors, beta agonists may stimulate these sites. Patients may experience nervousness, agitation, hand tremors, disturbed sleep, or muscle cramps. Men who have prostatic

Table 16-8 *Beta Agonists*

Relative Contraindications	Absolute Contraindications
Recurrent minor arrhythmias	Serious arrhythmias
Recent myocardial infarction	Accelerated angina
Angina associated with arrhythmias	Acute myocardial infarction with arrhythmias
Caution in patients with diabetes, hypertension, hyperthyroidism	Thyroid storm
Patients on MAO inhibitors	Active seizures Hypertensive crisis

enlargement may have difficulty in micturition. Most of these side effects are dose-related and tend to be worse in the elderly. They also improve after continued use of the drug in many patients. Beta agents should be used with caution in the psychiatric patient, as they can cause anxiety or nervousness and may interact with psychiatric medicines (MAO inhibitors).

Nonspecific Effects

One may see nonspecific effects of headache, dizziness, fatigue, weakness, sweating, and anxiety. There are reports of some patients with bronchospasm who decrease their arterial oxygen when they are treated acutely with beta agents. This is secondary to a worsening of ventillation : perfusion ratios since airways can dilate faster than perfusion can shift to the opened areas. This occurs despite increased alveolar ventilation and decreased airway resistance. This problem is not unique to the use of beta agents and may occur with other bronchodilator drugs such as theophylline and can be corrected by the administration of oxygen.

There has been concern that with long-term use of beta agonists a resistance might develop in their bronchodilator properties, although data for this are conflicting. In a recent review of this subject Patterson et al. (1979) state "the balance of evidence is against the hypothesis that significant 'tolerance' or 'resistance' to adrenergic drugs develops in asthmatic subjects who take the drugs on a long-term basis."

BETA-ADRENERGIC BLOCKAGE

In recent years beta-adrenergic blockade agents such as propranolol have come into widespread use for the treatment of angina, hypertension, and arrhythmias. Intraocular beta blocking agents are used for glaucoma since they can decrease intraocular pressure. Beta-adrenergic blockade can promote bronchoconstriction in the asthmatic patient as well as in other bronchospastic disorders. Severe wheezing, status asthmatics, and even death have been reported with oral, parenteral, and intraocular use of these medications. These drugs rarely cause bronchospasm in normal people but accentuate the process in the susceptible patient. Since the sympathetic nervous system plays a minor role in bronchodilation, it is not clear why beta blockade results in bronchoconstriction. Caution needs to be used with these drugs in the asthmatic. Selective $beta_1$ blocking agents have been developed that decrease the incidence and severity of $beta_2$ blockade, although these also are not without risk in certain patients. Should accelerated bronchospasm develop, treatment involves the use of theophilline and $beta_2$ agonists and withdrawal of the beta blockade agents.

SUMMARY

This chapter has reviewed the anatomy and physiology of the autonomic nervous system, particularly in relation to the use of beta agonists. Through modification of the basic catechol structure, epinephrine, selective $beta_2$ agonists are available that give greater bronchodilatation and less cardiac stimulation. Beta agonists are thus another important class of medications available to the physician who treats bronchospasm. These drugs provide additive effects when used with other bronchodilators such as theophylline. Hopefully in the future more selective beta agonists will be developed that totally eliminate undesirable $beta_2$ or $beta_1$ actions. The physician who treats asthma or other forms of bronchospasm should be well acquainted and experienced in the use of these selective $beta_2$ agonists.

Case History

A 15-year-old male patient has a history of episodic wheezing 1–2 times per year. These episodes are usually associated with a viral infection. He is on no daily asthmatic medications. On the day of admission to a local emergency room he developed wheezing associated with a sore throat, coryza, and a mild cough. Examination revealed a young male in moderate respiratory distress with audible wheezing. His blood pressure was 110/80 without paradox, and his pulse was 110. His lungs showed diffuse inspiratory and expiratory wheezing. His pulmonary functions showed a vital capacity of 3.0 liters at 65% of predicted and an FEV_1 of 1.8 liters (60%). His blood gases on room air were $p\text{O}_2$ 64, $p\text{CO}_2$ 28, and pH 7.52. His chest x-ray was normal.

On admission to the emergency room he was given 0.30 ml of aqueous epinephrine subcutaneously, and within 15 minutes his wheezing was improved but was still present. He was then given metaproterenol by nebulization, 0.3 ml in 2 ml normal saline with subsequent total clearing of his wheezing. His FEV_1 increased to 2.6 liters. He was discharged with a prescription for a long-acting theophylline preparation and an albuterol inhaler to use every 6 hours as needed for wheezing. Over the following 2 weeks he remained asymptomatic, with no return of asthma.

REFERENCES

Ahlquist, R. P. *Am. J. Physiol.* 1948, *153*, 586.

Lands, A. M., Arnold, A., McAuliff, J. P., Luduena, F. P., Brown, T. G. *Nature* 1967, *214*, 597.

Patterson, J., Woolcock, A., & Shenfield, G. *Am. Rev. Resp. Dis.*, 1979, *120*, 1149.

Wolfe, J., Tashkin, D., Calvarese, B., & Simmons, B. *New Engl. J. Med.*, 1978, *298*, 363.

SUGGESTED READING

Guyton, A. *Textbook of medical physiology*. Philadelphia: Saunders, 1981.

Inman, W. H. W., & Adelstein, A. M. *Lancet*, 1969, *2*, 279–285.

Jenson, D. *The principles of physiology*. New York: Appleton Century Crofts, 1980.

McFadden, E. R. *J. Allergy Clin. Immunol.*, 1981, *68*, 91.

Middleton, C., Reed, C., & Ellis, E. *Allergy, principles and practice*. St. Louis: Mosby, 1978.

Stein, M. *New directions in asthma*. Park Ridge, Ill: American College of Chest Physicians, 1975.

Webb-Johnson, D. C., Chir, B., & Andrews, J. L. *New Engl. J. Med.*, 1977, *297*, 476.

Weinberger, M., Hendeles, L., & Ahrens, R. *Pediatr. Clin. N. Am.*, 1981, *28*, 47.

Weinberger, P., & Patterson, R. *Ann. Intern. Med.*, 1978, *89*, 234.

Weiss, E., & Segal, M. *Bronchial asthma—mechanisms and therapeutics*. Boston: Little, Brown, 1976.

Zimet, I. *Respiratory pharmacology and therapeutics*. Philadelphia: Saunders, 1978.

QUESTIONS

1. Beta$_2$ stimulation results in all of the following except:
   a. relaxation of smooth muscle in bronchi
   b. glycolosis
   c. increased rate and force of cardiac contractility
   d. glycogenolysis
2. Which of the following is not a selective beta$_2$ agonists?
   a. isoetharine
   b. terbutaline
   c. isoproterenol
   d. albuterol
   e. metaproterenol
3. Beta agents are absolutely contraindicated in which one of the following?
   a. diabetes
   b. hypertension
   c. controlled angina
   d. serious ventricular arrhythmias
   e. pregnancy
4. Which of the following is a problem with the use of beta-blockade therapy?
   a. hypotension
   b. arrhythmias
   c. worsening of bronchospasm in the asthmatic
   d. precipitating wheezing in normal people
5. Aerosolized bronchodilators have the following advantages except:
   a. ease of administration
   b. good patient tolerance
   c. good bronchodilatory response
   d. lack of easy patient abuse
   e. several agents available

Answers can be found in Appendix B at the end of the book.

Peter Konig

17

Cromolyn Sodium

Cromolyn sodium (cromolyn) was first described in the medical literature in 1967 by Altounyan (1967), who demonstrated its protective effect against allergen-induced asthma initially in one patient, himself. This was an important discovery because it introduced a new class of drugs with purely prophylactic action into the management of asthma and a number of other illnesses.

MECHANISM OF ACTION

Cromolyn has a prophylactic action against asthmatic symptoms, but no direct bronchodilator, antihistamine, or anti-inflammatory activity; therefore, its unique mechanism of action raised a great deal of interest. Initial studies showed that cromolyn prevented or inhibited the liberation of mediators of anaphylaxis from sensitized and nonsensitized mast cells, after immunologic or nonimmunologic (e.g., Compound 48/80) challenge (Cox, 1967, 1971; Orr, 1977). These *in vitro* results have been confirmed by *in vivo* provocation tests and clinical trials. Thus cromolyn was shown to have a marked protective effect against the bronchospasm resulting from the inhalation of allergens, both in patients who had immediate and in those with dual (immediate and late) reactions (Booij-Noord et al., 1971) (Fig. 17-1).

In addition to its protection against allergen-induced asthma, cromolyn has a protective effect against a wide variety of nonimmunologic triggering mechanisms. These include cold-air hyperventilation, cold-air hyperventilation exercise and sulfur dioxide inhalation.

More recently, differences were noted between the protection against allergens, which clearly involves release of mediators from mast cells and against triggers in which mediator release probably is not involved. Thus the duration of protection against exercise provocation is much shorter than against allergen provocation (Fig.

ALLERGY: THEORY AND PRACTICE
ISBN 0-8089-1619-X

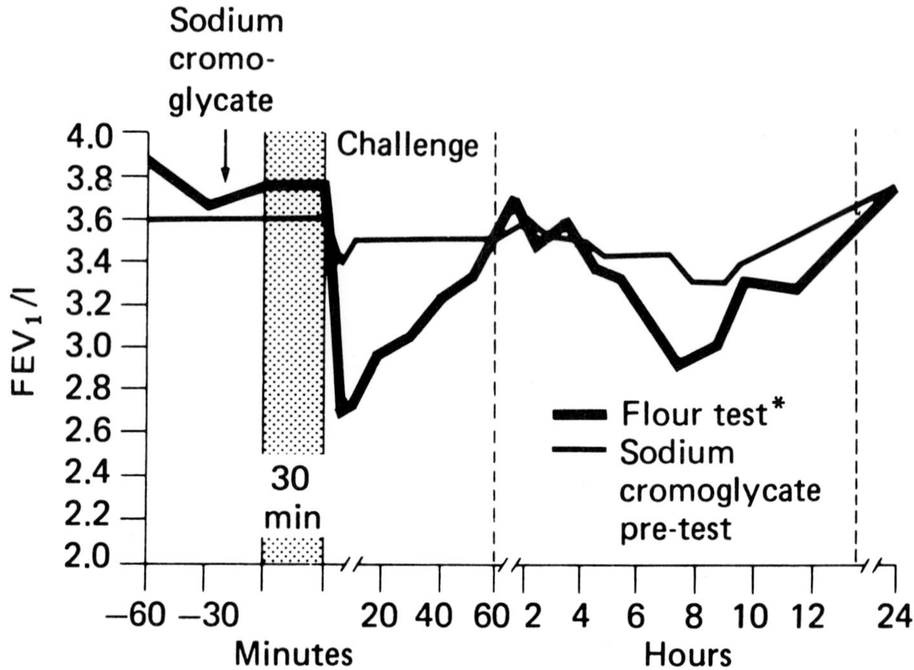

Fig. 17-1. Immediate and late asthmatic reactions to an occupational-type exposure test with wheat flour. Both reactions were blocked by pretest inhalation of 40 mg of cromolyn sodium. Altounyan, R. E. C. In J. Pepys & A. M. Edwards (Eds.). *The mast cell: Its role in health and disease*. Kent, England: Pitman Medical, 1979, p. 199. With permission.

17-2), and the dose response of the drug against allergen and sulfur dioxide is very different (Altounyan, 1979) (Fig. 17-3).

This suggests the existence of at least two different receptors for the drug and hence of another mechanism of action in addition to mast cell protection. The nature of this alternative mechanism is not known at this time, but it is presumed to be neurophysiologic.

A very interesting action of cromolyn is its long-term effect on nonspecific bronchial hyperreactivity. A number of studies have shown a considerable reduction of histamine-induced bronchospasm brought about by prolonged therapy with cromolyn (Altounyan, 1979; Dickson, 1979) (Fig. 17-4). The fact that all these studies were carried out during the allergen season of the patients whereas another study done outside the allergen season could not show the same effect casts some light on the possible mechanism of this phenomenon. It has been shown that allergen challenge, especially in patients who display a late (i.e., nonimmediate) reaction, increases nonspecific bronchial hyperreactivity. Cromolyn prevents the late reaction, and perhaps this could explain its effect on nonspecific hyperreactivity. As bronchial hyperreactivity correlates with clinical severity of asthma and drug regimes needed to control it (König, 1974), the ability of cromolyn to reduce airway reactivity could be a very important factor for long-term prognosis. It is possible that the carryover effect found in some clinical trials is due to this reduction in bronchial hyperreactivity,

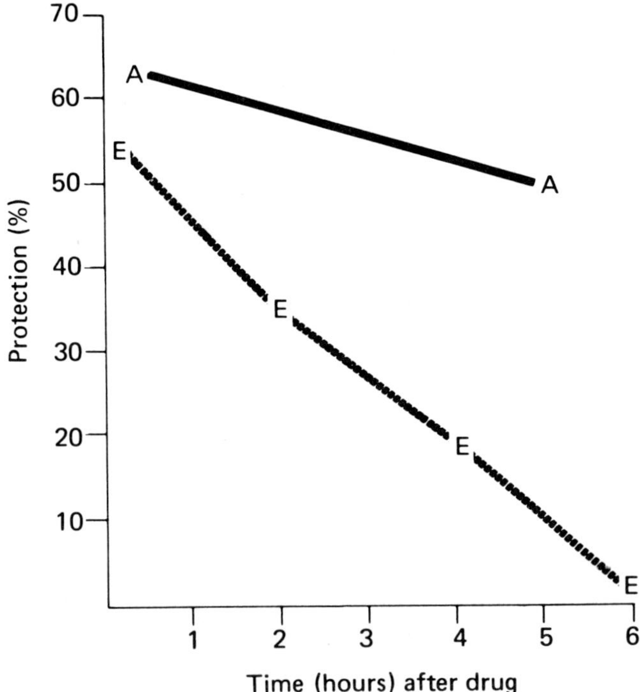

Fig. 17-2. Duration of protection afforded by cromolyn sodium against challenge with antigen and exercise in two groups of patients: (A) antigen challenge in 10 subjects and (E) exercise challenge in 80 children. Altounyan, R. E. C. In J. Pepys & A. M. Edwards (Eds.). *The mast cell: Its role in health and disease*. Kent, England: Pitman Medical, 1979, p. 203. With permission.

which then perhaps also explains the gradual improvement of patients taking cromolyn regularly sometimes with continuing improvement over weeks and months (Toogood et al., 1978).

CLINICAL TRIALS

Numerous clinical trials of cromolyn in patients with asthma have been described in the literature. These trials were generally very favorable, showing that approximately 60–80% of properly selected patients benefit from cromolyn prophylaxis. Silverman et al. (1972), in a year-long double-blind trial in children, found that 71% of those on cromolyn were doing well compared to only 24% on placebo.

Crisp et al., (1974) demonstrated an improvement in 87% of children treated with cromolyn, and the improvement was maintained in 80% for 2.5–4 years. Most of these studies were well controlled, and some of them involved follow-up of 1–10 years. No tolerance to cromolyn was found in a 3–5-year follow-up study in asthmatic children (Godfrey et al., 1975).

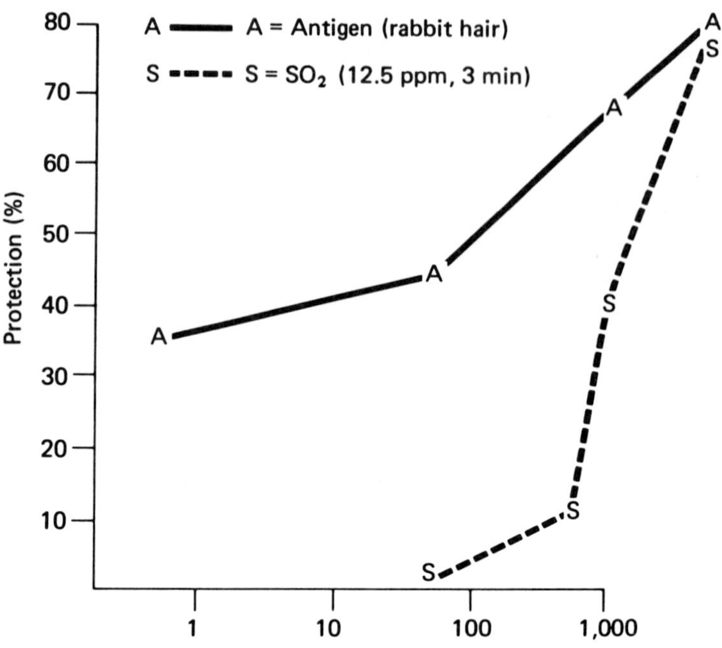

Fig. 17-3. Protective effect of cromolyn sodium against challenge with antigen or sulfur dioxide. Altounyan, R. E. C. In J. Pepys & A. M. Edwards (Eds.). *The mast cell: Its role in health and disease*. Kent, England: Pitman Medical, 1979, p. 205. With permission.

SAFETY

Cromolyn has been shown to be one of the safest drugs in use for the management of asthma. In a prospective multicenter study from Rhode Island, in 375 asthmatics the prevalence of side effects was 2% (1% in children); none of them was life-threatening, and they were all reversible (dermatitis, myositis, gastroenteritis) (Settipane et al., 1979). Toogood and his associates (Toogood, 1977) in a long-term, multicenter study based on chest radiographs, tests of lung diffusing capacity, and postmortem data, could not find evidence of fibrosis or other changes attributable to the chronic inhalation of cromolyn in the form of a fine, dry powder. Follow-up studies of up to 10 years have been reported in children, with no serious adverse reactions (Dickson & Cole, 1979).

A few cases of hypersensitivity, including at least two cases of anaphylaxis to cromolyn, have been described (Sheffer, et al., 1975; Brown et al., 1981), but the incidence is extremely low, considering the large numbers of patients treated with cromolyn since 1968.

Mild, transient side effects such as cough and sometimes wheezing due to the irritant effect of the dry powder inhalation are seldom sufficiently severe to warrant discontinuation of therapy. A dose of an inhaled adrenergic agent given before cromolyn inhalation can usually prevent these side effects.

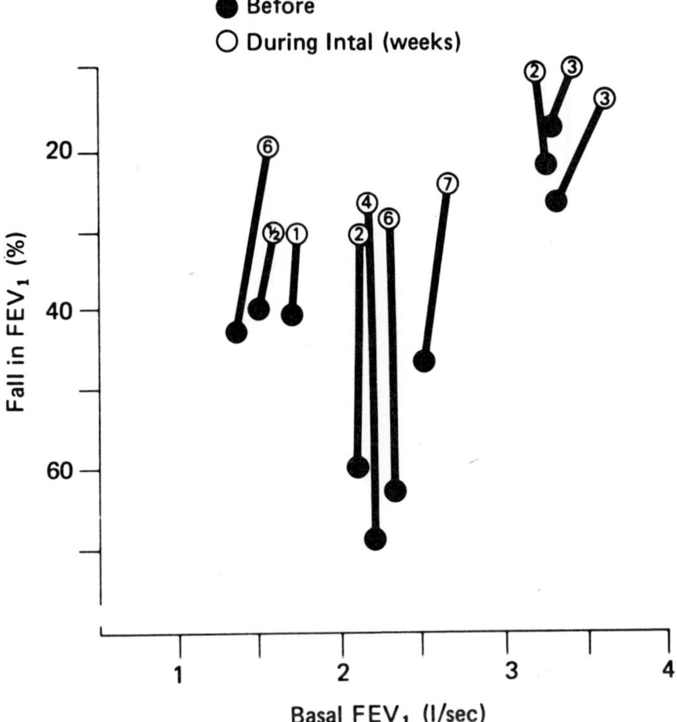

Fig. 17-4. Effect of a standard histamine challenge on FEV_1 in 10 allergic subjects before and during treatment with cromolyn sodium (Intal). Patients selected showed little or no change in basal FEV_1 values at times of histamine provocation tests. Altounyan, R. E. C. In J. Pepys & A. M. Edwards (Eds.). *The mast cell: Its role in health and disease*. Kent, England: Pitman Medical, 1979, p. 207. With permission.

INDICATIONS

Short-Term Use

In certain situations, such as the prevention of exercise-induced asthma, a single dose of cromolyn a few minutes before the exercise is generally very effective. Another situation in which occasional, as opposed to round-the clock, use of cromolyn can be useful is the anticipated short-term exposure to known allergens. Examples of this are visits to houses in which there are pets to which the patient is allergic and workers who occasionally have to work with laboratory animals. Cromolyn is dramatically effective in blocking the antigen-induced bronchospasm in such cases.

Long-Term Use

The following are the most important indications for cromolyn:

1. Perennial asthma, causing symptoms most of the time, not satisfactorily controlled by bronchodilators given on an "as needed" (prn) basis.

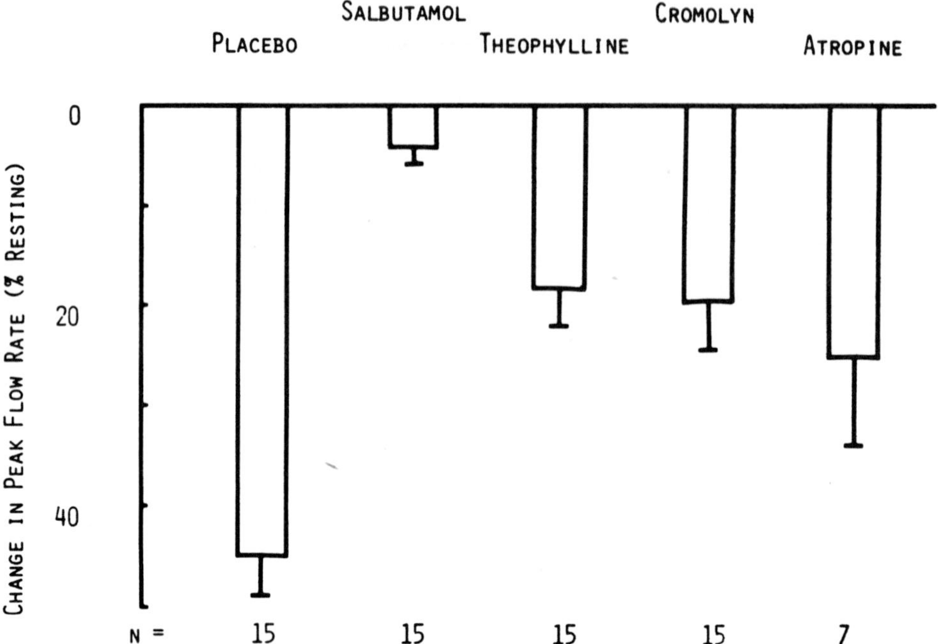

Fig. 17-5. Bronchoconstriction after exercise expressed as percent change from resting value immediately before exercise but after receiving the drugs indicated. The bars show ±SEM. Albuterol (Salbutamol) was given as pressurized aerosol in all but two patients who had tablets; theophylline was given in tablets, cromolyn by turboinhaler (Spinhaler), and atropine was nebulized. From König, P. *Adv. Asthma Allergy Pulm. Dis.*, 1978, 5(3), p. 2-8. With permission.

2. Seasonal asthma, not controlled by prn bronchodilators and immunotherapy (when indicated). Cromolyn can be used concomitantly with immunotherapy to protect the patient until the hyposensitization injections take effect.
3. Exercise-induced asthma in a patient who is very active and needs continuous protection. For occasional exercise, an inhaled beta$_2$ agent, given a few minutes before exercise, is likely to be more effective (Godfrey & König, 1976) (Fig. 17-5).

SELECTION OF PATIENTS

Many of the clinical trials sought to define those patients who were most likely to benefit from cromolyn.

Extrinsic versus Intrinsic Asthma

In 1967 it was believed that cromolyn was a specific anti-allergic drug, and thus it was assumed that allergic patients with extrinsic (atopic) asthma would do better on cromolyn therapy than intrinsic asthmatics. Although some studies have shown better results in extrinsic asthma, the difference was slight and other studies could not find any difference in the relative response rates. Thus in a study in adults (Brompton Hospital/Medical Research Council Collaborative Trial, 1972) the failure rate for cromolyn was 15% in extrinsic asthmatics and 44% in intrinsic asthmatics. This difference was *not* statistically significant, possibly because of relatively small numbers of patients. The American Academy of Allergy Drug Committee, in a controlled study in 252 asthmatics, found patient preference for cromolyn to be 58.6% in extrinsic and 40.9% in intrinsic patients. Some studies revealed no benefit in intrinsic asthmatics, whereas another controlled study actually found that intrinsic patients did better than extrinsic cases.

The degree of atopy also does not seem to be clearly associated with cromolyn success or failure. Toogood and collaborators (1978) found a marginally significant correlation of cromolyn success with a number of positive skin tests, but not with total IgE levels. A study in children, total IgE level, number of positive skin tests, and family history of atopy revealed no difference between cromolyn successes and failures. On the other hand, Charpin and associates (1971) found a success rate of 93% in patients with positive skin tests correlating with positive bronchial challenge tests, as compared with 64% success rate in skin-test-negative asthmatics.

Effect of Age on Response to Cromolyn

There seems to be a slight tendency for children placed on cromolyn therapy to do better than adults, although in a study involving patients of ages 11–60 years, no correlation was found between age and the steroid-sparing effect of cromolyn (Toogood et al., 1978). Among adult patients, younger adults seem to do slightly better than older ones. The possible slight differences in success rates in favor of younger and more allergic asthmatics are not sufficient to exclude any individual patient from the benefit of an adequate trial with cromolyn.

Other Criteria

Patient selection should be based on frequency and severity of symptoms rather than age or type of asthma. Patients having symptoms most of the time, limited in their exercise tolerance, missing a significant number of school or work days, or having disturbed nights despite adequate bronchodilator therapy given on a prn basis, are candidates for a trial of cromolyn.

Best results are obtained when it is used as a "first-line" prophylactic drug, before round-the-clock theophylline, adrenergic agents on a continuous basis, or corticosteroids are tried. Many disappointments in the past were due to the selection of intractable cases, those in whom round-the-clock treatment with theophylline and possible other drugs also, already had been tried unsuccessfully.

The decision as to whether cromolyn or theophylline should be the drug of choice as the first-line prophylactic agent should be based on a number of criteria: efficacy, safety, minor side effects, cost, and convenience.

Regarding efficacy, there are at this time four studies in the literature comparing cromolyn and theophylline. In a collaborative study performed in children in London, England and in Denver, Colorado, a significant advantage to theophylline was found in only one out of three criteria used. On the other hand, our study found cromolyn better in one out of three criteria (no difference in the other two), and two further studies revealed no difference at all between the two drugs.

In terms of safety, cromolyn clearly is superior. Cost is lower for theophylline, but if the cost of blood level determinations is added, which are necessary from time to time for the safety of theophylline therapy, the difference in cost is not very great. The convenience factor favors theophylline especially when controlled release formulations are administered twice daily. Cromolyn is usually given 3–4 times daily, although some patients can be controlled on a twice-daily (bid) regimen. Compliance is a problem with both drugs, as it is for any long-term medication.

The concept of a topical drug, such as cromolyn, delivered directly to the lung, with virtually no other pharmacologic effects, as opposed to the systemic administration of theophylline, a drug with multiple effects on many other organs, is attractive. The long-term reduction in nonspecific bronchial reactivity is another advantage for cromolyn. Using a bronchodilator round the clock, reduces the options one has for treating breakthrough attacks. This is even more of a problem in patients treated with theophylline plus adrenergic agents continuously.

PRACTICAL CONSIDERATIONS FOR CROMOLYN THERAPY

Starting a Patient on Cromolyn

Because cromolyn is an inhaled medication, one must achieve a certain patency of the airways. Even in ideal conditions, only about 8% of a 20-mg dose reaches the lungs; the remainder is swallowed and eliminated through the gut, without any effect on the lungs. The amount that is inhaled into the airways can be correlated with pulmonary function; therefore, airways obstruction should be reversed with bronchodilators and if necessary, a short course of systemic corticosteroids before initiating cromolyn therapy.

Probably the most frequent cause of treatment failure with any kind of inhaled medication including cromolyn is lack of adequate patient instruction about the proper technique of inhalation. The patient must be shown how to use the special turboinhaler (Spinhaler), and the technique must be rechecked on subsequent visits, especially if clinical results are not satisfactory. Improper technique will result in very little or no cromolyn reaching the lungs. Patient education should also include an explanation of the purely prophylactic nature of cromolyn, so that the patient does not expect instant relief.

Dosage

The starting dose is four capsules daily at regular intervals. A trial should last at least 6 weeks. Initially, other therapy, such as bronchodilators, should be continued unchanged. If results are not satisfactory, raising the dose of cromolyn to six capsules daily has been shown to change failure to success in about 50% of patients. Up to 8 capsules daily have been used without increasing the side-effects.

Progressive improvement starts in the first days or weeks and can continue for up to 6 months. After the first 6 weeks, if the symptoms of asthma are well controlled, the dose can be reduced to three and sometimes to two capsules daily. A patient who remains asymptomatic for 6 months may not need round-the-clock drug prophylaxis any longer, and a gradual withdrawal of cromolyn can be tried, reducing the dose by one capsule daily, at weekly or longer intervals.

Breakthrough Attacks

These should be treated promptly with bronchodilators, added to the cromolyn, which should *not* be discontinued, except if the patient is too dyspneic to be able to use the Spinhaler. An inhaled beta-adrenergic agent, given a few minutes before the cromolyn, will aid in dilating the bronchi and allowing the cromolyn to penetrate deeper and will also help to reduce the transient irritant effects of the fine powder.

Modes of Administration

The commercially available cromolyn in the United States is in capsules of 20 mg of cromolyn with 20 mg of lactose, given by a turboinhaler (Spinhaler) and capsules of solutions for nebulization 20 mg per 2 ml.

Most children 4 years or older can be taught to use a Spinhaler, and some as young as 2.5 years have been successfully treated (Geller-Bernstein, 1979). A whistle that can be attached to the Spinhaler can help to teach young children, and the intensity of the sound it emits indicates whether the inspiratory effort is adequate. For those too young to use the Spinhaler, the solution for nebulization can be administered by a power-driven nebulizer.

In Europe cromolyn has become recently available as a pressurized aerosol, which could be very useful for patients (especially adults) in whom inhalation of the dry powder causes cough or wheezing.

Failure of Cromolyn Prophylaxis

If a patient's symptoms are not adequately controlled on cromolyn, one can either add another drug or drugs on a round-the-clock basis or replace the cromolyn.

Replacement of cromolyn with inhaled beclomethasone (after an initial overlap of 1–2 weeks) is usually sufficient to control the symptoms. The combination of the two does not seem to offer any advantage over beclomethasone alone in the majority of patients. However, Altounyan has reported that there are some asthmatics who do better on a combination of cromolyn and a corticosteroid than on either drug alone (Altounyan & Howell, 1969). This is not unexpected considering the very different modes of action of these two classes of drug.

USE OF CROMOLYN IN OTHER DISEASES

Nasalcrom (Cromolyn Sodium) has recently been released in the U.S. for intranasal administration. Experimental studies have shown that cromolyn as a powder or 4% aqueous solution can inhibit reactions in the nose. Clinical trials in seasonal allergic rhinitis generally have produced favorable results, especially when intranasal cromolyn was administered as a micronized powder. In trials using a nasal spray, cromolyn was better than placebo in some but not all studies. The dosage was usually 10 mg in each nostril 4 times daily. Some, but not all, studies reported improvements of eye symptoms of hay fever, following the *nasal* administration of cromolyn.

Several studies revealed favorable results in perennial rhinitis, although results tend to be poorer than in seasonal allergic rhinitis. Interestingly, in perennial rhinitis, the presence of allergy does not seem to affect success or failure of cromolyn.

If the patient has marked nasal congestion or discharge, a topical decongestant (such as phenylephrine) and an antihistamine for the first days of cromolyn therapy, will increase the changes of a successful cromolyn trial.

In addition to rhinitis, in which the value of cromolyn as a therapeutic agent has been well established, there are a number of other diseases in which treatment with cromolyn has been tried, but the data are too inadequate or controversial to draw firm conclusions regarding the place of the drug in these diseases.

Oral administration of cromolyn was found useful in some cases of food allergy. In the form of 1–2% eye drops, cromolyn was found to be effective in vernal keratoconjunctivitis. Opticrom, a 4% solution of cromolyn sodium has recently been released for use in the eyes. In atopic eczema one investigator claimed good results with a 10% cromolyn ointment while another study could not reproduce these results. Other diseases in which cromolyn was tried with some degree of promise include ulcerative colitis (Mani, 1976), and systemic mastocytosis (Soter et al., 1979).

Case History

A 17-year-old white male presented with a chief complaint of shortness of breath when running.

The patient had been in excellent health all his life without atopic complaints. He had recently joined the high-school cross-country running club and stated that 10–15 minutes after he began to run he noted wheezing and dyspnea, which forced him to stop. On some occasions he was able to keep running and the symptoms disappeared.

Physical examination revealed a healthy white male. There was no wheezing, but workup revealed a normal CBC, urine analysis, and SMA-6, and his IgE was 35 IV/ml. Routine skin testing to common inhalant allergens was negative. Pulmonary function testing revealed normal FVC and FEV_1 at rest. The patient was exercised on a treadmill 15° elevation to a heart rate of 80% of maximum for 12 minutes. Following the exercise there was a 40% fall in FEV_1 accompanied by audible wheezing and subjective dyspnea. The patient was treated with an aerosolized $beta_2$ agonist with prompt resolution of symptoms. On the following day the patient was exercised 20 minutes after inhaling 20 mg of cromolyn sodium by Spinhaler. There was a 9% fall in FEV_1 and no wheezing or shortness of breath.

Accordingly, the patient was instructed to take 20 mg of cromolyn sodium 15–20 minutes before running. On this regimen he has done extremely well and is now engaged in competitive cross-country running without difficulty.

This case illustrates the efficacy of cromolyn sodium as a prophylactic agent in exercise-induced asthma.

REFERENCES

Altounyan, R. E. C. *Acta Allergol.*, 1967, *22*, 487–488.

Altounyan, R. E. C. In J. Pepys, & A. M. Edwards (Eds.), *The mast cell: Its role in health and disease*. Kent, England: Pitman Medical, 1979, pp. 199–216.

Altounyan, R. E. C., & Howell, J. B. L. *Respiration*, 1969, *26*(S), 131–140.

Booij-Noord, H., Orie, N. G. M., & de Vries, K. *J. Allergy*, 1971, *48*, 344–354.

Brompton Hospital/Medical Research Council Collaborative Trial. *Br. Med. J.*, 1972, *4*, 383–388.

Brown, L. A., Kaplan, R. A., Benjamin, P. A., Hoffman, L. S., & Shearer, W. T. Immunoglobulin E-mediated anaphylaxis with inhaled cromolyn sodium. *J. Allergy Clin. Immunol.*, 1981, *68*, 416.

Charpin, J., Gayrard, P., Orlando, J. P., & Razouk, H. *J. Franc. Med. Chir. Thorac.*, 1971, *25*, 679–689.

Cox, J. S. G. *Nature (Lond.)*, 1967, *216*, 1328–1329.

Cox, J. S. G. *Br. J. Dis. Chest*, 1971, *65*, 189–204.

Crisp, J., Ostrander, C., Giannini, A., Stroup, G., & Deamer, W. C. *JAMA*, 1974, *229*, 787–788.

Dickson, W., & Cole, M. Severe asthma in children—a 10 year follow-up. In J. Pepys, & A. M. Edwards (Eds.), *The mast cell: Its role in health and disease*. Kent, England: Pitman Medical Publishing Co., Ltd., 1979, p. 343.

Dickson, W. In J. Pepys, & A. W. Frankland (Eds.), *Disodium cromoglycate in allergic airways disease*. London: Butterworths, 1979, pp. 105–119.

Geller-Bernstein, C. An assessment of the effect of Lomudal spin-inhaler treatment in young children. In Pepys, J., & Edwards, A. M. (Eds.) *The mast cell: Its role in health and disease*. Kent, England: Pitman Medical Publishing Co., Ltd., 1979, p. 249.

Godfrey, S., Balfour-Lynn, L., & König, P. *J. Pediatr.*, 1975, *87*, 465–473.

Godfrey, S., & König, P. *Thorax*, 1976, *31*, 137–143.

König, P. Ph.D. thesis, University of London, 1974.

Mani, J., Green, F. H. Y., Lloyd, G., Fox, M., & Turnberg, L. A. Treatment of ulcerative colitis with oral disodium cromolycate. A double-blind controlled trial. *Lancet* 1976, *1*, 439.

Maider, S. A. Treatment of atopic eczema in children: Clinical trail of 10% sodium cromolycate ointment. *Br. Med. J.* 1979, *1*, 1570.

Orr, T. S. C. Mode of action of disodium cromoglycate. *Acta Allergol. Suppl.*, 1977, *32* (13), 9.

Settipane, G. A., Klein, D. E., Boyd, G. K., Sturan, J. H., Freye, H. B., & Weltman, J. K. *JAMA*, 1979, *241*, 811–813.

Sheffer, A. L., Rocklin, R. E., & Goetzl, E. J. *New Engl. J. Med.*, 1975, *293*, 1220–1224.

Silverman, M., Connolly, N. M., & Balfour-Lynn, L. *Br. Med. J.*, 1972, *3*, 378–381.

Soter, N. A., Austen, K. F., & Wasserman, S. I. Oral disodium cromolycate in treatment of sytemic mastocytosis. *N. E. J. M.*, 1979, *301*, 465.

Toogood, J. H. *Acta. Allergol.* (S13), 1977, *32*, 44–54.

Toogood, J. H., Lefcoe, N. M., Wonnacott, T. M., McCourtie, D. R., & Mullin, J. K. *Adv. Asthma Allergy Pulm. Dis.*, 1978, *5*, 2–15.

Zachariae, H., Afzeliush, & Laurberg, G. Topically applied sodium cromolycate in atopic dermatitis. Transact. Int. Mast Cell Symposium. Davos, 1979.

SUGGESTED READING

Bernstein, I. L., Siegel, S. C., Brandon, M. L., Brown, E. B., Evans, R. R., Feinberg, A. R., Friedlander, S., Krumholz, R. A., Hadley, R. A., Handelman, N. I., Thurston, D., and Yumate, M. *J. Allergy Clin. Immunol.*, 1972, *50*, 235–245.

Pepys, J., & Frankland, A. W. (Eds.). *Disodium cromoglyciate in allergic airways disease*. London: Butterworths, 1979.

Pepys, J., & Edwards, A. M. (Eds.). *The mast cell: Its role in health and disease*. Kent, England: Pitman Medical, 1979.

Toogood, J. H., Lefcoe, N. M., Wonnacott, T. M., McCourtie, D. R., & Mullin, J. K. *Adv. Asthma Allergy Pulm. Dis.*, 1978, *5*, 2–15.

QUESTIONS

1. Which of the following are direct actions of cromolyn sodium?

   a. Antihistaminic
   b. Anti-inflammatory

c. Inhibit mediator release from mast cells
d. Direct bronchodilator
e. All of the above

2. Cromolyn inhibits mediator release from mast cells or basophils *in vivo* induced by which of the following?

a. Inhibition of specific antigen
b. Exercise
c. Inhalation of sulfur dioxide
d. Hyperventilation with cold air
e. All of the above

3. In contrast to corticosteroids or beta-adrenergic agents cromolyn:

a. Is very effective in patients in status asthmaticus
b. Prevents both the immediate and late response following bronchial inhalation challenge
c. Cannot be used in children less than 6 years old
d. Is ineffective in patients with intrinsic asthma
e. All of the above

4. Cromolyn is effective in each of the following situations except:

a. Seasonal asthma not controlled by prn (as-needed) bronchodilators
b. Perennial asthma
c. Prophylactically in exercise induced asthma
d. As an adjunct to therapy in the wheezing asthmatic with extreme bronchospasm.
e. All of the above

5. With respect to cromolyn therapy which of the following are true?

a. The major cause of cromolyn treatment failure is inadequate patient instruction.
b. Cromolyn therapy should be reserved for use in steroid-dependent asthmatics.
c. Under any circumstances no more than four 20-mg capsules/day should be prescribed.
d. Cromolyn should be used with great caution since the incidence of side effects is extremely high.
e. Because of its solubility properties cromolyn cannot be used for allergic disorders other than asthma.

Answers can be found in Appendix B at the end of the book.

Arnold Dankner

18

Steroids

The pharmacologic use of glucocorticosteroids (steroid) results in suppression of the manifestations of allergic disease, but the association of potentially serious side effects necessitates a careful assessment of probable patient benefits and risks. This chapter reviews the current understanding of the therapeutic mechanisms of steroid action, potential adverse reactions, and recommended modes of administration. Steroid treatment of asthma may include administration by oral, parenteral, and topical (inhalation) routes and may be required briefly or on a long-term basis. Since dose, route, and duration of therapy markedly influence the effects of steroids, their use in the therapy of asthma is presented to exemplify generally applicable principles.

MECHANISM OF ACTION

The mechanisms by which steroids suppress the manifestations of allergic disorders are complex and certainly not fully understood. Species differences in steroid sensitivity and the questionable validity of equating many *in vitro* observations to *in vivo* events has retarded our understanding of how steroids work. Humans are relatively resistant to steroid effects as compared to some laboratory animals (mouse, rat, and rabbit) (Claman, 1972). A failure to recognize this distinction resulted in the erroneous application of observations made in many of the earlier animal studies to human physiology (Claman, 1975). It is difficult to interpret observations *in vitro* on the effects of steroids at concentrations that *in vivo* are only fleetingly, if at all, achievable (Fauci, 1979). Since steroids cause a significant redistribution of leukocytes and alter the opportunity for cell interaction, the impact on cell function resulting from steroid induced cell redistribution cannot be reflected in most *in vitro* studies.

ALLERGY: THEORY AND PRACTICE
ISBN 0-8089-1619-X

Intracellular Mechanics

Investigations of the intracellular mechanisms of steroid activity have resulted in observations strongly supporting the following hypothesis (Baxter, 1972; Baxter & Funder, 1979); steroids diffuse through cell membranes and reversibly combine with and activate intracytoplasma-specific receptors. The active steroid-receptor complex becomes bound to nucleoproteins and induces messenger RNA to direct enzyme or other protein synthesis, resulting in various effects. Steroids presumably act in additional ways since some observed effects occur too rapidly to be explained by a model requiring protein synthesis.

Anti-inflammatory and Immunosuppressive Effects

It is customary to catagorize therapeutic steroid effects as those that are anti-inflammatory and those that are immunosuppressive; however, few effects fall exclusively into either category. The beneficial effects of steroids in the treatment of the allergic states are believed to be almost entirely the result of anti-inflammatory effects.

Cell Movement

It has been known for many years that steroids cause neutrophil leukocytosis and a reduction in the number of circulating lymphocytes, monocytosis, eosinophils, and basophils (Table 18-1). In recent years the movement of these cells has been extensively studied and reviewed (Fauci, 1979). Thymus-derived (T) lymphocytes are redistributed to extravascular compartments, primarily the spleen, lymph nodes, thoracic duct, and bone marrow. Single bolus administration of steroid results in maximum lymphopenia in 4–6 hours with return to normal in 24 hours. The effects

Table 18-1 *Steroid Effect on Leukocyte Distribution*

Circulating cells increased	
Neutrophils	Increased release from bone marrow; prolonged circulatory half-life; inhibited movement to inflammatory sites
Circulating cells decreased	
Lymphocytes	Greater effect on T- than B-cell migration; cells move to extravascular sites*
Eosinophils, basophils	Probably redistributed to extravascular sites
Monocytes	Decreased release from bone marrow; reduced migratory response to lymphokines; probably redistributed to extravascular sites

*Primary extravascular sites are spleen, lymph nodes, thoracic duct, and bone marrow.

on lymphocyte counts are similar in degree with a small dose (15 mg) or a large dose (100 mg) of prednisone, but larger doses have a greater effect on cell function. The effects of steroids on circulating B lymphocytes appear limited compared to their effects on T cells and the differential depletion of T cell subsets has led to the speculation that a mechanism by which steroids modulate immunologic reactivity may be by altering the balance between suppressor and helper T cells (Fauci, 1979).

Steroids cause a monocytopenia that is probably due primarily to cell redistribution similar to that observed with lymphocytes. In addition, monocytopenia results from decreased release of these cells from the bone marrow and inhibition of their migratory response to lymphokines. Neutrophilia after steroid administration results from a combination of inhibition of neutrophil dispersion to inflammatory sites, increased release from bone marrow stores, and a prolonged half-life of the circulating cells. Eosinopenia was originally thought due to cell lysis but is now believed to be the result of redistribution. Basophil counts fall in response to steroid administration, but, perhaps because sparcity makes then difficult to track, there is little in the literature regarding their disposition.

Humeral Mediators

The details of steroid effect on lymphokine production and function is generally unclear. Studies concerning the action of steroids on the lymphokine, macrophage migration inhibition factor (MIF), indicate a decreased antigen induced production *in vivo* and, in most studies, an *in vitro* decrease in macrophage response to MIF (Stevenson & Fauci, 1981). High-dose steroid administration significantly depresses IgG and IgA blood levels with minimal or no effect on IgM levels (Posey et al., 1978), whereas IgE levels may transiently rise (Posey et al., 1978). Most important is the absence of any evidence that these alterations in immunoglobulin level significantly affect antibody response (Claman, 1975; Fauci, 1979).

Steroids decrease histamine synthesis release and rate of skin binding (rat) but not tissue stores. Steroids do not significantly effect wheal-and-flare allergy skin tests (Slott and Zwieman, 1974). There is a steroid-induced reduction in whole blood histamine probably directly related to the fall in the number of circulating basophils. High steroid doses suppress complement titers in animal experiments, but it is unknown whether this is immunologically relevant for steroid-treated patients (Atkinson & Frank, 1973).

Steroids inhibit formation of prostaglandins and slow-reacting substance by preventing their precursor, arachidonic acid, from being released from phospholipids (Blackwell et al., 1980; Hirata et al., 1980). Treatment with steroids may require several days to achieve maximal inhibition of prostaglandin synthesis (Metz, 1981).

Lysosome Membrane Stabilization

Steroids stabilize membranes, including those of the lysosomes (Claman, 1975; Fauci, 1979; Greaves, 1976). Evidence of this stabilization is based largely on *in vitro* observations at high concentrations; therefore, the significance of this action in therapeutic doses is debatable. Concentrations of steroid that are clearly attainable *in vivo* do effect the function as well as the migration of monocytes (Fauci, 1979). Steroids impair monocyte bacteriocidal and fungicidal activity by mechanisms not well understood but possibly by interference with lysomal function.

Beta-Adrenergic Responsiveness

It has been demonstrated that steroids are required for a normal adrenergic response. The leukocytes of asthmatic patients have reduced responsiveness to isoproterenol stimulation; responsiveness can be restored by steroids (Parker et al., 1973). The beta-adrenergic receptors in cell membranes are continuously being synthesized and degraded. Exposure to hydrocortisone results in a marked increase in the rate of their synthesis in human lung cells (Fraser & Venter, 1980). Clinical studies have confirmed the enhancement of response to catecholamines in steroid-treated asthmatics (Holgate et al., 1977).

Cyclic 3′,5′-Monophosphate (cAMP)

It is believed that cyclic nucleotides regulate many of the functions of cells involved in immunologic reactions including the release of mediators of the allergic and inflammatory responses. Steroids increase the level of lymphocyte cAMP, which occurs in response to beta-adrenergic drugs (Parker et al., 1973) and also amplifies the increase of cAMP produced in lymphocytes by prostaglandin E_1 (Mendelsohn et al., 1973). The observed cAMP increases may be partially the result of steroid inhibition of the cyclic nucleotide phosphodiesterase (Lee & Reed, 1977).

Vascular Effects

Steroids diminish the extravasation of fluids and cells through the vascular walls probably because of direct effects on the blood vessel endothelial cells and their effects on the migratory leukocytes and modulation of the mediators of inflammation described above (section on humeral mediators). In addition, studies indicate a vasoconstrictor effect of steroids attributable to antagonism of the vasodilating effects of prostaglandin E and bradykinin (Greaves & Hanissian, 1976).

TRANSPORT AND METABOLISM

Cortisol (hydrocortisone) is the principal glucocorticosteroid in humans. Only 8% of circulating hydrocortisone is free to interact with cells. Of the remainder, 22% is bound with low affinity to albumin and 70% with high affinity to an α-2-globulin (transcortin). There is no evidence that transcortin is necessary for biologic activity of steroids. The transcortin-bound cortisol seems to act as a steroid reservoir, and equilibrium is rapidly achieved between bound and free steroid. The synthetic analogs of hydrocortisone, with the exception of prednisolone, are poorly bound to transcortin (Morris, 1980).

Steroids are degraded principally in the liver but also by other tissues and are then excreted by the kidneys and in the feces. Reported plasma half-life in minutes for hydrocortisone is 80–115, prednisone 60, prednisolone 115–252, and dexamethasone 110–210 (Axelrod, 1976). Effects of steroids persist long after steroids leave the plasma, and there is little correlation of plasma half-life to relative duration of action among the various steroid analogs. Duration of biologic activity is influenced by dose and varies with tissue type. Biologic half-life of steroids is customarily denoted by measurement of the duration of hypothalamic-pituitary suppression.

Since a large percentage of circulating steroid is attached to albumin, hypoalbuminemia increases the unbound steroid free for tissue effect. Metabolic state also influences steroid biologic effects, with hyperthyroidism causing more rapid plasma clearance and the reverse noted in hypothyroidism. Accordingly, there is a decreased effect from a given steroid dose in the hyperthyroid state and an increased effect in the hypothyroid state. Concomitant administration of certain drugs results in a decrease in steroid effect; this has been demonstrated with phenobarbital, diphenylhydantoin, ephedrine, and rifampin. These drugs accelerate hepatic clearance of steroids by microsomal enzymes.

SIDE EFFECTS

Steroids administered in pharmacologic doses may cause a multitude of well-known undesirable effects. For a more detailed consideration of these side effects, the reader is referred to comprehensive reviews (Streeten & Phil, 1975). The major adverse effects may be classified as those that occur with relative predictability (Table 18-2). Also to be considered are the adverse effects associated with steroid withdrawal.

Predictable

The predictable side effects will gradually occur in most patients receiving pharmacologic doses of steroids for long periods of time. Larger doses accelerate the appearance and increase the severity of these adverse effects. Included are the steroid effects commonly associated with Cushing's syndrome. There is a redistribution of fat leading to central obesity and moon facies. Hypertension develops frequently. High doses of hydrocortisone result in sodium retention and potassium loss, but these mineral effects are less significant with the synthetic steroid analogs. Hypothalamic and pituitary suppression results in the decreased formation of adrenocorticosteroid hormone (ACTH), causing adrenal insufficiency and eventually adrenal

Table 18-2 *Steroid Side Effects*

Predictable	Unpredictable
Central obesity and moon facies	Psychiatric reactions
Hypertension	Pseudotumor cerebri
Sodium retention and potassium loss	Glaucoma
Hypothalamic-pituitary-adrenal insufficiency	Postcapsular cataracts
Skin atrophy	Peptic ulcer
Hirsutism	Pancreatitis
Acne	Avascular bone necrosis
Delayed wound healing	Increased infections
Retarded linear bone growth in children	
Osteoporosis	
Glucose intolerance	
Muscle wasting	

cortical atrophy. The skin gradually atrophies, becoming increasingly fragile with consequent tearing and bruising from minor trauma. Hirsutism and acne develop frequently. Wound healing is delayed. There is retardation of the linear bone growth of children. Osteoporosis, glucose intolerance, and muscle wasting occur, commensurate with the known metabolic steroid actions.

Unpredictable

Sporadically and unpredictably occurring side effects are less frequent and associated with predisposing factors either poorly identified or totally unknown. An increased incidence of certain complications associated with the disease process being treated may also be attributable to steroid therapy, but the increment of increase is very difficult to determine and speculative.

Among the unpredictable adverse effects are psychiatric reactions, including inappropriate euphoria and frank psychosis. In a study of acute adverse reactions to prednisone in 718 hospitalized patients there was a striking correlation of the occurrence of psychiatric reactions with dose, a correlation not observed with other reactions (Boston, 1972).

There is a marked difference of sensitivity within the population to the rise of intraocular pressure induced by steroids (Schwartz, 1978) and risk of precipitation of glaucoma. Postcapsular cataracts may develop in both children and adults and are associated mostly with long-term administration. Pseudotumor cerebri occurs more frequently in children, and its mechanism is unknown.

Peptic ulcer disease as a complication of steroid therapy was described from the earliest days of cortisone therapy. Analysis of the combined data of many clinical reports indicates peptic ulcer is a rare complication of steroid therapy except with prolonged use, high dose or previous ulcer history (Conn & Blitzer, 1976; Messer et al., 1983).

Steroid associated with clincially diagnosed pancreatitis is rare but has been reported. Pancreatitis at autopsy is much higher in steroid-treated patients than in matched patients not treated with steroids (Dojovne & Azrnoff, 1975; Walton, 1975).

Avascular bone necrosis has been reported in association with steroid therapy, but primarily in patients receiving high doses and for relatively long periods of times (Richards et al., 1980). The mechanism is unknown, and since it occurs in patients not receiving steroids, particularly as a part of the course of rheumatoid arthritis, the significance of the role of steroids is still debated (Dojovne & Azrnoff, 1975).

Increased susceptibility to bacterial, fungal, viral, and parasitic infection is well established. What is uncertain is the magnitude of risk to the patient. With the doses generally used for treatment of the allergic state, and particularly with short-time use, the risk appears to be very small. Even in long-term use, when the dose is small or moderate, the increased risk of infection is not readily descernible to the clinician. Studies that are available suggest that infections become more common in patients receiving greater than 20–40 mg of prednisone daily (Fauci, 1979).

It has been recommended that patients with positive tuberculin tests on prolonged steroid therapy receive prophylactic isoniazid (INH). However, observations of asthmatics on long-term steroid treatment, even with positive tuberculin tests, have not indicated an increased incidence of active tuberculosis (Schatz et al., 1976). Since INH is hepatotoxic it has been recommended for prophylactic use in steroid treated asthmatics only when there is a documented history of previous tuberculosis (Schatz et al., 1976). It should be noted that daily administration of more than 15 mg of prednisone will suppress intermediate strength tuberculin reactivity (Schatz et al., 1976) but that this reactivity will be retained on very high steroid doses (80 mg) administered on an alternate-day schedule (McGregor, 1969).

Contrary to early fears based primarily on rodent experiments, steroids do not seem to present a teratogenic risk to the human fetus (Wilson, 1973). However, babies of women on 10 mg of prednisone daily throughout pregnancy have been found to have a significant decrease in birth weight (Reinish et al., 1978). Steroid therapy does not seem to increase the risk of maternal or fetal complications and should not be withheld when required to control asthma during pregnancy (Schatz et al., 1975; Snyder & Snyder, 1978).

Withdrawal

Signs and symptoms of withdrawal observed in steroid-dependent patients may include adrenal insufficiency, fatigue, weakness, arthralgia, anorexia, nausea, desquamation of skin, orthostatic hypotension, syncope, and hypoglycemia (Byyny, 1976). Treatment consists of steroid replacement followed by more gradual dose reduction. More serious is the potential for stress-related collapse and death in the adrenopituitary suppressed patient no longer supported by exogenous steroid. Various protocols have been devised to test adrenal sufficiency by comparing plasma cortisol basal levels with those in response to exogenous ACTH (Byyny, 1966; Thorn, 1974). In the absence of such testing it is prudent to assume that adrenopituitary insufficiency may continue for 1 year or longer. Potentially adrenal-insufficient patients should be promptly supported with steroid administration during or, when anticipation is possible, before stress. These patients should have appropriate medical alert tags and wallet cards.

MINIMIZING SIDE EFFECTS

General Measures

Any consideration of reducing the occurrence and intensity of side effects must begin with the assumption that suitable control with alternate therapeutic methods alone is unsatisfactory. A continuation of adjunctive therapeutic measures is indicated to minimize both the dose and the duration of steroid administration. Prolonged systemic administration of steroids is associated with fewer side effects when given on an alternate-day basis. Topical administration of steroids is almost always less hazardous than oral or parenteral administration.

Alternate-Day Administration

When steroids became available for therapy it soon became evident that short-term or intermittent use of steroids was not associated with the severe side effects of long-term use. The control of chronic disease such as severe asthma by intermittent, rather than daily, administration of steroids presented an appealing goal. Trial with various intervals and with different steroid analogs resulted in the current clinically established method of administering morning doses of relatively short-acting steroids every 48 hours (Thorn, 1974). An ample body of literature indicates that alternate-day steroid therapy diminishes the adverse effects of steroids.

Morning administration of short-acting steroid preserves the normal diurnal cortisol secretory pattern. The tissues are normally exposed to the highest concentration of plasma cortisol in the early morning hours, and the addition of exogenous steroid in the morning therefore adds least to hypothalamic-pituitary suppression. Reduction in the adverse steroid effect of increased infection may in part be attributable to the return of normal numbers of inflammatory cells on the "off" day. Explanation for the reduction of the other side effects is not apparent. The beneficial therapeutic effects induced by the steroid seem to decay at a slower rate than do most of the detrimental effects.

The mechanics of initiating alternate-day steroid therapy are: (a) control the patient's manifestations with the least amount of short-acting steroid on a multiple-dose daily schedule; (b) combine and administer the total as a single morning dose; (c) double or, if necessary for control, triple (Thorn, 1974) the morning dose and administer every 48 hours; and (d) further reduce the alternate-day dose gradually as tolerated.

Each of these steps is often associated with breakthrough attacks of the underlying allergic problem. Patience and persistance are usually required for success. It must not be assumed that the method can safely and satisfactorily be used for all steroid-dependent patients. An every morning schedule of short-acting steroid is preferable to a daily multiple-dose schedule if an alternate-day regimen does not adequately suppress symptoms. There is some evidence that, at low doses, alternate-day therapy may be no more effective in reduction of side effects than daily morning doses (Shapiro et al., 1976). Alternate morning administration will reduce but not eliminate adverse effects of steroid therapy, and its adoption does not justify complacency.

Topical Administration

Targeting the maximal steroid action on the affected tissue by local application or injection has proved effective in the treatment of dermatologic, opthalmic, orthopedic, and respiratory problems. Consideration in this chapter is restricted to the topical use of steroids in the treatment of asthma. The use of topical steroids in the treatment of allergic rhinitis is described in Chapter 6.

A review of the early use of inhaled steroids for the treatment of asthma reveals investigations in the 1950s of nebulized cortisone, hydrocortisone solutions, and powder and aerosolized freon-propelled prednisolone. In the 1960s steroid inhalation for asthma was focused largely on the utilization of dexamethasone. Efficacy for the treatment of asthma with inhaled cortisone and hydrocortisone seemed dubious, but prednisolone and dexamethasone were demonstrably effective, probably as a result of absorption rather than any significant selective topical effect.

In recent years triamcinalone (Sly et al., 1978; Williams et al., 1974) flunisolide (Slavin et al., 1980), budesonide (Ellul-Micallef, 1980) and beclomethasone have been demonstrated to control asthma by inhalation. Only beclomethasone dipropionate aerosol (BDA) is currently available for nonexperimental treatment of asthma in the United States. The effectivity of BDA in the treatment of asthma and its high topical and low systemic activity have been well established (Williams, 1981).

The selection of BDA for the control of asthma was encouraged by the discovery that its topical activity by skin test was 5000 times that of hydrocortisone. Most of an inhaled steroid is ultimately swallowed, and the ingested dose of BDA is rapidly methabolized in the liver and excreted through the bile and feces. The significant portion of BDA that is available for systemic side effects is thus limited to that amount absorbed from the respiratory tract.

The effectiveness of inhaled BDA is dose-related (Brompton Hosp., 1974), with recommended daily doses (divided) for adults of 0.40–1.0 mg and children 6–12 years of age up to 0.50 mg. In adults significant hypothalamic-pituitary-adrenal suppression is not expected unless the daily dose exceeds 1.6 mg (Clark, 1980). Daily prednisone reduction of 5–10 mg has been observed in numerous studies utilizing 0.40–0.80 mg of BDA daily (Clark, 1980), and presumably somewhat greater reductions occur with larger BDA dosage, but probably not more than 15 mg. Use of BDA results in the complete elimination of oral steroid dependency in a very significant proportion of severe asthmatics. The reduction of oral steroid dose by the addition of BDA is desirable even when the complete conversion to inhaled steroid is impossible. Toogood and associates report that a large percentage of severe steroid dependant asthmatics are better controlled on combined aerosol-oral therapy than on either alone (Toogood et al., 1977, 1978).

Candidiasis of the oropharynx and larynx occurs in approximately 5% of BDA users (Clark, 1980), but colonization of the tracheobronchial tree has not been described. A simple mouth rinse after each inhalation treatment may diminish the incidence of symptomatic oral candidiasis, but if annoying symptoms occur, response to antifungal mouthwash is usually rapid and satisfactory.

Steroid withdrawal symptoms may occur during the transfer to BDA from oral steroids. The transferred patient, previously dependent on long-term systemic steroid administration, must be considered at risk of adrenal insufficiency during stress and protected accordingly.

Bronchodilators should be continued after the patient is transferred to BDA (Nassif et al., 1981), and when breakthrough asthmatic attacks occur, a prompt return to the temporary use of oral steroid is indicated. Rhinitis and nasal polyps, suppressed by long-term use of oral steroid, reappear after transfer to BDA. Administration of intranasal topical steroid is usually helpful in controlling these problems.

USE IN STATUS ASTHMATICUS

The early observation that severe asthma is controllable by steroid administration resulted in the recommendation that it be administered IV in high doses in addition to other therapeutic measures for life-threatening status asthmaticus. The risks associated with the administration of very high steroid doses for short time periods are usually relatively minor. Correlation of patient response with plasma steroid levels resulted in dose recommendations of 4-mg/kg bolus administration of hydrocortisone approximately every 4 hours or continuous infusion at the rate of 3 mg/kg every 6 hours (Collins, 1975). These doses of hydrocortisone, or equivalent doses of methylprednisolone, are currently considered conventional, and massively higher doses are not more effective (Britton et al., 1976; Harfi et al., 1978).

In severe asthma the beneficial effects of steroids may not be apparent for many hours (Collins, 1975). Because of the general belief in the efficacy of steroids in the treatment of very severe asthma, ethical considerations have limited the number of double-blind studies. In a double blind study McFadden et al. (1976) were unable to demonstrate any beneficial effect of a single IV bolus of 1.0 mg of hydrocortisone during 6 hours of observation (McFadden et al., 1976). McFadden and associates emphasized that in severe asthma the long latency between the onset of steroid therapy and beneficial effects indicates a need for continuation of vigorous bronchodilator therapy. A double blind study by Fanta et al. (1983) demonstrated a markedly more rapid improvement in FEV_1 percent in steroid treated patients after a 6 hour delay (Fonta et al., 1983). In another randomized study carried out for 24 hours in children, the steroid-treated group was found to have higher arterial oxygen tensions at the end of 24 hours but not other significant differences in clinical or spirometric assessments (Pierson et al., 1974). The authors concluded that witholding steroid treatment in status asthmaticus needlessly expose patients to prolonged hypoxemia. However, a 36-hour randomized study of children hospitalized with "moderately severe acute asthma" revealed a response to aminophylline and Salbutmol that was not increased by the addition of steroids (Kattan et al., 1980). These authors concluded that not all children hospitalized with asthma require steroid therapy.

Since the initiating of steroid therapy seldom results in a rapid resolution of life-threatening status asthmaticus, continued intense utilization of other therapeutic measures is required. Children hospitalized with moderately severe asthma may not additionally benefit from corticosteroid therapy, but the more the attack is perceived as life-threatening, the greater is the urgency to start conventional-dose IV steroid therapy in both children and adults.

SHORT-TERM USE

Steroid therapy for long periods of time at even low pharmacologic doses is associated with a high incidence of serious adverse reactions. In contrast, short-term administration even of very high doses of steroid is associated with a low incidence of serious side effects. Occasional treatment with moderate steroid doses for a few weeks is associated with a minimal risk of serious adverse reactions. Moderate dosage can be considered equivalent to 80 mg of prednisone or less on the initial day of therapy with appropriate tapering of dose during the remainder of the course. The tapering method is utilized in short-term therapy to allow for a resolution of the underlying disease process and not because of significant risk of adrenal insufficiency on withdrawal. Short-term courses of steroid are very useful in controlling the manifestations of the allergic state and should be considered when other therapeutic programs alone are unsatisfactory. During the management of asthma short steroid courses may be indicated to reduce morbidity and the risk of a progression toward status asthmaticus.

In the past, unrealistic fear of steroid side effects resulted in unnecessary discomfort for patients with self-limiting allergic reactions. Moderately extensive contact dermatitis, drug-induced urticaria, and marked symptoms of seasonal allergic rhinitis uncontrolled by other measures are examples of self-limited allergic reactions for which judiciously administered short courses of steroid usually results in a dramatic reduction of morbidity.

CONCLUSIONS

The mechanisms by which steroids work are not completely known; however, our knowledge continues to accumulate and, particularly in the past decade, at an accelerated rate. The adverse effects of steroid therapy are well documented, and, despite the sparsity of precise incidence rates, many years of clinical observation have provided perspective about the extent of patient risk associated with steroid therapy. It is certainly clear that long-term use of steroids is associated with high risks that can be reduced by selecting favorable modes of administration. It is also clear that brief courses of steroid administration are associated with only a low incidence of adverse reactions. The use of topically potent steroids for the treatment of respiratory tract disorders has proved to be very effective in providing beneficial steroid actions without systemic side effects and has very significantly increased the clinician's ability to safely utilize steroids to suppress the manifestations of asthma and rhinitis.

Case History

A 37-year-old woman with severe asthma of 20 years' duration remained steroid-dependent despite immunotherapy and daily sustained-release theophylline and beta agonist administration. Her minimum dose of prednisone, when administered as a single dose every morning, was established as 25 mg. Her prednisone dose had to be markedly increased and administered on a multiple-dose schedule approximately 6 times a year because of exacerbations of her asthma. Repeated attempts to control her asthma with alternate-day administration of prednisone were unsuccessful. She developed a cushingoid appearance. When beclomethasone became available it was found that inhalation of five breaths 4 times daily (approximately 1 mg daily) resulted in better control of her asthma and permitted a reduction of her morning prednisone dose to 12.5 mg. Alternate-day administration of 25 mg of prednisone was then found to be sufficient to control her asthma. She regained her normal appearance. Periodic exacerbations of her asthma, requiring a return to daily multiple dose steroid administration, have been reduced to approximately twice a year.

REFERENCES

Atkinson, J. P., & Frank, M. M. *J. Immunol.*, 1973, *111*, 1061–1066.

Axelrod, L. *Medicine*, 1976, *55*, 39–59.

Baxter, J. D., & Forsham, P. H. *Am. J. Med.*, 1972, *53*, 573–589.

Baxter, J. D., & Funder, J. W. *New Engl. J. Med.*, 1979, *301*, 1149–1161.

Blackwell, G. J., Carnuccio, R., DiRosa, M., Flower, R. J., Parente, L., and Persico, P. *Nature*, 1980, *287*, 147–149.

Britton, M. G., Collins, J. V., Brown, D., Fairhurst, N. P. A., & Lambert, R. G. *Br. Med. J.*, 1976, *2*, 73–74.

Brompton Hospital Medical Research Council Collaborative Trial. *Lancet*, 1974, *11*, 303–307.

Byyny, R. L. *New Engl. J. Med.*, 1976, *295*, 30–32.

Claman, H. *J. Allergy Clin. Immunol.*, 1975, *55*, 145–151.

Claman, H. N. *New Engl. J. Med.*, 1972, *287*, 388–397.

Clark, T. J. H., N. Mygind & T. J. H. Clark (Eds.), in *Asthma and rhinitis*. London: Bailliere Tindall, 1980, pp. 94–106.

Collins, J. V., Clark, T. J., Brown, D., and Townsend, J. *Q. J. Med.*, 1975, *44*, 259–273.

Conn, H. O., & Blitzer, B. L. *New Engl. J. Med.*, 1976, *294*, 473–479.

Dojovne, C. A., & Azrnoff, D. L. *Steroid therapy*. Philadelphia: Saunders, 1975.

Ellul-Micallef, R., Hansson, E., & Johansson, S. A. *Eur. J. Respr. Dis.*, 1980, *61*, 167–173.

Fauci, A. S. *J. Immunopharmacol.*, 1979, 1–25.

Fonta, C. H., Rossing, T. H., and McFadden, E. R. Jr., *Am. J. Med.*, 1983, *74*, 845–851.

Fraser, C. M., & Venter, J. C. *Biochem. Biophys. Res. Commun.*, 1980, *94*, 390–397.

Greaves, H. *Postgrad. Med. H.*, 1976, *52*, 631–633.

Harfi, H., Hanissian, A. S., & Crawford, L. V. *Pediatrics*, 1978, *61*, 829–831.

Harter, J. F. In *Steroid Therapy, A Clinical Update for the 1970's*. Kalamazoo, MI: MEDCOM, 1974, pp. 42–48.

Hirata, F., Schiffmann, E., Venkatasubramanian, K., Salomon, D., and Axelrod, J. *Proc. Natl. Acad. Sci. USA.*, 1980, *77*, 2533–2536.

Holgate, S. T., Baldwin, C. J., & Tattersfield, A. E. *Lancet*, 1977, *2*, 375–377.

Kattan, M., Gurwitz, D., & Levison, H. *J. Pediatr.*, 1980, *96*, 596–599.

Lee, T. P., & Reed, C. E. *Biochem. Biophys. Res. Commun.*, 1977, *78*, 998–1004.

MacGregor, R. R., Sheagren, J. N., Lipsett, M. B., and Wolff, S. M. *New Eng. J. Med.*, 1969, *280*, 1427–1431.

McFadden, E. R., Jr., Kiser, R., deGroot, W. J., Holmes, B., Kiker, R., & Viser, G. *Am. J. Med.*, 1976, *60*, 52–59.

Mendelsohn, J., Multer, M. M., & Boone, R. F. *J. Clin. Invest.*, 1973, *52*, 2129–2137.

Messer, J., Reitman, D., Sacks, H. S., Smith, H., & Chalmers, T. C. *New Engl. J. Med.*, 1983, *309*, 21–24.

Metz, S. A. *Med. Clin. N. Am.*, 1981, *65*, 713–756.

Morris, H. G. *Allergy Clin. Immunol.*, 1980, *66*, 343–346.

Nassif, E. G., Weinberger, M., Thompson, R., & Huntley, W. *New Engl. J. Med.*, 1981, *304*, 71–75.

Parker, C. W., Huber, M. G., & Baumann, M. L. *J. Clin. Invest.*, 1973, *52*, 1342–1348.

Pierson, W. E., Bierman, C. W., & Kelley, V. C. *Pediatrics*, 1974, *54*, 282–288.

Posey, W. C., Nelson, H. S., Branch, B., & Pearlman, D. S. *J. Allergy Clin. Immunol.*, 1978, *62*, 340–348.

Reinish, J. M., Simon, N. G., Karow, W. G., & Gandelman, R. *Science*, 1978, *202*, 436–438.

Richards, J. M., Santiago, S. M., & Klaustermeyer, W. B. *Arch. Intern. Med.*, 1980, *140*, 1473–1475.

Schatz, M., Patterson, R., Kloner, R., & Falk, J. *Ann. Intern. Med.*, 1976, *84*, 261–265.

Schatz, M., Patterson, R., Zeitz, S., O'Rourke, J., & Melam, H. *JAMA*, 1975, *233*, 804–807.

Schwartz, B. *New Engl. J. Med.*, 1978, *299*, 182–184.

Shapiro, G. G., Tattoni, D. S., Kelley, V. C., Pierson, W. E., & Bierman, C. W. *J. Allergy Clin. Immunol.*, 1976, *57*, 430–439.

Slavin, R. G., Izu, A. E., Bernstein, L., Blumenthal, M. N., Bolin, J. F., Ouellette, J. J., Reed, C. E., & Oren, J. *J. Allergy Clin. Immunol.*, 1980, *66*, 379–385.

Slott, R. I., & Zweiman, B. *J. Allergy Clin. Immunol.*, 1974, *54*, 229–234.

Sly, R. M., Imseis, M., Frazer, M., & Joseph, F. *J. Allergy Clin. Immunol.*, 1978, *62*, 76–82.

Snyder, R. D., & Snyder, D. *Ann. Allergy*, 1978, *41*, 340–341.

Stevenson, H. C., and Fauci, A. S. In *Clinical Immunology Update*, 1981, (E. Franklin, Ed.) Elsevier, North Holland.

Streeten, D. H. P., and Phil, D. *JAMA*, 1975, *232*, 944–947.

Thorn, G. W. *Steroid Therapy: A Clinical Update for the 1970's*, 1974, MEDCOM, Kalamazoo.

Toogood, J. H., Lefcoe, N. M., and Haines, D. S. M., Jennings, B., Errington, N., Baksh, L., & Chuang, L. *J. Allergy Clin. Immunol.*, 1977, *59*, 298–308.

Toogood, J. H., Lefcoe, N. M., Haines, D. S., Chuang, L., Jennings, B., Errington, N., Baksh, L., & Cauchi, M. *J. Allergy Clin. Immunol.*, 1978, *61*, 355–364.

Walton, J., and Ney, R. *Current Concepts of Corticosteroids—Uses and Abuses*, 1975, Year Book Medical Publishers, Inc., Disease-a-Month.

Williams, M. H., Kane, C., & Shim, C. S. *Am. Rev. Resp. Dis.*, 1974, *109*, 538–545.

Williams, M. H. *Ann. Intern. Med.*, 1981, *95*, 464–467.

Wilson, J. G. *Teratology*, 1973, *7*, 3–16.

SUGGESTED READINGS

Harter, J. F., In Steroid Therapy, A clinical update for the 1970's. Kalamazoo: MEDCOM, 1974, pp: 42–48.

Sheen, A., Anderson, K., Holbrook, P., & Sly, R. M. *Ann. Allergy*, 1980, *45*, 34–46.

Spector, S. L., Katz, F. H., & Farr, R. S. *J. Allergy Clin. Immunol.*, 1974, *54*, 367–379.

Zeiger, R. S., Schatz, M., Sperling, W., Simon, R. A., & Stevenson, D. D., *J. Allergy Clin. Immunol.*, 1980, *66*, 348–446.

QUESTIONS

1. Alternate-day administration (ADA) of steroid diminishes adverse reactions associated with long-term use. If satisfactory suppression of symptoms cannot be achieved with ADA, the next best alternative is:
   a. The smallest controlling dose of long-acting steroid administered every morning.
   b. The smallest controlling dose of short-acting steroid administered bid.
   c. The smallest controlling dose of short-acting steroid administered every morning.
   d. A small dose of short-acting steroid administered every morning supplemented with P. M. doses on a prn basis.

2. A second-strength tuberculin test was performed on a patient receiving 60 mg of prednisone on an ADA schedule. Interpretation of the test reaction would be:
   a. The same as for a patient not on steroids.
   b. Invalid because prednisone suppresses delayed hypersensitivity at this dose, preventing the tuberculin reaction.
   c. Valid only if "read" on the "off" steroid day.
   d. Valid if positive but not if negative.

3. A 16-year-old non-steroid-dependent asthmatic was admitted with status asthmaticus and responded to bronchodilators, oxygen, and conventional-dose IV steroids. After 72 hours his chest was almost free of wheezes. The most prudent way to eliminate steroids from his therapeutic program would be to:
   a. Discontinue abruptly since steroids are no longer necessary.
   b. Transfer to oral steroid and very slowly taper dose over a period of at least 4 weeks to avoid steroid withdrawal symptoms and minimize dangers of adrenal insufficiency.
   c. Transfer to very brief period of bid short acting-steroid, then A.M. doses tapered daily as determined by clinical observations.
   d. Transfer to oral short-acting steroid and after a few days start ADA.

4. Uncontrolled asthma during pregnancy presents a hazard to both mother and fetus. If steroids are required to control asthma during pregnancy, it should be recognized that current evidence indicates that:

a. Use during the first trimester is teratogenic.
b. Use in the last trimester is likely to cause adrenal insufficiency of the newborn child.
c. Increased birth weight of the newborn is to be expected.
d. Steroid therapy does not increase fetal or maternal complications.

5. Beclomethasone dipropianate aerosol (BDA) was successfully substituted for prednisone in an asthmatic previously steroid-dependent for 3 years. One month later, while on his regular bronchodilator program of theophylline and albuterol, the patient reported the onset of mild wheezing associated with symptoms typical of a common cold.

a. Prednisone should be started promptly.
b. The dose of BDA should be doubled, and if improvement is not observed after a 24-hour period, prednisone should be started.
c. Prompt hospitalization is indicated with the hope that IV aminophylline, aerosolized bronchodilators and oxygen may obviate the need for reinstituting systemic steroid therapy.
d. Adrenocorticotrophic hormone (ACTH) might serve the dual function of stimulating the probably insufficient adrenal cortex and controlling the asthma until the cold subsides.

Answers can be found in Appendix B at the end of the book.

James H. Day

19

Allergies in Pregnancy

There is no reason to believe that the frequency of allergies in pregnancy is significantly different from that seen in nonpregnant women of this age group. Most allergic disease states, including rhinitis, urticaria, and drug and food sensitivities, are likely to occur with the same incidence and severity and are mainly problems of medical management. These problems must be considered in pregnancy from the standpoint of causation, investigation, and ultimately treatment, all of which are likely influenced to some degree by the pregnant condition.

The exception is asthma, which is one condition that deserves special attention. It is an ongoing process occurring in 0.4–1.3% of pregnant women. Asthmatic symptoms may change during pregnancy, but for the most part they remain the same. When there is improvement, it tends to be early in pregnancy with return of symptoms at parturition. Pregnancies in individuals tend to respond alike; thus a pattern can usually be established by the nature of the first pregnancy. Nevertheless, the consensus is that fetal maternal complications in the pregnant asthmatic, even those receiving corticosteroids, are similar in the general population. Diagnostic tests for asthma are essentially the same as those in the nonpregnant population, but radiography and invasive measures should be limited in the investigation and where possible, medication should be restricted. Nevertheless, it is inappropriate to withhold treatment in the pregnant woman automatically on the basis of general principles.

PHYSIOLOGY OF PREGNANCY

Fetal Oxygenation

The uteroplacental circulation is in place by the 12th week. It acts as an atrioventricular (AV) shunt, which decreases systemic circulatory resistance and elicits maternal responses of increasing cardiac output. Despite the large maternal blood

ALLERGY: THEORY AND PRACTICE
ISBN 0-8089-1619-X

flow through the placenta, the fetus normally survives in relative hypoxia, and the average umbilical vein Po_2 is 28.5 mm Hg. The fetus compensates for the lower Po_2 through the special qualities of fetal hemoglobin, which absorbs oxygen more fully than adult hemoglobin and releases it more completely, especially at an acid pH. In addition, shunting of blood through the ductus venosus, ductus arteriosus, and foramen ovale increases the flow of the fetal circulation through the placenta.

Maternal Physiology

Pregnancy is accompanied by several alterations in maternal pulmonary physiology. Minute ventilation is consistently increased during pregnancy. This is the result of a rise in tidal volume rather than a change in respiratory rate, which is unaltered or only slightly increased. In addition, it would appear that progesterone, which occurs in high levels in the second and third trimesters, has the effect of decreasing airway resistance. Despite these two alterations, the breathing capacity and dynamic lung functions are unchanged in pregnancy. As might be expected, oxygen consumption is increased. A syndrome of dyspnea of pregnancy is observed in 60–70% of normal pregnancies during the first and second trimesters. It is postulated that these patients tend to have a high $Paco_2$ prior to pregnancy.

Endocrine and Metabolic Changes

A number of endocrine alterations occur during pregnancy. Cortisol metabolism is greatly increased by pregnancy, but there is evidence that levels of biologically active free cortisol are not elevated except during the third trimester, when there is an increase in the concentration of unbound cortisol. Although the fetal adrenal glands are capable of producing corticosteroids, most fetal cortisol appears to be of maternal origin. Human chorionic gonadotropin (HCG), progesterone, and estrogen predominate in the second and third trimesters. Additionally, a reported small but significant increase in cyclic adenosine monophosphate levels in urine and in serum, and an increase in diamine oxidase activity, which increases the histamine inactivating potency of the blood in the pregnant woman, could be of importance. The cause of these changes is not known, but it has been speculated that they are the results of the alterations in circulating hormonal levels.

Immunologic Changes

The immunology of pregnancy need be mentioned only in the context of the observation that pregnancy is associated with depressed maternal cell-mediated immunity, especially in the last trimester. There is a substantial reduction in maternal lymphocyte responses to specific antigens as evidenced by the fact that kidney allographs seem to do well or even better during pregnancy. In some women the dosage of immunosuppressive drugs can be decreased or even discontinued during this period. Interestingly, these changes do not seem to predispose the pregnant woman to infection or reactivation of tuberculosis. Moreover, there is no evidence of sufficient perturbations in humoral response to antigens to expect specific problems relative to immunotherapy; indeed, IgE levels tend to fall during pregnancy.

ASTHMA AND PREGNANCY

General Considerations

Most of the studies (Greenberger and Patterson, 1978; Weinstein, et al., 1979) considering the effects of pregnancy on asthma support the principle that asthmatic women have no increased risk of important obstetric or perinatal complications and that the pregnancy itself produces equal numbers of those who are worse, remain the same, or improve. However, some workers have indicated a statistically significant increase in prematurity, low birth weight, and hypoxia in infants of asthmatic mothers. Additionally, there is evidence that since IgE tends to fall in pregnancy, and those who have unchanged or increased IgE levels during pregnancy have more severe symptoms.

A greater risk exists for those in whom preexisting asthma is severe. There is a tendency for those whose conditions were worse before pregnancy to be worse during pregnancy. However, previously well-controlled patients may develop status asthmaticus during pregnancy with progressive deterioration until delivery.

During an acute exacerbation that is reflected in a decrease in fetal Po_2, pregnant women with severe asthma may develop a combination of hypoxemia and respiratory alkalosis. Alkalosis is more important than the hypoexamia in causing the depressed fetal Pao_2 since it prevents complete release of oxygen from fetal hemoglobin. For this reason treatment of the pregnant asthmatic patient should include maintaining Pao_2 at high levels as long as significant maternal alkalosis is present, particularly when the pH is greater than or equal to 7.60 or the Pco_2 is less than or equal to 17 mm Hg. Vigorous treatment aimed at relieving airway obstruction tends to reduce the stimulus to hyperventilation and the resultant tendency toward respiratory alkalosis (Turner et al., 1980).

Medical Management of Asthma in Pregnancy

Environmental Control

Central to the management of the allergic patient is the need for meticulous environmental control in order to limit the requirement for alternative treatment. It would be inappropriate, for instance, to intensively manage a patient with either upper or lower respiratory symptoms who has become sensitized to house dust without dealing with all the measures to control such exposure or alternatively overlooking smoke actively or passively inhaled.

Drugs Contraindicated in Pregnancy

The protocols used in testing new drugs do not allow their administration to pregnant women. Thus quite frequently the physician is faced with the statement that the safety of a given drug in human pregnancy has not been established, and the use of the drug in pregnancy requires that the expected therapeutic benefit be weighed against possible hazard to the mother and child. With this in mind, the physician, certainly during the first trimester of pregnancy, should not prescribe any medication unless it is absolutely essential. In contrast, the physician must also recognize that the adverse affects of untreated or poorly treated disease may be life-threatening for both the mother and the fetus. Abortion at any stage, stillbirth, or a deformed fetus is a spectere that the physician faces once treatment is undertaken in pregnancy, even though the cause is totally unrelated to medication. A rational approach, therefore, is needed for any therapeutic program maximizing benefits and minimizing risk.

Some general guide for the use of therapeutic agents in pregnancies is outlined below. Medicines to be avoided include those that contain iodine. These drugs block fetal organic binding of elemental iodine, thereby reducing the synthesis of thyroid hormone and resulting in increased levels of thyroid-stimulating hormone (TSH) secretion producing congenital goiters that may, in turn, block the infant's airways. Avoidance of iodine preparations should continue postpartum since iodine may be passed into the breast milk as well. Aspirin and tartrazine should be avoided in those patients who have demonstrated idiosyncracy to them in the production of either asthma or urticaria. Aspirin can be an important factor in the continuation of chronic urticaria. Prostaglandin F_2-alpha, which is injected intra-amniotically, or its methyl analog injected intramuscularly for induction of labor may lead to severe exacerbations and are contraindicated in the asthmatic.

The safety of terbutaline and metaproterenol in early pregnancy has not been established, but a single study of antenatal terbutaline revealed decreased incidence of hyaline-membrane disease in premature infants. Albuterol (Salbutamol) is teratogenic in mice. Albuterol and terbutaline have been used in the management of premature labor to delay delivery with no apparent adverse affects aside from moderate tachycardia. Terbutaline has been shown to inhibit uterine activity at term, when it may be contraindicated. There are reports of pulmonary edema in mothers treated with corticosteroids and beta adrenergics during premature labor.

Local anesthesia is preferable over general anesthesia. As a general anesthetic agent, halothane is favored since it will function as a bronchodilator. Halothane, however, has been associated with serious idiosyncratic reactions. Sedatives should be avoided because of their depressant effect on the medulla, whereas hydroxyzine hydrochloride has been reported to have teratogenic effects. Promethazine hydrochloride is known to decrease neonatal T-cell number and function. Additionally, there is some suggestion that epinephrine may cause temporarily decreased uterine perfusion with resultant fetal distress. There is concern as well that phenobarbitol may cause fetal abnormalities.

Bronchodilators

THEOPHYLLINE COMPOUNDS. These appear to be the mainstay of therapy for patients with asthma. It has been demonstrated that theophylline can cross the placenta. This may result in potentially dangerous serum theophylline concentrations in the neonate and can be of practical importance. The requirement for theophylline is likely to increase during the latter part of pregnancy since then the total weight also increases. Since the theophylline clearance (half-life $T_{1/2}$) remains the same as in the nonpregnant individual, the milligram per kilogram (mg/kg) dose remains unchanged. Therapeutic but nontoxic levels of 10–20 μg/ml should be maintained. Fixed combinations with other drugs such as ephedrine should be avoided in order to adjust the theophylline to an optimum level.

BETA AGONISTS. Beta stimulators such as albuterol, isoetharine, terbutaline, and metaproterenol, have proved to be effective in the management of asthma. Because beta bronchodilators such as albuterol are teratogenic in mice (Table 19-1), terbutaline metaproterenol should be utilized when possible.

In addition, other beta-adrenergic agonists may have undesirable side effects as pointed out above. Anticholinergic atropine-like compounds ipratropium (SCH 1000) have multiple actions. They have been demonstrated to decrease cyclic guanosine monophosphate levels, block vagal stimulation, and decrease irritant effects. This has led to consideration of this class of drug in management of asthma. Although these drugs may cross the placenta and potentially cause fetal tachycardia, this has not proved harmful. With the exception of atropine, these drugs are not available in the United States.

CROMOLYN SODIUM. Eight percent of a 20-mg dose of cromolyn is absorbed into the circulation. No human fetal damage has been known to occur clinically. Even though no teratogenicity occurred in animals after large daily IV doses throughout pregnancy, safety in human pregnancy has not been established. Its use is not recommended during pregnancy, nor is it necessary.

Corticosteroids

Corticosteroids may be needed to control moderately severe asthma uncontrolled by bronchodilators. Although maternal corticosteroids cross the placenta, a large proportion of the cortisol crossing the placenta is converted to inactive cortisone by enzymes within the placental villi. In contrast, prednisone and prednisolone cross the placenta poorly. The concentrations in maternal blood are 8–10 times higher than that in fetal blood. As a result, neonatal adrenal suppression in infants whose mothers are on pharmacologic doses of prednisone or prednisolone has rarely been documented. Such does not hold true with the maternal fetal gradients of other corticosteroids such as hydrocortisone (5.8 to 1) or betamethasone (3 to 1). A number of studies of patients treated with prednisone or prednisolone have not shown any untoward effect that can be attributable to maternal steroid treatment during pregnancy. Women treated with prednisone during pregnancy may have low urinary estriol secretion; again, no associated fetal distress or intrauterine growth retardation has been seen. Antenatal steroids used to prevent respiratory distress syndrome in premature infants have appeared to decrease the incidence of respiratory distress syndrome. No adverse fetal affects in the immediate postnatal period have been reported.

Beclomethasone diproprionate aerosol administration during pregnancy has been insufficiently studied, but limited evidence so far has not demonstrated any fetal abnormalities. It would seem that this form of corticosteroid administration would

Table 19-1 *Summary of Safety of Drugs for Asthma and Other Allergic States During Pregnancy*

Category Questionable	Agent	Safe	Unknown Effects	Questionable Effects
Antihistamines	Chlorpheniramine maleate			
(Chlor-Trimeton)		S*		
Pheniramine maleate		S		
Diphenhydramine HCl (Benadryl)		S		
Tripelennamine (PBZ)		S		
Brompheniramine maleate (Dimetane, Puretane)				Q†
Hydroxyzine HCl (Atarax, Vistaril, Marax, Enarax, Cartrax)			C‡	
Promethazine HCl (Phenergan)			C	
Cimetidine (Tagamet)				Q
Cyproheptadine (Periactin)				Q
Sympathomimetics	Phenylephrine HCl	S		
Phenylpropanolamine HCl				U
Ephedrine sulfate		S		
	Pseudoephedrine HCl (Sudafed, Novafed)		U§	
	Epinephrine (Adrenalin)			Q
	Epinephrine suspension 1 : 200 (Sus-Phrine)			Q
Beta Agonists	Terbutaline Sulfate (Brethine, Bricanyl)		U	
	Albuterol (Salbutamol, Ventolin, Proventil)			Q
	Isoproterenol (Isuprel, Medihaler, Norisodrine, Aerolone)		U	
	Metaproterenol sulfate (Alupent, Metaprel)		U	
	Anticholinergics			Q
Methylxanthines	Theophylline (Theolair, Elixophyllin, Theophyl, Theo-Dur)	S		
	Aminophylline (Somophyllin, Aminophyllin)	S		

Category Questionable	Agent	Safe	Unknown Effects	Questionable Effects
Cromoglycates	Cromolyn sodium (Intal, Aarane)			Q
Corticosteroids Systemic	Prednisone (Deltasone, Meticorten, Orasone)	S		
	Prednisolone (Delta-Cortef)	S		
	Dexamethasone (Decadron, Hexadrol, Dexone)		U	
Inhaled	Beclomethasone dipropionate (Vanceril, Beclovent, Beconase, Vancenase)	S		
	Dexamethasone (Decadron, Turbinaire)		U	
Expectorants	Iodine-containing (SSKI, Mudrane tablets, Isuprel Compound Elixir, Elixophyllin-KI Elixir, Pima Syrup, Iodo-Niacin Tablets)			Q
Antibiotics	Ampicillin (e.g., Amcill, Omnipen, Penbritin, Polycillin)	S		
	Penicillin (e.g., Pen-Vee, Omnipen, Unopen, Pentid)	S		
	Erythromycin (e.g., E.E.S., Erythrocin)	S		
	Tetracycline (e.g., Achromycin, Mysteclin-F, Robitet)		C	
Established immunotherapy	Stable antigen dose	S		

*S = safe for judicious use when indication is definite.
†Q = questionable adverse effects based on sporadic case reports or animal studies.
‡C = contraindicated.
§U = unknown effects; insufficient data (see text).

be appropriate in pregnant women who are not responding to conventional programs, the next alternative being oral corticosteroids.

Other Medications

Of the antihistamines, diphenhydramine, tripelennamine, pheniramine, and chlorpheniramine are safe for use during pregnancy. Cimetidine is a potent H_2 receptor antagonist that has not been carefully studied. Current evidence suggests that at doses of 100 mg/kg or greater cimetidine crosses placental barrier, thus affecting the fetus. There is a suggestion that it may interfere with hepatic function, such as hepatic bile acid transport in the fetus. Brompheniramine and hydroxyzine hydrochloride should not be used.

Antibiotics

Penicillin and its derivatives are safe. However, the sensitization ratio is 3–18%, with ampicillins having at least twice the rate of sensitization of other types. Thus anaphylaxis is always a possibility, even to the cephalosporins in the pregnant woman. A careful allergic history is an absolute necessity before utilizing these drugs. In the penicillin allergic individual rapid desensitization to penicillin should be undertaken only in situations where alternative medication or other forms of treatment are clearly unsuccessful in life-threatening situations. Erythromycin is inadequately studied, but probably a safe alternative drug for the penicillin-allergic patient. As mentioned above, tetracyclines should not be used because of their effects on the fetal teeth and bones.

Immunotherapy

Immunotherapy during pregnancy has been retrospectively studied by Metzger et al. (1978) using physician or maternal questionnaires along with obstetric records. The study disclosed that in the pregnancies of 90 atopic mothers who had received immunotherapy during pregnancy, the incidence of prematurity, toxemia, abortion, neonatal death, and congenital malformation was no greater than that for the general population. The offspring of treated mothers developed allergic diseases as frequently as did children born into allergic families.

A group of 147 untreated pregnancies of atopic mothers were similarly studied, and an equal incidence of those parameters were observed, except for possibly a greater incidence of abortions. There remains some doubt about actual differences since drug and alcohol intake, smoking, and severity of asthma between the treated and untreated groups were not taken into consideration. These findings confirm those of others who generally conclude that immunotherapy of IgE-mediated disease during pregnancy appears to present no added risk to the mother or fetus.

Immunotherapy should not be initiated during pregnancy because of uncertainties of vaccine tolerance. It should be discontinued if untoward reactions to injections become a problem in spite of dose reduction. The same principle applies to venom immunotherapy. As long as it is not producing reaction, the dose should be held constant and administered on the same schedule.

Summary

In summary, it may be concluded that most antiasthmatic drugs are safe to use during pregnancy. Ideal management would be one free of medications, and all attempts should be made to control factors that lead to or exacerbate asthma. If medications are required, the benefit : risk ratio must be considered for both mother and fetus. The effect of severe uncontrolled asthma with associated hypoxia must be weighed against the possible side effects of drugs on the developing fetus and the mother. Immunotherapy should not be initiated but if established should be continued with the recommendation that the level of antigen concentration be maintained throughout pregnancy to avoid anaphylactic reactions. Problems relative to immunotherapy may be an indication for discontinuation until the termination of pregnancy. At any rate there appears to be no evidence of increased risk to the fetus or the mother when the immunotherapy programs are properly administered.

It would appear that of the antiasthmatic drugs, epinephrine should be avoided certainly in the earlier stages of pregnancy. However, it is apparent that its use would override a threatened situation such as anaphylaxis. Sus-Phrine because of its prolonged action, should not be used. Although safety of $beta_2$ agonists such as terbutaline and metaproterenol is not established, their use may be required and preferable to the introduction of corticosteroids. Prednisone in its lowest effective dose, preferably alternate days, may be needed to minimize or abolish bronchospasm and is to be justified if conventional treatment is unsuccessful. Although the impact of high doses of corticosteroids used to treat severe status asthmatics is not known, the obvious risk to the fetus and mother of maternal hypoxemia, alkalosis or acidosis is greater. Beclomethasone aerosol can be utilized as a means to reduce or eliminate the need for systemic corticosteroids.

Management of Asthma in Specific Situations

Acute Asthma Attacks

Metaproterenol aerosol delivered as a nebulizer or from a pressurized unit 2–4 puffs should be effective in managing mild episodes of wheezing. Epinephrine probably should be withheld early in pregnancy and restricted in patients with hypertension and cardiac arrythmias later on.

Patients who do not promptly respond to aerosolized metaproterenol should receive IV theophylline. A patient not currently on theophylline should receive a loading dose of 6 mg/kg followed by 0.7 mg/kg hr^{-1} for the first 12 hours and then 0.5 mg/kg hr^{-1} on a regular basis. Theophylline levels should be monitored and the IV infusion adjusted to obtain an adequate, nontoxic theophylline blood level.

Patients presenting with severe attacks should receive aerosolized beta agonists and theophylline as described above, along with humidified oxygen at 4–6 l/min. Corticosteroids in the form of hydrocortisone may be administered first at 7 mg/kg IV as a bolus dose and a maintenance program established thereafter. Oral prednisone should be given as soon as practically possible. Corticosteroid dosage should be manipulated according to recognizable response rather than on a predetermined dose schedule of a set declining program.

The progress of the attack should be followed with arterial blood gases, spirometry, and blood pressure evaluation for pulsus paradoxus. If the PCO_2 is greater than 35 mm Hg in the pregnant patient and the arterial pH less than 7.35, the patient should be considered for transfer to an intensive care setting and, possibly, assisted ventilation. If the PO_2 drops below 60 despite all therapy, the fetus may be in jeopardy, and delivery by cesarean section considered, especially if the pregnancy is at term. It is suggested that in any asthmatic when pregnancy endangers life such pregnancy should be terminated as a life-saving procedure (Topiski et al., 1974). Patients who have an acute attack during labor may benefit from forceps delivery to shorten the second stage.

Management of Asthma During Delivery

There are many factors that may effect asthma during delivery. Increased respiratory effort is needed on the part of the mother, and medications used by obstetricians during and after labor may influence the asthmatic state, whereas antihistaminics may affect the course of labor. Steroid-dependent asthmatic patients need to be prepared to prevent serious exacerbations of asthma or addisonian crisis during delivery. Prostaglandins used to produce therapeutic abortion during the second trimester of pregnancy and to induce labor after incomplete spontaneous abortion or after fetal death has occurred can have significant bronchospastic affects with hypoxemia even in mild asthma.

Oxytocin, used frequently in obstetrics, causes uterine smooth muscle contractions but has no affect on smooth muscle elsewhere, including bronchial smooth muscle. Narcotic analgesics sometimes administered because of anxiety and pain during labor, may depress respiration, reduce cough reflex, dry secretions, release histamines, and provoke bronchospasm.

Terbutaline may have an inhibitory affect on labor and thus would be contraindicated near term. It would be optimal for both the mother and fetus in the presence of well-controlled maternal asthma to use nonmedicated forms of childbirth. Local anesthesia is preferable over general anesthesia, but when general anesthesia is required such as for cesarean section, those such as halothane, which possess bronchodilator activity, will be more desirable. Nitrous oxide has no apparent specific bronchial effects, but cyclopropane will cause bronchospasm. Diethylether, although having bronchodilating properties is very irritating to the bronchial mucosa. When corticosteroids are indicated and delivery times are impossible to predict, 100 mg of hydrocortisone may be administered IM at the time of admission to the labor room followed by 100 mg of hydrocortisone IM every 8 hours for 24 hours postpartum.

Anaphylaxis

Anaphylaxis, when it occurs, presents similarly to that in nonpregnant women, but the placenta appears to play an important protective role for the fetus. The placenta prevents crossing of high-molecular-weight IgE antibodies to the fetus. High diamine oxidase activity of the maternal decidua, will catalyze the oxidative deamination of histamine and other related endogenous amines released during anaphylaxis. The management, therefore, of such reactions need not be different. Emphasis should be directed on epinephrine. Rapid administration of parental fluid may be life-saving. Additional medications including antihistamines and corticosteroids should be added where appropriate.

CUTANEOUS RESPONSES IN PREGNANCY THAT MIMIC ALLERGY

Allergic skin reactions occur similarly in pregnant and nonpregnant women. These must be differentiated from papular dermatitis of pregnancy and prurigo of pregnancy. Other complications are not so commonly observed but may be confused with allergy.

Herpes Gestationis

Urticarial-type lesions developing during pregnancy may be herpes gestationis, which is an intensely pruritic, polymorphous eruption occurring in pregnant and postpartum women. It almost always resolves within several months and is likely to occur in succeeding pregnancies. The eruption may be isolated or confluent erythematous, edematous papules and plaques. Papular vesicles, grouped vesicles on erythematous bases, tense bullae, or a combination of some or all of these lesions may be seen.

The entire body may be involved although the abdomen, extremities including palms and soles seem to be preferred sites. It can be verified immunopathologically by *in vivo* bound C_3 with or without IgG in a band-like distribution along the basement membrane zone and complement fixation at the same region. It is highly responsive to prednisone in the range of 40 mg per day in divided doses.

Major clinical differentiating points include *bullous pemphigoid,* which presents as numerous tense blisters distributed over much of the skin surface, arising on normal skin or erythematous edematous areas that develops usually in childhood or old age; *dermatitis herpetiformis,* which is a disease of all ages characteristically affecting the extensor surfaces with grouped vesicles on erythematous plaques and may show erythematous papules and isolated vesicles as well; and *erythema multiforme,* which is a widespread but predominantly acral, polymorphous eruption with a range of lesions from papules to bullae tending to affect all ages.

Pruritic Urticarial Papules and Plaques of Pregnancy (PUPP)

This is a self-limited disease generally seen in the third trimester of the first pregnancy. It presents as an intensely pruritic cutaneous eruption featured by erythematous urticarial papules and plaques that begin on the abdomen and spread to involve the thighs, and occasionally, the buttocks and arms. Mucous membranes are seldom involved. Some are probably misdiagnosed as drug eruptions or categorized as unusual cases of erythema multiforme. Many are likely missed because of late occurrence in pregnancy and remission shortly after delivery. The etiology is unknown, and there is no evidence of increased fetal mortality or embryologic malformation. Unlin reported a similar eruption in the newborn son of a 19-year-old mother who had diagnosed pruritic urticarial papules and plaques of pregnancy. It too, resolved over a period of 10 days.

Autoimmune Progesterone Dermatitis

An interesting but rare condition of autoimmune progesterone dermatitis of pregnancy coming on the first trimester has been described. It is characterized by severe acneiform eruption, eosinophilic dermatitis and panniculitis, peripheral eosinophilia, hyperglobulineamia, transient inflammatory arthritis, and spontaneous abortion. This appears to be due to cell-mediated immunity against endogenous progesterone produced in pregnancy.

Case Report

A 32-year-old gravida-3 para-3 schoolteacher, a nonsmoker, presented for assessment of asthma in March 1982. Her asthma began in early childhood resolving by age 7 years. She was asymptomatic throughout her first pregnancy, which was delivered at term March, 1976. During the second and third trimesters of her second pregnancy, she had intermittent nocturnal cough and wheezing. Contributing factors included frosty air and a variety of irritants. In addition, there was an exertionally induced element. Pulmonary function tests revealed an FEV_1 of 70% predicted and an FEF of 25–75%, 40% predicted, indicating both large and small airways involvement. Management with a sustained-release theophylline preparation 250 mg every 12 hours effectively controlled symptoms. Within the first month postpartum (May 1979) she had a significant exacerbation of asthma. No differences in environmental factors could be determined.

Salbutamol inhaler 2 puffs (200 μg) 4 times daily in addition to the theophylline was necessary over a period of several weeks to achieve and maintain adequate control of symptoms. She was asymptomatic by December 1979.

She became pregnant once more in May 1981. Asthmatic symptoms became troublesome early in the second trimester and were treated with oral theophylline, again producing good clinical response. An acute exacerbation in November 1981 necessitated hospitalization. No specific triggering factors were identified. Intravenous aminophylline, nebulized metaproterenol, humidified oxygen, and adequate fluid intake were required to keep symptoms under control. She improved on this program and was discharged home 4 days after admission to continue on a sustained-release theophylline preparation 250 mg every 12 hours. She remained well-controlled for the duration of the pregnancy. Labor onset occurred spontaneously at term in January 1982. Because of failure to progress, an oxytocin drip was established. Labor and delivery under local anesthesia proceeded without incident.

Three weeks postpartum she was rehospitalized with an acute exacerbation of asthma. This time she required IV hydrocortisone in addition to IV aminophylline, nebulized salbutamol, oxygen, and fluids. She was discharged after 4 days following establishment of long-acting anhydrous theophylline 200 mg every 12 hours and salbutamol inhaler 2 puffs 4 times daily. Symptoms were inadequately controlled. The addition of beclomethasone 2 puffs (100 μg) 4 times daily taken 15 minutes after the salbutamol was required in order to produce optimum results.

ACKNOWLEDGMENTS

The author gratefully acknowledges the typing excellence of Mrs. Linda Sellery, and the literature search and editorial assistance provided by Dr. Margaret Gibson, Resident in Allergy and Immunology, Department of Medicine, Queen's University.

REFERENCES

Greenberger, P., & Patterson, R. *Ann. Intern. Med.*, 1978, *89*, 234–237.

Metzger, W. J., Turner, E., & Patterson, R. *J. Allergy Clin. Immunol.*, 1978, *61*, 268–273.

Topilsky, M., Levo, Y., Spitzer, S. A., Lewinski, U., & Atsmon, A. *Ann. Allergy*, 1974, *32*, 151–153.

Turner, E. S., Greenberger, P. A., & Patterson, R. *Ann. Intern. Med.*, 1980, *6*, 905–915.

Weinstein, A. M., Dubin, B. D., Podleski, W. K., Spector, S. L., & Farr, R. S. *JAMA*, 1979, *241*, 1161–1165.

SUGGESTED READINGS

Gluck, J., & Gluck, P. A. *Ann. Allergy*, 1976, *37*, 164–168.

Miller, R. K. *Am. Soc., Pharm. Expr. Ther.*, 1981, *15*, 1–8.

QUESTIONS

1. Immunotherapy in pregnancy:
   a. Should be continued using the regular schedule.
   b. Should be discontinued but reinstated immediately postpartum.
   c. Should be continued at exactly the same dose.
   d. Should not be established if the patient is known to be pregnant, but if already established should be maintained without increasing the dose, as long as there are no untoward reactions.
2. Which of the following medications are generally recognized to be safe to take during pregnancy:
   a. Brompheniramine
   b. Prednisone
   c. Potassium iodide solution
   d. Tetracycline
3. Theophylline may be administered during pregnancy:
   a. Only orally as the IV route may be dangerous to both the fetus and the mother.
   b. At less than the usual dose because of possible fetal toxicity.
   c. The same dose (mg/kg body weight) as in the nonpregnant woman.
   d. At more than the usual dose because of tendency to excess fluid accumulation in the third trimester.
4. The following obstetric medications are known to influence asthma:
   a. Oxytocin
   b. Prostaglandin F_2 Alpha

c. Demerol
d. Diethylether

5. Pregnancy may:

a. Have no effect on preexisting asthma
b. Worsen preexisting asthma
c. Improve preexisting asthma
d. Worsen, improve, or have no effect on preexisting asthma

Answers can be found in Appendix B at the end of the book.

PART 5

Allergic Lung Disease

Stephen S. Lefrak
Robert M. Senior

20

The Pathophysiology of Acute Asthma

Asthma is more easily described than defined. There are five hallmarks of asthma:

1. Asthma occurs in a tracheobronchial tree that displays hyperreactivity to many stimuli.
2. Asthma is manifested clinically by paroxysms of cough, dyspnea, chest tightness, and wheezing. It should be stressed that not all of these symptoms need be present together at one time. They may occur singly or in any combination.
3. Asthma is an obstructive disease of the airways. The severity and sites of obstruction to airflow may vary widely within the same patient at different times.
4. Asthma is a chronic disease. The evidence for this is both anatomic and functional. For example, highly sensitive tests of the pulmonary function of healthy asthmatics, including those who have "outgrown" asthma, demonstrate abnormalities in airway function. On the other hand, asthma is not progressive and thus is unlike emphysema and chronic bronchitis.
5. Many factors can trigger asthmatic attacks.

In spite of the diversity of features and causes of asthma, acute asthmatic episodes have characteristic pathophysiologic manifestations. This chapter attempts to concisely summarize the principal pathophysiologic abnormalities of the respiratory system and the heart during asthmatic obstruction to airflow and to correlate the pathophysiologic abnormalities of asthma with the observed symptoms and signs.

PATHOLOGY

The pathologic abnormalities in asthma reside exclusively in the airways, affecting the entire airway from lumen to smooth muscle. Based mainly on postmortem studies, there is qualitatively little difference in the airway pathology between the patient with quiescent asthma who has died of other causes and the asthmatic who

ALLERGY: THEORY AND PRACTICE
ISBN 0-8089-1619-X

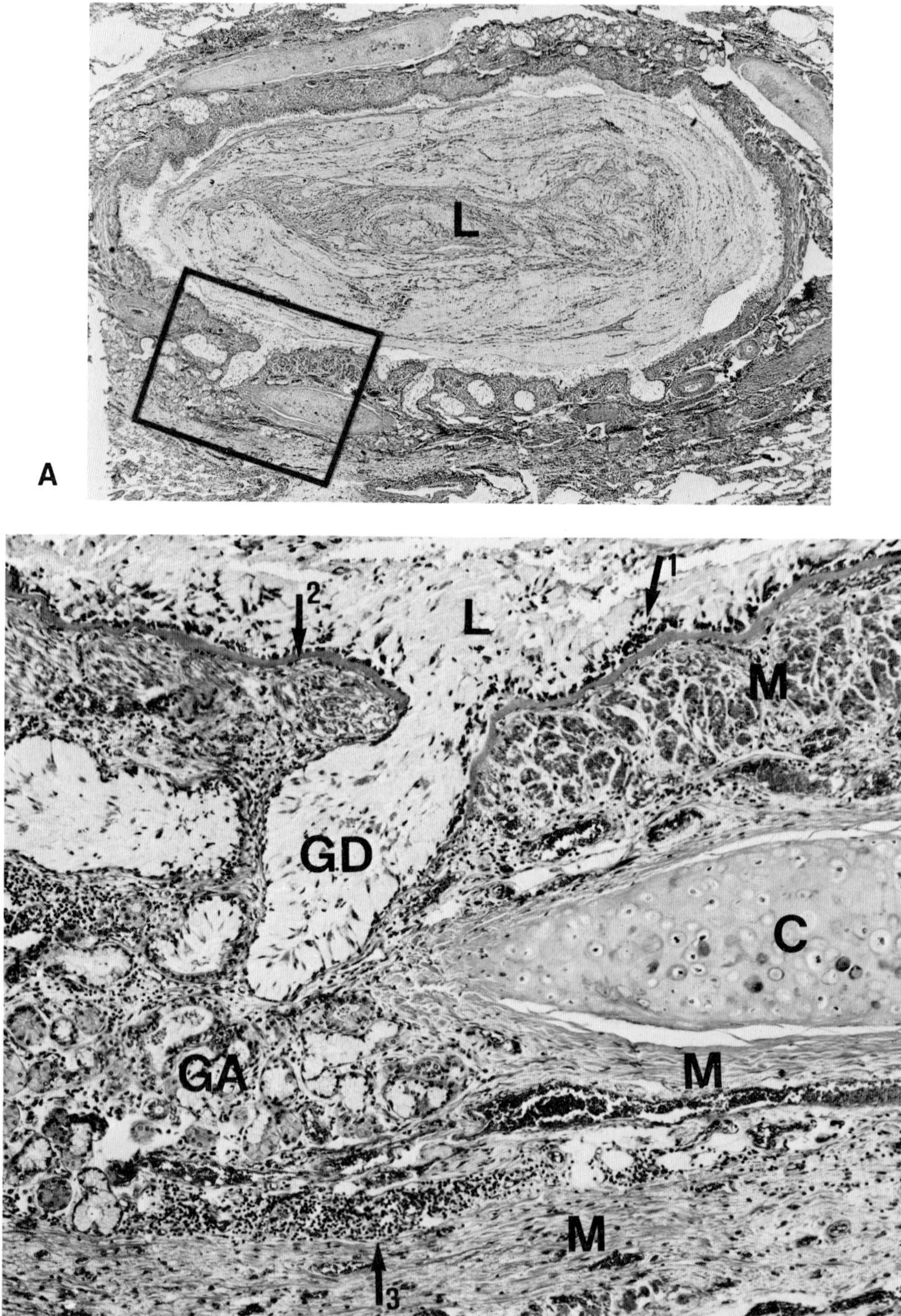

Fig. 20-1. Typical abnormalities of a bronchus in asthma: (A) the lumen (L) is occluded by organizing secretions and the entire wall is thickened (magnification 14×); (B) higher magnification (90×) of the area in the square in part A. The epithelium (arrow 1) is denuded and the basement membrane (arrow 2) is markedly thickened. A glandular duct (GD) containing mucus opens in to the bronchial lumen (L). There is marked increase of the glandular acini

has died in status asthmatacus. However, there is much more extensive and severe involvement in the tracheobronchial tree in the latter person. The airway pathology includes the following features (Fig. 20-1). The lumen of the airway is occluded with tenacious, eosinophil-containing plugs. In the patient with status asthmatacus large segments of airway from trachea to the periphery are frequently occluded, whereas in the "healthy" asthmatic there may only be small plugs in the peripheral airways. The mechanisms for formation of plugs are still unclear with evidence favoring both abnormal mucus production and faulty mucociliary function. The bronchial epithelium may be denuded if the patient has died during an acute episode; otherwise it is intact, although showing increased numbers of glandular cells. A markedly thickened basement membrane is one of the pathologic hallmarks of asthma. This finding has led to speculation of altered airway permeability allowing exudation of material from the vascular bed across the bronchial mucosa. There is marked edema in the submucosa, especially if the patient has died during an acute asthmatic attack. Inflammatory cell infiltrates, frequently eosinophilic, but sometimes of a mixed cellular type develop. Submucosal mucous gland hypertrophy and hyperplasia are marked. In fact, the mucous gland hypertrophy in asthma may even outstrip that present in chronic bronchitis. Also present is an excess of smooth muscle in the airway walls.

The airway obstruction occurring in asthma then must be related to mucous secretions, bronchial edema, and bronchoconstriction. In view of the pathology, asthma should not be regarded as a bronchospastic process alone. The spectrum of abnormalities in the airways must be considered and vigorously treated to effectively manage asthma. This point is important because the severity and duration of an asthmatic episode may well depend on the severity and relative amounts of each of these pathologic processes present.

PATHOPHYSIOLOGY

Regardless of the inciting events or of the pathologic anatomy producing an asthmatic episode, once the asthmatic attack is ongoing the pathophysiological events that follow are similar. The normal pressure–flow and pressure–volume interrelationships of the lung are disturbed, and these, in turn, have effects on pulmonary mechanics, alveolar gas exchange, respiratory muscle function, and the systemic and pulmonary circulation.

Pressure–Flow Changes

The pathologic changes associated with asthma increase the resistance to pulmonary airflow. The increase in airway resistance, whether due to mucous plugging, edema, or bronchoconstriction, results in a abnormally low air*flow* for any driving *pressure* compared to normal and reduces the flow that can be achieved with maximal driving pressure. The impaired airflow with maximum pressure is most evident during forced expiratory maneuvers. Airflow during maximum inspiration will not be as reduced because the pressure surrounding the airways during inspiration is negative favoring airway dilation, rather than positive as during expiration.

(GA). Inflammatory cells are present (arrow 3). There is marked muscular hyperthrophy and hyperphasia (M). A segment of cartilage is in view C. (Courtesy of Charles Kuhn, III, M.D.)

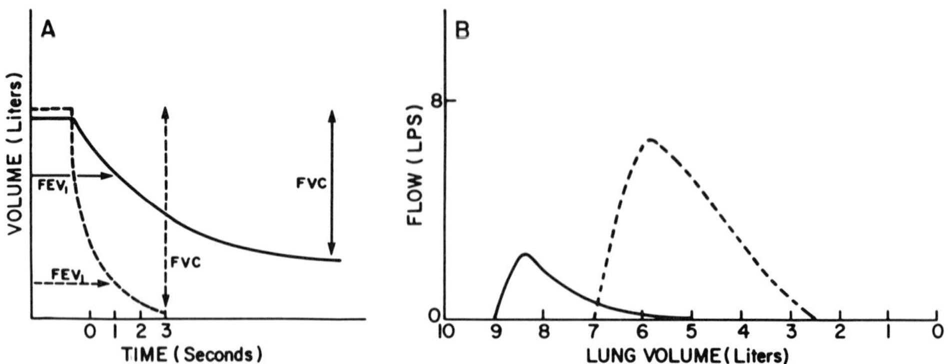

Fig. 20-2. The forced vital capacity (FVC) is recorded as an exhalation with maximal effort from total lung capacity. A timed spirogram is shown in part A in which exhaled volume is recorded over time. From this the forced expiratory volume in the first second (FEV_1) may be measured as well as other indices of expiratory flow. The FEV_1 and FVC of the asthmatic subject (solid lines) are all smaller than these of the normal subject (dashed line). A flow–volume recording is shown in part B. The patient performs a forced vital capacity maneuver, and the FVC is recorded as flow rate over lung volume. The flow–volume loop demonstrates that the maximum expiratory flow rate of asthmatic subject (solid line) is less than that of the normal subject (dashed line) despite the asthmatic's markedly increased lung volume. Also, the flow–volume loop in the asthmatic patient assumes a convex shape at low lung volumes.

Reductions in expiratory flow rates are usually demonstrated with timed spirometry or flow–volume measurements (Fig. 20-2). Both methods utilize a forced expiratory maneuver and contain essentially the same information, although the format is different. The main advantage of timed spirometry is that it is easier to perform in the emergency room or at the bedside and the equipment required is less expensive than that needed for flow–volume recordings. The advantage of flow–volume recording is that it relates flow to vital capacity with which it is closely related and generally allows detection of the distinctive configuration of the flow–volume loop seen with airway obstruction.

The reactivity of the airway obstruction in asthma may be demonstrated by provocation or bronchodilator testing. Airway obstruction may be provoked in many ways in asthmatic patients, whose initial pulmonary function studies are normal. These include exercise, inhalation of nebulized distilled water, methacholine, histamine, exposure to cold air, or ingestion of drugs such as aspirin or tartrazine. Such testing must be performed with great care and under controlled conditions using forced vital capacity maneuvers with appropriate measurements before and after the challenge.

Aerosolized bronchodilators may be used when pulmonary function testing demonstrates airway obstruction. The characteristic abnormality reverts partially or completely toward normal. An improvement in forced vital capacity or FEV_1 of 20% or greater is usually considered significant.

Pressure–Volume Changes

During an acute asthmatic attack, the normal pressure–volume relationships of the respiratory system are disturbed. The lung assumes a higher than normal resting volume (functional residual capacity) at a correspondingly more negative intrathoracic pressure. In addition, more air remains in the lungs after a maximum exhalation (increased residual volume).

Increases of the functional residual capacity and residual volume during an asthmatic episode occur primarily for two reasons: (a) there is an increased drive to breathe, apparently as a result of stimulation from central respiratory centers as well as from receptors in airways and the chest wall—the ensuing tachypnea, together with the increased airway resistance, leads to insufficient time to complete exhalation to the normal resting lung volume and air becomes "trapped" in the lungs; and (b) the pathology in the airways leads to closing of airways at higher than normal lung volumes, thus increasing the residual volume and contributes to the increase in functional residual capacity.

The increase in functional residual capacity (hyperinflation) has several important

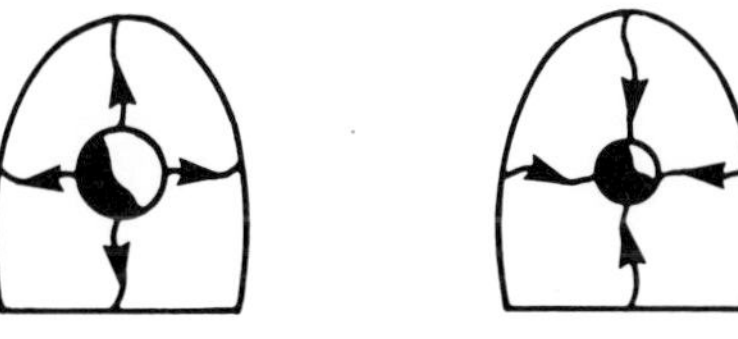

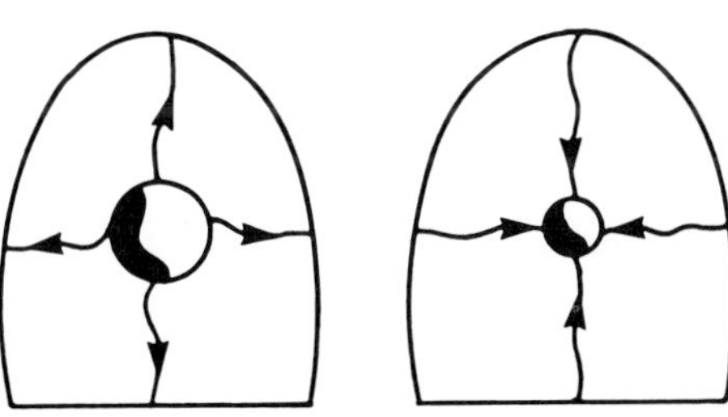

Fig. 20-3. Effect of hyperinflation on airway caliber during inspiration and expiration is shown schematically. The top of the figure depicts the situation at a normal functional residual capacity (no hyperinflation) and demonstrates the smaller cross-sectional diameter of the airways in asthma, which decrease even further during expiration. The bottom of the figure depicts the situation with an increased functional residual capacity (hyperinflation). The cross-sectional diameter of the airways is increased compared to the diameter existing without hyperinflation, and the effect is especially significant during expiration.

consequences favorable and unfavorable. The enlarged resting lung volume helps to distend the airways, providing relatively larger airway lumens through which air can move. The result is that airway resistance will be less than it would be if breathing occurred at the normal, lower, functional residual capacity (Fig. 20-3). On the other hand, the work of breathing increases because breathing at high functional residual capacity requires increased inspiratory pressure (Fig. 20-4). In addition, receptors in the chest wall and muscles recognize the increased functional residual capacity, and this is interpreted as inappropriate. Thus the feeling of dyspnea will increase at the larger functional residual capacity in spite of the fact that expiratory resistance may be relatively decreased. Furthermore, the hyperinflation and air-trapping adversely effect the cardiovascular system as explained below.

It should be noted that although lung volumes may be measured during an acute asthmatic episode and demonstrate the marked increase in residual volume and functional residual capacity, it is generally not necessary or practical to do so. A measurement of the vital capacity and a chest radiograph, which is obtained at total lung capacity, provides a semiquantitative judgment of the degree of hyperinflation present.

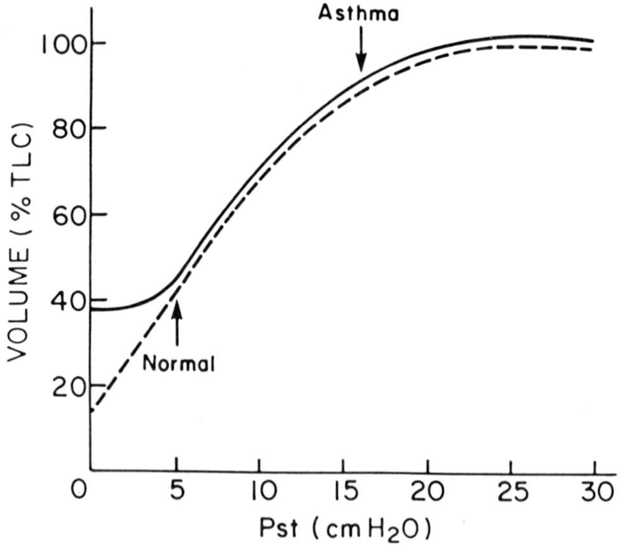

Fig. 20-4. A schematic representation of the static pressure–volume recordings of the lungs of a normal subject (solid lines) and a patient with an acute asthmatic episode (dashed lines) is shown. Total lung volume as a percentage of total lung capacity is recorded over static recoil pressure measured as esophageal pressure. The arrows delineate the position where tidal breathing occurs. The patient with an acute asthma attack tidally breathes at a much higher lung volume than the normal individual. This results in higher elastic recoil pressures with resultant increased work of breathing. It should be noted that during an acute asthmatic attack the entire pressure–volume curve may be shifted upward.

Distribution of Ventilation

Normally, inspired gas is distributed relatively homogeneously throughout the 300 million alveoli of the adult lungs. The evenness of the distribution depends on the fact that the distribution of the resistance of the small airways and the compliance of the alveoli are similar in all regions of the lungs. Frequently in diseases affecting the lungs, the abnormalities are not evenly distributed, so there is an increase in resistance in some airways but not in others; the affected areas of the lung empty and fill slower than the more normal areas. Such is the case in asthma, in which the abnormalities in pressure–flow and pressure–volume in the airways are distributed unevenly throughout the lungs.

The uneven distribution of the increased resistance in the airways during an asthmatic episode has two predominant effects: (a) the lung becomes more difficult to ventilate, and (b) arterial oxygenation decreases. Ventilating areas of the lung with increased airways resistance becomes progressively more difficult with higher respiratory rates. This is termed *frequency dependence*. During an acute asthmatic exacerbation, both tachypnea and frequency dependence are present; as a consequence, more effort must be expended to ventilate the lungs. In addition, areas with regionally increased resistance have decreased ventilation and produce mismatching of inspired gas and blood flow leading to hypoxemia.

Mechanisms of Dyspnea

A number of factors, all culminating in a greater effort associated with breathing, seem to cause the sensation of dyspnea in asthma. These include (a) an increase in overall airway resistance; (b) hyperinflation, resulting in increased pressures required to move a normal tidal volume and a sensation of inappropriateness of length–tension relationships in the chest wall; (c) regional increases in resistance that tend to make the lung progressively more difficult to ventilate at rapid respiratory rates; and (d) increased ventilatory drive producing increased respiratory rates. These abnormalities not only produce shortness of breath, but also increase the work of breathing required of the respiratory muscles.

Respiratory Muscles

The abnormalities produced by the abnormal pressure–flow and pressure–volume relationships of the respiratory system during an acute asthmatic episode increase the work performed by the respiratory muscles and decrease their efficiency. The increased work relates directly to the increased airway resistance, hyperinflation, and frequency dependence of the lung. The decreased efficiency is produced by the abnormal position of the diaphragm when hyperinflation occurs, especially when associated with rapid respiratory rates.

Alveolar Gas Exchange

The mechanical disturbances occurring in the respiratory system are accompanied by abnormalities in alveolar gas exchange. However, the correlation between the severity of the obstruction and the abnormality in gas exchange is not exact. There is a general correlation between the FEV_1 and the arterial oxygen tension, as the FEV_1 decreases, arterial oxygenation tends to decrease. A marked decrease in arterial oxygen tension probably indicates a severe asthmatic episode. However, this relationship is highly variable. Airway obstruction may be severe with a relatively well preserved arterial oxygen tension. Thus measurement of oxygen tension may be misleading in evaluating the severity of an asthmatic episode and should not replace spirometry.

Carbon dioxide production and elimination are also affected during an acute asthmatic episode. The increased work of the respiratory muscles increases production of carbon dioxide. Initially, however, and even through moderately severe attacks, the arterial tension of carbon dioxide is less than normal and respiratory alkalosis is present. This is a result of increased ventilatory drive. If the asthmatic episode worsens or becomes prolonged, however, lung function may deteriorate and respiratory muscles may fatigue. Both of these factors adversely effect carbon dioxide elimination, especially in the setting of increased carbon dioxide production. The net effect is for the arterial carbon dioxide tension to rise, reaching normal or higher levels. This development is omnious and occurs when the FEV_1 decreases below 25% of the predicted value. Endotracheal intubation with institution of mechanical ventilation may be a necessary life-saving measure.

Hemodynamics

An acute asthmatic episode may have profound hemodynamic effects. The high lung volumes, together with marked intrathoracic pressure changes, lead to a marked increase in the pressure distending the alveoli (transpulmonary pressure). Capillaries in these distended alveoli become attenuated. As a result, pulmonary vascular resistance increases and pulmonary artery pressure rises. Right ventricular pressure and wall tension must rise concomittantly. Increased right ventricular afterload may explain the electrocardiographic findings of "P" pulmonale and even right axis deviation during an acute asthmatic episode.

In addition to the effects on the pulmonary circulation and right ventricular function, acute asthma may also alter the systemic circulation and left ventricular performance. The change is readily observed with a blood pressure cuff; the normal decrease (less than 10 mm) in blood pressure during inspiration (pulsus paradoxus) is exaggerated. The reason for the pulsus paradoxus in asthma is not entirely clear but appears to involve both the increased airway resistance and increased functional residual capacity. In an acute asthmatic attack, extreme negative pleural pressure swings are generated. These large negative pressures outside of the left ventricle increase the presure across the left ventricle (transmural pressure). As a result, left ventricular wall tension, and thus afterload, increases. As the pleural pressures are most negative during inspiration, afterload will increase during inspiration. This results in a decrease in the volume of blood ejected from the left ventricle during inspiration. This effect may be exaggerated by the simultaneous abnormalities produced in the pulmonary circulation and in right ventricular function. The magnitude of pulsus paradoxus correlates in a general way with the severity of the asthmatic episode. If respiratory muscles fatigue and less negative pleural pressures are generated, however, pulsus paradoxicus may decrease, in spite of the fact that the patient's condition is deteriorating.

CORRELATION OF FUNCTION WITH CLINICAL MANIFESTATIONS

During acute asthma of moderate to marked severity the patient generally demonstrates wheezing, tachypnea, use of the accessory respiratory muscles, and increased pulsus paradoxus. The chest will appear hyperinflated by clinical and radiological examination. There is a marked reduction of expiratory flow, with a measured FEV_1 approaching 25% of its predicted value. The FEF_{25-75} and other parameters of flow are similarly reduced. The residual volume is markedly increased. Arterial blood gases show moderate reductions in the arterial tensions of both oxygen and carbon dioxide and respiratory alkalosis.

As treatment is initiated, the patient's symptoms and signs improve more rapidly than the objective measurements of disordered physiology. When the accessory muscles are no longer in use and retractions have ceased, expiratory flow is still markedly impaired, and the FEV_1 approaches only 40% of predicted. When the effects of treatment progress to the point at which wheezing subsides and the patient becomes asymptomatic, the FEV_1 is likely to be only about 60% of predicted. Marked impairment of the FEF_{25-75} persists. The residual volume will still be approximately twice the predicted value and the arterial oxygen tension will remain reduced, and it may not return to its baseline normal value until 1 week following the acute episode. The point to be made is that when an acute asthmatic episode has resolved to the point where the patient is comfortable and free of adventitious breath sounds, there is still significant airway obstruction, hyperinflation, and abnormalities in alveolar gas exchange.

The divergence between improvement in clinical manifestation and altered physiology may best be explained by an understanding of airway geometry. The total cross-sectional area of the peripheral airways is great when compared to the more proximal airways. The initial improvement in symptoms and signs correlates with relief of bronchoconstriction in the proximal airways where small changes may have dramatic effects. However, there are still significant abnormalities that persist in the more distal airways in which small changes in airway size may be less noticeable. It is these abnormalities that account for the continued hyperinflation, decrease in flow rates, and defects in gas exchange in spite of clinical improvement.

These observations have great clinical significance: (a) measurements of expiratory flow obtained by bedside spirometry are critical in judging the severity of an asthmatic episode; (b) objective measurements are helpful in evaluating the response to therapy; (c) in spite of initial improvement, significant abnormalities in airway function linger following an acute episode; (d) these abnormalities require prolonged treatment (at least 1 week) to avoid recurrent attacks and to restore airway function to normal; and (e) there are patients with "asymptomatic" asthma, who may be detected only by spirometry and who will improve markedly with bronchodilator therapy.

SUGGESTED READINGS

Dunnill, M. S. The pathology of asthma. In *Transactions of World Asthma Conferences*. London: Heart & Elect Association, March 1965.

Mayfield, J. D., Paez, P. N., & Nicholson, D. P. *Thorax*, 1971, *26*, 591.

McFadden, E. R., Jr., & Lyons, H. A. *New Engl. J. Med.*, 1968, *278*, 1027.

McFadden, E. R., Jr., & Lyons, H. A. *J. Appl. Physiol.*, 1968, *25*, 365.

McFadden, E. R. Jr., Kiser, R., & de Groot, W. J. *New Engl. J. Med.*, 1973, *288*, 221.

Meisner, P., & Hugh-Jones, P. *Br. Med. J.*, 1968, *1*, 470.

Rosenthal, R. R. (Ed.). *J. Allergy Clin. Immunol.*, 1979, *64*(6, P. 2), 561.

Roussos, C., & Macklem, P. T. *New Engl. J. Med.*, 1982, *307*, 786–797.

Wise, R. A., Robotham, J. L., Summer, W. R. *Lung*, 1981, *159*, 175–186.

QUESTIONS

1. As an acute asthmatic episode begins to resolve and the patient becomes asymptomatic, which of the following statements are true?

   a. Arterial oxygenation has returned to normal.
   b. The residual volume has returned to normal.
   c. Significant airway obstruction is still detectable by spirometry.
   d. Abnormalities in small airways will be nondetectable.

2. Acute airway obstruction in asthma may include all the following effects on the circulation except:

   a. Increased left ventricular afterload.
   b. Increased pulmonary vascular resistance.
   c. Increased right ventricular afterload.
   d. Increased left ventricular preload.

3. Dyspnea in acute asthma is a result of all the following except:

   a. The increased airway resistance.
   b. The marked hyperinflation.
   c. The marked hypoxemia that is a usual accompaniment of moderate asthma.
   d. The frequency dependence of terminal respiratory units.

4. All the following is true of the marked hyperinflation occurring with an acute asthmatic episode except:

   a. It leads to inefficiency in diaphragmatic function.
   b. It increases the work required of the respiratory muscles.
   c. It produces a relative decrease in airway resistance.
   d. It decreases the pulmonary vasculator resistance.

5. The severity of an asthmatic attack is best evaluated by (choose only one):

   a. Arterial blood gases.
   b. Pulsus paradoxus.
   c. Measurement of expiratory flow rates.
   d. The character of wheezing present.
   e. Chest radiograph.

6. All the following are true of the alveolar gas exchange abnormalities which occur during an acute asthmatic episode except:

a. Carbon dioxide tension in arterial blood is usually low except when the FEV_1 is less than 25% of predicted.
b. Hypoxemia correlates only in a general way with the degree of airway obstruction present as measured by the FEV_1.
c. An elevated carbon dioxide tension in acute asthma results from decreased ventilatory drive.
d. Respiratory alkalosis is the most common acid–base abnormality detected.

Answers can be found in Appendix B at the end of the book.

Phillip E. Korenblat

21

Asthma Management

Asthma, as defined by the American Thoracic Society (1962), is a disease characterized by an increased responsiveness of the trachea and bronchi to various stimuli and manifest by a widespread narrowing of airways that changes in severity either spontaneously or as a result of therapy. This increased responsiveness may lead to a diversity of airways obstruction over variable lengths of time. Asthmatics have pulmonary hyperreactivity, regardless of whether the eliciting factors are allergic (hyperresponsive) or nonallergic (hyperirritable).

DIAGNOSIS

An etiologic classification of asthma includes the following divisions: allergic, infectious, aspirin-sensitive, allergic bronchial pulmonary aspergillosis (APBA), exercise-induced, occupation-related, and idiopathic. Often the same patient has multiple etiologic factors.

Differential Diagnosis

The proper management of patients with symptoms suggestive of asthma requires the physician to consider that the symptoms are not in fact due to asthma. When the patient is seen initially, an accurate diagnosis requires a careful, intensive, inquiring history and an alert and suspicious attitude toward findings on physical examination. The diagnostic differential must be fully considered with each patient (Table 21-1).

Causative and Contributory Factors

A description of the first episodes of asthma and the events surrounding them must be completely elicited since they often reveal the best evidence of the condition's etiology. We have seen a child for whom long-range immunotherapy and a

ALLERGY: THEORY AND PRACTICE
ISBN 0-8089-1619-X

Table 21-1 *Differential Diagnosis of Airways Obstruction*

Obstructive lesions
Endobronchial tumor
Endobronchial foreign body
External bronchial compression
Laryngeal obstruction
Congenital anomaly
Chronic obstructive lung disease in exacerbation and/or cystic fibrosis
Congestive heart failure
Pulmonary embolus

meticulous environmental control program had been outlined who was cured of his "asthma" by removal of a peanut from his bronchus. In this patient there were obvious clues to the correct diagnosis through both history and physical examination. The child had eaten peanuts and was noted to cough. Several days later wheezing began and persisted for several years, remaining appreciably unaltered by the use of multiple medications. There was no history of a causative infection or inhalant antigen exposure that would explain the occurrence of asthma. Further evidence to rule out asthma was apparent on physical examination. Wheezes were audible primarily on inspiration, and inhaled bronchodilators were ineffectual. A chest roentgenogram during full expiration revealed a localized area of air trapping and bronchoscopy demonstrated the peanut, which was extracted. Attention to the history and physical examination in this child, previously evaluated, and in whom an inappropriate management plan had been recommended, was rewarding. In a similar case, a 42-year-old man was treated with bronchodilators for 2 years for wheezing until it was appreciated that his wheeze was focal and mainly inspiratory. Following resection of a bronchial adenoma, his symptoms disappeared.

Just as other conditions marked by wheezing can simulate asthma, symptomatic asthma may appear without wheezing. Asthma may thus be expressed as persistent nonproductive cough, breathlessness, or chest discomfort often worsened by exercise.

Once satisfied that there are no other operative etiologies and asthma is diagnosed, the physician must elicit causative and contributory factors (Table 21-2).

MANAGEMENT

General Approach

In contrast to a few decades ago, when therapy of asthma stressed the desperately ill patient and the relief of acute attacks, attention is currently directed at preventing asthmatic episodes by reducing the hyperreactivity of the airways. There is appreciation now that the asthmatic patient is most effectively treated at a stage when asthma is only minimally apparent clinically. If prophylactic therapy is stressed and treatment is accelerated promptly with increasing symptoms, life-endangering episodes of status asthmaticus are largely preventable. The physician must make certain that the patient understands that daily medication on a round-the-clock basis will

Table 21-2 *Causative and Contributory Factors in Asthma*

Immunologic	
Type I allergic sensitivity (IgE-mediated)	
Type III allergic sensitivity (antigen-IgG-complement, i.e., allergic alveolitis)	
Infectious	
Viral URI-induced infection	
Post lower respiratory viral infection (followed by persistent asthma)	
Bronchitis	
Sinusitis	
Miscellaneous	
Aspirin sensitivity	Beta–adrenergic blocking drugs
Exercise-induced bronchospasm	Metabisulfite sensitivity
Occupational exposure	Monosodium glutamate sensitivity
Esophageal reflux	
Emotional stress	
Irritant sensitivity	

cause less harm than "toughing it out" with frequent asthmatic attacks. It is preferable to prevent wheezing rather than tolerate even a small degree of frequent symptoms. Simply stated, asthma begets more asthma.

The pathophysiology and chemical mediators of asthma have been presented in Chapters 20 and 3. Each pharmacologic agent used in the care of asthma has been discussed in Chapters 15 through 18. This information is integrated in this chapter and a scheme for the clinical management of asthma presented.

Careful attention to the emotional factors involved is a prerequisite to proper care. Environmental control is fully discussed in Chapter 12 and will, therefore, not be discussed in this chapter.

A comprehensive approach to the care of the asthmatic involves careful consideration of the problems and needs of the individual patient. Therefore, the recommendations made in this chapter should be applied to each patient only insofar as they are individually adaptable. A clinician must carefully consider the concerns of the patient and the immediate family, being flexible when possible and rigid only when necessary.

Pharmacologic Principles

The overreliance on a single medication often results in abuse of that medication and the development of side effects when it is necessary to increase the dosage to control exacerbating symptoms. Therefore, multiple medications thoughtfully introduced in a stepwise fashion are appropriate in the care of most asthmatics. Recent concern has been expressed regarding cardiotoxicity resulting from combination theophylline and beta agonist therapy[1,2] (Wilson, et al., 1981; FDA, 1981). There is not adequate evidence to abandon concomitant utilization of these two medications in the asthmatic (Novey, 1983). Often, however, adjunctive instructions and monitoring by the physician are called for. For example, theophylline, a mainstay in the care of asthma, should be administered according to blood theophylline levels to assure therapeutic and safe treatment. Therapy with cromolyn sodium, inhaled beta-adrenergic agonist, or beclomethasone dipropionate requires that the patient be well versed in the proper use of these agents. In fact, patients should be asked to demonstrate the extent of their expertise.

Although extensively covered in Chapter 18, corticosteroids deserve special mention to emphasize their importance in asthma. As a result of concern about side effects, clinicians are often too resistant to the early introduction of corticosteroids; however, it *is* proper that these medications ordinarily be the last included in a cumulative regimen, and they should be the first to be removed when symptoms have abated. Certainly, inclusion of corticosteroids in the treatment plan is appropriate for most patients requiring hospital admission because of asthma. In addition, outpatients who have persistent symptoms while on adequate doses of bronchodilators will usually need either inhaled or oral corticosteroids.

The therapy of the asthmatic patient is guided by the severity and chronicity of symptoms. Asthma may be sorted into mild, moderate, and severe classifications. This chapter presents a schema for managing asthma according to these categories.

Mild Asthma

Patients with mild asthma have episodic bouts of wheezing or cough, with or without dyspnea, and the symptoms are promptly relieved by medication. These patients do not need continuous medication. Between episodes, they are asymptomatic without bronchodilators and have good ventilatory function (e.g., FEV_1 and peak flow of at least 75% predicted). Suggested treatment regimens for acute and chronic mild asthma are given below.

Acute Mild Asthma

REGIMEN

Inhaled $beta_2$ agonist
Oral theophylline (add if needed)
Oral $beta_2$ agonist (add if needed)

EXAMPLE. A 13-year-old boy has a history of episodes of wheezing occurring 4–6 times a year. These episodes are relatively mild and do not interfere with his normal activity or sleep.

COMMENT. The physician must document that pulmonary function is normal during the "symptom-free interval." This may be accomplished by routine pulmonary function testing or by providing the patient with a peak flow meter (e.g., Mini-Wright) for self-examination periodically.

RECOMMENDATION. The initiation of an inhaled $beta_2$ agonist (metaproterenol or albuterol) 2 puffs 4 times daily (qid) under parental supervision for a brief period would be indicated in general for patients whose asthma occurs as discrete episodes at intervals of weeks to months and lasts only minutes to a few hours. If symptoms do not totally abate, oral theophylline and/or oral $beta_2$ agonist (i.e., albuterol, metaproterenol, or terbutaline) should be given as well.

Chronic Mild Asthma

REGIMEN.

Cromolyn sodium or oral theophylline
Inhaled $beta_2$ agonist (add if needed)
Oral $beta_2$ agonist (add if needed)

EXAMPLE. A 17-year-old girl presents with a history of asthma in the early and late spring. During the remainder of the year she is asymptomatic. She resides in the Midwest, where spring is punctuated by the presence of tree and grass pollen. Positive skin tests to trees and grasses are obtained.

COMMENT. This patient's symptoms are present to a variable degree for several weeks and thus require continuous medication during that period of time rather than medication taken "as needed" (prn) in episodes of acute mild asthma.

RECOMMENDATION. An immunotherapy program to protect against reactions to tree and grass pollen should be considered. Environmental control should be recommended (Chapter 12). Until a satisfactory response from the immunotherapy program has occurred, medications will be necessary. Initial therapy may be with either cromolyn sodium or theophylline. Cromolyn sodium offers the advantage of possible prophylaxis without the need of a blood level of the drug being determined, and it also has significantly less potential for side effects. Cromolyn sodium may be begun by inhalation (1 capsule qid) beginning 1 or 2 weeks prior to the season. If the prophylactic use of cromolyn sodium does not prevent the emergence of symptoms, it may be discontinued (although it may be increased to six or eight capsules daily before halting). Regardless of whether cromolyn sodium is discontinued, theophylline should be begun, with blood theophylline levels obtained to assure proper dosing. Should symptoms persist, an inhaled $beta_2$ agonist can be added. [If cromolyn sodium alone or in combination with theophylline does not prevent the emergence of asthma, inhaled beclomethasone dipropionate (Vanceril or Beclovent) beginning 2–4 weeks prior to the following implicated season would be an appropriate prophylactic measure.] If these modalities are not totally successful, the patient probably has moderate or severe asthma.

Moderate Asthma

Patients with moderate asthma are those whose symptoms linger somewhat between attacks, reflected by spirometry values always well below normal. Suggested treatment regimens are given below.

Acute Moderate Asthma

REGIMEN. The following therapy is provided in the emergency room:

Parenteral epinephrine and/or terbutaline (in addition to nasal O_2 and adequate hydration)
Inhaled $beta_2$ agonist (add if needed)
Intravenous aminophylline (add if needed)
Intravenous corticosteroids (add if needed)

EXAMPLE. A 36-year-old woman with a 7-year history of asthma requiring daily theophylline and oral $beta_2$ agonist presents to the emergency room with increasing symptoms of bronchospasm. Pulmonary hyperreactivity, however, is moderately severe, and symptomatic wheezing limits her activity and renders her lungs unresponsive to her usual oral bronchodilators. On physical examination there is a paradoxic pulse of 20 mm Hg and inspiratory as well as expiratory wheezes. The complete blood count (CBC) reveals a mild leukocytosis with 15% eosinophilia. Sputum demonstrates 90% polymorphonuclear leukocytes (PMN) and 10% eosinophils (eos) along with gram-positive cocci in pairs. Hyperaeration is noted on chest roentgenogram. Sinus tachycardia is the only electrocardiographic abnormality. The FEV_1 is 1.2 l/min, with a peak flow of 100 l/min (40% of predicted normal). Initial blood gases are reported: $Paco_2$, 56 mm Hg; Pco_2, 38 mm Hg, and pH, 7.38.

COMMENT. Upper respiratory tract infections, usually viral in origin, often are responsible for the exacerbation of symptoms in patients with asthma. The care of the moderately severe asthmatic with acute respiratory symptoms is essentially the same regardless of whether the increased symptoms are secondary to infection, untoward physiologic events, or immunologic factors, except for the addition of antibiotics in those instances with accompanying infection.

RECOMMENDATION. The patient is begun on nasal O_2 at 5 l/min, and blood gases are repeated in 20 minutes. Aqueous epinephrine 1:1000, 0.30 ml, or terbutaline 0.25 mg is administered subcutaneously and, if necessary, repeated in 20 minutes. Metaproterenol 0.30 ml added to 2.5 ml sodium chloride is inhaled by nebulization. A theophylline blood level is obtained. Since the patient has already received theophylline and there is no history of theophylline intoxication, aminophylline 2.5–3.0 mg/kg is given IV over 20 minutes as a loading dose followed by 0.6–0.9 mg/kg hr^{-1}. Intravenous fluids are calculated to deliver 2 liters in the first 6 hours. After 45 minutes the paradoxic pulse is no longer present and chest examination demonstrates only a prolonged expiratory phase. The FEV_1 increases to 2.5 l/min, peak flow to 250 l/min, and Po_2 to 65 mm Hg; the Pco_2 is reported as 28 mm Hg with a pH of 7.42. Because of historic and laboratory evidence of infection (purulent sputum and gram-positive cocci on gram stain) appropriate antibiotics are begun. When the patient is discharged from the emergency room, she should be instructed to continue the oral theophylline, oral beta agonist and inhaled beta agonist as well as antibiotics. She is given an appointment to be seen in the physician's office in 48–72 hours. Had the pulmonary functions and blood gases not demonstrated an adequate response within 30–45 minutes, then intravenous (IV) corticosteroids would have been administered and the patient admitted to the hospital. The presence of eosinophils in the sputum does not necessarily imply allergic asthma, but is an indicator of reversible airways disease, regardless of the etiology. In pure allergic asthma, the sputum reveals ciliated columnar epithelial cells and 5–85% eosinophils. When infection is playing a prominent role in the asthmatic episode, there may be up to 20% eosinophils, but most of the cells are PMN. Antibiotics were included in the management of this patient because there was evidence of infection. Antibiotics should not be given routinely to all asthmatics who present with increasing symptoms. In patients with moderately severe asthma, there are ample data to demonstrate that the combination of $beta_2$ agonist and theophylline is more effective in relieving symptoms than either agent used alone.

It may be difficult to determine which emergency room patient should be admitted to the hospital and which discharged. Too often, only the findings on physical examination (i.e., relief of obvious dyspnea, diminished wheezing, lessened auxiliary chest muscular contraction) and improvement in blood gases are the major considerations. Although a pulsus paradoxus of 10 mm Hg or greater will be present only if the FEV_1 is 1.2 liters or less (Rebuck & Read, 1971), pulmonary function studies are still necessary to render proper judgment as to how well the patient will fare after leaving the emergency room. The FEV_1 is a satisfactory representation of pulmonary function and can be used to make this judgment (Kelsen et al., 1978). If the pretreatment FEV_1 is less than 0.6 l/min or if the maximally achieved posttreatment FEV_1 is not equal to or greater than 1.6 l/min, hospital admission will probably be required (Nowak et al., 1979). A second guideline is to plan admission to the hospital if the FEV_1 does not rise at least 0.4 l/min from the initial FEV_1 after treatment (Kelsen et al., 1978). To disregard these predictors and not admit the patient to the hospital will, more often than not, result in recurrent emergency room visits because of the patient's increasing respiratory difficulty. It is specifically at this juncture of management that the physician often has a last opportunity to prevent the occurrence of status asthmaticus. Most patients who develop status have made several trips to a physician's office or an emergency room within the preceding few days and been discharged either after inadequate treatment or after an inadequate response to proper treatment.

Chronic Moderate Asthma

REGIMEN

Cromolyn sodium and/or oral theophylline
Oral $beta_2$ agonist (add if needed)
Inhaled $beta_2$ agonist (add if needed)
Oral corticosteroids (add if needed)
Inhaled beclomethasone dipropionate (add if needed)

The removal of oral corticosteroids and any of above not felt to be beneficial.

EXAMPLE. A 47-year-old man with a history of perennial wheezing for three years is seen in the physician's office. His asthma began after a severe bout of bronchitis. He has a normal hemoglobin, hematocrit, and white blood cell count. There is an elevated absolute eosinophil count of 535 mm^3. A chest roentgenogram demonstrates only hyperaeration. The patient has a normal erythrocyte sedimentation rate (ESR) and normal immunoglobulins, including IgE. Spirometry reveals mild to moderate airways obstruction with a 20% improvement following inhalation of a $beta_2$ agonist. Blood gases are normal. Allergy skin testing demonstrates no significant positive reactions.

COMMENT. Before the availability of corticosteroids, the emergence of asthma after the age of 40 carried with it a dramatically poor prognosis. At present, the armamentarium of drugs and philosophy of management makes this type of asthma relatively easy to treat, with a much improved prognosis.

Cromolyn sodium is an appropriate drug to consider initially in treating moderate asthma. However, in those patients with an exacerbation of symptoms theophylline and beta agonist are ordinarily indicated first to establish prompt relief of symptoms. Once the symptoms of bronchospasm have been controlled, cromolyn sodium can be included to take advantage of its prophylactic effect.

RECOMMENDATION. The stepwise introduction of theophylline, with blood levels of the drug monitored to assure proper dosage, together with inhaled and oral beta_2 agonist comprise the initial therapy. Once symptoms have abated, the inclusion of cromolyn sodium should be considered. Compliance with medication is stressed on each office visit. If symptoms continue, oral steroids are begun at doses of 40–60 mg/day with a decreasing dose schedule (Table 21-3). Once airway function has improved, and prior to the cessation of oral steroids, beclomethasone dipropionate is begun at 3–4 puffs 3 or 4 times daily (tid or qid). If the need for long-term beclomethasone dipropionate is established, some feel that cromolyn sodium will not enhance the patient's care (Togood et al., 1981).

Pulmonary function testing is essential to conduct proper follow-up of this patient and others with asthma requiring daily medication. Many feel that the total eosinophil count can be used as a guide in regulating oral corticosteroid dosage in steroid-dependent adult patients (Horn et al., 1975). In Europe, where ipratropium bromide (Atrovent), an atropine-like parasympathomimetic, is available, it is often included in therapy if because of recurrent symptoms oral corticosteroids are needed continuously. This drug is given in addition to the theophylline, beta agonist, and beclomethasone dipropionate. Ipratropium bromide may also lower or halt the requirement for oral corticosteroids. However, ipratropium bromide is indicated only when inhalation challenge has demonstrated its effectiveness by improving FEV_1 by 20% or greater. If corticosteroids must be continued, they should be adjusted to allow for alternate-day dosing if possible.

For patients who comply with this full regimen of bronchodilators and beclomethasone dipropionate and who continue to require greater than 10 mg/day of prednisone, one must consider the possibility of other diseases or complicating factors, such as exposure to environmental or occupational causative agents, vasculitis, cystic fibrosis, immunodeficiency, and emotional interplay. There are asthmatics who have concomitant sinusitis. For reasons not well understood, correction of the sinus disease, either by appropriate antibiotics or, if necessary, surgery, may lead to easier control of asthma.

Table 21-3 *Suggested Steroid Schedule for Outpatient Acute Moderate Asthma*

Each dose is given for 2 days:	
Prednisone:	20 mg bid
	15 mg bid
	10 mg bid
	5 mg tid
	5 mg bid
	5 mg od

EXAMPLE. A 13-year-old boy presents with a history of late spring and fall wheezing. The episodes last one to several days during which the child feels uncomfortable and limits his activities.

COMMENTS. This child is classified as having moderate asthma because of both the duration of asthma and the degree of discomfort incurred.

RECOMMENDATION. A trial of preseasonal inhaled cromolyn sodium 4 times daily beginning one or two weeks before the onset of the usual season of involvement should be undertaken. If this does not prevent symptoms, theophylline is added to the treatment regimen, preferably in the form of a sustained-relief preparation (to aid in compliance). A blood theophylline level should be obtained to demonstrate a therapeutic concentration of drug. If cromolyn sodium is ineffectual and the child continues to wheeze while being treated with the theophylline preparation, an oral $beta_2$ agonist should be added to the treatment regimen. The theophylline is readjusted if necessary to maintain a therapeutic blood level, and if there is continued difficulty, an inhaled $beta_2$ agonist can be made available to the patient's parents. It is preferable not to give the child an inhaled $beta_2$ agonist to have at the child's ready disposal because of the possible psychological dependence on the rapid relief obtained from this form of therapy. Persistent wheezing should be managed with oral corticosteroids, and if it is felt that steroids will be necessary for several months, an attempt should be made to convert the therapy with oral steroids to treatment with beclomethasone dipropionate 3–4 puffs tid or qid. The beclomethasone dipropionate dosage may be decreased, depending on the patient's response. Oral $beta_2$ agonist and theophylline (monitored to assure therapeutic levels) are continued until the season of involvement has ended, as is beclomethasone dipropionate if it has been part of the therapy.

Appropriate skin testing and an immunotherapy program should be outlined for the next year. In addition, if corticosteroids were required this season, consideration should be given to prescribing prophylactic beclomethasone dipropionate aerosol several weeks prior to the next season of involvement.

Many clinicians would not necessarily begin the patient's therapy with cromolyn sodium but would use this agent as a steroid-sparing drug for those patients taking theophylline and $beta_2$ agonist who have continued difficulty and require steroids. Although it has been usual to include cromolyn sodium in the care of allergic and exercise-induced asthma, it has not been advocated for nonallergic wheezing [except with some occupational exposures, i.e., toluene diisocynate (TDI sensitivity)]. Recent data suggest that cromolyn sodium has a role in the treatment of other forms of asthma (Harris, 1981).

Severe Asthma

Patients with severe asthma have symptoms that vary from episodic wheezing and cough with dyspnea while on continuous therapy to hypercapnea requiring mechanical ventilation. Often pulmonary functions are significantly diminished, and during bouts of difficulty, spirometry shows severe decrease in airflow; an example would be an FEV_1 of 1 liter or less and a peak flow of 80 l/min or less (in an average adult). Suggested treatment regimens are given below.

Acute Severe Asthma

REGIMEN

Parenteral epinephrine and/or terbutaline (in addition to nasal O_2 and adequate hydration)
Inhaled $beta_2$ agonist (add if needed)
Intravenous aminophylline (add if needed)
Intravenous corticosteroids (add if needed)
Assisted mechanical ventilation (add if needed)

EXAMPLE. A 14-year-old boy with a history of mild perennial asthma went to a local emergency room for increasing symptoms of bronchospasm. Pulmonary function studies and blood gases were not obtained. He was given an injection of epinephrine. Prior to discharge from the emergency room, he received an injection of epinephrine (Sus-Phrine). The next morning, after a sleepless night, he returned to the emergency room where he received epinephrine, aminophylline, inhaled $beta_2$ agonist, and oral steroids. Later that day, because of continued symptoms, he presented to another emergency room.

Physical examination revealed a tired, breathless young man who was diaphoretic and unable to complete even short sentences without stopping to catch his breath. There was a pulsus paradoxus of 30 mm Hg, and chest examination revealed a hyperresonant chest with brief, high-pitched diffuse wheezing. Pulmonary studies showed that his FEV_1 was 0.6 l peak flow 60 l/min. Blood gases were $Pa{O_2}$, 48 mm Hg; $P{CO_2}$, 38 mm Hg; and pH, 7.32. His chest roentgenogram demonstrated hyperaeration without infiltrates, and the ECG showed only sinus tachycardia. He was admitted immediately to the Respiratory Care Unit and given nasal oxygen, epinephrine, a nebulized $beta_2$ agonist, IV aminophylline, and IV steroids. Over the next 2 hours there was continued deterioration in his clinical appearance and his $P{CO_2}$ rose to 55 mm Hg with a pH of 7.25. In spite of nasal oxygen, the $Pa{O_2}$ remained at 48 mm Hg. An endotracheal tube was inserted, and the patient was begun on assisted mechanical ventilation. Additional laboratory data included CBC, chemistry profile with electrolytes, urinalysis, sputum culture, gram stain, and Wright stain for eosinophils. A repeat chest roentgenogram was done after intubation to document that the endotracheal tube was positioned properly.

COMMENT. In addition to adequate history, physical examination, and routine laboratory data, proper care of the asthmatic interviewed in the emergency room requires that a spirogram or peak flow measurement and a chest roentgenogram be obtained. Those patients who do not respond to emergency medication should be admitted promptly to the Respiratory Care Unit.

Hospitalized Patients

The primary care of hospitalized patients with acute asthma involves three spheres of management (Senior et al., 1975), discussed as follows.

ALVEOLAR GAS EXCHANGE. Hypoxemia is an expected occurrence in asthma. It is necessary to provide nasal oxygen to maintain a desired $Pa{O_2}$ of 60–80 mm Hg. This is usually accomplished without difficulty via nasal prongs at 2 liters or by using a 28% Venturi mask. In keeping with the oxygen dissociation curve, a Pa_{O_2} of 60 mm Hg allows almost 90% oxygen saturation. One must remember that alveolar hyperventilation is typical in asthma. Therefore, most symptomatic asthmatics have a P_{CO_2} of 30–35 mm Hg. In severe asthma the patient's effectiveness of ventilation is impaired and the P_{CO_2} may rise to 40 mm Hg, ordinarily a normal value, but in this setting a sign of impending catastrophe. A normal or slightly elevated P_{CO_2} in a severely symptomatic patient is cause for great concern (Fig. 21-1). Combined with an assessment of the patient's overall condition and trend, a rising P_{CO_2} is an indication for strongly considering intubation and ventilatory support. On occasion, particularly in children, a trial of IV isoproterenol has been advocated. This mode of therapy is attempted when the physician feels it will control the rise in P_{CO_2} and prevent the need for intubation. However, IV isoproterenol is used for only 6–8 hours, and if not fully successful, intubation is carried out. *This manner of therapy is discussed primarily in an effort to be complete and the author would discourage its use. If attempted, however, IV isoproterenol should be used only in a respiratory care unit by persons familiar with its use and during close cardiac monitoring.* In-

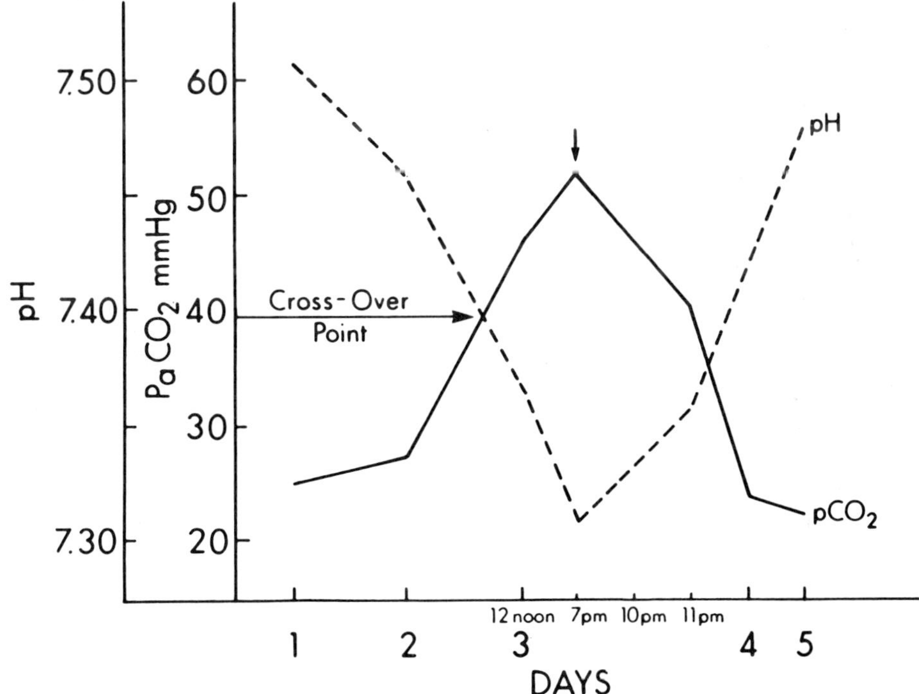

Fig. 21-1. Crossover stage in status asthmaticus. Initial hypocapnia and respiratory alkalosis deteriorating to frank respiratory acidemia. Note the normalization of Pa_{CO_2}–pH relationships as an index to such frank hypoventilation. The P_O value was 80 mm Hg because of supplemental oxygen. The patient recovered fully after intubation and mechanical ventilation were instituted at point of vertical arrow. Adapted from Weiss E. B., & Faling, L. J. *Ann. Allergy*, 1968, *26*, p. 889. With permission.

appropriate delay in instituting mechanical ventilation can be disastrous, although mechanical ventilation itself carries hazards such as pneumothorax and pneumomediastinum. Details of ventilator care in the asthmatic, such as the use of paralyzing agents, should be sought in the appropriate literature.

DRUGS. Unless the patient requires mechanical ventilation, sedation is categorically contraindicated. Anxiety is a natural response to asthma and will cease when airflow improves. Although by definition the severely ill asthmatic is not responsive to $beta_2$ agonists, these agents should be continued, either subcutaneously or orally, because there is evidence that the introduction of corticosteroids will improve airway responsiveness to beta agonists. Nebulized $beta_2$ agonist is administered every 4 hours. However, IPPB machines, which were often used in the past, no longer are advocated because there is an increased incidence of pneumothorax with their use in addition to the problem of delivering adequate tidal volumes at flow rates that will satisfy the patient's air hunger. Aminophylline is maintained IV after an initial loading dose of 5.6 mg/kg in a person not presently taking the drug. The aminophylline is continued at 0.6–0.9 $mm/kg/hr^{-1}$. A loading dose of corticosteroids in the form of 1–2 mg/kg of IV methylprednisolone sodium succinate is followed by 1 mg/kg every 4 hours for several days. High-dose corticosteroids may cause significant hypokalemia; therefore, supplemental potassium chloride will often be necessary. Antibiotics are not included unless there is evidence of infection. Once the bronchospasm has halted and pulmonary functions have improved adequately, $beta_2$ agonist, aminophylline, and corticosteroids may be administered orally. They must be continued for several weeks following hospital discharge. Sodium bicarbonate is rarely indicated for respiratory acidosis. (When acidosis is in need of correction, then intubation is indicated and the ventilatory rate can be adjusted to increase CO_2 elimination.)

CLEARANCE OF MUCOUS SECRETIONS. Obstruction of the airways by impacted, tenacious mucus rather than bronchospasm is usually responsible for death in the asthmatic. The most appropriate approach to helping removal of secretions is the administration of adequate amounts of fluids (2.5–4 l/day in adults) combined with chest physiotherapy. Mucolytic agents and bronchial lavage are rarely indicated. Ultrasonic nebulization tends to increase irritability of the airways and is not recommended. It is useful to have a sputum cup at the bedside to provide the physician with another way of judging the patient's progress. Initially, there will be little or no sputum production. Coincident with improvement mucus plugs may then appear, followed by a gradual thinning of sputum.

Chronic Severe Asthma

REGIMEN

Cromolyn sodium and/or oral theophylline
Oral $beta_2$ agonist (add if needed)
Inhaled $beta_2$ agonist (add if needed)
Oral corticosteroids (if needed)
Inhaled beclomethasone dipropionate (add if needed)

Removal of oral corticosteroids and any of above not felt to be beneficial
Trial troleandomycin (TAO) (add if needed)

EXAMPLE. A 25-year-old man with perennial asthma of 15 years' duration was found to have an elevated IgE of 700 IU (normal: 20 IU or less), 40% eosinophils, and 60% PMN in his sputum along with a 15% peripheral eosinophilia. His ESR, chest roentgenogram, $alpha_1$ antitrypsin level, sweat chlorides, and other immunoglobulins were normal. Spirometry revealed a significant decrease (less than 60% predicted) in airflow, which improved more than 20% with inhaled albuterol. There was no evidence of a restrictive component. Hypersensitivity pneumonitis panel and *Aspergillus* precipitating antibody were negative, sinus roentgenograms were normal, and nasal brush biopsy did not demonstrate evidence of immotile cilia syndrome (see Chapter 31). Although the patient was taking 25 mg of prednisone per day, his absolute eosinophil count was $100/mm^3$. Skin testing had revealed positive reactions to house dust, dust mite, molds, trees, grasses, and ragweed. The patient had been following an immunotherapy program for 2 years with proper antigens and adequate doses. Environmental control was optimal, and there were no suspected occupational factors in his condition. His theophylline blood level was 18 mg/l, and he was taking terbutaline 5 mg tid and albuterol 2 puffs qid followed 20 minutes later by 2 puffs of beclomethasone dipropionate qid, in addition to the 25 mg prednisone/day. In spite of adherence to the above regimen, he had daily wheezing and limitation of his activities.

Initially, the patient's beclomethasone dipropionate was increased to 4 puffs qid; however, there was no improvement. Prednisone was then switched to equivalent amounts of methylprednisolone in preparation for a planned trial of troleandomycin (TAO), a macrolide antibiotic chemically similar to erythromycin estolate. (It has been shown that corticosteroids other than methylprednisolone do not give comparable reduction in airways hyperirritability when used in combination with TAO.) The methylprednisolone could not be lowered below 20 mg/day without the emergence of increased bronchospasm. A clinical trial with TAO was thus indicated and was carried out in accordance with the suggested protocol due to Zeiger et al. (Appendix I). There was significant improvement and the patient was maintained on oral and inhaled $beta_2$ agonist, round-the-clock theophylline, TAO 250 mg along with methyl prednisolone 8 mg every other day, and inhaled beclomethasone dipropionate.

COMMENT. This patient represents an unusual case and a challenge to even the most experienced clinician. Ordinarily, the symptoms of even the relatively severe chronic asthmatics can be controlled without the necessity of daily steroids in doses greater than 20 mg of prednisone per day.

Although the beneficial effect of TAO on chronic asthma has been known for two decades, its use has been tempered by a fear of its side effects. These side effects, which occur frequently, can be divided into steroid and nonsteroid varieties. The steroid-induced side effects diminish or halt (except in older patients who may exhibit osteoporosis, cataracts, and increased extraocular pressure) if the TAO trial is successful and culminates in alternate-day low-dose TAO and steroids. Non-steroid-related difficulties during TAO administration are usually mild and transient. They include gastrointestinal (GI) tract symptoms of nausea, pyosis, and cramps, along with theophylline intolerance and hepatic enzyme elevation. These side effects usually halt spontaneously or with reduced TAO dosage.*

SUMMARY

After interviewing and examining the patient who presents with bronchospasm, the physician should be able to answer a series of questions, beginning with:

1. Do I fully comprehend the patient's problem?
2. Does this patient have asthma, or is the presenting symptom another disease process?

If asthma is in fact the diagnosis, one should be able to answer the following questions:

1. What is the etiology of the asthma?
2. What precipitates or worsens the episodes? What diminishes the wheezing?
3. What diagnostic studies are indicated to establish the diagnosis and prepare a therapeutic tract to be followed?
4. Does the patient and the immediate family have a full and proper understanding of the illness?
5. Does the therapeutic program give due consideration to the individual needs of the patient? Have the simplest modalities of management been included first?
6. Does the patient and the immediate family understand the therapeutic goals and what is expected of them as participants in their own care?

Finally, all physicians should be prepared to ask themselves one additional question when caring for another human being, and that is, simply, "Has my patient been treated by me as I would wish to be treated by others?"

REFERENCES

American Thoracic Society. *Am. Rev. Respir. Dis.*, 1962, *85*, 762.

FDA, *Drug Bull.*, 1981, *11*, 19.

Harris, M. G. *Ann. Allergy*, 1981, *46*, 156.

Horn, B. R., Robin, E. D., Theodore, J., & Van Kessel, A. *New Engl. J. Med.*, 1975, *292*, 1152.

Kelsen, S. G., Kelsen, D. P., Fleegler, B. F., Jones, R. C., & Rodman, T. *Am. J. Med.*, 1978, *64*, 622.

Novey, H. S., *Immunology and Allergy Practice*, 1983, *V*, 208.

Nowak, R. M., Gordon, K. R., Wroblewski, D. A., Tomlanovich, M. C., & Kvale, P. A. *J. Am. Coll. Emer. Phys.*, 1979, *8*, 9.

Rebuck, A. S., & Read, J. *Am. J. Med.*, 1971, *51*, 788.

Senior, R. M., Lefrak, S. S., & Korenblat, P. E. *JAMA*, 1975, *231*, 1277.

Togood, J. H., Jennings, B., & Lecope, N. M. *J. Allergy Clin. Immunol.*, 1981, *67*, 317.

Weiss, E. B., & Faling, L. J. *Ann. Allergy*, 1968 *26*, 545.

Wilson, J. D., Sutherland, D. C., & Thomas, A. C. *Lancet*, 1981, *1*, 1235.

Zeiger, R. S., Schatz, M., Sperling, W., Simon, R. A., & Stevenson, D. D. *J. Allergy Clin. Immunol.*, 1980, *66*, 438.

*Suggested TAO administration protocol adapted from Zeiger, R. S., Schatz, M., Sperling, W., Simon, R. A., & Stevenson, D. D. *J. Allergy Clin. Immunol.*, 1980, *66*, p. 438. With permission.

QUESTIONS

1. Emotional stress is an etiologic classification of asthma. True or false.
2. Asthmatics should have one reliable drug to use so as not to confuse them with too many drugs. True or false.
3. Inhaled beta$_2$ agonist should not be used. True or false.
4. Patients dying of asthma usually die because of:
   a. dehydration
   b. arrhythmias
   c. acidosis
   d. mucus impaction
5. A normal or slightly elevated P_{CO_2} in asthma should cause concern. True or false.

Answers can be found in Appendix B at the end of the book.

Appendix 21-1 *SUGGESTED PROTOCOL FOR USE OF TROLEANDOMYCIN IN CORTICOSTEROID-DEPENDENT ASTHMATICS*

A. Initiation phase
   1. Select only severe, chronic, steroid-dependent and resistant asthmatics
   2. Optimize conventional asthma therapy (medical and psychological)
B. Methylprednisolone trial phase
   1. Switch to methylprednisolone at corticosteroid equivalent dose that maintains maximal clinical status and pulmonary function
   2. Attempt to reduce methylprednisolone
   3. Add TAO only if there is:
      a. Absence of liver disease
      b. Absence of drug allergy to macrolide antibiotics
      c. No response to methylpredinisolone
      d. Favorable response to methylprednisolone *but*
         1. Methylprednisolone required daily in children and adolescents
         2. Methylprednisolone required in doses greater than 10 mg daily in adults
         3. Methylprednisolone required in frequent high-dose bursts
         4. Adrenal suppression persists
         5. Patient remains poorly functional
C. TAO trial phase
   1. Inform and educate patient (i.e., about side effects and compliance)
   2. Obtain baseline studies (spirometry, liver function tests, theophylline and cortisol levels, eye examination)
   3. Reduce theophylline dosage by 25–50% depending on baseline levels
   4. Consider reducing high-dose daily methylprednisolone (32 mg) by 25% both at initiation of TAO and again at end of first week if patient is doing well

(*continued*)

Appendix 21-1 (continued)

---

5. Add TAO
   a. Week 1, TAO dose: 250 mg qd (or 14 mg/kg/daily)
   b. Week 2, TAO dose: 250 mg td (or 10 mg/kg/daily)
   c. Determine weekly liver and pulmonary function tests and theophylline levels
   d. Determine responsiveness to TAO at the end of second week by clinical well-being and/or spirometric improvement
      1. If unfavorable, discontinue TAO
      2. If favorable, continue TAO and follow tapering guide

D. TAO-methylprednisolone tapering phase
   1. Week 3, TAO dose: 500 mg qd (or 7 mg/kg/daily)
   2. Week 4, TAO dose: 250 mg qd in morning (or 3.5 mg/kg/daily)
   3. Determine weekly liver enzymes, spirometry, and theophylline levels until TAO dose of 250 mg or less per day is reached
   4. Reduce daily methylprednisolone dose by 4 mg weekly if possible (PFTs stable, patient asymptomatic) to 4 mg/day
   5. Switch to methylprednisolone 16 mg qod
   6. Then, in 1–2 weeks, switch to TAO 250 mg qod (administered on the same day as methylprednisolone)
   7. Taper methylprednisolone slowly by 2-mg qod decrements every 1–2 weeks to 0.10 mg qod, then every 2–4 weeks to lowest possible dose
   8. May try cromolyn sodium when PFTs are maximal
   9. Consider trial of beclomethasone dipropionate when lowest effective methylprednisolone dose is established
   10. Obtain morning cortisol level when doses of methylprednisolone 16 mg qod (or less) and TAO 250 mg qod are reached

---

Adapted from Zeiger, R. S., Schatz, M., Sperling, W., Simon, R. A., & Stevenson, D. D. *J. Allergy Clin. Immunol.*, 1980, *66*, 438.

*Abbreviations: PFT = pulmonary function test; qid = four times a day; tid = three times a day; qd = every day; qod = every other day.

Jack Barrow

22

Occupational Asthma

"When you come to a patient's house, you should ask what sort of pains he has, what caused them, how many days he has been ill, whether the bowels are working and what sort of food he eats," so says Hippocrates in his work Affections. *I may venture to add one more question: What occupation does he follow?*

Bernardino Ramazzini
De Morbis Artificum, 1713
(Diseases of Workers)

The first description of true asthma due to occupational exposure was probably written by Ramazzini, who is recognized as the father of occupational medicine. He is also responsible for the change in the procedure of classic Hippocratic history-taking to include questions about the patient's job. From the early eighteenth century to the present, asthma has been associated with an increasing number and variety of occupations, and today asthma is a leading cause of work loss. Despite this, the United States does not gather sufficient data to show what proportion of the 8–10 million asthmatic Americans are so afflicted because of their occupations. Estimates from other industrial nations suggest that 2% of asthma cases are of occupational origin. If that figure is applicable in the United States, up to 200,000 Americans have occupational asthma. Several good reviews on occupational asthma have been published (Dosman et al., 1981; Pepys, 1980; Salvaggio, 1979; Weill, 1979). The purpose of this chapter is to bring together the most significant concepts, to update the tables of causes and mechanisms by which many specific substances produce asthma and the industries wherein exposure to these substances may occur, and to provide current information on diagnosis and management of occupational asthma.

ALLERGY: THEORY AND PRACTICE
ISBN 0-8089-1619-X

MECHANISMS OF OCCUPATIONAL ASTHMA

Three basic mechanisms are believed to operate singly or together to cause occupational asthma (Fig. 22-1). Substances induce acute bronchial obstruction by acting as an irritant, by causing an allergic reaction, by a pharmacologic process, or by a combination of these mechanisms. More than 200 substances had been identified as causes of occupational asthma by 1980, and more have been added to the list since then.

Irritants

Irritative substances such as sulfur dioxide, ammonia, or chlorine cause acute airway narrowing by sensitizing rapidly adapting epithelial receptors in the bronchial mucosa (Salvaggio, 1979). Further inhalation of the irritant causes these sensitized receptors to induce bronchoconstriction via a vagal reflex. Whereas initially a sufficient concentration of an irritant will affect almost all persons exposed, repeated exposure to far lower concentrations will induce asthma in those who have acquired bronchial hyperirritability.

Immunologic Mechanisms

Substances inducing asthma via allergic mechanisms require a latent period of exposure during which antibodies often, but not always, of the immunoglobulin E (IgE) type are produced. Once they are produced in sufficient quantity, further exposure causes asthma by way of type I immunologic mechanisms leading to the release of histamine and other chemical mediators from the mast cells, the classic allergic reaction. Some industrial compounds have been demonstrated to cause pro-

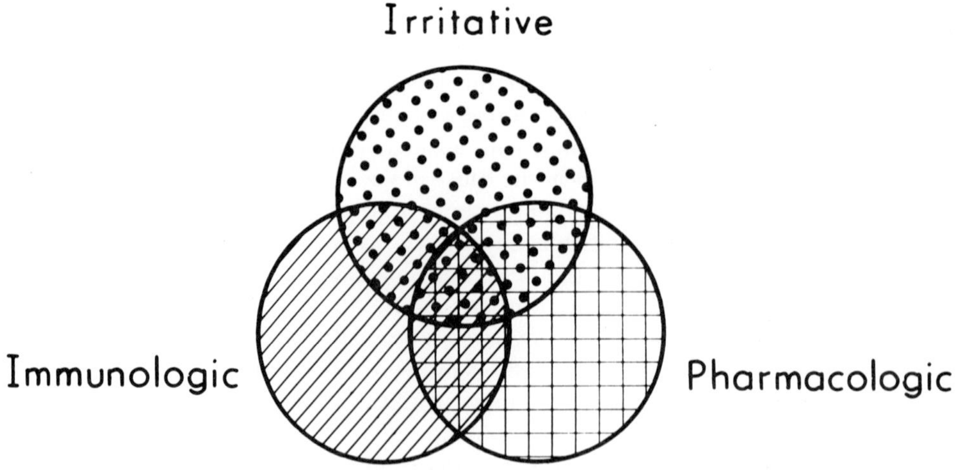

Fig. 22-1. The mechanisms responsible for occupational asthma may have significant overlap in an individual patient.

duction of immunoglobulin G antibodies (IgG); subsequent exposure induces symptoms by way of type III antigen–antibody complex production.

An extremely important cause of occupational asthma, trimellitic anhydride (TMA) does so chiefly via immunologic means. Used extensively in manufacture of epoxy and other resin-type plastics and as the "hardener" in epoxy glues, TMA is a small but active organic compound. Exposure to TMA may occur by inhalation of fumes while it is molten or after exposure to dust particles generated from TMA in granular form. Workers inhaling TMA in sufficient concentration develop lacrimation, rhinorrhea, and cough as an irritant response. TMA readily binds to respiratory tract proteins to produce a hapten-protein complex capable of inducing antibody formation. After a latent period, exposed workers may develop a variety of symptoms. Some may have rhinitis and asthma immediately on exposure. When skin-tested with a trimellitic-human serum albumin (TM-HSA) conjugate, these patients show an immediate wheal-and-flare response as seen in classic type I allergies, and a similar preparation can be used to demonstrate anti-TMA IgE antibody in their blood (Zeiss et al, 1977). Other workers may begin to wheeze and cough 4–8 hours after exposure. In addition, they complain of malaise, fever, and joint pain; the workers' name for this syndrome is "TMA flu." These workers have negative TM-HSA skin tests but have anti-TMA IgG antibodies in their blood; theirs is a type III immune reaction. Many TMA-exposed workers also have anti-TM-HSA antibodies of the IgA class, but the role of these IgA antibodies in humans is presently unclear. Antibodies against epoxy resins or resin-HSA complexes have not been found (Sale, et al, 1981).

Pharmacologic Substances

Finally, some substances induce asthma through direct pharmacologic mechanisms. For example, several organic pesticides have potent anticholinesterase activity, and farm workers spraying crops with these compounds may develop acute asthma from inhalation or from skin absorption. These compounds induce asthma by causing increased local concentration of acetylcholine in bronchial airways.

Occupational exposure to toluene diisocyanate (TDI) and other isocyanate compounds (Malo & Zeiss, 1982) can result in the development of severe immediate or late asthmatic reactions, or both. These reactions can be reproduced by inhalation challenge with or exposure to extremely low concentrations— as little as 0.005 ppm, compared to the threshold level of 0.05 ppm. Immunoglobulin-E antibodies against TDI and isocyanate analogs have been identified in only 9 out of 55 symptomatic workers in one study (Baur & Fruhmann, 1981). On the other hand, TDI at a concentration of 10^{-4} *M* has been found to inhibit release of cyclic adenosine monophosphate in human lymphocytes in vitro (Butcher et al, 1977) and to inhibit adenylate cyclase activity in frog erythrocytes stimulated with isoproterenol (McKay & Brooks, 1981), a standard model for study of beta-agonist activity. The relative lack of demonstrable antibodies against TDI in the majority of workers who react to TDI inhalation, along with these *in vitro* studies, suggests that TDI plays a significant beta-agonist-inhibiting, pharmacologic role more often than an immunologic role in causing asthma. However, Malo and Zeiss were able to use antigen prepared by attaching diphenylmethane diisocyanate to human serum albumin (MDI-HSA) to demonstrate anti-MDI antibodies of the IgG type in a foundry worker who had developed hypersensitivity pneumonitis after being exposed to MDI at work. Ultimate elucidation of the mechanism of action of TDI may depend on immunologic techniques not yet applied in its study.

Other substances known to cause asthma may do so via yet another pharmacologic mechanism, that of direct histamine release. Experimental inhalation of cotton dust may lead to airway constriction in healthy, previously unexposed persons as well as in affected workers. A substance, not as yet characterized, found in the plant bract can stimulate histamine release when incubated with nonsensitized chopped human lung (NIAID, 1979). Convincing evidence of the existence of immune mechanisms has not been found in byssinosis.

Table 22-1, adapted from the National Institute of Allergy and Infectious Diseases Task Force Report on Asthma and Other Allergic Diseases (NIAID, 1979) and amended to incorporate information accumulated since 1979, lists industrial occupations presently known to cause asthma, as well as the materials responsible and the test data derived from related case studies. Table 22-2 lists the material and the various industries allowing exposure to occur. It will be noted that comparatively few substances are listed solely as irritant causes of asthma. The fact that many industrial materials may cause asthma through more than one mechanism operating sequentially or simultaneously, or via one mechanism in one patient and another in the next, is made apparent by these tables and is implied schematically by the areas of overlapping in Figure 22-1. It seems likely that as knowledge of the lungs' mechanics of response to injury increases, the number listed as "irritant" causes will diminish further.

Clinical suspicion is increasing that occupational exposure to such diverse causes as raw cotton and colophony resin may induce asthma via direct histamine release. In each example, acidic materials of low molecular weight have been extracted and found to be histamine liberators.

Table 22-1 *Materials Reported to Cause Occupational Asthma*

	Pathogenesis††			Diagnostic Tests††			
Material	I	P	A	Brr	ST	PT	IgE
Amprolium HCl	*	†					
Animal, bird, fish, and insect sera; dander; secretions and excreta			†	+	+	+	+
Antistatic agents	*			+			
Castor beans			†	+	+		+
Cotton dust		*	*	+	+		
Diisocyanates (TDI, HDI, MDI)	*	*	*	+			+
Enzymes from *B. subtilis*			†	+	+		

Table 22-1 *(Continued)*

Material	Pathogenesis††			Diagnostic Tests††			
	I	P	A	Brr	ST	PT	IgE
Ethanolamines			†	+	+	+	
Ethylenediamine			†	+	+	+	
Flour			†	+	+		+
Formaldehyde	*		*	+			
Furans**			*	+			
Grain (including insect and related contaminants)		*	*	+	+		
Green coffee beans		*	†	+	+		+
Hog trypsin			†	+	+	+	
Molds			†	+	+	+	
Natural resins (colophony)		*	*	+	+		
Nickel and chromium compounds		*	†	+		+	
Organic dusts			†	+	+	+	
Organophosphorous compounds		†					
Pancreatic extracts			†	+	+	+	
Papain			†	+	+		+
Phenylglycine HCl			†	+	+	+	
Phthalic anhrydride			†	+	+		+
Piperazine			*				
Platinum and platinum salts		*	†	+	+	+	+
Pyrolysis products of polyvinyl chloride and of price labels and adhesives	*		*				
Sulfone chloramines			†	+	+	+	
Sulfur dioxide	*			+			
Trimellitic anhydride			†	+	+	+	+
Vegetable gum, acacia			*		+	+	
Vegetable gum, karaya§			*		+	+	
Wood dusts, especially western red cedar		*	*	+	+		

*Mechanism suspected but not proven.
†Known mechanism (Kagen et al., 1981).
§Anaphylactic reaction to powdered karaya gum applied around colostomy site; asthmatic reaction likely in personnel doing "ostomy dressings" (Karr et al., 1978).
**Cockcroft et al. (1980).
††Abbreviations: I = irritant; P = pharmacologic; A = allergic; Brr = Bronchial provocation; ST = skin test; PT = passive transfer.

Table 22-2 *Industrial and Occupational Exposure to Asthma-Inducing Materials*

Industry	Material
Adhesives	Diisocyanates, trimellitic anhydride
Agriculture	Animal, bird, fish, and insect sera; dander; secretions and excreta; grain (including insect and related contaminants; molds, organic dusts; and organophosphorous compounds
Animal and poultry breeders, fishermen, laboratory workers, and veterinarians	Animal, bird, fish, and insect serum; dander; secretions and excreta; grain (including insect and related contaminants); molds; organic dusts; and organophosphorous compounds
Auto workers	Diisocyanates, formalin, nickel and chromium, platinum and platinum salts
Bakers and millers	Flour, grain (including insect and related contaminants)
Brewers	Grain (including insect and related contaminants), hog trypsin, organic dusts, sulfone chloramines, sulfur dioxide, vegetable gum, acacia
Cabinet makers, carpenters, sawmill workers	Wood dusts, especially western red cedar
Cotton gin and textile workers	Cotton dust
Detergents	Enzymes from *B. subtilis*
Electrical workers	Ethanolamines, natural resins
Exterminators	Organophosphorous compounds
Food processors	Green coffee beans, organic dusts, papain, vegetable gum, acacia, and karaya
Foundry workers	Diisocyanates and furans
Grain elevators	Grain (including insect and related contaminants), molds, and organic dusts
Laundry workers	Antistatic agents and sulfur dioxide
Meat wrappers	Pyrolysis products of polyvinyl chloride and of price labels and adhesives
Medicinal substances	Formalin, vegetable gum, karaya
Metal plating	Nickel and chromium
Metal refining	Nickel chromium, platinum and platinum salts
Oil extraction	Castor beans and cotton dust
Ostomy teams	Vegetable gum, karaya
Painters	Diisocyanates and formalin
Petroleum refining	Platinum and platinum salts and sulfur dioxide
Pharmaceutical	Amprolium HCl, pancreatic extracts, phenylglycine HCl, piperazine, sulfone chloramines, vegetable gum, karaya and acacia

Table 22-2 *(Continued)*

Industry	Material
Photofinishing	Platinum and platinum salts
Plastics	Diisocyanates, ethylenediamine, formalin, phthalic anhydride and trimellitic anhydride
Rubber	Diisocyanates, formalin and sulfur dioxide
Welders, solderers	Ethanolamines and natural resins (colophony)
Winemaking	Molds, organic dusts, sulfone choramines, sulfur dioxide, vegetable gum, acacia

Of the commercially important woods, western red cedar *(Thuja plicata)* has been found to cause occupational asthma far more commonly than any other species. The cause of western red cedar asthma was attributed to immune mechanisms when the disorder was first described in 1969. Attention has since focused on two pharmacologic mechanisms, histamine liberation (NIAID, 1979) or beta-adrenergic receptor blocking agents (Pepys, 1979). Sosman et al. (1969) reported four cases of asthma due to sawdust—one to oak, one to mahogany, and two to western red cedar. Using aqueous extracts of the specific woods, these authors detected precipitin bands with immunodiffusion studies, and in the two western red cedar cases, late reactions with bronchial provocation tests as well, but no skin test reactions. They concluded that the sawdust must cause asthma via an immunologic mechanism. In 1971, Chan-Yeung et al. reported on four cases of western red cedar asthma, each having positive bronchial provocation tests, but with negative skin tests and no demonstrable precipitins. Chan-Yeung's group noted that reports that volatile "tropolones," including plicatic acid from western red cedar, could act as beta-receptor blockers, only to discard that as a possible mechanism since in their series the bronchial provocative reaction could only be induced with the nonvolatile fractions from western red cedar. They concluded that immune mechanisms must be involved. Brooks et al. (1981) demonstrated positive dose–response relationships in various groups exposed to western red cedar dust and suggested that nonimmunologic mechanisms were to blame. Obviously, the last word on the subject of the mechanism involved in western red cedar asthma has yet to be written.

Meat wrappers' asthma, tentatively described in 1973, was quickly and widely discussed in the communications media of butchers' and meat cutters' unions. This disease was held to be caused by inhalation of fumes generated when a sheet of polyvinyl chloride (PVC) film is cut by being passed over a hot wire, a procedure usually conducted in a cold, poorly ventilated room. Additional fumes, probably of a different nature, are generated when price and weight labels are heated so that they will stick to the package, but the majority of affected workers blame the PVC film and the hot wire cutter. By 1980 "meat wrappers' asthma" was so thoroughly accepted as a syndrome that one medical report used it to describe asthma in a worker who wrapped and sealed tin cans in polyethylene film (Skerfving et al, 1980). Meanwhile, questions have been raised as to whether pyrolysis products of PVC film actually cause asthma, "meat wrappers'" or otherwise. Studies by two groups have failed to show significant changes in pulmonary function on bronchial provocational challenge with PVC fumes as generated by the hot wire method, in workers otherwise diagnosed as having meat wrappers' asthma (Butler et al., 1981). The problem may become of academic interest only as "hot wire" cutters are replaced with "cold wire" cutters that generate less fumes.

HOST FACTORS

Atopy

Host factors are important in determining who gets occupational asthma. Atopic persons, that is, those with a past history or a family history of allergy, seem to be at greater risk, not only when the causative substance is clearly allergenic, but also in situations where allergic mechanism are less clearly operative.

Whether the worker smokes cigarettes is the third host factor. It is evident that smoking plus occupational exposure, regardless of type, results in pulmonary dysfunction in excess of that produced by smoking alone or occupational exposure alone.

CLINICAL FEATURES

The chief clinical feature of occupational asthma is wheezing related to work. Similarities exist regardless of the operative mechanism or the substance involved. Initially, there is a symptom-free interval that may vary from weeks to years in length, during which sensitization develops. Thereafter, symptoms begin to occur in relation to work. They may begin during the work shift—the "immediate" reaction, or at night or hours after the work shift is over—the "late" reaction. Some workers may have both reactions, and some causative agents can provoke fever, myalgia, and arthralgia along with the late reaction. Symptoms typically, but not always, diminish over weekends, or during vacations, but it is not rare for symptoms to recur for weeks after exposure has ended, and this may obscure the work-related nature of the problem. Identification and termination of exposure results in improvement that is usually complete, but in some workers asthmatic symptoms and evidence of bronchial hyperreactivity may persist indefinitely. On occasion, permanent fixed airways resistance may develop (Dosman et al, 1981). It is a rare patient who cannot tell what work procedure causes symptoms, and whenever a worker does blame working conditions for respiratory illness, the complaints should be carefully evaluated. Most examples of occupational asthma have been identified by appropriate investigations of such complaints.

Examination in the doctor's office may reveal nothing significant; examination at work or shortly thereafter is more likely to be significant but is often impractical. Measuring and recording the peak expiratory flow rates (PEF) at regular intervals during and after work may be useful. This can be done with instruments such as the mini-Wright peak flowmeter, which is accurate, sturdy, and inexpensive so that it can be lent to individual workers and patients under study. Peak flow rates falling at least 15% below symptom-free or preemployment rates are significant. Bronchial provocational challenge in pulmonary medicine laboratories with special cubicles wherein the subject may be exposed to inhalation of low dosages of suspected substances under controlled conditions is a method of study that is becoming increasingly available (Pepys. 1981). Other pulmonary function tests are less helpful in diagnosis but may be needed to monitor the effects of exposure or treatment over a long period of observation. Skin tests are of no help if negative and must be carefully evaluated if positive. Radioallergosorbent tests (RAST) may be useful in study of the mechanism of action of suspected causative agents, but RAST for the agents presently known to induce occupational asthma by immunologic means are not generally available. In the end, diagnosis of occupational asthma depends heavily on the clinical history, augmented as needed by regular, frequent measurement of ventilatory function over adequate periods of time, and on occasion, with bronchial provocational challenge studies.

Case Histories

Two case histories will indicate the variety of exposures and responses to TDI.

CASE 1. The first patient, T. M., is a 25-year-old nonsmoker with no past or family history of allergy. He was seen in 1981 with complaints of breathlessness and wheezing on exertion beginning in 1975. He had worked since 1974 on the production line in a small factory where plastic parts were made. In early 1975, he was accidentally drenched with a mixture of TDI and polyurethane. He was rinsed in the emergency shower, but he became feverish and dyspneic that evening. The initial chest roentgenogram was unremarkable, but a second made the next day revealed "chemical pneumonitis, right lower lobe." He received IV hydrocortisone, and a third chest roentgenogram 3 days later revealed "substantial clearing." He returned to work but became aware of heightened ability to smell TDI, followed by dyspnea and coughing, which caused him to leave the building. He was transferred to another work area, where he handled only finished products but eventually returned to the production line, where early in 1976 he was again accidentally soaked with a mixture of TDI and polyurethane. He again felt feverish and noted increasing dyspnea. By avoiding exposure to TDI, he was able to work in the same factory until 1978, when he decided to return to school. Nocturnal cough and exertional dyspnea persisted. Evaluation elsewhere in early 1980 revealed no physical abnormalities. At that time, the following studies were normal: routine complete blood counts; chemical profile; urinalysis; immunoglobulins IgA, IgG, and IgM; arterial blood gases; and chest roentgenograms. Pulmonary function tests were normal except for reduced total lung capacity and forced vital capacity (FVC) and a marked reduction in peak expiratory flow.

In late 1981 the patient reiterated complaints of exertional dyspnea. Reductions were noted in FVC and forced expiratory volume in one second (FEV_1), plus continued reduction of PEF to 55% of the predicted value. After inhalation of a bronchodilator, his FEV_1 increased to 86% and PEF to 79% of predicted values. Subjective and objective evidence of bronchial hyperreactivity have persisted for more than five years after the last known exposure to TDI.

CASE 2. The second case, K. B., age 22, was seen in early 1978 for complaints of nighttime cough and wheezing. He had had seasonal allergic rhinitis in childhood with complete resolution. He began working as a spray painter in an auto repair shop in 1976. He had never smoked. By late 1977, he began to have the above symptoms at night after he had used a specific acrylic enamel containing a "polyurethane conversion material," in other words, TDI. Gradually, he became so sensitive to TDI that he would cough and wheeze at night despite the use of a mask equipped with charcoal filters. He was relieved of spray-painting duties but continued to wheeze whenever auto bodies were spray-painted even though he was at the opposite end of the shop.

The patient's lungs were clear on each of three office visits. Prednisone 10 mg daily prevented both immediate and delayed symptoms, whereas bronchodilators did not. Eventually, he had to quit his job; thereafter, he continued to have episodes of asthma usually associated with respiratory infections despite a lack of known TDI exposure since 1979.

DISCUSSION. These two case histories illustrate several points common to TDI sensitivity, if not to all examples of occupational asthma. The fact that one patient was nonatopic and the other atopic fits the picture of TDI sensitivity. Sensitivity may follow occasional exposure to high concentrations or frequent exposure to low concentrations. Symptoms in both cases began after a latent period of exposure. Once bronchial hyperreactivity became established, one worker exhibited immediate symptoms, during periods of exposure; the other had late symptoms developing at night. One has mild evidence of restrictive pulmonary disease as well as exertional dyspenea; the other has more severe but reversible bronchial constriction. In both cases evidence of bronchial hyperreactivity has persisted for more than 2 years after the last known exposure to TDI.

MANAGEMENT

Management of occupational asthma is like that of any other asthma (see Chapter 21). Along with prescribed medication, measures should be taken to avoid further exposure to the causative substance. Wearing masks or respirators is usually acceptable only when the exposure is intermittent. Disodium cromoglycate or beclomethasone inhalations may block asthmatic responses to many occupational agents. Thiel and Ulmer (1980) reported satisfactory prevention of asthma in a group of 36 bakers with flour-dependent asthma by use of a regimen that included preventive use of cromolyn inhalations. In the United States sending the patient back to work with medical management raises an ethical question, "Should such individuals with occupational asthma be sent back, on medication, for further exposure on the job?" If occupational asthma is generally to be prevented, industry has some obligation to provide an acceptable quality of air in the environment. The establishment of threshold limit values for harmful inhalants has been done for some substances but needs to be done for many more. Preemployment testing for evidence of hyperreactive airways by bronchial challenge with methacholine, histamine, or cold air could be utilized as a screening procedure when workers are being selected for employment involving exposure to substances known or suspected to cause asthma. The creation of a social, legal, and political environment wherein all the information thus generated might be uniformly, effectively applied, rather than the present haphazard system, would do much to minimize the problem of occupational asthma.

REFERENCES

Baur, X., & Fruhmann, G. *Chest*, 1981, *80*, 73–76.

Brooks, S. M., Edwards, J. J., Jr., Apol, A., & Edwards, F. E. *Chest*, 1981, *80*, 30–32.

Butcher, B. T., Salvaggio, J. E., O'Neil, C. E., & Davies, R. J. *J. Allergy Clin. Immunol.*, 1977, *60*, 223–229.

Butler, J., Culver, B. H., & Robertson, H. T. *Chest*, 1981, *80*, 71–73.

Chan-Yeung, M., Barton, G.M., McLean, L., & Grzybowski, S. *Can. Med. Assoc. J.*, 1971, *105*, 56–61.

Cockcroft, D. W., Cartier, A., Jones, G., Tarlo, S. M., Dolovich, J., & Hargreave, F. E. *J. Allergy Clin. Immunol.*, 1980, *66*, 458–463.

Dosman, J. A., Cockcroft, D. W., & Hoeppner, V. H. *Med. Clinics N. Am.*, 1981, *65*, 691–706.

Kagen, S., Fink, J., Schleuter, D., Cohen, S., Kidd, J., & Arkins, J. *J. Allergy Clin. Immunol.*, 1981, 67, 30(A).

Karr, R. M., Davies, F. J., Butcher, B. T., Lehrer, S. B., Wilson, M. R., Dharmarajan, V., & Salvaggio, J. E. *J. Allergy Clin. Immunol.*, 1978, *61*, 54–65.

Malo, J. L., & Zeiss, C. R. *J. Allergy Clin. Immunol.* 1982, *69*, 133(A).

McKay, R. T., & Brooks, S. M. *Chest*, 1981, *80*, 61–63.

NIAID Task Force Report *NIH Publication*, 1979, *79-387*, 330–366.

Pepys, J. *J. Allergy Clin. Immunol.*, 1980, *66*, 179–85.

Pepys, J. *Bull. N.Y. Acad. Med.*, 1981, *57*, 608–616.

Sale, S. R., Roach, D. E., Zeiss, R., & Patterson, R. *J. Allergy Clin. Immunol.*, 1981, *68*, 188–93.

Salvaggio, J. E. *J. Allergy Clin. Immunol.*, 1979, *64*, 646–649.

Skerfving, S., Akersson, B. S., & Simonsson, B. G. *Lancet*, 1980, *1*, 8161, 211.

Sosman, A. J., Schleuter, D. P., Fink, J. N., & Barboriak, J. J., *New Engl. J. Med.*, 1969, *281*, 977–980.

Thiel, H. and Ulmer, W. T. *Chest*, 1980, *78*, 400–405.

Weill, H. *J. Allergy Clin. Immunol.* 1979, *64* 662–664.

Zeiss, C. R., Patterson, R., Pruzansky, T. J., Miller, M. M., Rosenberg, M., Suszko, I., & Levitz, D. *J. Allergy Clin. Immunol.*, 1977, *60*, 96–103.

SUGGESTED READINGS

Becklake, M. R., *Chest*, 1981, *80*, 73–76.

O'Byrne, P. M., Ryan, G., Morris, M., McCormack, D., Morse, J., Jones, N. & Hargreave, F. E., *J. Allergy Clin. Immunol.*, 1982, *69*, 104(A).

QUESTIONS

1. A worker in a plant where TMA powder is mixed with epoxy resin for molding into small electric appliance parts reports that he begins to cough and "ache all over" in the evening and into the night. Which of the following statements is true and which is false?
   a. This is his second day of work and already he's blaming the job. Is he likely to be correct?
   b. He's been there a year. He's found to have antibodies against TM-HSA protein conjugates in his blood.
   c. His job is to pack the finished plastic parts for shipment. He has anti-TM-HSA antibodies in his blood.
   d. He has a high level of IgG anti-TM-HSA in his blood.

2. A worker in a plant wherein polyurethane foam is blown into flotation compartments in canoes begins to cough and wheeze on the job, after working there for 6 months. Are the following statements true or false?
   a. Hourly checks on his peak expiratory flow rates would provide useful information.
   b. He's granted 2 months' leave, and his symptoms disappear. When he applies polyurethane varnish to his sailboat in his closed garage, the symptoms return.

c. His blood has a high level of IgE antibodies against TDI.
d. He returns to work in the plant's "front office," where fumes occasionally waft through from the plant and he begins wheezing again.

3. A worker in a large flour mill begins to wheeze at work after 10 years' employment there. Which of the following is likely to be true?

   a. She sneezes repetitively at work, as well as wheezing.
   b. Prophylactic inhalations of cromolyn effectively prevent the wheezing.
   c. She can eat bread and other baked wheat products without having any symptoms.
   d. All the above are false.

4. Data on threshold limit values (TLV) for all industrial dusts and volatile substances are:

   a. Established and readily available.
   b. Desirable but difficult to obtain.
   c. Usually based on the amount required to induce coughing or sneezing in most workers while on the job.
   d. Likely to become available from the Occupational Health and Safety Administration (OSHA) by 1984.

5. A self-employed cabinet maker finds that he wheezes after sawing one variety of wood but not others.

   a. Is it oak or mahogany?
   b. Is it western red cedar?
   c. Would skin tests with extracts of the various woods provide the correct answer to a and b?
   d. He learns which wood causes his asthma but can't avoid some exposure to that wood. Could cromolyn inhalation prevent his symptoms?

Answers can be found in Appendix B at the end of the book.

Raymond G. Slavin

23

Hypersensitivity Diseases of the Lung

The lung is being increasingly recognized as a superb immunologic shock organ. Certainly, all of the ingredients for an immune response are present. There is ready access to a host of airborne antigens, and there are, in the lung, a battery of cells, including mast cells, antibody-producing plasma cells, macrophages, and lymphocytes, both of the T and B series that are well equipped to respond to an antigenic onslaught. In the past decade there have been tremendous advances in the definition and characterization of an important group of disorders termed *hypersensitivity disease of the lung*. These diseases offer a reminder to all clinicians to extend their scope of immunologically mediated pulmonary diseases beyond IgE-mediated bronchial asthma and cell-mediated diseases such as tuberculosis.

The present era of interest in hypersensitivity lung disease began almost 50 years ago with the first description of "farmer's lung," a disease caused by exposure to moldy hay; however, a renewal of recent interest based on more widely available immunologic techniques has stirred a great deal of study on a wide variety of similar diseases associated with different antigens and different exposure situations. The physician's index of diagnostic suspicion in dealing with this group of diseases must remain high for several reasons: (a) these diseases are being recognized with increasing frequency and a variety of new antigens responsible for hypersensitivity lung disease are being described with regularity; (b) the inexorable outcome of these disorders is irreparable tissue damage; thus it is vital to recognize the disease early before irreversible changes take place; and (c) a clearer definition of hypersensitivity lung diseases will further our understanding of immunologic diseases in general.

The first of these conditions to be described is hypersensitivity pneumonitis. Synonyms for this entity include pulmonary hypersensitivity syndrome and extrinsic allergic alveolitis. This latter term is perhaps the best and most descriptive. "Extrinsic" refers to an exogenous antigen or allergen; "allergic" indicates that the disease is of a hypersensitivity origin; and "alveolitis" refers to that part of the lung that is most affected.

ALLERGY: THEORY AND PRACTICE
ISBN 0-8089-1619-X

HYPERSENSITIVITY PNEUMONITIS

Morbidity and Mortality

Little is known about the natural history and prognosis of the disease in the instance of chronic exposure. One study of farmer's lung revealed a 5-year morbidity of 30% and a mortality of 10%. If acute hypersensitivity pneumonitis is left unrecognized, the disease may assume an insidious, subacute form that resembles progressive, chronic bronchitis. Prolonged and intense exposure or low level, but continuous exposure, may lead to chronic disease and irreversible lung damage, resulting in pulmonary fibrosis and far-advanced ventilatory insufficiency.

Basic Mechanisms (Pathophysiology)

Several factors determine the response of an individual to an organic dust inhalation. First, is the basic immunologic reactivity that of the host; in other words, is the host atopic or nonatopic? In general, inhalation of an organic dust by an atopic individual result in an immediate Type I IgE-antibody response. A nonatopic person will tend to respond with a Type III reaction characterized by precipitating antibody. Another important host factor may be the association of HLA haplotypes with disease. In patients with farmer's lung, HLA-B8 has been noted with increasing frequency, and in "pigeon-breeder's disease," a common form of hypersensitivity pneumonitis, HLA-B8 and HLA-BW40 have been reported with increased frequency. A second factor that determines the response to an organic dust is the nature and source of the antigen. Can it be grown in the respiratory tract? Is it small enough to reach the alveoli? Can it induce the proper immune response? A third factor is the nature and circumstances of the exposure. Is it an isolated but heavy exposure to an antigen, or is it a low-grade chronic insidious type of exposure?

Table 23-1 lists some common antigens that may result in hypersensitivity pneumonitis. The list is by no means complete. Any organic dust of proper antigenicity and particule size can produce the identical syndrome. As physicians become increasingly aware of clinical features of hypersensitivity pneumonitis, other causes will undoubtedly be discovered.

One can divide the antigens that cause hypersensitivity pneumonitis into three general categories. The first is the thermophilic organisms. Diseases caused by these agents are associated with environmental exposure to materials that are subjected to high temperatures and high humidity. This is a fertile source for the growth of the thermophilic organisms; unicellular, branching organisms that resemble true bacteria. An important recent finding is that an occupational exposure need not be incriminated. The disease has been described by a number of investigators in individuals who are exposed to the organism growing in home humidifiers or air-conditioning systems. The second general antigenic category is molds. Several examples are given in Table 23-1.

A third category is animal protein. Pituitary "snuff-taker's" lung is no longer common because of the substitution of synthetic pituitary (Pituitrin) for the pituitary powder of ox or pig that was used to treat patients for hypopituitarisim. "Bird-fancier's" lung is common and is due to sensitivity to avian antigen present in the

Table 23-1 *Causes of Hypersensitivity Pneumonitis*

Antigen	Disease
Thermophilic actinomycetes	
Micropolyspora faeni	Farmer's lung, mushroom worker's disease,
Thermoactinomyces vulgaris	humidifier lung,
Thermoactinomyces sacchari	bagassosis
Mold	
Cryptostroma corticale	Maple bark disease
Aspergillus clavatus	Malt-worker's lung
Alternaria	Wood pulp worker's disease
Pullularia	Sequoiosis
Penicillium	Suberosis
Animal	
Ox or pig	Pituitary snuff-taker's lung
Pigeon	Pigeon-breeder's disease
Dove, parakeet, parrot	Bird-fancier's lung
Rat	Rat-handler's disease
Gerbil	Gerbil-keeper's lung
Others	
Amoeba	
Toluene diisocyanate (TDI)	

droppings of a variety of birds, including pigeons, parakeets, parrots, and doves. Two other animal sources recently described are rats and gerbils.

Under "other" antigens are listed amoeba and toluene diisocyanate (TDI). There is evidence that amoeba may contaminate the residual water of humidification units and, in some cases, may be the cause of humidifier lung.

Toluene diisocyanate is a simple, low-molecular-weight, inorganic chemical commonly encountered in the manufacture of polyurethane foam, plastics, paints, and adhesives. Although more commonly incriminated as a cause of asthma, it may also result in extrinsic allergic alveolitis (see Chapter 22).

The precise immunologic mechanism responsible for extrinsic allergic alveolitis or hypersensitivity pneumonitis is presently unclear. A type I IgE-mediated reaction would seem to be excluded by the nonatopic status of most of the patients, the normal IgE levels, and the absence of eosinophilia and significant bronchospasm. Several features strongly suggest Type III immune complex mediated disease. These include the presence of precipitating antibodies in the sera of most patients against the offending organic antigen; an increase in antibody titers with increasing severity of the disease coupled with a decrease in titers on remission; the development of late Arthus-type skin reactions with some antigens; the time interval of 4–6 hours between exposure and development of symptoms; and the presence of antigen, immunoglobulin, and components of serum complement in lung lesions. Arguing against a pure precipitating antibody–immune complex mechanism is the relative absence of pulmonary vasculitis, the absence of serum complement depletion in acute disease, the presence of precipitating antibody to organic dust in a large percentage of asymptomatic exposed persons, and the failure to transfer the disease from humans to monkeys or from affected animals to nonaffected animals with serum.

There is a great deal of evidence to suggest that Type IV delayed hypersensitivity plays an important role in the pathogenesis of hypersensitivity pneumonitis. Certainly, the pathologic changes, including granuloma formation, in this disease are consistent with delayed hypersensitivity. Studies have been carried out in symptomatic and asymptomatic pigeon breeder's, both of whom had comparable titers of precipitating antibody. The results indicate that *in vitro* correlates of delayed hypersensitivity, including antigen-induced migration inhibition factor (MIF) production and lymphocyte transformation, can be found in symptomatic breeders, but not the asymptomatic breeders.

The role of serum complement in production of disease is presently unclear. Nonspecific activation of the alternate and perhaps the classic pathways of complement may be involved in some early inflammatory components of hypersensitivity pneumonitis. It has been demonstrated that some organic dust antigens can directly activate complement pathway.

Another factor in the pathogenesis of hypersensitivity pneumonitis concerns local immune mechanisms in the lung that operate independently of systemic mechanisms. It has been reported that bronchoalveolar cells obtained by bronchial lavage from patients with pigeon breeder's lung produce lymphokines in response to pigeon antigen, but peripheral blood lymphocytes from the same patient did not.

It would thus appear that at least three immunologic mechanisms as well as nonimmunologic factors are operative in the pathogenesis of hypersensitivity pneumonitis and that more information is needed to clarify this issue.

Clinical Manifestations

The characteristic history in acute hypersensitivity pneumonitis is repeated episodes of fever, chills, chest pain, cough, and dyspnea that occur 4–6 hours after exposure to the organic dust. Remission of symptoms on avoidance of the contaminated area is an important diagnostic feature. A common occurrence is the hospitalization of a patient with fever, cough, and a pulmonary infiltrate. Antibiotics are administered, and the patient is considerably improved in a few hours. This improvement may be attributed to the antibiotics when, in fact, the removal of the patient from the home or working environment accounts for the clinical improvement. In the more insidious form, progressively increasing malaise, dyspnea, and weight loss are the result of chronic exposure to smaller amounts of antigen.

The findings on physical examination are disproportionate to the patient's subjective complaints and the extent of parenchymal involvement observed roentgenographically. Examination of the chest usually reveals basilar, bilateral, crepitant rales. Wheezing may be heard in some instances of pigeon breeder's disease.

Differential Diagnosis

The symptoms mentioned above of fever, chills, chest pain, cough, and dyspnea together with a pulmonary infiltrate on chest x-ray, would obviously be mistaken most often for a bacterial or viral pneumonitis. In the chronic stage, hypersensitivity pneumonitis may be erroneously diagnosed as idiopathic pulmonary fibrosis or Haman-Rich disease.

Key Diagnostic Tests

Routine laboratory tests are of little value. Some IgE levels are normal, and, although leukocytosis is common, eosinophilia is seldom present. The findings on chest x-ray depend on the stage of the disease. The acute form is most often associated with diffuse, finely granular infiltrates characteristic of alveolar or interstitial pneumonitis. Micronodular deposits are common. In the chronic stage, the infiltrates become confluent. Chest roentgenographic findings generally resolve after 3–6 months but may become permanent in more severe cases.

Pulmonary function testing demonstrates a restrictive type of ventilatory impairment. In classical cases there is a decrease in forced vital capacity decreased pulmonary compliance and defects in alveolar gas exchange as demonstrated by a decrease in carbon monoxide diffusion capacity (DLCO). Arterial oxygen desaturation is often seen with a further fall after exercise.

Lung biopsy reveals the basic pathologic condition to be an inflammation of the alveoli and interstitial pulmonary tissue with bronchiolar involvement. In the acute stage, there is alveolar thickening with infiltration of mononuclear cells, lymphocytes, and plasma cells. Occasionally, foamy histiocytes are found in the alveolar walls or within the alveoli. In the chronic stage, noncaseating granulomas are seen with Langerhan's giant cells, epithelioid cells, and varying degrees of fibrosis.

The immunologic hallmark in the clinical workup of extrinsic allergic alveolitis is the presence of serum precipitating antibody to the extrinsic antigen. This is generally an IgG and can be detected by the double gel diffusion technique. The pressure of precipitins is evidence of exposure and sensitization and does not necessarily indicate that the clinical process is present. A substantial percentage of asymptomatic pigeon breeders and sugar cane workers have precipitating antibody to avian antigen and thermophilic organisms, respectively. Skin testing with the antigens responsible for extrinsic allergic alveolitis is of limited value. When antigens such as pigeon serum or mold are used, skin testing will generally result in a dual response, that is, an immediate wheal and erythema reaction followed by a late Arthus reaction occurring 6–8 hours later.

When the specific diagnosis is in doubt because of the question of the relevance of the particular exposure, bronchial provocation tests may be helpful. Under carefully controlled conditions, an aqueous extract of the particular antigen is delivered to the bronchial tree. A positive challenge consists of appropriate changes in pulmonary function, most notably a decrease in DLCO and worsening of symptoms after 4–6 hours. The provocative test should not be performed on a routine basis and must be used with great caution, limited to those with experience in performing the test. Patients may become quite ill and may even require hospitalization after a positive challenge.

Therapy

Patients with acute hypersensitivity pneumonitis will usually respond to bed rest and supportive care. Corticosteroids are indicated in more severely affected patients and generally provide excellent results. The most desirable treatment is removal of the patient from the offending environment. In some instances, a patient may be able to remain on the job if exposure is decreased. The wearing of masks, for example, by heavily exposed individuals, may be of some help. Alterations in the industrial processing of organic antigens may also be of some help. Bagassosis or Louisiana sugar cane worker's disease has essentially disappeared due to several industrial modifications. Wetting of compost before handling reduces the dissemination of thermophilic organisms, and the growth of these organisms is suppressed by spraying composts with a nontoxic solution of proprionic acid.

Prognosis

The prognosis of hypersensitivity pneumonitis is excellent, provided the disease is recognized in the early stage and the antigen avoided before irreparable tissue damage has taken place. In the acute case, further avoidance of the offending antigen will result in a return of pulmonary function to normal. In the subacute or chronic case in which an individual is exposed to a lower antigen challenge over a long period of time, however, pulmonary fibrosis and far-advanced ventillatory insufficiency may result.

Perspectives on New and Future Developments in the Field

In the future years, research will be directed to three different issues: (a) further characterization of the precise immunologic process that is involved in hypersensitivity pneumonitis; (b) the delineation of new antigens responsible for this disease; and (c) the preventive medicine measures to be undertaken by industry to prevent this disease from occurring—a fruitful issue.

ALLERGIC BRONCHOPULMONARY ASPERGILLOSIS

Aspergillus is a hardy and ubiquitous mold found in air, soil, and decaying vegetation. It is also common in swimming pool water, house dust, and bedding. Many species of aspergillus may infect humans, but the most common one is *Aspergillus fumigatus*.

The most common form of pulmonary aspergillosis is the aspergilloma, or fungus ball. In this state the organism colonizes existing anatomic abnormalities, such as a bronchiectatic cavity or congenital cyst, with only a superficial invasion of tissue. Aspergillomata can develop outside the lung as well.

Several other lung diseases may be caused by aspergillus. Invasive or septicemic aspergillosis occurs in patients whose immune function has been compromised, either naturally by a disease such as leukemia or lymphoma, or iatrogenically by immunosuppressive agents. This opportunistic form of aspergillosis may result in bronchitis, mycotic abscesses, and pneumonia. Bronchial asthma on an IgE-mediated basis may also be due to aspergillus, and this organism can also cause extrinsic allergic alveolitis or hypersensitivity pneumonitis as discussed previously.

Finally, aspergillus may cause a hypersensitivity lung disease characterized by pulmonary eosinophilia, that is, by pulmonary infiltrates seen roentgenographically and by eosinophilia of the sputum and peripheral blood. This condition is termed *allergic bronchopulmonary aspergillosis*.

Morbidity and Mortality

Patients with bronchial asthma who develop allergic bronchopulmonary aspergillosis will generally have a marked worsening of their asthmatic states. Among the complications of allergic aspergillosis are atelectasis, destructive bronchiectasis, and ultimately chronic pulmonary fibrosis with resultant, marked pulmonary disability.

Basic Mechanisms (Pathophysiology)

The pathogenesis of allergic aspergillosis begins with the inhalation and trapping of the short-chain spores of *A. fumigatus* in the viscid secretions of the asthmatic. The size of the spores and the broad temperature at which *A. fumigatus* grows makes this organism ideally suited for colonization of the human bronchial tree. Most other fungus spores will not survive at human body temperature, but *A. fumigatus* germinates and forms mycelia at that temperature.

A cardinal feature that distinguishes allergic aspergillosis from other hypersensitivity responses to inhaled allergens is that the organism grows in the respiratory tract and continually sheds antigens into the tissues. Antigens released from the mycelia combine with IgG and IgE antibodies to set in motion a chain of immunologic reactions circulating in bronchial wall damage and the surrounding pulmonary eosinophilic consolidation.

Both IgE skin-sensitizing antibody and IgG-precipitating antibody are thought to play a major pathogenetic roles in allergic aspergillosis, and their necessity in mediating tissue damaging effects has been demonstrated in passive transfer experiments in monkeys. Transfusion of serum from a patient with allergic aspergillosis to a monkey, followed by aerosol challenge with aspergillus antigen, results in the development of pulmonary lesions in the monkey consistent with the picture of human allergic aspergillosis. Transfusion of human serum containing only skin-sensitizing antibodies, however, causes no pulmonary lesions.

In another series of experiments, monkeys that had developed precipitating antibody following immunization with *A. fumigatus* received intravenous (IV) infusion of human serum rich in IgE antibody against *A. fumigatus*. Following an aerosol of *A. fumigatus*, monkeys demonstrated lung findings characteristic of allergic aspergillosis. Infusion of normal human serum into monkeys with precipitating antibody or infusion of allergic human serum with IgE against *A. fumigatus* into monkeys without precipitating antibody resulted in no pulmonary changes.

The presence of granulomata and a mononuclear cell infiltration in lung biopsies of patients with allergic aspergillosis would seem to implicate cell-mediated immunity in pathogenesis. A large percentage of patients with allergic aspergillosis demonstrate *in vitro* lymphocyte transformation in response to aspergillus antigen using the whole blood method. This has been attributed to the presence of immune complexes.

It would appear, therefore, that both T and B cells may play roles in the response to aspergillus. Patients with allergic aspergillosis do not manifest a positive delayed skin test reaction to aspergillus. This is probably due to the fact that histamine locally released as a result of the immediate skin test reaction inhibits lymphocyte production of lymphokines, substances that mediate delayed skin test reactivity.

The final immunologic mechanism that may be operative in allergic aspergillosis is complement activation. Circulating immune complexes and evidence of activation of the classic complement pathway have been demonstrated during the acute phase of allergic aspergillosis. Aspergillus antigen also activates the alternate complement pathway *in vitro*.

In summary, the pathogenesis of allergic bronchopulmonary aspergillosis probably represents the sum total of a number of immunologic processes.

Clinical Manifestations

There are seven basic criteria for diagnosis of allergic aspergillosis:

Bronchial asthma
Eosinophilia
Positive immediate skin test
Positive serum precipitins
Elevated IgE
Pulmonary infiltrates
Central bronchiectasis

The presence of the first six makes the diagnosis of allergic aspergillosis highly likely; all seven make it certain. Patients uniformly have a history of bronchial asthma. Indeed, this disease can be considered a complication of bronchial asthma. In a recent study, 42 corticosteroid-dependent asthmatics were evaluated for underlying allergic aspergillosis. Twelve were found who were suspect, and of these, three had definite and three probable allergic aspergillosis.

Pulmonary and blood eosinophilia are marked. Peripheral blood eosinophils generally exceed 1000/mm^3. Levels greater than 3000/mm^3 are quite commonplace.

A skin test with aspergillus is a good screen for allergic aspergillosis in that a positive, immediate wheal-and-erythema reaction indicating the presence of skin-sensitizing antibody is a requisite finding. The standard aspergillus mixture from some suppliers does not contain *A. fumigatus*, and one should test separately. If the immediate skin test is negative, it is highly unlikely that *A. fumigatus* is responsible for the pulmonary eosinophilia.

An intradermal aspergillus skin test immediate reaction is occasionally followed by a later Arthus-type reaction, reaching a peak at 6–8 hours and resolving within 24 hours. This constitutes the dual skin test response.

A positive immediate skin test reaction to aspergillus is not unique to patients with allergic aspergillosis. It is also commonly found in atopic individuals and occurs in 14–33% of asthmatic patients.

Circulating, precipitating antibody to aspergillus is generally present in allergic aspergillosis. It is an IgE immunoglobulin and can be easily detected with the double gel diffusion technique. As in the case of immediate skin test reactions, precipitins to aspergillus are found in other situations—2.5% of the general hospital population and 25% of extrinsic asthmatic patients. A. Fumigatus growing in the bronchial tree is a potent stimulus of specific and nonspecific IgE. Serum IgE levels are markedly elevated in patients with allergic aspergillosis and are significantly higher than in patients with uncomplicated bronchial asthma. This marked elevation results from nonspecific stimulation of IgE-producing plasma cells. One recent case report described a cystic fibrosis patient with all the characteristics of allergic aspergillosis except for a low serum IgE.

A variety of roentgenographic shadows may be seen in patients with allergic aspergillosis. The most common abnormality is a homogenous shadow without fissure displacement that usually appears in the upper lobes. These opacities frequently shift rapidly from one side to another in serial films. A recurrence in the same area suggests previous bronchial damage, which may predispose local bronchi to further episodes. A rather inconspicuous roentgenographic finding can represent extensive tissue damage. A frequently seen abnormality is "tram-line" shadowing which consists of 2 parallel hairline shadows extending out from the hilum in the direction of the bronchi. This sign is thought to represent edema of the wall of an anatomically normal bronchus.

Parallel line shadows are similar to tram-line shadows, but the width of the transparent zone is wider. These shadows appear to be due to bronchial damage. A common complication of allergic aspergillosis is atelectasis of a segment or a lobe or even total collapse of the whole lung. This is due to occlusion of a bronchus by a mucus plug.

A distinctive type of bronchiectasis is seen in allergic aspergillosis. It appears saccular, with pronounced proximal or center involvement and peripheral or distal sparing. This suggests a localized toxic reaction in the bronchial walls resulting from the presence of the fungus, rather than the usual sequence of events leading to bronchiectasis; that is, bronchial obstruction, atelectasis, and infection.

A normal chest x-ray does not preclude early or minimal bronchiectasis. Chest tomograms may reveal the presence of central bronchiectasis, making bronchography unnecessary. Bronchography has been reported to cause adverse reactions, including an increase in asthma and toxic reactions, in patients with allergic aspergillosis. It should be performed only after careful consideration of the risks and benefits.

Differential Diagnosis

Bacterial pneumonia, carcinoma, tuberculosis, eosinophilic pneumonia, and extrinsic allergic alveolitis constitute the differential diagnosis of allergic bronchopulmonary aspergillosis. In a patient who presents with asthma and pulmonary shadows on x-ray, the main diagnostic considerations are bacterial pneumonia, carcinoma, and tuberculosis. The frequently seen roentgenographic findings in allergic aspergillosis of upper lobe shrinkage and cavitation are particularly suggestive of tuberculosis.

Eosinophilic pneumonia consists of migratory pulmonary infiltrates, usually accompanied by an excess of eosinophiles in the peripheral blood. It is also called *pulmonary eosinophilia* or the PIE syndrome; that is, pulmonary infiltrate with eosinophilia.

The clinical findings of eosinophilic pneumonia include cough, anorexia, and weight loss. The chest infiltrates are roentgenographically migratory and transient. On x-ray, a peripheral density adjacent to the pleura with a clear zone located centrally is quite characteristic and has been called a "photographic negative of pulmonary edema." The characteristic histologic picture is the filling of alveoli with

Table 23-2 *Differential Characteristics of Extrinsic Allergic Alveolitis (Hypersensitivity Pneumonitis) and Allergic Bronchopulmonary Aspergillosis*

	Extrinsic Allergic Alveolitis	Allergic Bronchopulmonary Aspergillosis
Basic nature of patient	Nonatopic	Atopic
Physical examination	±	Wheezing
Skin test	±*	Dual positivity
Roentgenography	Pulmonary infiltrates (interstitial)	Pulmonary infiltrates (lobar)
Complications	Pulmonary fibrosis	Atelectasis, bronchiectasis
Blood	Normal	Eosinophilia
Sputum	Normal	Eosinophilia, mycelia
IgE	Normal	Elevated
Pulmonary function	Restrictive	Obstructive (restrictive late in course)
Antibody	Precipitating (IgG)	Precipitating (IgG) and nonprecipitating (IgE)
Proposed immunologic basis	Immune complexes and delayed hypersensitivity (types III and IV)	Immediate hypersensitivity and immune complexes (types I and III)

*Positive reaction is immediate and late in some patients with pigeon-breeder's lung.
(Adapted from Slavin, R. G. Allergic bronchopulmonary aspergillosis, in E. Middleton, Jr., C. E. Reed, & E. F. Ellis (Eds.), *Allergy: Principles and practice*, St. Louis: Mosby, 1978, p. 851. With permission.

eosinophils and large mononuclear cells and an interstitial infiltrate of eosinophils, lymphocytes, and plasma cells.

A confusion exists in many minds between allergic bronchopulmonary aspergillosis and extrinsic allergic alveolitis (hypersensitivity pneumonitis). Table 23-2 points out the distinctive features of each. Extrinsic allergic alveolitis occurs almost exclusively in nonatopic individuals and is not associated with eosinophilia, increased levels of serum IgE, immediate skin reactivity, or marked bronchoconstriction. It is, instead, as stated before, a restrictive lung disease, the pathogenesis of which is quite different from that of allergic aspergillosis.

Key Diagnostic Tests

The diagnosis of allergic bronchopulmonary aspergillosis can be suspected strongly in an asthmatic whose bronchospasm has increased and who has pulmonary infiltrates, a markedly elevated IgE with positive immediate skin test reactivity, and positive serum precipitins to *A. fumigatus*. Tomography indicating central bronchiectasis is further evidence of the disease.

Pulmonary function testing in patients with allergic aspergillosis shows a significant decline in total lung capacity, vital capacity, forced expiratory volume in one second (FEV_1), and carbon monoxide diffusion during clinical flares, with a return to baseline values during remission. A reduction in carbon monoxide diffusion probably relates to the presence of bronchiectasis and is the best pulmonary function index of disease severity since ordinary bronchial asthma is associated with a normal carbon monoxide diffusion.

Production of brown mucus plugs is an important diagnostic clue. Direct examination of the plugs will reveal fungal mycelia and large numbers of eosinophiles in a majority of patients. The mycelia show good preservation of cytoplasm, indicating active growth of the fungus. Because aspergillus is commonly inhaled and expectorated by the population at large, a positive sputum culture is not diagnostic of aspergillosis.

Therapy

The aim of therapy for allergic aspergillosis is to prevent the continued release of antigenic material by the aspergillus organism trapped in the bronchial secretions. Early and strenuous treatment is important, for it is extremely difficult to clear the damaged bronchial tree of the fungus once it has become entrenched. If permanent bronchial damage can be prevented, the nidus of fungus can be more easily expectorated during subsequent clinical exacerbations. Corticosteroids are the most effective drugs in the treatment of allergic aspergillosis. The decrease in the allergic inflammatory response, the decrease in the amount of viscid secretion, and the relief of airway obstruction all lead to more effective removal of the fungus.

Corticosteroids must be given in sufficiently large doses over a sufficient period of time to accomplish these aims. A large daily dose of prednisone, 45–65 mg or more in adults, may be required for complete clearing of the chest x-ray. A daily dose of approximately 0.5 mg/kg of body weight should be continued for 2 weeks, with the drug then given every other day for 3 months. This alternate-day dose is then tapered and discontinued over another 3-month period (see flow sheet in Fig. 23-1).

Follow-up and Prognosis

A long-term follow-up study of 50 patients with untreated bronchopulmonary aspergillosis has been reported. All followed a chronic course with airway obstruction, recurrent pulmonary consolidation, and in many instances, severe lung destruction. A third of the patients with recurrent pulmonary consolidation were asymptomatic; that is, episodes could recur without gross functional deterioration. Therefore, the use of symptoms as a guide to therapy bears no relationship to the activity of the disease. Patients with allergic aspergillosis can continue to have clinically unrecognized pulmonary consolidation capable of progressing insidously and causing severe lung damage and thus must be carefully monitored. Total serum IgE levels mirror disease activity. A rising level is predictive of a clinical flare, whereas a stable or declining value implies remission. Since a rise in IgE and the extent of pulmonary infiltrate may be associated with minimal symptoms, serial chest x-rays and serial IgE measurements are extremely useful for monitoring treatment. Chest x-rays should

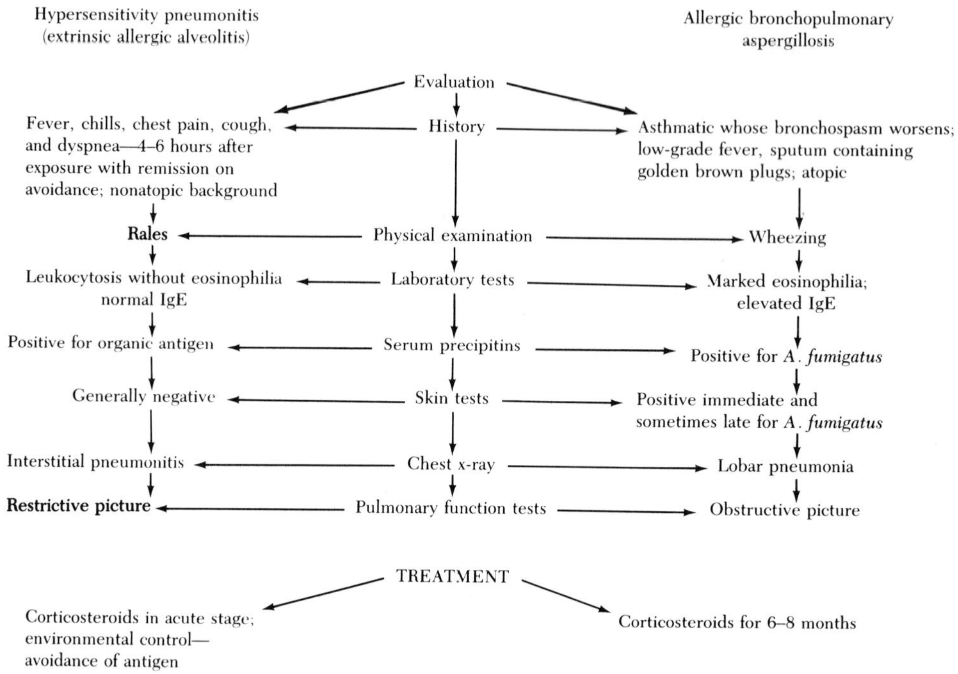

Fig. 23-1. Flow sheet for evaluation and treatment of hypersensitivity diseases of the lung.

be obtained 4 months for 2 years, then every 6 months for 2 years, then once a year thereafter. Serial IgE levels should be obtained monthly for 2 years, then every 2 months thereafter. A rise in this level should prompt the institution of a regimen of systemic corticosteroids.

New and Future Developments in the Field

Perhaps the most important development in this disease is the increasing recognition of the process. The diagnostic index of suspicion must be kept high, for failure to recognize this complication of bronchial asthma may result in severe pulmonary disability. Patients who had developed allergic aspergillosis were, until recently, thought to require systemic steroids for the rest of their lives. As stated earlier, it is now possible through the aid of IgE levels and chest x-rays to markedly limit the duration of steroid therapy. This is particularly important since the great majority of patients with allergic aspergillosis are under the age of 20 years. It is not clear as yet whether aerosolized corticosteroids are adequate. A long-term controlled clinical trial is needed to properly evaluate these agents for treating allergic bronchopulmonary aspergillosis.

Histories

CASE 1. A 29-year-old accountant had a long history of bronchial asthma. In the past 6 months he had wheezed a great deal more and was producing brownish plugs in his sputum. He is now hospitalized with his third episode of pneumonitis in 6 months. Physical examination revealed a temperature of 101°F. Examination of the chest showed generalized expiratory wheezes. Laboratory evaluation revealed a WBC of 11,200 with 34% eosinophils. Serum immunoglobulin data were as follows: IgG 1300 mg%, IgA 300 mg%, IgM 250 mg%, and IgE 11,000 ng/ml. Sputum examination revealed many eosinophils and mycelia. Chest x-ray showed a solid infiltrate in the right upper lobe. In pulmonary function testing, the FEV_1 was 50% of normal. Allergy skin testing revealed a 4+ immediate reaction to a prick test of 1 : 10 *Aspergillus fumigatus*. Serum precipitins were positive for *A. fumigatus*. Tomograms showed central bronchiectasis in the right lower lobe. The diagnosis was allergic bronchopulmonary aspergillosis.

CASE 2. A 22-year-old college student, whose main interest was birds, lived in a small apartment with his wife and 14 birds who flew around freely. The birds included parakeets and finches. His chief complaint was cough, increasing shortness of breath, malaise, and weakness. He had been hospitalized twice before with pneumonitis and had responded promptly to antibiotics. However, shortly after returning to his apartment, he experienced the above symptoms. Physical examination showed a temperature of 100.6°F, and examination of his chest revealed bilateral basilar crepitant rales. Laboratory evaluation revealed a WBC of 7000 with a normal differential. Serum immunoglobulin levels were IgG 1200 mg%, IgA 275 mg%, IgM 300 mg%, and IgE 150 ng/ml. The sputum examination was negative. Chest x-ray showed patchy infiltrates in both lower lung fields. Pulmonary function testing showed an FEV_1 of 70% of normal, a vital capacity decreased by 20%, and a DLCO that was 30% below expected. Serum precipitins were positive to pigeon serum. The diagnosis was extrinsic allergic alveolitis (bird fancier's lung).

SUGGESTED READINGS

Farmer's lung and related disorders. NIAID Task Force Report: Asthma and other allergic diseases. (1979). Washington, D.C.: NIH Publication No. 79–387, U.S. Department of Health, Education, and Welfare, 1979, pp 292–330.

Imbeau, S. A., Nichols, D., & Flaherty, D. *J. Allergy Clin. Immunol.*, 1978, 62, 243.

Karr, R. M., & Salvaggio, J. E. Infiltrative hypersensitivity disease of the lung. In C. W. Parker, (Ed): Philadelphia: Saunders, 1980, pp. 1336–1371.

Lopez, M., Salvaggio, J. E. *Ann. Rev. Med.*, 1976, 27, 453.

Rosenberg, M., Patterson, R., & Mintzer, R. *Ann. Intern. Med.*, 1977, *86*, 405.

Rosenberg, M., Patterson, R., Roberts, M., & Wang, J. *Am. J. Med.*, 1978, *64*, 699.

Salvaggio, J. E., *Hosp. Pract.*, 1980, 93.

Salvaggio, J. E., & Karr, R. M. *Chest*, 1979, 75, 270S.

Schwartz, R. H., and Hollich, G. E. Allergic bronchopulmonary ampergillosis with low serum immunoglobulin E. *J. Allergy Clin. Immunol.*, 1981, *68*, 290.

Slavin, R. G., Allergic bronchopulmonary aspergillosis. In E. Middleton, Jr., E. E. Reed, & E. F. Ellis, (Eds.), *Allergy: Principles and practice*, St. Louis: Mosby, 1978, pp. 843–855.

Wang, J. L. F., Patterson, R., Roberts, M., & Ghory, A. C. *Am. Rev. Resp. Dis.*, 1979, *120*, 87.

QUESTIONS

1. Which of the following is *not* an example of extrinsic allergic alveolitis?

   a. Farmer's lung
   b. Bagassosis

c. Silicosis
d. Pigeon breeder's lung

2. A 35-year old farmer complains of low-grade fever, cough, and dyspnea. A chest film shows evidence of interstitial pneumonitis. He is hospitalized, and within 2 days the symptoms disappear and a second chest film is normal. However, the symptoms recur after he returns to the farm. The results of a precipitating antibody test to thermophilic organisms are positive. Which of the following statements related to this case is (are) false?

   a. The pulmonary function abnormality is largely one of restriction.
   b. Fever, chills, chest pain, cough, and dyspnea 4–6 hours after exposure could be expected to result from appropriate bronchial challenge.
   c. The presence of serum precipitating antibody is pathognomonic of farmer's lung.
   d. Further episodes of exposure to thermophilic organism may result in pulmonary fibrosis.

3. Characteristic symptoms of hypersensitivity pneumonitis include:

   a. Cough, wheezing, and dyspnea within minutes after inhalation of the offending antigen.
   b. Cough, dyspnea, and myalgia 24–48 hours after removal of contact with the offending antigen.
   c. Progressive and insidious dyspnea, cough, and weight loss.
   d. Anaphylactic symptoms.

4. Which of the following laboratory pictures are most characteristic of allergic bronchopulmonary aspergillosis?

   a. IgE 200 ng/ml, positive immediate skin test to *A. fumigatus*, positive precipitating antibody to *A. fumigatus*.
   b. IgE 3600 ng/ml, positive immediate skin test to *A. fumigatus*, positive precipitating antibody to *A. fumigatus*.
   c. IgE 1800 ng/ml, positive immediate skin test to *A. fumigatus*, negative precipitating antibody to *A. fumigatus*.
   d. IgE 1000 ng/ml, negative immediate skin test to *A. fumigatus*, positive precipitating antibody to *A. fumigatus*.

5. Which of the following would *not* be characteristic of allergic bronchopulmonary aspergillosis?

   a. Marked eosinophilia
   b. Nonatopic background
   c. Profound elevation of serum IgE
   d. Transient pulmonary infiltrates

Answers can be found in Appendix B at the end of the book.

PART 6

Allergies to Specific Agents

Walter H. Lewis

24

Pollen Allergy

The pollen wall consists of three layers: an outer resistant exine separable into an external sexine, an internal impervious nexine, and an inner nonresistant intine. The outer surface of the sexine is normally permeated by many micropores, but the major gap in the wall is the aperature, either a pore or furrow, from which a pollen tube emerges following successful pollination. What is important in immediate hypersensitivity is that proteins and other compounds—perhaps recognition molecules typical of species—stored in the sexine and intine are released through these pores and apertures when the pollen contacts mucosal surfaces, giving rise in sensitized atopic individuals to allergic rhinitis, allergic sinusitis, and bronchial asthma.

POLLEN DIVERSITY

With a few notable exceptions, all pollen found in the ambient air is potentially allergenic. The major exception is the widely dispersed pollen of many gymnosperms, particularly of the pine family that includes fir, larch, spruce, hemlock, and Douglas fir, as well as pine.

About 60 families of higher plants found in North America are implicated in pollinosis (Lewis et al., 1983), but only about one-half of these are of general significance. Pollen grains of these plants are mostly *aperturate* (with pores and/or furrows) or occasionally nonaperaturate as for poplars. Pores may be one per grain as typical of grasses; two per grain as for members of the mulberry and stinging nettle families; three per grain as for hops, birches, hazelnuts, barberries, hickories, and Osage Orange; four to six pores as for alders, walnuts, plantain, hackberries, and elms; or with many pores as found in the pigweed and goosefoot families. Other grains are characterized by furrows, usually three or four, as found for maples, oaks, ashes, sycamores, and willows. Sometimes pores and furrows are combined in a single aperture to form mostly 3-colporate aperatures without (mugwort, olive, dock,

ALLERGY: THEORY AND PRACTICE
ISBN 0-8089-1619-X

tree-of-heaven) discernible spines or with spines as characteristic of many members of the aster family. Representative examples of trees and shrubs (Fig. 24-1) and of weeds and grasses (Fig. 24-2) show that size, shape, wall thickness, and aperture type and number often are sufficiently variable to allow determination of pollen to family and sometimes to genus (Lewis et al., 1983).

POLLEN DISPERSAL

When mature, anthers release pollen that functions to transmit the male genetic material in sexual reproduction. Pollen may be wind-dispersed (anemophilous), and, depending on its bouyancy, sculpturing, shape, and stickiness, as well as environmental conditions, can be carried some distance from the immediate vicinity of the parent. Wind-pollinated species are the source of the vast majority of pollen allergens. The flowers of these species possess a set of adaptive characteristics that includes reduction in the size and number of perianth parts; little or no nectar or aromatic compounds; small, dry, and smooth pollen (20–40 μm in diameter) with slow terminal velocities (2–6 cm/sec), a complex feathery stigma with a relatively large surface area, and a large number of pollen grains released per ovule (Adams et al., 1981). Exceptions exist for each of these adaptations, however, as the spiny pollen of the wind-pollinated ragweeds illustrates.

The majority of flowering plants have maintained a vector-mediated pollination system. Such plants are of little general concern in pollinosis, not because their pollen lacks antigens, but because exposures are so limited that sensitization rarely occurs. Yet some animal-pollinated species produce abundant pollen, have an open

Fig. 24-1. Pollen grains of representative trees and shrubs: (a) *Acer negundo* (box-elder), SEM near-equatorial view showing two or three apertures (magnification ×2050); (b) *A. rubrum* (red maple), SEM equatorial view showing two or three apertures (magnification ×1800); (c) *Betula nigra* (river birch), polar views showing the three apertures (magnification ×360); (d) *Corylus avellana* (European hazelnut), polar view of the three apertures and three large intinous onci (magnification ×915); (e) *Quercus marilandica* (blackjack oak), polar views showing the three apertures (magnification ×360); (f) *Q. prinoides* (chiquapin oak), SEM equatorial view showing one of three apertures (magnification ×1600); (g) *Q. virginiana* (live oak), one equatorial view and three polar views (magnification ×360); (h) *Carya* × *laneyi* (hickory hybrid), polar views magnified 360 times (acetolyzed); (i) *Juglans nigra* (black walnut), views showing many or no pores at poles (magnification ×360) (acetolyzed); (j) *Caclura pomifera* (Osage orange), equatorial and polar views showing the three apertures magnified 360 times (acetolyzed); (k) *Morus alba* (white mulberry), equatorial views showing the two apertures magnified 360 times; (l) *Comptonia peregrina* (sweet fern), polar views showing the three apertures (magnification ×360); (m) *Fraxinus pennsylvanica* (green ash), mostly polar views showing four apertures (magnification ×360); (n) *Salix caroliniana* (coastal plain willow), equatorial view showing one of three apertures (magnification ×915); (o) *S. exigua* (coyote willow), equatorial view showing one of three apertures (magnification ×360); (p) *Ailanthus altissima* (tree-of-heaven), SEM polar view showing the three apertures (magnification ×2100); (q) *Celtis tunuifolia* (Georgia hackberry) showing many pores (magnification ×360); (r) *Ulmus parvifolia* (chinese elm), SEM of pore and adjacent sexine (magnification ×5500). Light micrographs unless indicated as SEM (scanning electron micrographs) and stained untreated grains unless indicated as acetolyzed.

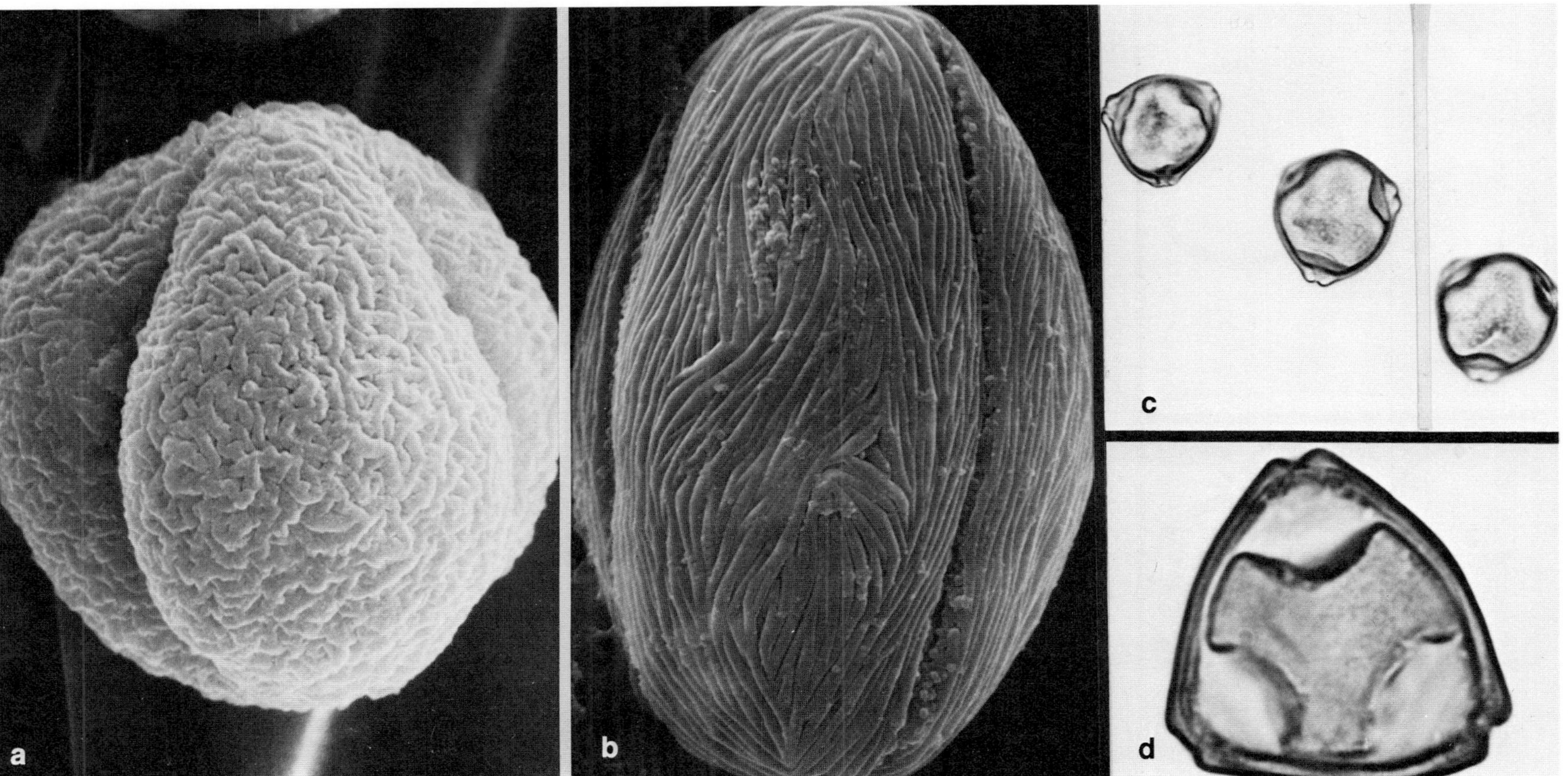
a
b
c
d

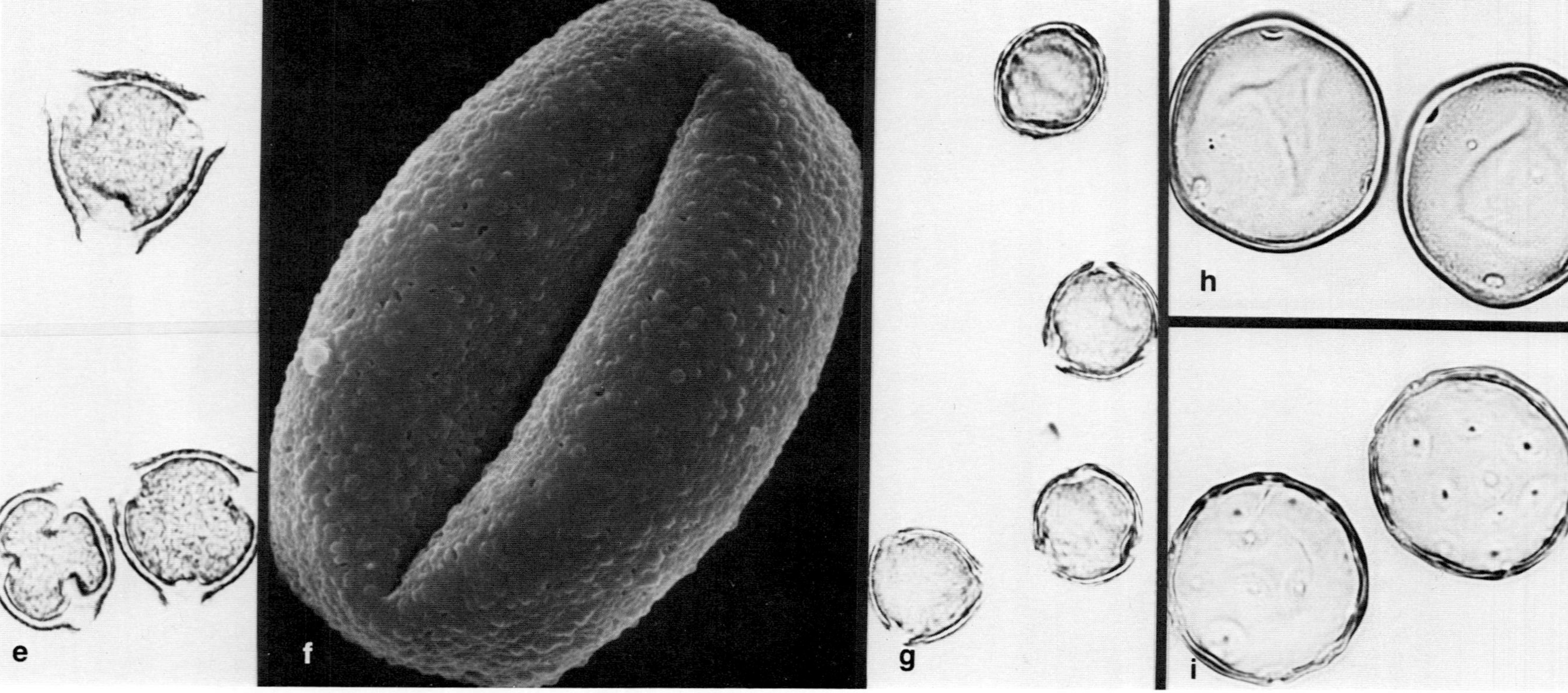
e
f
g
h
i

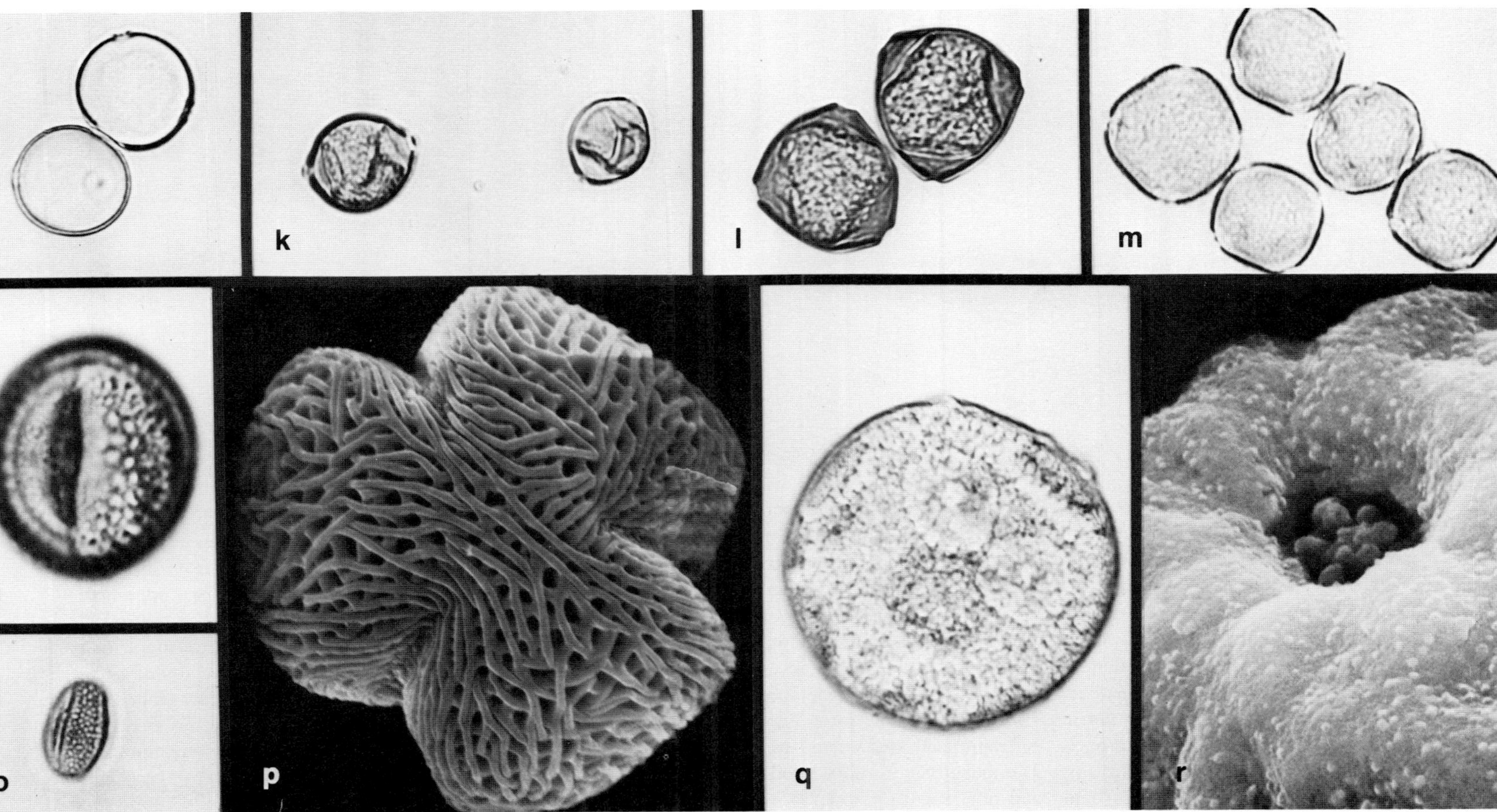
j
k
l
m
n
o
p
q
r

Fig. 24-2. Pollen grains of representative weeds and grasses (m–o). (a) *Amaranthus retroflexus* (redroot pigweed) with many pores (magnification ×360); (b) *Ambrosia artemisiifolia* (short ragweed) showing two equatorial (upper) and one polar (lowest) views magnified 360 times; (c) *A. bidentata* (southern ragweed) showing various but mostly polar views (magnification ×360); (d) *A. trifida* (giant ragweed) (magnification ×360); (e) *Artemisia absinthium* (common wormwood), near-polar views (magnification ×360); (f) *A. ludoviciana* (western mugwort) showing polar (right) and equatorial (bottom) views magnified 360 times (acetolyzed); (g) *Cichorium intybus* (chicory) magnified 360 times (acetolyzed); (h) *Iva annua* (rough marsh-elder) magnified 360 times (acetolyzed); (i) *Parthenium integrifolium* (American feverfew), SEM polar view with long spines and many sexinous micropores (magnification ×1500); (j) *Humulus lupulus* (hops), near-polar view showing two of three apertures and three onci (magnification ×915); (k) *Atriplex truncata* (wedgescale) with many pores magnified 360 times (acetolyzed); (l) *Salsola kali* (Russian thistle) with many pores magnified 915 times (acetolyzed); (m) *Poa practensis* (Kentucky bluegrass) magnified 915 times; (n) *Hordeum jubatum* (foxtail barley) showing the one pore typical of all grasses (magnification ×360); (o) *Dactylis glomerata* (orchard grass) magnified 915 times; (p) *Rumex crispus* (curly dock) magnified 360 times; (q) *Boehmeria cylindrica* (bog-hemp) showing the two pores magnified 915 times (acetolyzed); (r) *Pilea pumila* (clearweed) showing the two pores magnified 915 times (acetolyzed); (s) *Urtica dioica* (stinging nettle) showing the two pores and one of two onci magnified 915 times. Light micrographs except part i (SEM) and stained untreated grains unless indicated as acetolyzed.

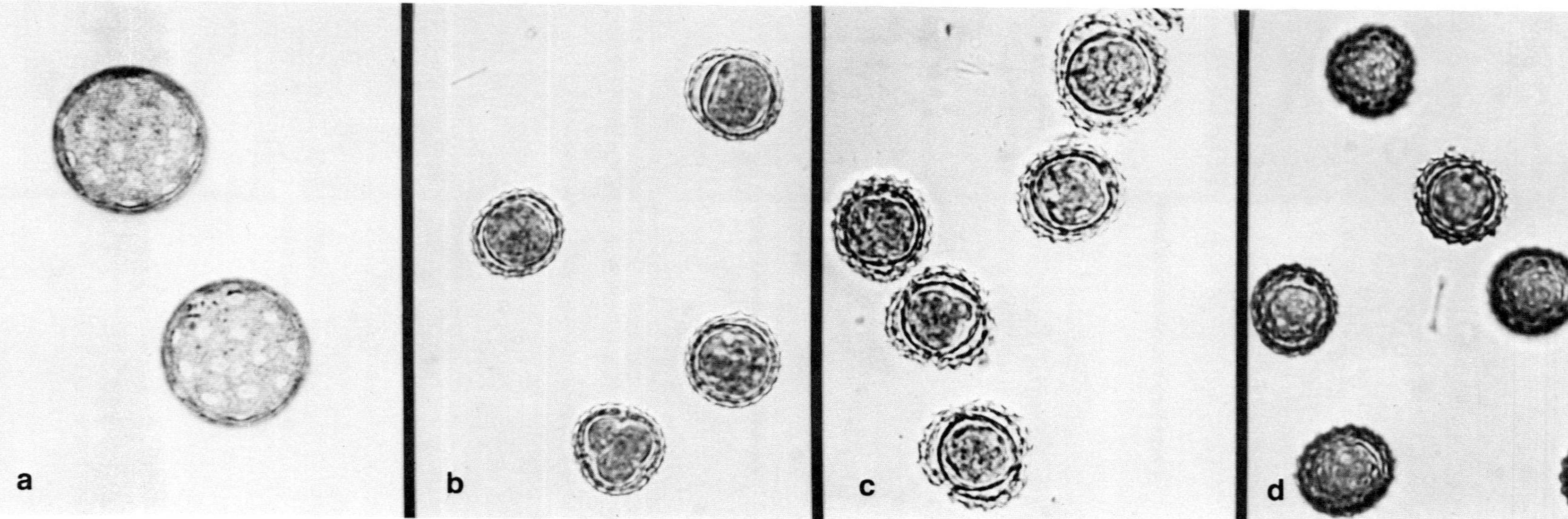

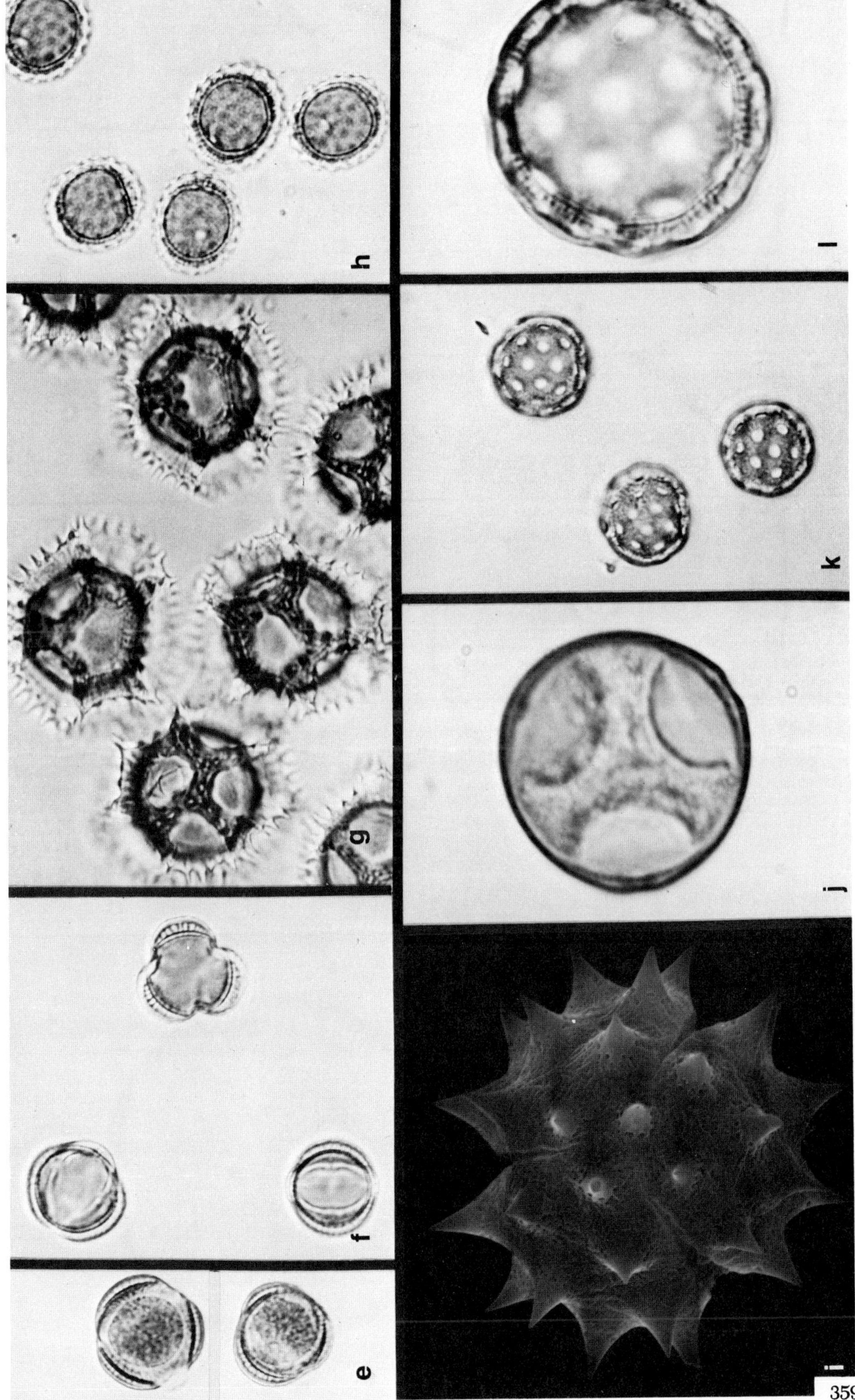
e
f
g
h
i
j
k
l

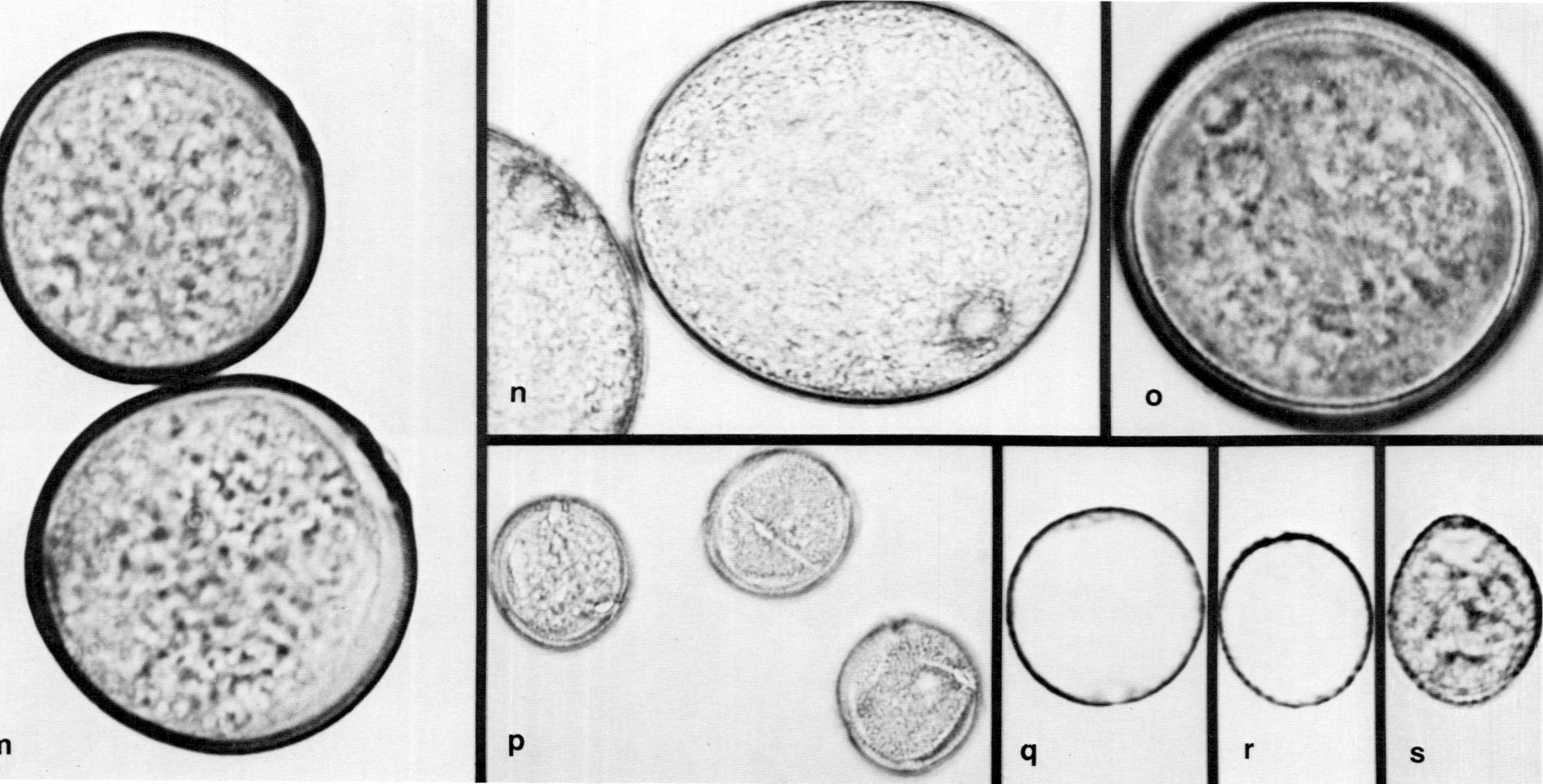
m
n
o
p
q
r
s

floral morphology with exposed anthers, produce few lipids giving rise to less sticky pollen, and release at least moderate amounts of pollen that is carried by the wind (Lewis & Vinay, 1979). These entomophilous species are sometimes partially adapted to wind dispersal as a secondary mode of pollination and are thus facultatively anemophilous, whereas others release pollen incidental to pollination merely as an accidental event. Because of either facultative anemophily or incidental release of pollen, it is fallacious to ignore all entomophilous species as potential offenders in localized cases of inhalant allergy.

In temperate areas allergenic plants are traditionally grouped as trees, grasses, and weeds, a useful grouping because it follows a generalized flowering sequence from spring to autumn. Trees and shrubs flower primarily from late winter to late spring, grasses from late spring to midsummer, and weeds from midsummer to autumn. Exceptions are noteworthy—particularly the woody *Ricinus* (castor bean), *Albizia* (mimosa tree), *Castanea* (chestnut), and *Tilia* (basswood or linden), which often flower during summer months; some *Ulmus* (elm) species that are late summer and autumn flowering; and the herbaceous *Rumex* (dock or sorrel) and *Thalictrum* (meadow-rue), which flower during the late spring and summer. Some grasses begin flowering in spring after a mild winter and continue flowering until autumn during a wet summer. Still other grasses do not begin flowering until late in the summer thus in certain localities a secondary release of pollen with subsequent grass pollinosis is not unusual. Additionally, in more southern areas of the continent, flowering does not necessarily follow this traditional pattern; rather, it may be multiseasonal or year-round, or it may occur during a totally different season from a temperate counterpart.

POLLEN ALLERGENICITY

Allergic reactions to pollen are discussed briefly for genera of a few gymnosperms and 33 angiosperm families. A more detailed discussion can be found in Lewis et al. (1982).

Trees and Shrubs

Some allergenic trees and shrubs are as follows:

GYMNOSPERMS. *Juniperus* (juniper, red and mountain cedar) pollen has been implicated in late autumn, winter, and early spring pollinosis. In the foothills of the Rocky Mountains it is often a serious concern in pollinosis, but in eastern North America it is rarely implicated as a factor in inhalant allergy. Pollen of *Taxodium* (bald cypress) is morphologically similar and may be a minor offender in winter.

ACERACEAE (MAPLES). All species of maple are potentially allergenic, but different modes of pollination vary the extent of pollen exposures and subsequent sensitizations. The wind-pollinated and ubiquitous *Acer negundo* (box elder) is perhaps the most troublesome species in inhalant allergy (Lewis & Imber, 1975).

ARECACEAE OR PLAMAE (PALMS). The most common palms in the United States are *Phoenix* (date) and *Cocos* (coconut). In Florida, California, and Hawaii they are cultivated commercially for fruit or are grown for street plantings. Reports of allergenicity are sharply localized to those persons living near areas where street plantings are heavy and among those employed in palm plantations.

BETULACEAE (ALDERS, BIRCHES, HAZELNUTS). Pollen of *Alnus* (alder) is a major offender west of the Rocky Mountains, whereas that of *Betula* (birch) is more serious in the northeastern United States and adjacent Canada. Exposure to other betulaceous pollen is much more limited, although sensitivity to *Corylus* (hazelnut) has been reported in the Pacific Northwest. High cross-reactivities on skin testing have been reported to pollen extracts from these three genera, as well as between them and members of the Fagaceae (oak family), which are related to the Betulaceae (Dalen & Voorhorst, 1981).

BIGNONIACEAE (BIGNONIAS). Pollen is largely insect-pollinated, but the large showy flowers of *Catalpa* (cigar tree) shed some pollen incidentally that can be caught airborne in the vicinity of the trees. Strong allergic reactions have been elicited among individuals sensitized by repeated exposure to *Catalpa* pollen (Swineford, 1940), illustrating the importance of the patient's microenvironment in understanding the course of some allergic reactions.

CASUARINACEAE (AUSTRALIAN PINES). In Florida and California, where *Casuarina* has been introduced, a few patients have been sensitized following exposure to its pollen.

EUPHORBIACEAE (CASTOR BEAN). Even though well documented elsewhere, there is no reported case of allergenicity to *Ricinus* (castor bean) pollen in North America. This is perhaps an example of not recognizing the allergenic potential of a plant occasionally cultivated and naturalized, particularly in southern regions of the United States.

FABACEAE OR LEGUMINOSAE (LEGUMES). Occasional allergenicity has been associated with three woody genera of mimosoid legumes: *Acacia* (wattle) in the southwest, *Albizia* (mimosa tree) in Flordia, and *Prosopis* (mesquite) in the southcentral and southwestern regions. Wherever exposure to their pollen is sufficient, limited cases of sensitivity are possible.

FAGACEAE (BEECHES, CHESTNUTS, OAKS). Only pollen of *Quercus* (oak) is a major offender in the family; pollen dispersal of the other genera is reduced or primarily entomophilous, and exposure is limited. Oak pollen, however, is responsible throughout the continent for many cases of moderate to severe spring pollinosis and is invariably considered a potential incitant of tree inhalant allergy.

GARRYACEAE (SILK-TASSELS). As abundant pollen is dispersed, *Garrya* may be responsible for some undiagnosed cases of silk-tassel pollinosis wherever plants are common in the southwest.

HAMAMELIDACEAE (SWEET GUM). Occasional spring pollinosis results from exposure to the abundant pollen shed by *Liquidambar* (sweet gum). Reports of allergenicity are rare, but where sweet gums are common their role in inhalant allergy should be considered.

JUGLANDACEAE (HICKORIES, WALNUTS). *Carya* (hickory, pecan) pollen is a serious concern in pollinosis in eastern North America, whereas *Juglans* (walnut) is of greater significance west of the Rocky Mountains. In California and Oregon, for example, symptoms of pollinosis are so acute that walnut allergens are considered among the most serious spring offenders there.

MORACEAE (MULBERRIES, OSAGE ORANGE). Where common, the wind -pollinated mulberries (*Morus*) are capable of causing severe spring pollinosis. They tend to be weedy trees and shrubs, with frequencies sometimes rising rapidly in neglected urban and suburban areas and exposures to their abundant pollen suddenly increasing. Occasionally Osage orange (*Maclura*) is also a serious offender.

MYRICACEAE (BAYBERRIES, WAX-MYRTLES). Severe allergic reactions to *Myrica* pollen is well documented by a case of sensitivity to *Myrica cerifera* (southern bayberry). Prince & Meyer (1977) found that following exposure their patient suffered from sneezing, severe ocular irritation, profuse rhinorrhea, and nasal occlusion. He responded favorably to hyposensitization using *M. cerifera* pollen extracts. Other species of *Myrica* and *Comptonia,* where common in coastal regions of the continent, may be equally as important in pollinosis. Unfortunately for sufferers of spring allergies, these sources of allergens are not often recognized.

MYRTACEAE (BOTTLEBRUSHES, EUCALYPTS). *Melaleuca* (Lockey et al., 1981), and probably *Eucalyptus* and *Callistemon,* are of only minor significance in terms of allergy because of limited pollen shed.

OLEACEAE (ASHES, OLIVES, PRIVETS). Wind-dispersed pollen of *Fraxinus* (ash) is an important source of allergens where trees are common. The facultatively wind-pollinated pollen of *Ligustrum* (privet) and *Olea* (olive) is of more local concern where cultivated.

PLATANACEAE (SYCAMORES). Even where common, pollen of *Platanus* is only moderately allergenic and of secondary importance in pollinosis.

SALICACEAE (POPLARS, WILLOWS). The incidence of sensitivity to wind-dispersed pollen of *Populus* (poplar) is far greater throughout North America than to the pollen of *Salix* (willow). This reflects reduced exposure to *Salix* pollen, which is primarily insect-pollinated and either facultatively or incidentally wind-dispersed. However, willow pollen tends to be more allergenic (Lewis & Imber, 1975).

SIMAROUBACEAE (TREE-OF-HEAVEN). Modest levels of positive skin test reactions and moderate incidences of sensitivity to the secondarily wind-dispersed *Ailanthus* pollen are typical of exposure to this late spring and early summer flowering tree of weedy urban habitats.

TAMARICACEAE (TAMARISKS). Pollen of *Tamarix* is dispersed by vectors and only facultatively by wind. Consequently, limited pollen exposures have resulted in only a few reported cases of pollinosis from California and Arizona.

TILIACEAE (BASSWOODS, LINDENS). Although anemophily is secondary to insect pollination, sufficient pollen of *Tilia* becomes airborne to be a major inhalant offender where trees are common (Derbes, 1941). Pollinosis due to *Tilia* should receive greater consideration than it does east of the Rocky Mountains during June and July.

ULMACEAE (ELMS, HACKBERRIES). Spring and autumn pollinosis is commonly attributed to the wind-dispersed pollen of *Ulmus* (elm). The trees release abundant pollen, although exposures have been much reduced in recent years in eastern North America with the loss of many American elms to the Dutch elm disease. In southern California, however, exposures to *autumn flowering* species have resulted in many reports of severe allergic reactions.

Grasses and Grass-like Plants

Grasses and grass-like plants that elicit allergic reaction include the following:

POACEAE OR GRAMINEAE (GRASSES). The largest and most important of the temperate grass subfamilies (Pooideae) includes many allergenically significant genera, such as *Agrostis* (redtop), *Anthoxanthum* (vernalgrass), *Bromus* (bromegrass, chess), *Dactylis* (orchard grass), *Festuca* (fescue), *Holcus* (velvetgrass), *Lolium* (darnel, ryegrass), *Phleum* (timothy), and *Pao* (bluegrass, June grass). They illustrate a high degree of immunologic similarity. Pollen antigens from members of other subfamilies differ substantially from these pooids (Watson & Knox, 1976) with below average cross-reactivities between them and the chloridoid *Cynodon* (Bermuda grass) and the panicoid *Sorghum* (Johnson grass, cultivated sorghum). In all instances, the level of cross-reactivity was insufficient to justify the clinical use of a single genus as a dependable indicator of allergenicity.

CYPERACEAE (SEDGES) AND JUNCACEAE (RUSHES). Considering the volume of airborne pollen released by sedges and rushes and their close relationship to the grasses, it is surprising that so few reports of pollen sensitivity exist. This may be due simply to limited exposure, for few of these plants are closely associated with population centers.

Weeds and Herbs

Some weeds and herbs found to be allergenic are as follows:

AMARANTHACEAE (AMARANTHS, PIGWEEDS). In central and western regions of North America numerous reports of severe pollinosis from midsummer to September have been reported from *Amaranthus* pollen. Allergenicity of pollen from other genera is poorly known, but predominantly wind-pollinated species of *Iresine* (bloodleaf) and *Tidestromia* are likely candidates for eliciting allergic reactions. Morphologically and perhaps allergenically, Amaranthaceae and Chenopodiaceae pollen are very similar.

ASTERACEAE OR COMPOSITAE (RAGWEEDS, MARSH-ELDERS, SAGEBRUSHES). Members of the Asteraceae, together with the grasses, are responsible for more cases of pollinosis than all other plants combined. The major offenders by far are *Ambrosia* (ragweed),

Iva (marsh-elder), and *Artemisia* (sagebrush, wormwood), the pollen of which is wind-dispersed in large quantities during late summer. Pollen sensitivity to one species in any genus implies some degree of sensitization to the pollen of other species. Thus care must be exercised when travelling to or living in southern latitudes of the continent so as to anticipate exposure to ragweed and other pollen "out of season" during the winter and spring months. For example, *Ambrosia hispida* (coastal ragweed), native to southern Florida and the Caribbean, flowers year-round, although commonly from January to March, during the height of the tourist season. Other significant, mostly wind-pollinated offenders in the family include *Baccharis* (groundsel-tree), *Dicoria, Hymenoclea* (burro-brush), *Parthenice,* and *Xanthium* (cocklebur). Occasionally the primary insect-pollinated *Anthemis* (dog fennel), *Solidago* (goldenrod), *Taraxacum* (dandelion), and others have been implicated in pollinosis (Lewis & Vinay, 1979).

BRASSICACEAE OR CRUCIFERAE (MUSTARDS). Limited sensitivity to the incidentally wind-dispersed pollen on *Brassica* (mustard) has been reported where common in California and Oregon.

CANNABACEAE (HEMPS, HOPS, MARIJUANA). Shedding abundant pollen, *Cannabis* (hemp, marijuana) and *Humulus* (hops) are probably underestimated as incitants of inhalant allergy. This is particularly true of *Humulus,* which is often a common urban weed. Commercially pistillate plants are largely cultivated and are not sources of pollen allergens.

CHENOPODIACEAE (GOOSEFOOTS). Allergenically important genera are *Atriplex* (saltbush), *Bassia* (smother weed), *Beta* (sugar beet), some *Chenopodium* species (goosefoot, pigweed), *Kochia* (burning bush), and *salsola* (Russian thistle), for they release sufficient wind-dispersed pollen for sensitizations to occur where common, particularly in the western half of the continent. Cross-reactions occur between members of the goosefoots and the Amaranthaceae.

EUPHORBIACEAE (SPURGES). Although pollen of *Mercurialis* (mercury) is known to be allergenic in Europe, there is no report of pollen allergenicity in North America, either of the introduced *Mercurialis* or the common indigenous *Acalypha* (three-seeded mercury). Their pollen, and particularly that of *Acalypha*, probably contributes to pollinosis in North America but is an unrecognized source of allergens.

FABACEAE OR LEGUMINOSAE (LEGUMES). Cases of pollinosis have been reported among agricultural workers exposed to dried hay containing *Medicago* (alfalfa), *Melilotus* (sweet clover), *Trifolium* (clover), and/or *Vicia* (vetch), because dried pollen from broken flowers may become airborne when the hay is disturbed.

PLANTAGINACEAE (PLANTAINS). *Plantago* pollen is responsible for modest levels of allergenicity and frequencies of pollinosis throughout the continent, but particularly in the eastern coastal states, the northwest, and California.

POLYGONACEAE (DOCKS, SORRELS). Most species of *Rumex* (dock or sorrel) and the rare *Oxyria* (mountain sorrel) release wind-dispersed pollen at about the time grass allergenicity is paramount. Although *Rumex* pollen sensitivity is known (Solomon,

Table 24-1 *Pollen-Producing Plants of Allergic Significance in Continental United States*

Geographic Area	Trees	Grasses	Weeds	Major Pollen
Northeastern New England, New York, New Jersey, Pennsylvania	Birch, elm, maple and box elder, oak, poplar	Annual bluegrass, June, orchard, sweet vernal, timothy	Short and giant ragweeds, plantain	Ragweeds, grasses
Middle Atlantic Delaware, Maryland, Washington D.C.	Birch, elm, hickory, maple and box elder, oak, mulberry, sycamore	Orchard, timothy	Short and giant ragweeds, plantain	Ragweeds, orchard grass
Virginias and Carolinas	Beech, elm, maple and box elder, oak, pecan, red cedar	Annual bluegrass, Bermuda, June, orchard	Short ragweed, dock	Short ragweed, Bermuda grass, pecan
Southern Florida and Georgia to eastern Texas, Arkansas, and southern Missouri	Bayberry, beech, cottonwood, elm, oak, mulberry, pecan, poplar, privet, red cedar	Bermuda, orchard, timothy	Giant and short ragweeds, pigweed, Russian thistle, water hemp	Bermuda grass, pecan, ragweeds
North Central Ohio and Kentucky to northern Missouri, Iowa, Wisconsin, Michigan	Ash, cottonwood, elm, hickory, maple and box elder, oak, willow, mulberry	Bluegrass, June, orchard, timothy	Dock, short and giant ragweeds	Ragweeds

Plains and Prairies Minnesota, Dakotas, eastern Montana, Nebraska, Kansas	Elm, maple and box elder, oak, willow	Bermuda, bluegrass, orchard, redtop, timothy	Giant, short and western ragweeds, Russian thistle, hemp, marsh-elder	Ragweeds, Russian thistle
Rocky Mountains Idaho, western Montana, Wyoming, Colorado, Utah	Birch, box elder, cottonwood, Rocky Mountain cedar	Fescue, June, orchard, redtop, timothy	Ragweed, sagebrush, Russian thistle, plantain	Plantain, Russian thistle, sagebrush
Pacific Northwest Washington, Oregon, Nevada, northern California	Acacia, alder, hazelnut, birch, cottonwood, maple, oak, walnut	Bluegrass, fescue, oats, orchard, redtop, timothy, velvet, western rye	Burning bush, dock, pigweed, plantain, Russian thistle, saltbush, sagebrush	Plantain, Russian thistle, sagebrush
Southwest Western Texas, New Mexico, Arizona	Ash, cottonwood, Rocky Mountain cedar, mulberry, oak, olive	Bermuda, Johnson	Amaranth, canyon ragweed, Russian thistle, saltbush	Amaranth, Bermuda grass, goosefoot, Rocky mountain cedar
Southern California	Ash, elm, oak, olive, walnut	Bermuda, salt grass	Dock, lamb's quarters, pigweed, Russian thistle, sage, saltbush, sea blite, stinging nettle	Bermuda grass, saltgrass

1969), possibly it has been overshadowed by the effects of the more frequent grasses and its significance in pollinosis underestimated.

RANUNCULACEAE (MEADOW-RUES). *Thalictrum* is wind-pollinated, and its pollen is a suspected candidate in undiagnosed cases of pollinosis during late spring and early summer.

URTICACEAE (NETTLES). As incitants of inhalant allergy, pollen of this family, which includes such genera as *Boehmeria* (false nettle), *Laportea* (wood nettle), *Parietaria* (pellitory), *Pinea* (clearwood), and *Urtica* (stinging nettle), remains virtually unknown and unexplored in North America. A few American reports of *Urtica* pollen allergenicity (Lewis et al., 1982) and *Parietaria* in Europe exist, but generally the pollen remains unrecognized as potentially allergenic. There are a number of reasons for this: the pollen is very small and somewhat resembles fungal spores and usually remains undetermined in aerosamples (Fig. 24-2), the plants (except for *Urtica*) are not common near population centers, and the plants flower at the peak of the ragweed season in eastern North America and some allergic reactions may be unrecognized because of the overwhelming frequency of ragweed-induced pollinosis.

A regional summary of pollen allergenicity is given in Table 24-1.

Case Histories

CASE 1. A 23-year-old opera student presented with complaints of severe rhinitis and ophthalmitis in spring and fall. The patient's symptoms began in mid-March and lasted until the end of April. He was then symptom-free until mid-August, when his symptoms recurred. He continued to be symptomatic until the first frost. The patient's symptoms included perfuse rhinorrhea, nasal occlusion, and intense nasal pruritus. In addition, he had severe occular pruritus and intense lacrimation. Because of his symptoms he was considering giving up his singing career. The patient stated that he was much better indoors than out of doors, especially in air conditioning. He also was significantly better when he went to the West Coast for a vacation in late August. The patient received modest benefit from antihistamines but was loath to utilize them because of excessive somnolence.

Laboratory investigation revealed an IgE of 540 IU/ml but was otherwise normal. Skin testing using a Multitest apparatus revealed a 4+ reaction to giant ragweed (*Ambrosia trifida*) and oak (*Quercus*) pollen. All other skin tests were negative.

Immunotherapy was instituted with ragweed and oak pollen extracts and was carried through to 2500 PNU/injection of each extract. On this regimen he had a marked reduction in both spring and fall symptoms. He was able to continue to pursue his singing career.

CASE 2. The following is a case report of hayfever from *M. cerifera* (southern bayberry or wax-myrtle). *Myrica* (bayberries and wax-myrtles) consists of six species that are particularly common in northern latitudes and along the Pacific and Atlantic-Gulf coasts. The monotypic *Comptonia* (sweet fern) is very closely allied to *Myrica*. All species flower by spring, but extending to summer in northern regions, and shed enormous amounts of pollen.

A 39-year-old forester consulted Prince & Meyer (1977) on March 14, 1974 for acute hay fever, an attack that had begun the day before while working in the woods. Symptoms included sneezing, severe irritation of the eyes, profuse rhinorrhea, and nasal occlusion. He had had similar severe attacks in the early spring of 1965 and 1966 when living in northern Florida, and also during the spring from 1967 to 1973 when stationed in Arkansas, although the attacks were less severe there. He was transferred to eastern Texas in 1974, where he again manifest acute rhinitis. Physical examination was entirely within normal limits, except for a reddened appearance of the sclerae, edema, and redness of the conjunctivae and of the nasal turbinates, which were covered with clear mucus. Oral temperature was 98.6°F.

Pressure puncture skin tests revealed a 3+ reaction to southern bayberry pollen; tests for other trees and grasses were completely negative.

Myrica species and probably *Comptonia* release abundant allergenically significant pollen grains that should be recognized as important factors in spring pollinosis wherever plants are common.

REFERENCES

Adams, D. E., Perkins, W. E., & Estes, J. R. *Am. J. Bot.*, 1981, *68*, 389–394.

Dalen, G. van, & Voorhorst, R. *Ann. Allergy*, 1981, *46*, 276–278.

Derbes, V. J. *J. Allergy*, 1941, *12*, 502–506.

Lewis, W. H., & Imber, W. E. *Ann. Allergy*, 1975, *35*, 42–50.

Lewis, W. H., & Vinay, P. *Ann. Allergy*, 1979, *42*, 309–318.

Lewis, W. H., Vinay, P., & Zenger, V. E. In Airborne and Allergenic Pollen of North America, Baltimore, Johns Hopkins University Press, 1982.

Lockey, R. F., Stablein, J. J., & Binford, L. R. F. *Proc. Melaleuca Symp., Agriculture, Tallahasee*, Geiger, R. K. (Ed.), 1981, pp. 101–115.

Prince, H. E., & Meyer, G. H. *Ann. Allergy*, 1977, *38*, 252–254.

Solomon, W. R. *J. Allergy*, 1969, *44*, 25–36.

Swineford, C., Jr. *J. Allergy*, 1940, *11*, 398–401.

Watson, L., & Knox, R. B. *Ann. Bot.*, 1976, *40*, 399–408.

QUESTIONS

1. Potentially allergenic proteins are released through pollen
   a. nexine and sexine
   b. nexine and exine
   c. micropores and apertures
   d. micropores and nexine

2. Where may ragweed allergies be found during the winter months in the United States?
   a. Midwest
   b. Florida
   c. Pacific Northwest
   d. New Mexico

3. The least allergenic of major airborne pollen includes the
   a. pines
   b. insect-pollinated shrubs
   c. ragweeds and marsh-elders
   d. grasses

4. Members of the stinging nettle family (Urticaceae) are probably an unrecognized source of pollen allergens in the

   a. spring
   b. late summer
   c. winter
   d. year round

5. A common summer flowering urban weed that is probably underestimated as an incitant of inhalant allergy is

   a. *Ambrosia* (ragweed)
   b. *Carya* (hickory)
   c. *Humulus* (hops)
   d. *Plantago* (plantain)

Answers can be found in Appendix B at the end of the book.

H. James Wedner

25

House Dust and Other Perennial Antigens

Perhaps the most frustrating of all allergic patients are those with year-round or perennial symptoms. In contrast to patients with well-defined seasonal symptoms, the perennial allergic patient, to a greater or lesser extent, suffers year round. It is incumbent on the physician to demonstrate whether the symptoms are the result of interaction between the patient and an allergen continuously present in the environment or a reaction on a nonallergic basis. This is not to say that the patient with perennial allergies has symptoms of the same severity throughout the year. Their symptoms tend to wax and wain and, depending on the allergen, may in some instances have a seasonal increase in symptoms that tempts one to implicate a seasonal allergen. This is best exemplified by the patient with mold sensitivity who has a marked increase in symptoms in late fall, a time when the mold counts become particularly high. Indeed, in one study of asthmatic patients with increased symptoms in the fall, there was a better correlation of disease with airborne mold spores than with ragweed pollen (Salvaggio & Aukrust, 1981). Similarly, dust sensitivity tends to be significantly worse in the winter, when patients spend more time indoors, than in the spring or summer. Nonetheless, the hallmark of perennial allergic disease is that when questioned closely, there is some degree of disease all year round.

Perennial allergic disease has been recognized for many years and has led to the search for the agents that cause this disease. A by no means complete list of the agents that have been implicated in perennial allergic disease is presented in Table 25-1. Of these agents house dust, most probably the house dust mite, and molds are the most important offending agents and are the subject of the remainder of this chapter.

HOUSE DUST

Of all antigens used for the diagnosis and treatment of allergic disease, house dust is by far the most complicated. House dust is an amalgam of simple dust, human and animal danders, mold spores, decayed and decaying vegetable material, dried Arthropoda parts and excreta, bacteria, food remnants, and a variety of inorganic

ALLERGY: THEORY AND PRACTICE
ISBN 0-8089-1619-X

and synthetic organic substances. The concept that this heterogeneous material was a unique allergen was first suggested by the studies of Cooke and Kein in the early 1930s. These workers were the first to demonstrate that a crude extract of house dust was capable of inducing a classical wheal-and-flair reaction when injected into the skin of patients with suspected dust sensitivity. Subsequently, the true allergenicity of house dust has been shown using a variety of both *in vivo* and *in vitro* test systems.

The incidence of positive skin tests to house dust among allergic patients is very high. However, the exact prevalence varies among studies due to differencies in the extract of house dust utilized, the concentration of the extract used, and the method of skin testing (prick vs intradermal). In general, the more concentrated the extract, the higher the percentage of positive skin reactions seen. However, these concentrated solutions are capable of inducing a similar reaction in some, albeit significantly fewer, nonatopic individuals, suggesting that at least a portion of the reactions were the result of nonspecific histamine release. Nonetheless, there are series reporting as high as 80% of atopic patients with positive skin tests to dust, under conditions where nonspecific reactions were minimal. Thus on a percentage basis house dust may be the most prevalent allergen.

Despite the obvious complexity of house dust, it has been known for many years that house dust is a universal, worldwide antigen. Thus extracts made in many foreign countries are generally as efficacious for skin testing and treatment in this country as are those prepared here. This led many workers to suggest that there were one or more common antigens in house dust, and this suspicion (or concern) has resulted in large numbers of studies attempting to identify the common theme. These studies can in large part be divided into two groups: (a) Attempts to utilize complex extraction and purification schemes to isolate individual allergens and (b) examination of the allergens in individual components of house dust. The former techniques to a large extent have not yielded significant information. Those readers with an interest in this approach are referred to the excellent review article by Berrens (1970). The latter technique has been quite effective in defining the major allergen in house dust, the house dust mite.

Allergenic Components of House Dust

Mites

Shortly after the description of house dust as a major cause of perennial allergic symptoms, evidence accumulated suggesting that mites might be a major cause of asthma (Dekker, 1928). That this early finding was not pursued for over 30 years may seem a grevious oversight. However, it should be noted that although the house mite was first described by van Leeuwenhoek in 1694 (probably *Glycyphagus domesticus*), the genius responsible for the majority of mite allergy, *Dermatophagoides*, was not described as a constituent of house dust until 1954 (Baker, 1956). There are over 50,000 species of mite. The relevant mites belong to the family Pyroglychoid, which is comprised of 15 species. Within this family two members of the genus *Dermatophygoides* and one or more members of the genus *Euroglyphus (E. mayner)* are important contributors to human allergic problems.

Early studies by Voorhoist and his colleagues demonstrated a correlation between the prevalence of the mite *D. pteronyssinus* in dust and the allergenicity of the dust extract. These studies were confirmed in a number of countries, including the United States and Japan. In the United States the more prevalent species was *D. farinae,* and studies in this country have suggested that this species provides the major antigenicity. When skin test reactivity was assayed, the potency of a number of dust extracts was shown to be directly related to the concentration of mites in the house dust used for extractions. Differences in the correlation of dust reactive potency and mite count are to some extent related to the fact that much of the mite antigen is contained in decayed mite parts and mite feces. Indeed, a recent study suggested the mite fecal pellets contained the majority of the antigenic material.

This is not to say that all studies have demonstrated a correlation between mite content and house dust reactivity. Several studies that have demonstrated no correlation between mite and house dust sensitivity (Kawai et al., 1972). This discrepancy emphasizes the fact that although mites may provide the major allergen in house dust, they by no means provide *all* of the antigenic material, and other factors must be taken into account when evaluating the dust-sensitive patient (see Chapter 4).

The biology of the Pyroglychoid mites has been studied in extensive detail, and the reader is referred to the excellent review by van Bronswujk & Sinha (1971). As mentioned above, only a limited number of mites have been implicated as important in house dust sensitivity. The two important species are *Dermatophygoides pteronyssinus* and *D. farinae*; in addition, three members of the genus *Euroglyphus* have been implicated in European studies. These arthropods appear to be ubiquitous; they have been found in dust in every part of the world. In addition, they are less than finicky as to the type of dust they inhabit. For example, *D. farinae* has been isolated from furniture dust, floor dust, the nest of birds and mammals, stored products such as grain, human skin, and the skin of birds and mammals. *Dermatophygoides pteronyssinus* inhabits all of the above with the exception of stored products. Thus even though mite prevalence does vary greatly within the home, evaluation and control of these pests must take into account all areas of the home. For example, one study demonstrated that the density of mites is 100-fold greater in mattress dust than in living room dust, presumably because of the greater availability of human dander as a food source. In addition, there is marked seasonal differences in mite infestation, with fall levels being significantly higher than other seasons.

The principal food source for the dermatophygoid mite is human dander; however, these mites will feed on animal and bird dander, grain and foodstuff dust, pollen, and fungal spores, all of which are common constituents of house dust.

For optimum growth mites require relatively high temperatures and high humidity. Optimum growth is at temperatures of 22°–30°C (72°–86°F) and at relative humidities in excess of 75%. Although it may seem that these conditions may not be obtained in most home environments, certain areas of the home such as the mattress frequently attain this ecology. Relative humidity is a critical factor. In one study wet houses had ninefold more mites than did dry houses. This is because egg laying does not occur at relative humidity below 60% and is not maximal until 75% has been reached. However, these animals have remarkable defense mechanisms against drying, and the relative humidity need be raised only to an optimum level for short periods during the day for the normal life cycle to occur. Heavy infestation may thus be found in homes where the *average* humidity is well below 70%.

In light of these considerations some general measures for controling mite infestation can be presented (discussion of these is expanded in Chapter 12). First, the drier the house, the better, as this will be particularly effective in decreasing infestations in floor dust. Vacuuming is extremely important for environmental control protocols and is much more effective than washing since mites can survive quite well in warm soapy water. However, at least one recent study has pointed out that even vacuuming is relatively ineffective in removing mites from carpeting. In addition, vacuuming the mattress, and furniture is particularly effective. Indeed, van Bronswujk & Sinha (1971) report that the number of mites that become airborne is eightfold less during bed making if the mattress is vacuumed first. Washing clothes in *hot* water will destroy the mites, as will 2 hours of ultraviolet light or freezing temperatures for 24 hours. If measures are undertaken to kill mites, however, these must be followed by a thorough vacuuming to remove the dead mites and their excreta, both of which are highly allergenic.

Animal Danders

Proteins contained in the epithelial scales of a variety of animals, including humans, have been implicated as a cause of allergic symptoms. Indeed, these antigens can be some of the most potent that effect humans. In numerous sources the percentage of atopic patients who have reactivity to animal danders may be as high as 30%, and where exposure is high, such as workers who handle laboratory animals, the proportion of sensitive individuals may be higher. In these individuals, however, the allergic disease is *not* in the classic sense perennial, and a careful occupational history is usually sufficient to make the diagnosis. On the other hand, where animals are present in the home, these animals can be a cause of continuous allergen exposure and thereby causative of perennial symptoms. Thus accurate historic information about pets, both usual and unusual, is invaluable in pointing to the correct diagnosis. It is important to ask whether animals were present in the house since dander may persist for some period of time despite thorough cleaning. This may be important in cat sensitivity since these animals, because of their small size, agility, and curiosity, seem to seek out every nook and cranny of the house, including the heating ducts in some cases. The historic evaluation is all the more important because the presence of a positive skin test does not of itself confer the diagnosis of dander allergy.

There is some confusion as to the exact nature of the allergens in animal dander. Evidence from work with cats suggests that the major allergen, now called "CAT I," is not a serum protein. Other studies have indicated that in some species the major antigen is serum albumin. Whatever the exact antigen or better antigens are it is now clear that they are not limited to the skin. These antigens are found not only in internal organs, but more importantly in excretions such as saliva or urine, and aerosolization of dried secretions is a potential cause of allergic sensitivity. Indeed, the CAT I protein is in highest concentration in saliva and is most probably deposited on the fur by the incessant preening common to all cats.

There have been a number of studies examining the breed specificity of allergies to dog dander. Using radioallergosorbent test (RAST) testing, Fagerberg & Wide (1970) demonstrated that there was considerable differences in the reactivity of various dog-sensitive sera with dander from a variety of breeds. On the other hand, a more recent study demonstrated that the majority of patients reacted to both single and mixed breed extracts. They suggested that previous differences might be due to the type of antigen extracted (pelt vs skin) or the extraction procedure (Mercney et al., 1979). These studies were largely confirmed by Moore & Hyde (1980). This later study used extracts from long- and short-haired as well as shedding and nonshedding breeds, putting to rest dogmatic statements concerning the lack of allergenicity of the nonshedding breeds (poodles, kerry blue, and airedale terriers).

The best treatment for dander sensitivity is avoidance of the offending animal and its removal from the home. However, there are instances when the animal exposure is work related or where allergic individuals are either unwilling or unable to remove pets from the home. Several studies have shown the efficacy of immunotherapy to laboratory animals, and at least one report of effective immunotherapy for cat sensitivity has appeared. Thus in highly selected cases immunotherapy to animal danders may be attempted (Taylor et al., 1978).

The problem of human dander antigen and its role in allergic symptoms is difficult to assess. There are several reports indicating that many atopic individuals have skin reactivity to extracts of human dander. However, the relationship between these reactions and human disease states is not clear.

The importance of sensitivity to other animal danders has decreased with the use of nonanimal products. Nonetheless, an historic examination of this possibility is always warranted, and cow or horse products in carpet matting or horse hair stuffing in antique furniture should not be overlooked. Sensitivity to wool is more likely to be an irritant effect of the wool rather than a true allergic reaction.

Feathers

Feathers of any type, but more commonly chicken, goose, or duck, have been implicated in perennial allergic symptoms. However, the exact nature of the antigen in feathers is not clear. It has been known for some time that extracts of fresh feathers do not induce skin reactivity whereas extracts of aged feathers do (Solomon & Mathews, 1978). As a result it was proposed that the antigen is either feather specific, a degradation product (Berrens, 1968) or resulted from mite infestation (Voorhorst et al., 1969). The weight of the evidence seems to be in favor of the mite as the source of the antigen. Virtually 100% of patients with feather skin reactivity are also sensitive to mite; in contrast, isolated feather sensitivity is quite rare.

The treatment of feather sensitivity like other perennial allergen is avoidance. Thus feather quilts and comforters should be avoided. As recently demonstrated by Shatz et al., (1982), the use of so-called feather- or down-proof coverings are useless and provide no protection to the sensitive individual.

It is also important to note that the antigen(s) in feathers, irrespective of their origin, does *not* cross-react with egg proteins. Thus the feather-sensitive individual is *not* at risk if given a viral vaccine that was prepared from viruses grown in eggs. This is not true for patients sensitive to egg (see Chapter 26).

Vegetable Proteins

A variety of vegetable products have been implicated in perennial allergic symptoms. These include kapok and cotton batting as well as other fibrous products that are used mainly in furniture. As with feathers, extracts of "aged" material seems to be significantly more allergenic than fresh material, suggesting that mite allergens may contribute to these sensitivities as well. Nonetheless, these products are becoming less and less important as their use is being supplemented by synthetic products.

Vegetable grains may also be a problem, but this is less important as a cause of perennial symptoms.

Insect Products

A number of insects have been implicated in perennial allergic disease. Of these the cockroach is by far the most important. Several studies have indicated that cockroach antigen is a major cause of bronchial asthma among inner-city dwellers. A recent study by Hulett & Dockhorn (1979) demonstrated that 50% or more of house dust sensitivity in the Kansas City, Missouri population was the result of cockroach infestation. Thus skin testing with cockroach antigen is warranted in patients with perennial allergic disease.

The antigenic material in cockroach sensitivity has not been identified. By analogy to mite and other insects, however, it is reasonable to assure that crumbled insect parts, decaying insects, and excreta all contribute to the problem. Since these insects tend to live in relatively inaccessible areas, a program of extermination followed by extensive vacuuming and cleaning is warranted. Nonetheless, it may take some time to remove all the antigenic material, and since new insects are continually introduced into the home, continued vigilance is necessary (see Chapter 12).

MOLDS

Like house dust, molds as a group represent a perennial antigen. Patients sensitive to molds generally have symptoms continually with exacerbations and remissions based on such diverse factors as time of the year (simulating seasonal pollenosis) or relative humidity, and whereas the individual who is mold-sensitive may be reacting to only a single species, the vast majority are allergic to multiple molds, and thus some of the peaks and valleys of symptoms are blunted. In addition, many mold sufferers are also sensitive to house dust (mite) and/or other perennial antigens that mask alterations in symptomatology that might give clues to mold sensitivity. Patients with perennial symptoms should thus be questioned closely for historical clues (Chapter 4). On the other hand, seasonal symptoms do not rule out mold sensitivity.

It has been known since the 1930s that molds are the cause of significant allergic problems. The reader is referred to the work of Van der Werff (1958) for a thorough review of the relationship of molds to asthma and other allergic diseases. Although it has been clear for over 50 years that molds, or more importantly mold spores, were a major source of allergic disease, studies of the actual proteins that are responsible for the allergic response have been sparse. This is the result of several factors: (a) the large number of molds that have been shown to be allergenic and (b) the bewildering complexity of mold proteins. Whereas three to five or less are important in allergic pollenosis, at least 10 times that number have been found in a single species of mold (e.g., 56 in *Alternaria*). For this reason, sophisticated techniques have been developed to explore the relevant proteins, and appropriate studies are only now being performed. In addition, molds may cause disease by mechanisms that are not IgE-related or where factors other than type I hypersensitivity is important, thus complicating the analysis. These considerations are important for the study of allergic diseases and the practical treatment of allergic individuals. Nonetheless, standard extracts of whole mold spores have been shown to be effective reagents for the identification of sensitive individuals.

Classification

All molds belong to the phylum Thallophyte (lacking roots, stems, and leaves), and since they lack chlorophyll most allergenic molds are saprophytes. In general, the allergenic mold can be classifed in two groups: the smaller are several classes that are "true fungi"; that is, they can reproduce sexually and in many cases asexually. The larger group are the deuteromycetes or fungi imperfecti, which produce spores only asexually. The number of molds species that cause allergies is probably not known, but if the rarer varieties are taken into account, it probably exceeds 100. A simplified list containing 28 genera and/or species is given in Table 25-2. There are a variety of other classifications or tables, both longer or shorter, and the reader is referred to standard allergy texts for these. Most of the fungi in this list cause allergy rarely and under special conditions. For example, members of the class Basidiomycetes include dry rot, which is rarely an allergic problem but a major cause of wood destruction. Smuts and rusts are also members of the class Basidiomycetes, and these two latter groups are responsible for significant destruction of grain, particularly wheat but also corn, and have been shown to cause allergic reactions in individuals who are in contact with grain, such as farmers and grainery workers. It would be of value to evaluate these groups if the history incriminates them but is no value in other individuals.

As noted above, the majority of allergenic molds belong to the fungi imperfecti, and the majority of the important fungi fall in the order Moniliales in two families, Monilialceae and Dematiaceae. These two families contain many allergic species; several other families have one or two allergenic varieties (Table 25-2).

Although one can discuss these fungi anatomically, for the allergist it is better to classify mold according to where they are most prevalent. Thus one can speak of outdoor and indoor molds or in some texts "field fungi" and "storage fungi." However, these classifications are *not* absolutes and give only a general idea. Field fungi are found indoors, and sensitive patients may encounter indoor molds outdoors.

Outdoor Molds

The two most common outdoor molds are *Alternaria* and *Cladosporium* genera (often referred to incorrectly in the allergy literature as *Hormodendrum*). *Helminthosporium, Spondylocladium,* and *Fusarium* are other common field fungi. As a group, these molds grow in or on plants, and decaying plant products in the soil, they tend to be most prevalent, beginning in the spring, when the snow uncovers decaying vegetation and provides the appropriate moisture content. Sporulation continues into the fall and decreases but *does not stop* with the first frost. Rain or high humidity will decrease the spore count temporarily, but a rapid rise in the

Table 25-1 *Factors Implicated in Perennial Allergic Disease*

True allergens
House dust (mites)
Molds
Human dander
Animal dander
Upholstery materials
Gums
Insects (cockroach)
Vegetable material
Nonspecific irritants
Tobacco smoke*
Air pollutants
Chemical fumes
Perfumes
Changes in temperature
Upper respiratory infections

*In most cases but may be a true allergen.

count follows since these molds require high moisture content, which increases sporulation markedly.

A number of studies have shown that the spore counts for *Alternaria* and *Cladosporium* are significantly higher outdoors than indoors, and measures that are utilized to decrease pollen counts indoors are also effective in patients sensitive to the field fungi. These include (a) keeping windows closed, (b) air conditioning, (c) frequent cleaning of air-conditioning filters, and (d) electrostatic air cleaners. Compost piles or piles of decaying grasses or leaves should be removed or kept to an absolute minimum. It should also be remembered that some patients who complain of symptoms when cutting grass may be mold-sensitive, not grass-sensitive.

Indoor Molds

The indoor or storage molds include *Aspergillus, Penicillium,* and *Rhizopus,* of which the two former are the most important. *Penicillium* is the green growth seen on a variety of articles in wet basements. It is commonly called "mildew." *Rhizopus* is the circular fluffy black growth seen on old bread. *Aspergillus* is a unique mold allergen since it will grow on substrates with low moisture content but grows better if the relative humidity is high. These organisms are commonly found in dusty, wet basements and crawl spaces. They are particularly fond of stored vegetable products and may be found in the home in vegetable bins. They may also be contained in bedding and thus may be confused with house dust. Control measures are similar to those for house dust. Areas that might harbor molds should be removed; the relative humidity should be kept to a minimum; and if the house has a crawl space, it may have to be lined with a moisture barrier. Cleaning should be frequent and done with fungicidal agents. Vegetables should be stored cold or in airtight bins.

Table 25-2 *Mold Species*

Class	Order/Family	Genus	Species	Common Name
Phycomycetes	Zygomycetes	*Mucor*	*racemosis*	Black bread mole
		Rhizopus	*nigricans*	
Ascomycetes		*Saccharomyces*	*cervevisiae*	Baker's yeast
		Chaetomium	*indicum*	
Basidiomycetes		*Merulius*	*lacrymans*	Dry rot
		Ustilaginales	"Many"	"Smut"
		Uredinales	"Many"	"Rust"
Deuteromycetes (fungi imperecti)	Sphaeropsidales	*Phoma*	*herbarium*	Slime mold
	Moniliaceae	*Aspergillus*	"Many"	
		Penicillium	"Many"	
		Botrytis	*cinerea*	
		Monilia		
		Mycogone		
		Paecilomyces	*varioti*	
		Trichoderma	*viride*	Slime mold
		Gliocladium	*fimibriatum*	
	Dematiaceae	*Alternaria*	"Many"	
		Cladosporium (hormodendrum)	"Many"	
		Helminthosporium	*interseminatum*	
		Spondylocladium		
		Stemphylium	*botrysoum*	
		Nigrospora	*sphaerra*	
		Pullularia	*pullulane*	Slime mole
	Tuberculariaceae	*Fusarium*	*vasintectum*	Slime mold
		Epicoccum		
	Cryptococcaeae	*Rhodotorula*	*glutinis*	
		Cryptococcus		

Other Molds

The slime molds *Fusarium, Phoma, Pullularia,* and *Trichoderma* deserve some mention. They are unique in that their spores are spread by raindrops, and these may be the cause of some, but certainly not a major portion, of the increase in symptoms seen in mold-sensitive patients during the rain. The yeasts *Cryptococcus* and *Rhodotorula* grow on leaves, berries, or other fruit and are frequently cultured indoors. They are not generally considered to be important as allergens, but at least one author considers *Rhodotorula* sensitivity to be much higher than generally thought (Gutman, 1972).

Diagnosis and Treatment

Mold Surveys

It is possible to culture numerous molds from the home environment. Placing multiple plates containing Sabouraud's agar media in the home will allow the identification of species prevalent in that environment. Unfortunately, molds are so ubiquitous that unless the cultures are closely correlated with history, other diagnostic tests are of little value. We do *not* do routine home mold surveys.

Skin Testing

Skin testing has been shown to be extremely effective in the diagnosis of mold sensitivity. Because of the large number of allergenic molds it is not practical or necessary to skin test all of them. A limited number of genera make up the bulk of the clinically important fungi, depending on the area, and these should be utilized. At Washington University we use eight antigens tested individually. These include both outdoor molds *(Cladosporium, Alternaria, Spondilocladium, Helminthosporium, Fusarium)* and indoor molds *(Aspergillis, Penicillium, Phoma)*. Where indicated, other molds are also individually tested.

Treatment

Immunotherapy is discussed in Chapter 13. Suffice it to say that immunotherapy to molds has been shown, in limited studies, to be effective and should be pursued where history and skin testing indicate.

REFERENCES

Baker, E. W., Evans, T. M., Gould, D. J. *A manual of parasitic mites of medical or economic importance*. New York: National Pest Control Association, Inc., 1956.

Berrens, L. In P. Kallos and B. H. Waksman (Eds.), *Progress in allergy*. Vol. 14, S. Karger, 1970, pp. 259.

Berrens, L. On the composition of feather extracts used in allergy practice. *Int. Arch. Allergy Appl. Immunol.*, 1968, *34*, 81.

Dekker, H. Asthma and milben. *Munch. Med., Wochenschr*, 1928, *75*, 515. (translated in *J. All. Clin. Immunol.*, 1971, *48*, 251.

Fagerberg, E. and Wide, L. Diagnosis of hypersensitivity to dog epithelium in patients with asthma bronchiole. *Int. Arch. Allergy Appl. Immunol.*, 1970, *39*, 301.

Gutman, A. A. Allergens and other factors important to atopic disease. In Patterson, R. (Ed.) *Allergic Diseases-Diagnosis and Management,* Philadelphia: J. B. Lippincott, 1972.

Kawai, T., Marsh, D. G., Lichtenstein, L., Norman, P. S. The allergens responsible for house dust allergy. I. Comparison of *Dermatophygoides Pteronyssinus* and house dust extracts by assay of histamine release from allergic human leukocytes. *J. Allergy Clin. Immunol.*, 1972, *50*, 117.

Mercney, D. K., Waklace, D., Miller, J., Goel, Z. A., & Grieco, M. H. *Int. Arch. Allergy Appl. Immunol.*, 1979, *58*, 453.

Moore, B. S., & Hyde, J. H. *J. Allergy Clin. Immunol.*, 1980, *66*, 198.

Hulett, A. C., & Dockhorn, R. J. *Ann. Allergy*, 1979, *42*, 160.

van Bronswujk, J. E. M. H., & Sinha, R. N. *J. Allergy*, 1971, *47*, 31.

Salvaggio, J., and Aukrust, L. Mold induced asthma. *J. All. Clin. Immunol.*, 1981, *68*, 327.

Shatz, G., Sullivan, T. J., Kulczycki, A. Jr., Zull, D., Yecies, L. D., & Wedner, H. J. *JAMA*, 1982, *48*, 50.

Solomon, W. R., Mathews, K. P. Aerobiology and inhalant allergens. In Middleton, E., Reed, C. E., and Ellis, E. F. (Eds) *Allergy Principles and Practice*, St. Louis: The C. V. Mosby Co., 1978.

Taylor, W. W., Ohman, J. L., Jr., Lowell, F. C. Immunotherapy in cat-induced asthma. Double-blind trial with evaluation of bronchial responses to cat allergens and histamine. *J. Allergy Clin. Immunol.*, 1978, *61*, 283.

Tovey, G. R., Chapman, M. D., Platts-Mills, T. A. E. Mite feces are a major source of house dust allergens. *Nature*, 1981, *289*, 592.

Van der werff, P. J. *Mold fungi and bronchial asthma*, Springfield, Ill: Charles C. Thomas, 1958.

Voorhorst, R., Spiebraman, F. T. H., Varekamp, H. *House-dust atopy and the house dust mite*. Luden: Scientific Publishing, 1966.

QUESTIONS

1. A 14-year-old perennial asthmatic lives in the inner city. His asthma has been very refractory to treatment. You should:
   a. Skin test to house dust and mold as these are most likely the cause of this problem.
   b. Skin test to mite antigen since this is the major antigen in house dust.
   c. Skin test to perennial aeroallergens, including cockroach, since this may be a major offender in the inner city.
   d. Skin test to mold as these are the most important perennial antigens.
   e. Do not skin test because immunotherapy of perennial asthmatics does not work.
2. Which of the following is true of feathers:
   a. Feathers per se may not be allergenic, and the actual antigen in feathers may be mites.
   b. Patients sensitive to feathers should not be immunized with vaccines grown in eggs.
   c. Feather garments may be utilized if they are washed frequently.
   d. The only feather-filled articles of concern to sensitive patients are pillows.
   e. Pillows marked "feather- and down-proof" may be used in feather-sensitive individuals.
3. A 37-year-old white female has severe perennial rhinitis. She is skin-test-positive to house dust, mite, dog, cat, and penicillium. She has a wet basement and an old English sheep dog, and sleeps on a feather pillow. As part of environment control you would advise:
   a. She should get a new feather pillow and launder it frequently.
   b. She should keep the sheep dog out of doors or replace it with a poodle since nonshedding dogs are not allergenic.

c. She should try and dry out the basement, but this may not be effective since mold grows on substrate with low moisture content.
d. She should replace feather pillow with Dacron and cover it and mattress with allergy-proof casings.
e. She should try and clean up her home, but she shouldn't be disappointed if this doesn't help since patients with this much sensitivity are basically doomed.

4. A 44-year-old white male has rhinitis from early spring to late fall. There is no lull in midsummer, and his symptoms abate but do not disappear after the first frost. He is:

   a. Most probably sensitive to trees, grass, and weeds. If he were mold-sensitive, he would have perennial symptoms.
   b. Most likely sensitive to *Penicillium* or *Aspergillus*.
   c. Most likely sensitive to *Alternaria, Cladosporium,* or both, but not to trees or grasses.
   d. He is likely to be sensitive to *Alternaria, Cladosporium,* or both, but may also be sensitive to a seasonal allergen.
   e. He is obviously sensitive to *Rhodotorula*.

5. A 39-year-old farmer complains of perennial symptoms that worsen when he is working. His major crop is wheat. Skin testing to *Alternaria, Cladosporium, Fusarium, Spondylocladium,* and *Helminthosporium* is negative as is house dust. You would:

   a. Advise the patient that he has nonallergic rhinitis and must "learn to live with it."
   b. Tell the patient he is probably sensitive to house dust but the skin test didn't pick it up.
   c. Send off a RAST test for common molds since this is a more sensitive test.
   d. Advise the patient to move to the city to get away from farm-related antigens.
   e. Skin test the patient to smuts and rusts (class Basidiomycetes) since these may cause symptoms in this special situation.

Answers can be found in Appendix B at the end of the book.

Anthony Kulczycki, Jr.

26

Food Allergy and Adverse Reactions to Foods

A wide variety of adverse reactions may occur in certain individuals as a result of the ingestion of foods. One should only apply the term "food allergy" to the adverse reactions that are initiated by IgE antibody. In a given case food allergy might be an obvious diagnosis, or it might be a difficult diagnostic problem because foods may provoke a wide variety of reactions, from very local or mild reactions to serious systemic ones. Foods may trigger one or more of a wide variety of allergic symptoms: anaphylaxis, urticaria, angioedema, abdominal pain, nausea, vomiting, diarrhea, wheezing, and rhinitis. The foods commonly implicated in food allergy are milk, egg, peanuts and other nuts, fish and shellfish, and soy protein. Recent studies also suggest that immunologic reactions to foods may be associated with some cases of atopic eczema (Atherton, 1981) and migraine (Munro et al., 1980). Controversy and confusion often surrounds the topic of food allergy, in part because various non-allergic reactions have been inappropriately classified as "food allergy."

MORBIDITY AND MORTALITY

The mortality associated with food allergy is quite rare. Most fatalities have resulted from systemic anaphylaxis after ingestion of an allergenic food, but a few cases have been reported of fatal anaphylactic reactions during skin testing procedures and of fatal reactions in egg-allergic patients who received vaccines prepared from viruses grown in egg.

Food allergy is thought to be much more common in children than adults. For example, various reports estimate the incidence of cow milk "allergy" in children to be from 0.1–7%, although actually much of the acute gastroenteropathy caused by milk is not IgE-mediated. Patients with food allergy are often inconvenienced by dietary restrictions, but after a diagnosis is made most individuals do not experience

ALLERGY: THEORY AND PRACTICE
ISBN 0-8089-1619-X

severe morbidity. Patients allergic to a large number of common foods may require skillful management to avoid inadequate nutrition.

PATHOPHYSIOLOGY

Antigenic substances from food can penetrate the intestinal mucosa despite the barrier of mucus and local (IgA) antibody. Food antigens then react with local lymphoid cells to stimulate production of IgE antibodies, which become bound to mast cells and basophils. Food antigens may also stimulate production of antibodies other than IgE (such as IgG precipitating antibodies to cow's milk) or may stimulate cell-mediated immunity (as in gluten enteropathy or contact dermatitis).

CLINICAL MANIFESTATIONS

The most common symptoms associated with food allergy are gastrointestinal (GI), cutaneous, and respiratory. Food antigens may produce a greater variety of allergic symptoms than other types of allergen because their absorption allows exposure of many different tissues.

The most convincing allergic reactions are dramatic and occur shortly after eating a particular food. Most manifestations of food allergy appear within 2 hours of food ingestion. Eczema, which probably is not predominantly IgE-mediated, is reported to have a delayed onset (Atherton, 1981). Various other symptoms (e.g. the "tension-fatigue syndrome," hyperkinesis) are sometimes ascribed to food allergy, but they have not been confirmed scientifically by double-blind challenges.

The clinical manifestations of food allergy are not always as reproducible as manifestations of other allergic diseases (e.g., challenge with suspected food allergen compared to bronchial inhalation challenge). One potential explanation is that some food antigens might at times be digested completely and rendered non-allergic. At other times, the presence of large quantities of other foods might protect a given food antigen from digestion allowing it to remain antigenic in the small bowel.

Immunologic Reactions to Milk

Although milk provokes numerous diverse types of immunological reactions in children, only a small fraction of these can be attributed solely to IgE-mediated events (Bahna & Heiner, 1980). Thus only a minority of immunologic reactions should be termed "allergic." Symptoms such as anaphylaxis and urticaria occurring after milk ingestion are almost always IgE-mediated reactions to milk protein. (One exception is the allergic reaction to penicillin, which occasionally contaminates milk because mastitis in dairy cows is treated with penicillin injected into the udder.)

Immunologic reactions to milk most frequently involve the GI tract. Diarrhea occurred in 88% of children with adverse reactions to milk, vomiting in 44%, and abdominal pain in 39%. Of these reactions, vomiting is the most likely to involve solely IgE-mediated reactions especially when it occurs shortly after milk ingestion. Vomiting usually occurs within 1 hour of milk ingestion; vomitus may contain excessive amounts of mucus, and the differential diagnosis may include pyloric stenosis. In a review of children with adverse reactions to milk, 12% experienced anaphylaxis usually manifested by swelling of the lips and tongue within minutes of milk ingestion, and 13% had urticaria (Lebenthal, 1975). It is believed that delayed hypersensitivity and complement-mediated reactions may be involved in many of the adverse reactions to milk ingestion, especially when the symptoms occur long after milk ingestion. The diarrhea, characterized by frequent loose stools, often with excessive mucus, is not always strictly an "allergic" phenomenon, especially when blood-streaked stools are present. Milk has been proposed to play a major pathogenetic role in the abdominal "colic" of infancy, characterized by prolonged crying, flexion of thighs, and amelioration at about age 3 months. In older children milk-induced abdominal pain appears to be milder than in infancy and presents as epigastric or periumbilical stomach aches. Milk also appears to play a role in some cases of eosinophilic gastroenteritis.

Immunologic reactions to milk may also involve the respiratory tract, although only a few of the reactions appear to be IgE-mediated. Rhinitis, postnasal drip, and excess mucus production may result in breathing difficulty during sleep, chronic cough, or chronic throat-clearing in older children. Recurrent bronchitis, recurrent pneumonia, asthma, and pulmonary hemosiderosis have also been associated with milk-sensitivity.

Dermatologic manifestations of milk-sensitivity include atopic dermatitis, urticaria, and angioedema. In one study cow's milk was found to be the cause of atopic dermatitis in 27 of 41 children under 2 years of age.

The major milk proteins involved in immunologic reactions are β-lactoglobulin, casein, α-lactalbumin, albumin, and IgG. The latter two macromolecules are heat sensitive; thus some individuals will tolerate boiled milk. Milk-allergic children often appear to lose their sensitivity over a period of years (Bock, 1982). Frank milk allergy is rare in adults, and most milk intolerance in adults results from lactose intolerance.

Immunologic Reactions to Egg

Egg proteins are well established as a cause of allergic symptoms in children, and in some cases the allergy can be outgrown (Bock, 1982). There is controversy as to whether egg proteins might be a major factor in the pathogenesis of many cases of childhood eczema. It is claimed that two-thirds of eczematous children under age 8 benefit from avoidance of egg and milk (Atherton, 1981). Almost none of the patients had previously suspected the etiologic role of foods. There was *no* association between the clinical response to avoidance and the results of skin tests and RAST tests, however, raising the question of whether an IgE-mediated reaction was involved. On the other hand, in a group of 22 patients, mostly *adults*, who *reported* definite egg sensitivity, 18 did have positive skin tests to egg proteins (Davies & Pepys, 1976). Their symptoms included urticaria, swelling of lips and mouth, wheezing, sneezing, vomiting, and diarrhea. Seven of 22 patients had positive skin tests to influenza vaccine, and two of these seven had previously received influenza vaccine and encountered adverse reactions. It is recommended that egg-sensitive individuals *not* be given vaccines grown in embryos. If there are strong clinical indications for administering influenza vaccine, intradermal testing with the vaccine should be carried out first.

Fish Allergy

The most common symptom of fish allergy is urticaria. In one study 85% of fish-allergic patients had urticaria (Aas, 1966). The major antigen of cod (allergen M) is derived from muscle, has a molecular weight of 15,000, and is heat-stable and relatively resistant to acidic denaturation and proteolysis. Patients may also present with rhinitis, conjunctivitis, and/or asthma because the major antigen of fish muscle is not destroyed by cooking and is aerosolized during the cooking process. Asthma has been reported in 56% of fish-sensitive individuals and nasal symptoms in 28%. Other manifestations of fish allergy are believed to include vomiting, diarrhea, abdominal pain, and eczema. It has been noted that about two-thirds of fish-allergic patients are allergic to almost all species of fish; the other one third are allergic only to closely related species.

Allergy to Crustaceans and Mollusks

Acute urticaria is the most common manifestation of seafood allergy, particularly common after eating shrimp. Anaphylaxis and angioedema may also occur. One should document that an IgE-mediated reaction is involved by RAST testing because of the danger involved in skin testing to seafood antigens. Asthma as an isolated symptom of seafood allergy is unusual. If asthma is encountered alone, sensitivity to metabisulfites—used to prevent oxidation—or to spices such as pepper (which may contain cockroach antigen) should be considered. Patients who are allergic to a given crustacean (shrimp) often may have similar reactions to other crustaceans (crab, lobster) but will usually tolerate mollusks. Patients with allergies to bivalve mollusks (clam, oyster) may tolerate other mollusks (abalone, octopus, squid, etc.) and crustaceans.

Allergy to Nuts and Peanuts

In one patient series 13 individuals with peanut and/or nut hypersensitivity as well as appropriately positive RAST tests were studied (Gillespie et al., 1976). All but one had urticaria or angioedema. Six (46%) had throat tightness, and four (31%) had asthma. Five had positive histories and RAST tests, indicating allergy to peanut, which is a legume and might theoretically cross-react with peas and beans. Of "true nuts," Brazil nut was the most commonly allergenic, with RAST tests positive in nine individuals. Black walnut, English walnut, almond, cashew, pecan, filbert, and pistachio have also been documented to be allergenic. Peanuts, as legumes, do not cross-react with true nuts (except possibly with pecans). Antigens of peanuts and nuts are heat-stable (they remain after roasting) and can produce localized gum itching (because antigen is accessible to the gingival space).

Adverse Reactions to Soybean and Soy Protein

Milk-sensitive infants after transfer to soy formula may develop diarrhea. In most cases this is due to irritant and/or pharmacologic effects of soy protein. In one study of five children with soy sensitivity, three (those under $2\frac{1}{2}$ years) had diarrhea and were skin-test-negative to soy protein whereas two (ages 5 and 11 years) had positive skin tests, abdominal pain without diarrhea, and either wheezing and urticaria or rhinitis. Bahna & Heiner (1980) estimated that one quarter of milk-sensitive children may become allergic to soy protein after long exposure.

Soy protein allergy occasionally occurs in adults. Soybeans and peanuts are botanically related, and cross-allergenicity is suspected. The soybean is an economic source of protein, and soy protein is increasingly present in foods. In patients with apparent sensitivity to soy sauce one must also consider the possibility that the reaction was a nonimmunologic response to glutamate [e.g., monosodium glutamate (MSG)].

Adverse Reactions to Chocolate

Chocolate is frequently suspected as the cause of numerous adverse reactions, in part because it is a discretionary nonessential food. Often food and substances associated with chocolate such as milk, peanuts, almonds, sugar, caffeine, and phenylethylamine are responsible for observed reactions. Nevertheless, allergy to cocoa bean, with positive skin tests and angioedema, does occur. Because of the similarity of the cocoa bean and the cola nut, patients allergic to chocolate may have similar (but often less severe) reactions to cola drinks.

Immunologic Reactions to Grains and Corn

Individuals who experience anaphylaxis when exposed to traces of wheat flour in food are occasionally identified. Most individuals who suspect reactions to wheat usually have other immunologic reactions, such as gluten enteropathy.

Corn intolerance, as well as corn allergy, does occur. But in one study none of the 14 patients suspected to be allergic to wheat or corn had symptoms elicited by the appropriate food, and few had positive skin tests (Bock et al., 1978).

Adverse Reactions to Meat

Many suspected reactions to luncheon meats, frankfurters, and sausages are due to milk, egg, and other foods rather than meat. Some intolerances are due to physiologic mechanisms that are triggered by any fatty foods. Individuals sensitive to bovine serum components present in cow's milk (albumin, IgG) may have symptoms on eating beef (especially rare beef). True allergy to meat alone is rare.

Allergy to Fruit

Seeded fruits are alleged to be more frequently allergic than other fruits (banana). Lip erythema after eating oranges is frequently mislabeled "allergy." Actually, *limonene,* the oil found in citrus peels (and celery) initiates a delayed hypersensitivity reaction, and such individuals would tolerate peeled oranges.

Other Foods

Four cases of anaphylaxis to sesame seeds with positive RAST tests have been reported (Malish et al., 1981). Sesame seed products include oil (used in salad dressing), flour, and halvah candy. IgE-mediated anaphylaxis to millet seeds has been reported. Buckwheat flour has been shown to provoke explosive allergic symptoms. Fresh berries, strawberries, and fruits are frequently mentioned in the etiology of acutc urticaria. Thc difficulty in demonstrating IgE against these antigens probably arises because the allergic proteins of fresh fruits, berries, and strawberries may be easily denatured. In addition, at this medical center we have seen reactions to potato, tomato, and watermelon that we believe are IgE-mediated reactions.

NONIMMUNOLOGIC ADVERSE FOOD REACTIONS

An important problem in evaluating potential allergic reactions to foods is differentiating them from a multitude of nonimmunologic adverse reactions that may be elicited by foods and additives to foods. These are classified into four main groups:

1. Pharmacologic: caffeine, monosodium glutamate, tartrazine, sodium metabisulfite, tyramine, phenylethylamine
2. Toxic: ethanol, acidic juice, fava beans, quinine
3. Irritant-pharmacologic: prunes, onions, soybean protein
4. Intolerance: lactose, gluten, seeds, nuts, milk

Caffeine can induce in certain sensitive individuals anxiety, insomnia, and frequent urination as a result of its pharmacologic effects. Many patients would not require sedatives for sleep if their caffeine intake were decreased. Caffeine withdrawal can product anxiety and muscle tension as well as a variety of headache syndromes. Patients often take caffeine-containing analgesics (APC, Excedrin, Coricidin, etc.) or foods (cola drinks, coffee, tea, chocolate, etc.) for relief. Perhaps the ill-defined tension-fatigue syndrome is related more to caffeine in foods than to allergic mechanisms.

Monosodium glutamate, found in soy sauce, can pharmacologically induce the "Chinese restaurant syndrome" characterized by headache; palpitations; weakness; and numbness in the chest, neck, and face. The syndrome may occur almost immediately after starting an Oriental meal or up to 4 hours later and may last for several hours. A completely different problem with MSG has been recently documented. Severe asthma can be a late sequela of MSG ingestion (Allen & Baker, 1981).

Tartrazine (FDC yellow dye No. 5) is still widely used in foods and drugs. Tartrazine can pharmacologically release histamine and other mediators, resulting in asthma or urticaria. Only 5% of aspirin-sensitive individuals are estimated to have tartrazine sensitivity (Chapter 29). A tartrazine-free diet has been difficult to maintain, but recently adopted package labeling requirements should make this easier.

Sodium metabisulfite is an antioxidant commonly used by restaurants to prevent oxidation and discoloration of salads, seafoods, dips, and other foods. Metabisulfite, like sulfur dioxide in air pollution, can cause asthma in certain susceptible individuals (Stevenson & Simon, 1981). Sodium metabisulfite is extremely important because it is used very commonly in food processing, particularly in wine and restaurant foods, but also in dried fruits, baked goods, beet and corn sweeteners, beer, and some medications. Symptoms include anaphylaxis in extremely sensitive individuals, asthma, hives, flushing, nausea and diarrhea. Even though this commonly used food additive and processing agent has full FDA approval, the FDA has notified state agencies that supervise restaurants that metabisulfites should either be removed or notification of their presence be given to the consumer.

Tyramine, found in cheese and red wine, is contraindicated in patients taking monoamine oxidase (MAO) inhibitors because it may precipitate a hypertensive crisis. But even hypertensive individuals not taking MAO inhibitors may have increased blood pressure as a result of tyramine.

Phenylethylamine, which is quite similar to tyramine, is found in certain grades of chocolate. Phenylethylamine has no immediate adverse reaction but may produce headaches, sometimes quite intense, 6–12 hours after ingestion. Crude chocolate, like Baker's chocolate used in cakes, and semisweet chocolate, as in chocolate chips, contain significant amounts of phenylethylamine; milk chocolate in candy bars has relatively little.

Some adverse reactions to foods are toxic ones. Substances such as ethanol and acidic juices can be toxic if consumed in large amounts by normal individuals or in moderate amounts by certain individuals, such as patients with gastritis. Fava beans may be toxic for individuals with glucose 6-phosphate dehydrogenase (G6PD) deficiency. Quinine, in tonic water, may induce thrombocytopenia in rare individuals.

Some substances can exert a pharmacologic effect, an irritant effect, or both effects. Prunes, raw onions, soy beans, and soy bean "milk" may have a mild laxative effect, may induce loose stools, or in some cases may produce abdominal cramps and profuse diarrhea. Patients may be unaware that cramps and diarrhea shortly after a meal might result from salad containing onions well disguised by prolonged soaking.

In considering possible milk allergy in adults it is important to rule out lactose intolerance which occurs in 75% of adult blacks and 10–20% of adult Caucasians. In possible "milk allergy" in infants one must also consider glucose-galactose malabsorption and galactosemia.

A similar problem with intolerance to an unabsorbed sugar occurs commonly with *raffinose*, which is found in various types of bean. Other types of intolerance are suspected to be due to the physical properties of indigestible residues of foods.

DIAGNOSTIC PROCEDURES

After a careful review of the patient's dietary history and symptoms and family history, the following diagnostic measures should usually be undertaken:

1. Consider all nonallergic etiologies.
2. If severe or anaphylactic reaction, do RAST testing. If mild to moderate reaction, may do skin-testing.
3. If sporadic episodes, have patient keep a diet and symptom diary. If constant or regular episodes occur, have patient initiate an elimination diet.
4. Oral challenge with suspected foods should not be carried out in individuals with a previous history of severe reactions. Oral challenge (double-blind is preferred) may be undertaken in other cases.

Patients who experienced anaphylaxis should *not* receive diagnostic challenges with the suspected food and ordinarily should *not* be skin tested. If necessary, RAST testing would be most appropriate. In most other cases of suspected food allergy, however, skin testing followed by double-blind challenge with suspected foods is the appropriate sequence of diagnostic procedures. In the case of suspected cow's milk intolerance, milk avoidance for up to 1 month with appropriate dietary substitutions is the procedure of choice.

Skin Testing

Skin tests are often quite useful in the diagnosis of food allergy but have certain limitations: (a) the procedure may be hazardous to the patient since anaphylactic reactions can occur; (b) false positives may occur because some food extracts may contain histamine (e.g., spinach), and others may contain skin irritants; and (c) false-negative reactions may be encountered in cases where the food extract loses its antigenicity, and this is particularly a problem with fresh fruits and berries. Nevertheless, a battery of food antigens is often very helpful in avoiding or curtailing long and expensive diagnostic workups, provided common and fairly stable antigens are screened.

RAST Testing

The RAST test is, in selected cases, useful in the diagnosis of food allergy. It is an excellent way to document sensitivity to fish, seafood, and nut antigens because it eliminates the need for skin testing, which may be potentially dangerous. The RAST tests also avoid the problems posed by irritants and anti-histamines in skin testing. However, RAST testing appears to be less sensitive than skin testing (Chua et al., 1976). Furthermore, RAST testing is quite expensive (currently about $10–$15 per antigen tested), and one usually waits weeks for results. There is no justification for indiscriminate ordering of every available RAST test in patients with suspected food allergy.

Diet Diary

When patients have occasional symptoms suggestive of food allergy, a diet diary is the appropriate diagnostic tool, especially if episodes are infrequent and not severe. The diary records the time and severity of symptoms and lists all foods consumed in the previous 24 hours and the times of ingestion.

Elimination Diet and Food Challenge

In infants where cow's milk intolerance is suspected, the infant should receive no milk for 4 weeks. Then the infant should be challenged with milk using appropriate precautions (Bahna & Heiner, 1980).

There are numerous approaches to placing adult patients on elimination diets. My preference is to start hospitalized patients with severe and chronic problems, such as chronic urticaria, on the strictest possible diet of lamb, rice, and water (with dry "Puffed Rice" cereal for breakfast). Obviously, strict elimination diets are more easily set up and monitored in the hospital. An alternative elimination diet contains chicken, lettuce, carrots, olive oil, vinegar, salt, cane sugar, asparagus, sweet potato, oleomargarine, apples, and pears in addition to lamb and rice (May & Block, 1978). This alternative diet is often more accepted by patients, particularly outpatients.

Elimination diets should not last beyond 7 days. If hives, asthma or other reactions persist beyond this period then food allergy is very unlikely to be involved (except possibly for proteins of milk or meat which may persist for longer periods). Accordingly, we advocate a dairy product elimination diet for 3–4 weeks at this juncture. If symptoms resolve on either diet the best procedure is to test in a double-blind fashion whether food sensitivity is present (May & Block, 1978). One fills opaque dye-free capsules with dry foods such as cow's milk, soybean flour, whole wheat flour, whole egg, peanuts, and other nuts. Depending on sensitivity, an amount weighing 10 mg to 2 g is initially tested in a double-blind fashion. More commonly in practice, one common food is openly added each day to the patient's diet (e.g., egg, milk, baked potato, broiled steak, corn, wheat flour) in order to detect which one might be causing the problem. If addition of 8 g of a dried food in the capsule or an open challenge with food does not provoke recurrence of symptoms, the food should be incorporated into the allowed diet.

Other Procedures

If patients appear to be sensitive to specific groups of foods, they should be skin tested for sensitivity to certain related inhalant antigens. For example, patients who seem to have symptoms after eating mold-containing foods such as mushrooms, aged cheese, beer, and wine should be skin tested for the appropriate mold antigens. If patients appear to be allergic to honey, ragweed sensitivity should be considered since honey is easily contaminated with ragweed pollen. Individuals sensitive to spices, especially pepper, might benefit from skin testing to cockroach antigen. (A positive skin test would suggest that uncontaminated pepper might be tolerated.) Individuals with reactions due to milk may actually be sensitive to penicillin (Wicher et al., 1969). Individuals with reactions to chicken or veal may be sensitive to tetracycline.

THERAPY

The only currently acceptable therapy in food allergy is the avoidance of offending food antigens. Food avoidance may be a relatively simple procedure if a single readily identifiable food is involved (e.g., lobster, cashews, fresh berries).

Avoidance is more complicated when antigens occur in unexpected sources, and inspection of package labels is then essential. Patients highly sensitive to milk will recognize that butter, cheese, yogurt, and ice cream are milk products, but they may be less aware that milk products are in cakes, chocolate, custards, luncheon meats, hot dogs, sausage, breads, rolls, and waffles. Patients with egg allergy must avoid cakes, cookies, many candies, doughnuts, French toast, some ice cream, cake icings, some luncheon meats, marshmallows, mayonnaise, meringues, noodles, pancakes, pies, pretzels, salad dressings, and sausages. Individuals with egg allergy should not be given vaccines grown in chicken or duck embryos unless skin tested with the vaccine. Extremely egg-sensitive individuals may react to trace of egg albumin unexpectedly found in certain foods. Egg white can be used to clear wine and instant coffee of sediment and to produce foam in root beer. Patients with fish allergy need to avoid cod liver oil. Extremely allergic individuals may react to vitamins because some of the vitamins are derived from fish. Patients with chocolate allergy may not be able to tolerate cola drinks. Corn products such as starch, oil, and sugar are found in many foods, including syrups of preserved fruit and glazes on hams. Corn protein may be present in adhesives and envelope glue. Wheat flour is also quite difficult to avoid.

Food allergy may induce urticaria, asthma, gastrointestinal (GI) symptoms, and perhaps eczema and migraine, and symptoms might be suppressed by antihistamines, theophylline, steroids, or other drugs. Preliminary studies suggest that cromolyn may suppress food allergy symptoms. However, the use of drugs for treatment of food allergy is generally not recommended; avoidance is the treatment of choice.

FOLLOW-UP AND PROGRESS

In following patients with food allergy on avoidance diets one must ensure that they are receiving adequate nutrition. One must ascertain whether alternate diets are acceptable to the patient. Often infants switched from milk-based formulas (Enfamil, Similac) to soy-based formulas (Isomil, Mull-Soy, Neo-Mull-Soy, Pro-Sobee) may encounter new or recurrent problems (usually not allergic). Such infants must be switched again to casein hydrolysates (Nutramigen, Pregestimil) or meat-based formulas. Older children or adults with milk allergy can easily substitute imitation milk (e.g., Vita Rich) but should receive supplemental calcium and vitamin D (e.g., Os-Cal, 250-mg tablets bid).

It is often very helpful to enlist the support of professional dieticians for patients on avoidance diets. Patients may require help in identifying ingredients in specific foods and in planning adequate balanced diets. Patients may also benefit from books containing recipes free of the food to which they are allergic.

Case Histories

A 27-year old woman experienced profound dizziness, tightness in her throat and chest, cough, dyspnea, rhinorrhea, and skin pruritus 1 hour after eating turbot fish. Her blood pressure was 80/56 and her pulse, 104. She had urticarial lesions and wheezing. Symptoms were relieved by epinephrine, antihistamine, and intravenous (IV) fluid but recurred 4 hours later. A month previously, the patient noted conjunctivitis when cooking turbot fish. Scratch tests documented extreme sensitivity to most orders of fish. Patient has been asymptomatic on fish avoidance and carries epinephrine in case of accidental ingestion.

A 19-year old woman had severe chronic urticaria of 4 years' duration responsive only to steroids. A psychogenic cause was postulated and she was placed in a mental hospital for 3 months. Except for widespread urticarial lesions, physical examination was unremarkable. The patient was unable to maintain an avoidance diet. Subsequently, skin tests demonstrated large IgE-mediated reactions to potato and corn. On a diet free of potato and corn she has no urticaria. On occasion, she has french fries, potato chips, or corn chips with friends and experiences acute urticaria that responds to diphenhydramine hydrochloride (Benadryl).

REFERENCES

Aas, K. *Int. Arch. Allergy*, 1966, *29*, 346–363.

Allen, D. H., & Baker, G. J. *New Engl. J. Med.*, 1981, *305*, 1154–1155.

Atherton, D. J. *Clin. Exp. Dermatol.*, 1981, *6*, 317–325.

Bachman, K. D., & Dees, S. C. *Pediatrics*, 1957, *20*, 400–407.

Bahna, S. L., & Heiner, D. C. *Allergies to milk*. New York: Grune & Stratton, 1980.

Bock, S. A., Lee W.-Y., Remigio, L. K., & May, C. D. *J. Allergy Clin. Immunol.*, 1978, *62*, 327–334.

Bock, S. A. *J. Allergy Clin. Immunol.*, 1982, *69*, 173–177.

Chua, Y. Y., Bremner, K., Liobet, J. L., Kokubu, H. L., & Collins-Williams, C. *J. Allergy Clin. Immunol.*, 1976, *58*, 477–482.

Davies, R. & Pepys, J. *J. Allergy Clin. Immunol.*, 1976, *57*, 373–383.

Gillespie, D. N., Nakajima, S., & Gleich, G. J. *J. Allergy Clin. Immunol.*, 1976, *57*, 302–309.

Lebenthal, E. *Pediatr. Clin. N. Am.*, 1975, *22*, 827–833.

Malish, D., Glovsky, M. M., Hoffman, D. R., Ghekiere, L., & Hawkins, J. M. *J. Allergy Clin. Immunol.*, 1981, *67*, 35–58.

May, C. D., & Block, S. A. *Allergy*, 1978, *33*, 166–188.

Munro, J., Brostoff, J., Carini, C., & Zilkha, K. *Lancet*, 1980, *2*, 1–4.

Stevenson, D. D., & Simon, R. A. *J. Allergy Clin. Immunol.*, 1981, *68*, 26.

Wicher, J., Reisman, R. E., & Arbesman, C. E. *JAMA*, 1969, *208*, 143–145.

QUESTIONS

1. A 43-year-old man has acute urticaria and dizziness after eating dinners of either lobster and rice or shrimp and rice; however, he can eat salads without difficulty.

   a. He is probably allergic to rice.
   b. He is probably not allergic to other seafoods such as clams, oysters, abalone, and fish.
   c. He is probably sensitive to metabisulfites used to prevent discoloration of seafood.
   d. He is probably not allergic to crab.

2. A 9-year-old boy, following an upper respiratory infection (URI) at age 7, began to increasingly clear his throat up to 30 times an hour. The problem has persisted continuously for 2 years. He had colic as an infant. Evaluation by a pediatric allergist and an ear, nose, and throat (ENT) specialist demonstrates only enlarged tonsils. You would:

   a. Agree with the teacher and parents that this is a psychosomatic problem that is probably an attention-getting device in school.
   b. Have the boy's tonsils and adenoids removed.
   c. Eliminate milk and milk products from his diet.
   d. Try astringents and gargles or antihistamines to decrease mucus production.

3. A 45-year-old woman presents with allergic rhinitis secondary to dust and mold and frequently severe headaches from the vertex to the back of her neck in the morning. History reveals frequent ingestion of chocolate cake, chocolate chips, and chocolate chip ice cream. She is normotensive, and physical examination and sinus films are unremarkable. Allergic rhinitis is well controlled.

a. She has tension headaches.
b. She is allergic to chocolate.
c. Mold-containing foods may initiate headaches.
d. She should be placed on diet free of phenylethylamine.

4. A 52-year-old man with chronic obstructive pulmonary disease has avoided eggs because they induced swelling of his lips and throat, wheezing, and pruritus. Radioallergosorbent testing to egg white was negative. Skin tests were negative to egg white but positive to egg yolk and egg allantoic fluid. Recently he has had episodes of wheezing and mild urticaria. You would *not* recommend:

a. Reviewing diet for foods containing egg products, such as luncheon meat, sausage, pretzels, pancakes, and noodles.
b. Reviewing diet for drinks containing traces of egg such as wine, coffee, and root beer.
c. Trial avoidance of chicken and other poultry.
d. Receiving an influenza (flu) shot.

5. A healthy 32-year-old male has almost daily chronic urticaria of 2 years' duration. Antihistamines help somewhat but are soporific. He takes no other medications and has never been outside the continental United States. Physical examination and laboratory studies, including erythrocyte sedimentation rate (ESR), are normal. You would recommend:

a. Elimination diet, paraben avoidance, and skin testing (off antihistamines) to about 12 food antigens.
b. Diet diary and RAST testing to all available food antigens.
c. Trial of periactin and/or cimetidine.
d. Evaluation for occult infection and stools for ova and parasites.

Answers can be found in Appendix B at the end of the book.

J. Allen Thiel

27

Hymenoptera Sensitivity

Since the first recording of the death of an ancient Egyptian king from an insect sting, humans have been plagued by allergic reactions to hymenoptera (Fig. 27-1). Fatalities in the United States are estimated at 40–50 per year, but there is little doubt that many more go unreported. Retrospective studies indicate that 1–2 million people in this country are sensitive to insect stings, and some are at risk for life-threatening anaphylactic reactions. Fortunately, a new and effective preventive treatment for selected patients is now available in the form of venom immunotherapy. In the ensuing discussion, the offending insects, important characteristics of venom, and the clinical problem are addressed.

OFFENDING INSECTS

Although there are over 16,000 species of hymenoptera on the North American continent, the medically important species belong to the Vespidae, Apidae, and Formicidae families of these insects. Recognition of the offending hymenoptera is important in clinical evaluation. Certain distinguishing characteristics are discussed in the following sections.

Vespidae

The subfamily Vespidae includes two major genera: *Vespula* (concealed nesting yellow jackets) and *Dolichovesputa* (aerial nesting yellow jackets and hornets).

Vespula species approximate the size of the honeybee, have smooth bodies with bright yellow and black markings, and build their enclosed nests in the ground or in concealed spaces in human dwellings. They have a taste for sweets and meat and hence are often unwelcome guests at picnics and around garbage cans. They attack without provocation and are particularly aggressive in the early fall.

ALLERGY: THEORY AND PRACTICE
ISBN 0-8089-1619-X

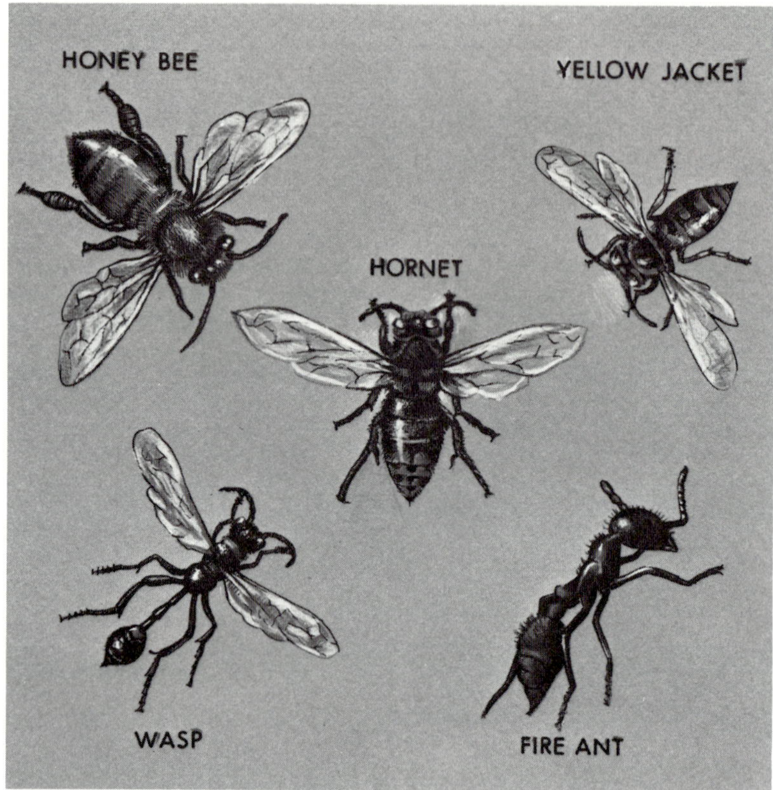

Fig. 27-1. Hymenoptera.

Dolichovespula, the yellow hornet and white-faced or bald-faced hornets are large, black, thick-bodied insects with yellowish-white markings. They hang their football-shaped nests from trees or shrubs or in the eaves of homes and out buildings. They are also quite aggressive and are often disturbed when patients are involved in household repairs.

Polistes, or paper wasps, have narrow, pinched waists and are generally black-brown or red in color. They build small, open-combed nests under eaves and rafters. It is fortunate that they are not very aggressive, since they often hibernate inside homes in the winter.

Apidae

The honeybee, *Apis mellifera,* is squat and hairy, and builds large nests in hollow trees or cavities of walls. The majority of colonies, however, are domesticated and live in artificially produced hives. Most stings, therefore, occur in beekeepers, or when children are barefoot in a field of clover. The honeybee sting is the easiest to identify since its barbed stinger is entrapped in human skin and is avulsed with the venom sac attached when the insect flies away. The sac continues to contract for 2–3 minutes, injecting more venom. Grasping or squeezing the sac would also serve to increase the amount of venom injected; hence it should be flicked away as soon as it is noticed.

Bumblebees, *Bombus* sp. species, are large (15–25 mm), hairy, black insects with yellow markings. They often make their homes in deserted rodent nests and sting only when their nests are disturbed.

Stings by the Halictids or sweat bees are occasionally described. These insects are small (5–15 mm) and are usually dark colored or brownish to metallic green. They nest in the ground and are attracted to perspiration. Venoms are not available for prevention of anaphylaxis caused by these genera.

Formicidae

In the late 1930s and early 1940s the imported fire ant (Figs. 27-2; 27-3), *Solenopsis invicta,* named for its painful sting, was introduced into the area of Mobile, Alabama from its native habitat in South America. Earlier fire ants, of the species S. *richteri,* have been confined largely to a small area in northern Mississippi. The species *invicta* is small to medium in size (3–6 mm) and brown to reddish-brown in color. This species has now heavily infested over 127 million acres in 13 southern states, limited only by heavy winters and desert conditions.

Colonies may reach 250,000 individuals in 3 years, and 1 acre of farm land may contain 100 colonies (Fig. 27-4). Loss in income from destruction of valuable agricultural land in the United States in 1972 was estimated at approximately 600 million dollars. The use of effective insecticides has been severely restricted because of environmental concern.

The medically important *invicta* species is responsible for 95% of the clinical

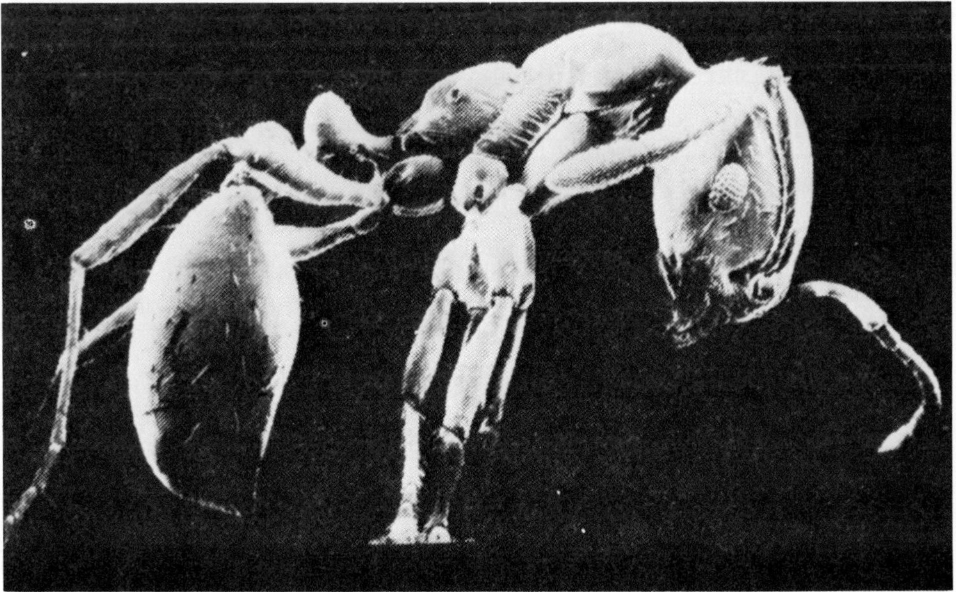

Fig. 27-2. Scanning photomicrograph of imported fire ant worker.

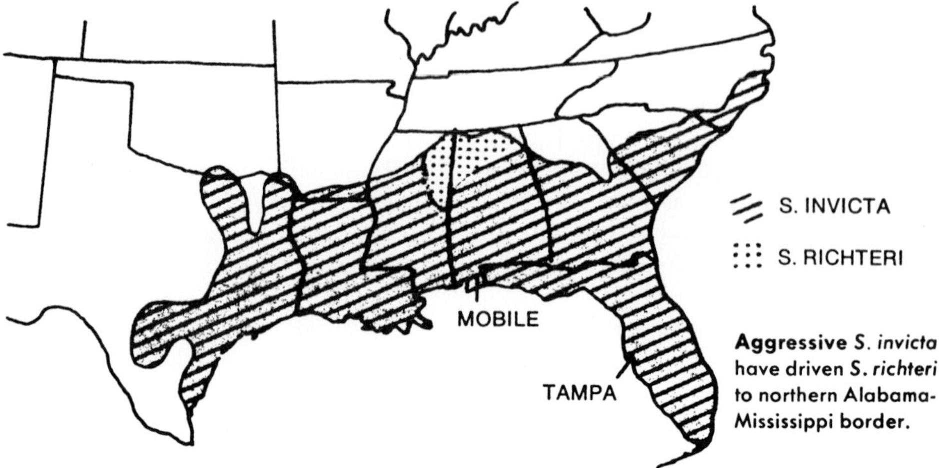

Fig. 27-3. Distribution of fire ant.

problems produced by ant stings. A survey by Florida allergists in 1974 revealed that the incidence of imported fire ant hypersensitivity exceeded the incidence of allergy reactions to the other hymenoptera combined.

The fire ant bites an individual with its jaws, then proceeds to pivot about its head, inflicting multiple stings with its abdominal stinger. The lesion becomes a sterile pustule within 24 hours and then resolves with a tendency to scarring (Fig. 27-5). The pustule is virtually diagnostic of a fire ant sting, although the absence of such a lesion does not completely exclude a sting by this insect.

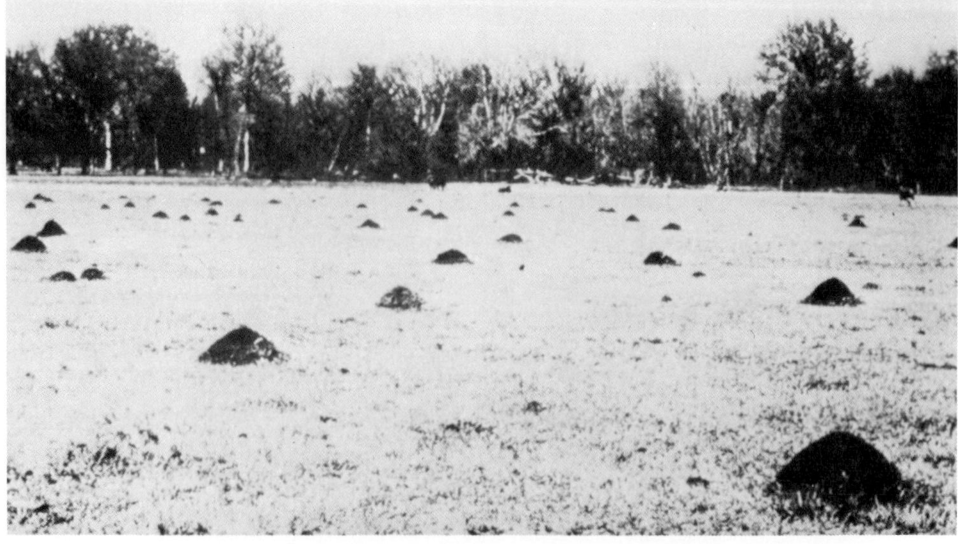

Fig. 27-4. Ant hills built by colonies of fire ants.

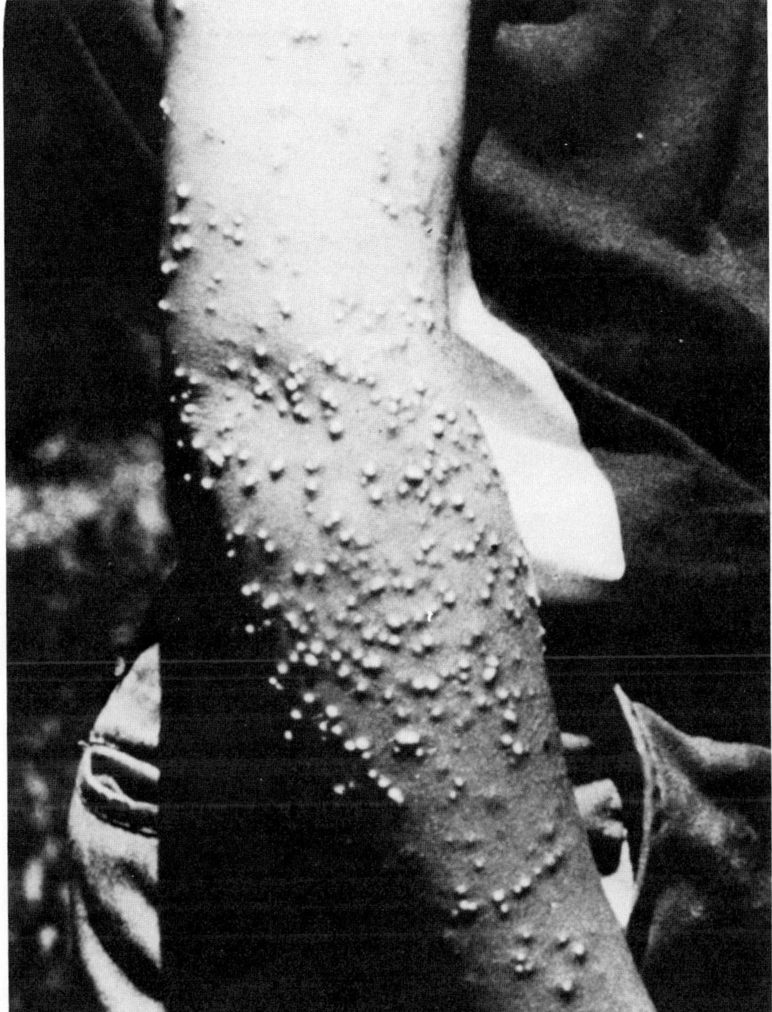

Fig. 27-5. Typical pustules produced by fire ants.

VENOMS

Most studies of venoms have been restricted to those of the honeybee, yellow jacket, yellow hornet, white-faced hornet, and more recently the fire ant. Venom is collected from the honeybee by electrical stimulation, from the vespids by dissection of the sacs, and from the fire ant by capillary tube from the stinger. Each venom is a complex mixture of enzymes, biogenic animes, and peptides, only a portion of which is antigenic (Table 27-1).

Honeybee venom, the most extensively studied, contains at least four major allergenic proteins: phospholipase A, hyaluronidase, acid phosphatase, and mellitin.

Table 27-1 *Identified Venom Contents*

Honeybee	Yellow Jacket	Hornet	Wasp*
Phospholipase A	Phospholipase A	Phospholipase A	Phospholipase A
Hyaluronidase	Phospholipase B	Phospholipase B	Phospholipase B
Acid phosphatase	Hyaluronidase	Hyaluronidase	Serotonin
Melittin	Acid phosphatase	Acid phosphatase	Histamine
Apamin	Kinin	Kinin (hornet)	Hyaluronidase
Mast cell degranulating peptide (MCD)	Histamine	Histamine	Kinin
	Serotonin	Serotonin	
	Dopamine	Acetylcholine	
Minimine?†	Norepinephrine	Dopamine	
Norepinephrine	Epinephrine	Norepinephrine	
Dopamine	Cholinesterase	Epinephrine	
Histamine	Histidine decarboxylase	Protease	
	Protease		

From Levine, M., & Lockey, R. (Eds.), *Monograph in insect allergy*. Hartland: Parker Printing, 1981, p. 29. With permission.

*Small number of identified components probably reflects limited studies.

†Minimine has been described as a minor polypeptide that retards the development of Drosophilia. Its existence has not been confirmed.

Ninety percent of IgE antibody from pooled honeybee-sensitive sera appears to be against the phospholipase A moiety.

Vespid venoms contain three major allergenic proteins: a phospholipase, a hyaluronidase, and a protein of unknown function, called *antigen 5*. The latter seems to be the most important allergen in humans.

Fire ant venom is basically alkaloid but contains a trace amount of at least three proteins that are allergenic. Hopefully, studies in progress will clarify their importance and cross reactivity with other hymenoptera venom.

Patients vary in their response to individual components of venom. Significant cross-reactivity exists among the vespid species, but little between bees and vespids. Further investigation is critical to resolve the problem of unique versus cross-reacting antigens in order to limit the amount and types of venom needed to treat patients.

CLINICAL PICTURE

The vast majority of reactions to insect stings are confined to minor local pain, redness, and swelling due to the venom's pharmacologic and enzymatic properties. The entire reaction rarely lasts more than a few hours.

In some patients, swelling progresses to involve much larger areas such as an entire limb. These large local reactions are usually immunologically mediated, but the incidence of subsequent systematic reaction is debated, and probably quite low. There is evidence to implicate a cellular as well as an IgE response in such cases. Patients who have a history of progressive local reactions should be informed of their potential increased risk. At present such patients are not considered candidates for immunotherapy, even if specific IgE can be demonstrated by skin test or RAST. They should be advised to immediately inject epinephrine from readily available kits or auto injectors if a systemic reaction occurs with a future sting and to contact their physicians.

Generalized reactions are life-threatening and can be toxic or allergic in nature. Toxic reactions are due to the direct destruction of membranes and cellular constituents by injected venom. Allergic reactions are due to the effects of many of the same chemical mediators. Upward of 100 stings are usually necessary for a toxic death in an otherwise healthy adult as compared to one to four stings when the reaction is due to allergy. A generalized allergic reaction or anaphylaxis may involve the skin with erythema, pruritus, urticaria, or angioedema; the respiratory tract, with laryngeal edema and bronchospasm; the cardiovascular system, with hypotension and shock; and the gastrointestinal (GI) system, with nausea, vomiting, and incontinence.

The susceptibility to anaphylaxis is enhanced, probably because of increased exposure, in family members of beekeepers and males over the age of 30. An atopic background does not increase that risk. Patients who have experienced generalized allergic reactions often manifest the same clinical picture with a characteristic aura minutes before. The latter premonitory symptoms are an indication for emergency care.

Less common reactions, often of a delayed nature, include serum sickness, vasculitis, nephrosis, neuropathy, and encephalopathy. These reactions are not felt to be indications for immunotherapy.

The possibility of infection should be remembered in evaluating hymenoptera reactions since 2% of deaths from insect stings are associated with septicemia. Infection is more common following wasp stings as vespids pick up virulent bacteria when foraging among decaying animal and vegetable matter. Appropriate aerobic and anaerobic culture should be obtained when confronted with possible cellulitis and fever.

TREATMENT

Treatment of allergic reactions is directed at the site of involvement. In a report on data collected from the study of 400 cases of hymenoptera sting deaths in the United States, Barnard (1973) showed that 60% died from respiratory obstruction, 24% from vascular complications and anaphylaxis, and 7% from neurologic involvement. Miscellaneous causes of death included 2% from bacterial septicemia. Ninety percent of fatalities in the respiratory and vascular cases occurred within the first few hours after one to four stings. It is significant, however, that 9% of fatal cases in this study had the onset of their symptoms greater than 24 hours after the sting (Barnard, 1973).

The importance of early treatment was underscored. Barnard (1973) compared the time from sting to the beginning of treatment in 100 nonfatal versus 50 fatal cases. Eighty seven percent of the recovered patients received treatment within the first hour compared to only 6% of the fatal cases. Patients should be made aware of these facts and advised to report immediately any untoward symptoms that occur within 2 weeks following a sting.

In the emergency situation, the first step is the injection of epinephrine. Even mild symptoms of apprehension and urticaria may progress to life-threatening anaphylaxis and should be treated. The usual dose of epinephrine 1 : 1000 is 0.01 ml/kg in children and 0.3–0.5 ml in adults. This dose may be repeated several times at 5–15 minute intervals if necessary. When the blood pressure fails to respond to the above treatment, measures to correct hypovolemic shock should be instituted. Cardiac complications are more frequent in the middle- to older-age population and are treated in the usual manner. Antihistamines and glucocorticoids are not effective in the acute reactions but may be helpful for relief of minor symptoms.

If laryngeal edema does not respond to epinephrine, tracheostomy may be necessary. Bronchospasm, in the absence of hypotension, may be treated with theophylline.

Most local reactions do not require treatment, but cold compresses, antihistamines, and aspirin may be helpful. For more extensive edema a short course of steroids is indicated, for example, 10 mg of prednisone every 6 hours until improved and then rapidly decreased over approximately 3–5 days.

A patient who has sustained a systemic reaction to hymenoptera should be carefully instructed in precautions to avoid future stings. It is helpful to review a check list of "do's and don'ts" with the patients. The habits of the insects and methods of minimizing exposure are detailed. A medical alert medal (Medic-Alert) should be obtained to ensure that emergency treatment will be prompt and efficacious should the patient be unconscious when discovered.

Avoidance Instructions for Venom-Sensitive Patients

- Do not go barefoot or wear sandals out-of-doors.
- Wear a hat, long sleeves, and pants when the presence of flying insects can be anticipated. Tie up long hair.
- Wear gloves when gardening or handling piled trash, lumber, stone, and similar material in which insects may hide or nest.
- Do not mow the lawn or trim trees, hedges, or bushes.
- Outdoors, avoid flowers (and flowering shrubs or trees).
- Do not use perfumes, shampoos, or other flower-scented cosmetics.
- Avoid bright-colored clothing.
- Use extreme caution near picnic areas, garbage cans, and other places where food may attract insect (e.g., roadside fruit stands, fruit trees).
- Have an exterminator eliminate bee, wasp, hornet, and yellow jacket nests in the vicinity of your house.
- Do not swat at a persistent insect. Stay calm. Move away slowly.
- Make sure that your emergency kit, containing antihistamines and epinephrine (Adrenalin), is always nearby and ready for use.

Kits containing a preloaded syringe with two doses of 0.3 ml of epinephrine, tourniquet, chewable antihistamines, and instructions are quite useful and should be carried by the sensitive patient at all times. Spring-loaded epinephrine auto injectors are also available if it is unlikely that the patient can, or will, self-inject.

IMMUNOTHERAPY

Initial attempts at immunotherapy for bee sting allergy involved the stepwise injection of extracts made from whole bodies of offending insects (WBE). This material was chosen for treatment by Benson and Semenov in 1930, based on studies involving a beekeeper (Benson, 1930). The latter individual probably became sensitized to bee body protein by the inhalant route, demonstrating respiratory symptoms when caring for his hives. Skin tests thus were positive to whole body extract as well as to venom. When the American Academy of Allergy Committee on Insects reported the combined experience of practicing allergists and endorsed the value of WBE, further impetus was given to its continued use (Insect Allergy Committee, 1965). Subsequently the validity of this report has been questioned, largely because of the lack of identification of the insect responsible for the initial and subsequent stings and failure to consider the effect of emergency treatment. Further investigations demonstrated that in many cases WBE did not contain venom-specific antigens and could not differentiate normal from allergic persons by skin test.

As early as 1956, Loveless and Fackler had demonstrated the effectiveness of pure wasp venom extract for the treatment of anaphylactic sensitivity, but their protocol was not generally accepted (Loveless, 1962). The modern era of venom immunotherapy was ushered in by the application of new immunologic techniques and venom collection procedures to study the hymenoptera-sensitive patients. Such patients were shown to have circulating specific IgE antibodies to venom by leukocyte histamine release, and RAST assays (Reisman et al., 1975; Sobotka et al., 1974, 1978). Since previous studies in ragweed pollen immunotherapy had indicated that there was some correlation between the levels of IgG-blocking antibody and clinical protection, it was reasoned that such antibodies might be even more effective in a system where they could react with injected antigens before they were exposed to tissue-bound IgE. That this indeed might be the case was suggested in two separate studies reported in 1974 by Busse and Lichtenstein (Busse et al., 1975). Relatives of beekeepers who continued to have systemic anaphylaxis after WBE treatment were protected by venom injections. Clinical protection was also associated with a rise in IgG-blocking antibody and a gradual decline in specific IgE or cell sensitivity by histamine release. These cases prompted Lessof et al. to administer gamma globulin from hyperimmune beekeepers to patients highly allergic to bee venom. On challenge, they were able to tolerate doses of venom higher than amounts that had previously caused reaction (Lessof et al., 1978).

These reports were extended by a now classic study by Hunt et al. (1978) at John Hopkins University. Sixty patients with a history of a generalized allergic reactions, positive venom skin tests, leukocyte histamine release, and RAST were divided into three groups. One group was placed on venom immunotherapy, one received whole body extract, and the remaining group received placebo. Following 6 weeks of therapy, most venom-treated patients had received 100 μg of venom for 2 weeks, and sting challenges were begun. Subjects in the other two groups were randomly selected for challenge. The protection rate in the venom group was 95%, whereas 60% of the WBE group and placebo group experienced systemic reactions after being restung. Levels of IgG-blocking antibodies rose significantly only in the venom-treated patients.

Sting challenges have now been done in greater than 500 venom-treated patients, and protection is demonstrated in approximately 97%. Failures are generally milder than the original reaction and usually respond to raising the dose of venom to 200 μg.

A characteristic response of IgE and IgG antibody level in successfully treated patients is shown in Figure 27-6. An initial rise in IgE level is followed by a gradual decline. Levels of IgG antibody rise over 3–6 months and remain elevated. Unfortunately, no absolute level of IgG or fall in IgE can predict with certainty the response of the individual patient to a sting.

Whereas the venom skin tests and/or RAST is necessary to demonstrate the IgE response to a specific hymenoptera, only the clinical history can select patients for testing and subsequent immunotherapy (see immunotherapy schedule in Table 27-2). In general, treatment is recommended only for those patients with a positive venom skin test and a history of a systemic reaction following an insect sting. Work at John Hopkins indicates that children with urticara only may be excluded from consideration for immunotherapy. Some patients with progressive local reactions and positive skin tests are at risk for subsequent systemic reaction, but the degree of risk is not known. At present these patients should be warned of their increased risk and encouraged to carry emergency medications at all times.

Once it has been decided that a patient has had a generalized allergic reaction to a stinging insect, venom skin testing is performed. Extracts are available to test for sensitivity to honeybee *(Apis mellifera)*, yellow jacket *(Vespula)*, yellow hornet or aerial yellow jacket *(Dolichovespula aernaria)*, white-faced hornet *(D. maculata)*, and paper wasp *(Polistes)*. Tests should be performed at least 3–6 weeks after the sting reaction to avoid the so-called refractory periods and take advantage of maximum IgE response. Because of the problem of cross-reactivity, all five venoms are tested by serial dilution to a maximum level of 1 μg/ml. Above this level nonspecific reactions

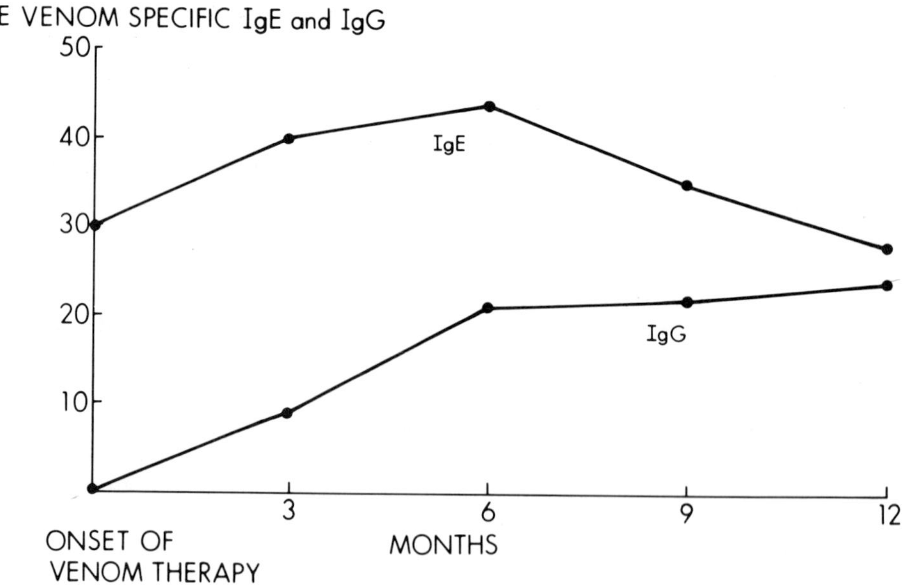

Fig. 27-6. Average, idealized IgE and IgG antibody response to bee venom Immunotherapy.

Table 27-2 *Standard Schedule for Venom Immunotherapy*

Week No.	Day No.	Dose No. Per Day at ½-Hour Interval	Concentration of Venom Used (μg/ml)	Volume Injected (ml)	Amount of Venom Injected (μg Protein)
1	1	1	0.01	0.1	0.001
		2	0.1	0.1	0.01
		3	1.0	0.1	0.1
2	8	1	1.0	0.1	0.1
		2	1.0	0.5	0.5
		3	10	0.1	1.0
3	15	1	10	0.1	1
		2	10	0.5	5
		3	10	1.0	10
4	22	1	100	0.1	10
		2	100	0.2	20
5	29	1	100	0.2	20
		2	100	0.3	30
6	36	1	100	0.3	30
		2	100	0.3	30
7	43	1	100	0.4	40
		2	100	0.4	40
8	50	1	100	0.5	50
		2	100	0.5	50
9	57	1	100	1.0	100
10	64	1	100	1.0	100
12	78	1	100	1.0	100
15	99	1	100	1.0	100
Monthly		1	100	1.0	100

occur. A positive test is considered to be a wheal of 5–10 mm and an area of erythema exceeding 11 mm.

Patients are often treated with all reacting venoms starting with solutions of 0.01 or 0.001 μg/ml until the average maintenance dose of 100 μg is reached. The standard schedule in the package insert can be followed in most cases, (Table 27-2) reaching a maintenance dose in 16–20 injections. "Rush" schedules are possible in less sensitive patients, reaching maintenance dose in 6 weeks. Very sensitive patients may take up to 1 year to reach 100 μg. The latter dose is then administered at increasing intervals until a 4-week interval is reached. Although preliminary data indicate that some patients may be safely increased to 6 weeks with demonstrated protection on sting challenge, it is probably safer to hold the four week interval (Golden et al., 1981). Doses less than 100 μg are associated with approximately 20% lower rates of protection, and 200 μg doses are necessary in 4–5% of patients.

Side effects consist largely of local reactions that are more extensive than with inhalant immunotherapy. They seldom impede the schedule and tend to peak at levels of 15–20 μg, receding at 100 μg. Systemic reactions vary greatly and tend to reproduce signs and symptoms of the original reaction. They occur at a frequency of approximately 15%, with half requiring treatment with epinephrine. Because of these reactions, the recommendation has been made that only physicians skilled in immunotherapy and those who are prepared to treat anaphylactic reactions should administer venom injections. Investigations are currently under way at Johns Hopkins and other medical centers to develop reliable assays utilizing IgG antibody levels against venom constituents in hopes of being able to confirm a status of immunity. No absolute contraindications exist, nor are long-term adverse effects seen in over 5 years of treatment.

Until better criteria are developed for assaying the status of immunity, it is recommended that venom injections be continued indefinitely.

Emergency kits should still be carried by venom-treated patients and epinephrine administered if more than two stings occur.

Immunotherapy for fire ant sensitivity is currently only available with WBE. Retrospective studies indicate 90–95% protection and suffer from the same criticism as did the original bee and vespid WBE reports. Failures certainly occur; in one study, 2 of 18 patients who were restung on fire ant WBE experienced generalized reactions (Rhodes & Schafer, 1977). Until appropriate immunologic studies with venom antigens are completed, no firm recommendations can be made regarding immunotherapy.

CONCLUSION

In conclusion, physicians can now offer their hymenoptera-sensitive patients a program of immunotherapy that offers virtually 100% protection in a potentially life-threatening situation. It is hoped that studies under way will define more precise criteria for selection of patients for treatment and provide the physician with reliable means for assaying loss of sensitivity.

Case History

A 27-year-old farmer's wife was stung twice on the leg while plowing a field. Within 5 minutes she noticed itching in the palms of her hands, axillae, and groin. This was rapidly followed by generalized urticaria, hoarseness, a tight feeling in the anterior chest, and a sensation of weakness. When she arrived in the local physician's office 45 minutes later, he noted the above signs and symptoms, together with hypotension. She rapidly responded to two injections of 0.3 ml of epinephrine 1 : 1000 subcutaneously and 50 mg of diphenhydramine intramuscularly (IM). She was hospitalized for observation and blood pressure monitoring. All symptoms cleared within a few hours. Swelling and erythema of the local sting extended from the ankle to the knee and gradually resolved over the next 2 or 3 days with the aid of oral prednisone. Before leaving the hospital, she was instructed in the self-administration of epinephrine, avoidance procedures and advised to wear a medical alert medal.

When seen in the allergist's office 2 weeks later, she gave a history of a previous uneventful sting 1 month before by a small "yellow-striped bee." There was no personal nor family history of atopy disease. Venom skin tests to honeybee, yellow jacket, white-faced and yellow faced hornet, and polistes were performed. Positive reactions were noted at 0.01 μg/ml intradermally (ID) to yellow jacket and both hornets.

Venom immunotherapy to the three reacting vespids was begun. Treatment was complicated by two mild systemic reactions characterized by throat itching and hoarseness and responding rapidly to a single injection of epinephrine. At approximately 10 months the 100-μg dose was achieved and she resumed working in the fields.

Three weeks after a maintenance injection, she was stung again and experienced local swelling and scattered urticaria, again clearing within 10 minutes of the self-administration of epinephrine. On this occasion, and on the advice of her physician, she brought the dead insect to the office. It was found to be a polistes species, and repeat skin testing documented positive reaction to polistes venom at 0.1 μg/ml. Immunotherapy with the latter vespid venom was added to her program and proceeded uneventfully. Subsequent field stings were without reaction.

This case illustrates a classic anaphylactic reaction to hymenoptera venom and the appropriate immediate and prophylactic treatment. Although most patients achieve maintenance doses of venom extract without difficulty, the risk of systemic reaction is always present. When such a reaction occurs, the next dose should be reduced, usually in half, and subsequent increases given at a more gradual pace. Eventually the 100-μg level can be reached in the majority of patients.

If the offending insect had not been examined by the physician after the second sting, he would have had to consider increasing the venom dose to 200 μg as well as shortening the maintenance interval of the original reacting venoms. Although cross-reaction between vespid venoms often occurs, individual antigens do exist and necessitate individual treatment.

REFERENCES

Barnard, J. H. *J. Allergy Clin. Immunol.*, *1973, 52,* 259.

Benson, R. L., & Semenov, H. *J. Allergy*, 1930, *1*, 105.

Busse, W. W., Reed, C. E., Lichteinstein, L. M., & Reisman, R. E. *JAMA*, 1975, *231*, 1154.

Golden, D. B., Sobotka, A. K., Valentine, M. D., & Lichtenstein, L. M. *J. Allergy Clin. Immunol.*, 1981, *67*, 482.

Hunt, K. J., Velentine, M. D., Sobotka, A. K., Benton, A. W., Amodio, F. J., & Lichtenstein, L. M. *New Engl. J. Med.*, *1978*, *299*, 157.

Insect Allergy Committee of the American Academy of Allergy. *JAMA*, 1965, *193*, 109.

Lessof, M. H., Sobotka, A. K., & Lichtenstein, L. M. *Johns Hopkins Med. J.*, 1978, *142*, 1.

Loveless, M. H. *J. Immunol.*, 1962, *89*, 204.

Reisman, R. E., Wypych, J. I., & Arbesman, C. E. *J. Allergy Clin. Immunol.*, 1975, *56*, 443.

Rhodes, R. B., & Schafer, W. L., Newman, M., (1977) *J. Fla. Med. Assoc.*, 1977, *64*, 247.

Sobotka, A. K., Valentine, M. D., Benton, A., & Lichtenstein, L. M. *J. Allergy Clin. Immunol.*, 1974, *53*, 170.

SUGGESTED READINGS

Levine, M., & Lockey, R., (Eds.) *Monograph on insect allergy*. Hartland: Parker Printing, 1981.

Lichenstein, L. M., Valentin, M. D., & Sobotka, A. K. *J. Allergy Clin. Immunol.*, 1979, *64*,5.

Rhoades, R. B. *Medical aspects of the imported fire ant*. Gainesville: University Presses of Florida, 1977.

QUESTIONS

1. The majority of deaths from stinging insects (70%) are due to:

   a. Shock
   b. Respiratory obstruction

c. Sepsis
d. Myocardial infarction

2. The most important therapeutic measure in the treatment of insect sting anaphylaxis is the administration of:

 a. Corticosteroids
 b. Antihistamines
 c. Epinephrine
 d. Oxygen

3. The following types of patient would be considered candidates for venom immunotherapy under presently accepted criteria:

 a. History of progressively increasing local reactions and positive skin tests or RAST
 b. History of severe systemic reaction, i.e., shock or respiratory involvement, and a positive skin test or RAST
 c. History of generalized urticaria and a positive skin test or RAST in an adult
 d. History of a systemic reaction with negative skin test and RAST

4. The following statements regarding antibodies involved in stinging insect allergy are generally accepted:

 a. IgE antibody titers reflect the degree of clinical sensitivity to insect stings.
 b. IgE antibody levels usually increase faster and peak earlier than IgG levels during venom immunotherapy.
 c. IgG levels usually double and IgE levels slowly fall during successful venom immunotherapy.
 d. RAST is a more sensitive test for venom specific IgE than the skin test.
 e. IgE and IgG levels can be used to determine the need for continuing or discontinuing venom immunotherapy.

5. Whole body extract (WBE) may:

 a. Be used for treatment of inhalant allergy in beekeepers
 b. Fail to distinguish between normal and allergic patients on skin testing
 c. Differ little from placebo in increasing IgG levels and protecting from a challenge sting
 d. Sensitize patients to body proteins resulting in weakly positive vespid skin tests.

Answers can be found in Appendix B at the end of the book.

Timothy J. Sullivan

28

Drug Allergy

Drug allergy, adverse reactions to drugs mediated by immune reactions or chemical activation of immune effector systems, is a common and serious problem in modern medicine. Excellent overviews of the many forms of immunopathology that can be induced by drugs have been published recently (Parker, 1975, 1980). This chapter focuses on the principles and practices applied to the clinical management of immediate hypersensitivity reactions to drugs. Therapy of acute allergic reactions is emphasized in other chapters of this book. Approaches to the identification and management of patients at risk for allergic reactions to drugs are emphasized in this chapter.

The diversity of mechanisms and specific stimuli leading to drug reactions in susceptible patients makes identification of patients at risk and methods to avoid reactions a difficult task. A careful inquiry into adverse reactions associated with previous exposures to an agent selected for therapy and immunologic assessments, when feasible, are used to identify allergic patients. Three general approaches are taken to bypass reactions in susceptible individuals: avoidance of specific agents or groups of agents, premedication, and desensitization.

The diversity of potential immunologic and nonimmunologic reactions triggered by drugs presents a formidable obstacle to effective general premedication or identification of patients at risk. Premedication and immunologic or genetic screening are not sufficiently developed to be applied to all drug therapy. As noted below, however, in some circumstances immunologic screening and premedication have proved effective.

ASSESSMENT

Assessment of History of Drug Allergy

Positive histories of adverse reactions to drugs should be scrutinized carefully to distinguish allergic reactions from untoward but nonallergic reactions. Isolated gastrointestinal complaints associated with ampicillin therapy, pain at the site of a drug injection, headache associated with nitroglycerine therapy, malaise and local

ALLERGY: THEORY AND PRACTICE
ISBN 0-8089-1619-X

discomfort for 2 days following a tetanus toxoid injection, and similar predictable untoward reactions to drugs do not indicate an allergic reaction. If a patient has experienced an allergic reaction during an earlier exposure, the role of the agent in question should be assessed. Identification of the offending agent may be difficult. Some patients have underlying illnesses such as systemic lupus erythematosus (SLE) that might cause symptoms resembling allergic reactions. In some instances primary allergic diseases are mistakenly treated as infections or other diseases; subsequent inflammatory or destructive reactions are mistakenly attributed to drugs. Often multiple drugs have been given simultaneously. Penicillin G, semisynthetic penicillins, cephalothins, and gentamicin are common causes of drug allergy (over 1 percent of treated patients). A diagnosis of IgE-mediated β-lactam antibiotic allergy often can be confirmed by skin testing. Indomethacin, heparin, nitrofurantoin, chloramphenicol, glutethimide, and barbiturates also provoke reactions in a significant fraction of patients (0.5–1 percent of those treated). Demonstration of positive immunologic tests for allergy to β-lactam antibiotics, insulin, and selected other agents may clarify the situation (see below). If prior adverse reactions are not indicative of an allergic reaction, the drug of choice can be used.

Alternative Drugs

If a reasonable likelihood of allergy to a current drug of choice is found, alternative approaches should be considered. Since immune reactions are highly specific, drugs with similar actions but distinctly different structures usually are appropriate alternatives. Structurally different antibiotics often can be used in place of β-lactam drugs. Alternative diagnostic maneuvers such as computerized tomographic (CT) scanning or ultrasound may prove adequate to delineate disorders usually assessed by radiocontrast studies. Some aspirin-sensitive patients can be treated with sodium salicylate or perhaps benoxyprophen, depending on the indication for aspirin. If clinically effective, relatively nontoxic alternatives are available, they should be selected.

Assessment of Relative Risks of Allergic Reactions and Alternative Drugs

If valid tests for allergy are unavailable, or if such tests are positive, but potential alternatives are not as effective as the drug of choice or carry serious potential hazards, consideration should be given to cautiously administering the drug of choice despite the risk of an allergic reaction. Determination of relative risks must be highly individualized. Attention should be given to the patient's age, clinical condition, concurrent therapy (particularly with beta-adrenergic blocking agents), the nature of the problem being treated, concurrent illnesses, and relative efficacies and toxicities of the alternatives.

DESENSITIZATION

Acute desensitization, or the cautious administration of progressively larger doses of a substrate, has been applied successfully with chemical activators of mast cells such as aspirin, haptens (e.g., penicillin), insulin, heteroantisera, and other preformed antigens. Insulin allergy, a relatively common problem, can be used as an exmple of the principles applied to desensitization to macromolecules. Patients with a history of immediate hypersensitivity reactions to insulin who are on insulin therapy are removed from insulin, and allergic reactions are allowed to subside (if possible). Prick and then intradermal skin tests are performed by using serial tenfold dilutions of U-100 regular bovine, porcine, or human insulin to identify the least reactive insulin species and to establish the highest concentration of insulin that does not cause an immediate intradermal wheal and flare response. This solution is administered subcutaneously beginning with 0.05 ml. Progressively doubled doses of insulin are administered at 30-minute intervals until therapeutic doses are achieved. If allergic symptoms appear during desensitization, a more gradual increase in dosage can be considered.

Aspirin sensitive patients can be desensitized if a compelling indication for a nonsteroidal anti-inflammatory agent is present (Stephenson et al., 1980, 1982) (see Chapter 29). If asthma is active, the patient should be treated vigorously to achieve maximal normalization of pulmonary function. Desensitization usually should not be attempted if a severe impairment of pulmonary function persists since asthmatic responses usually occur during desensitization. Pulmonary functions should be measured before the procedure and regularly during the procedure, using 3-hour intervals between doses of 10, 20, 40, 80, 160, 320, and then 650 mg of aspirin administered orally. If the schedule is interrupted at night, the procedure can be resumed the next morning beginning with the last tolerated dose. The patients should be monitored by clinical assessment and spirometry. A clinical reaction usually occurs at some point in this process. Such a response should be allowed to subside or if necessary conventional means should be used to suppress the reaction. The dose that provoked the response should be administered at least 3 hours later. In most instances no response occurs after rechallenge and the procedure can continue. Occasionally a second milder response appears. These reactions are addressed as described above. The desensitization procedure continues until full dose therapy is achieved. Once desensitization to aspirin is accomplished, any of the nonsteroidal anti-inflammatory agents can be used. The state of desensitization usually persists for days after the last dose. Caution should be exercised if more than a day elapses between doses, and the desensitization procedure should be repeated if more than 2 days elapse. In addition, at least one patient has been described (Dankner & Wedner, in press) who lost the desensitized state despite daily doses of aspirin or indomethicin. Thus an exascerbation of asthma in an aspirin-desensitized patient may demonstrate loss of tolerance and in this instance ASA should be discontinued.

SPECIFIC APPROACHES TO AVOIDANCE OF DRUG ALLERGY

Progress has been made in identifying patients at risk for some forms of anaphylaxis and for avoiding or minimizing the risk. Three representative situations and approaches are reviewed: (1) penicillin and related drugs—skin testing and densensitization, (2) local anesthetics—selection of a structurally dissimilar agent, and (3) radiocontrast medium reactions—premedication.

Penicillin and Other β-lactam Antibiotics

A history of an apparently allergic reaction to penicillin or closely related β-lactam antibiotics is offered by approximately 7 percent of the adults in this country. Acute allergic reactions to penicillin are noted in approximately 2 percent of courses of therapy with this agent. These drugs are a major cause of acute systemic allergic reactions and a dominant cause of fatal and nonfatal anaphylaxis.

Skin tests to detect IgE to penicillin were developed in the late 1950s and early 1960s by Charles W. Parker and independently by Bernard B. Levine (Parker, 1972). This was a very difficult task since antibodies react with drug determinants covalently coupled to endogenous proteins, not free drug. The immunochemistry of penicillin had to be established before tests could be developed. Since that time considerable experience with these techniques has been obtained [reviewed in Sullivan et al. (1981)]. The reagents commonly used include commercial Pre-Pen (peniciloyl-poly-L-lysine 6×10^{-5} *M*), Penicillin G, or any other β-lactam drug of interest (5000 units/ml or approximately 10^{-2} *M*, 3.3 mg/ml and penicilloic acid, 3.3 mg/ml, 10^{-2} *M*). The methods used and criteria for positivity are detailed in Sullivan et al. (1981). Clearly, immediate wheal-and-flare skin testing offers a potential bedside method for assessing current immunologic status with information sufficient to make therapeutic decision available within 40 minutes.

How useful is this technique? The incidences of acute allergic reactions in skin-test-positive patients treated with full therapeutic doses of penicillin have ranged from 39 to 73 percent with an aggregate of 27 of 54 or 50 percent (Green et al., 1977; Levine & Zolov, 1969; Parker et al., 1962; Shapiro, 1964; Solley et al., 1982). In these same series the incidences of acute reactions in skin-test-negative subjects ranged from 0 to 2.9 percent, with an aggregate of 12 reactions in 1967 treated patients or 0.6 percent. To date anaphylaxis has never been reported in a penicillin-treated, skin-test-negative patient. Thus penicillin skin testing is a very useful tool for identifying patients at risk for acute allergic reactions.

The issue of the risks of giving cephalosporins or semisynthetic penicillins to penicillin-allergic patients remains incompletely resolved. On one hand cross-reactions with IgE to penicillin as assessed by skin tests are common (Anfosso et al., 1979; Delafuente et al., 1979; Grieco, 1967; Levine, 1973; Petz, 1978; Solley, 1982; Sullivan et al., 1981) and clinical cross-reactions are well documented (Kabins et al., 1965; Petz, 1978; Rothschild & Doty, 1966; Scholand et al., 1968; Spruitt et al., 1974; Thoburn et al., 1966; Van Dellen & Gleich, 1970; Zeok & Tsueda, 1980). Our own experience is presented in Table 28-1. On the other hand, many physicians administer cephalosporins to patients with a history of penicillin allergy with an apparently low rate of cross-reaction. No studies have prospectively examined the fate of penicillin skin-test-positive patients given full doses of cephalosporins.

Two important features of this issue should be mentioned. Many patients who have had penicillin reactions years ago are skin-test-negative and could receive any β-lactam drug without incident (Sullivan et al., 1981). In addition, the likelihood that a true cross-reaction would be accurately identified in the context of acute serious infections is speculative.

Although an accurate estimate of the *degree* of risk of a cross-reaction is not possible, patients allergic to penicillin as determined by a positive skin test clearly are at some risk of anaphylaxis to cephalosporins or semisynthetic penicillins.

Table 28-1 *Skin-Test Reactivity to Ampicillin and Cephalothin in Patients Also Skin-Tested for Penicillin Reactivity*

Degree of Penicillin Reactivity	Skin Test Results*			
	Ampicillin		Cephalothin	
	+	−	+	−
Negative	0	14	4	45
Intradermal positive	25	15	26	35
Percutaneous positive	16	0	12	1

Reprinted with permission and modified from Sullivan, T. J., Wedner, H. J., Shatz, G. S., Yecies, L. D., & Parker, C. W. Skin testing to detect penicillin allergy. *J. Allergy Clin. Immunol.*, 1981, *68*, 171–180.
*Skin tests with these agents were performed with the same concentrations that were selected for skin tests with Penicillin G. Reactions to percutaneous or intradermal tests were combined as a total.

When β-lactam drugs are needed for therapy of allergic patients, an acute *desensitization* procedure can be considered (Brown et al., 1982; Sullivan, 1982; Sullivan et al., 1982). The rationale for the oral desensitization method is presented in Table 28-2 and in detail in Sullivan et al. (1982).

In most instances alternative antibiotics can be given; however, in rare cases the risk of not using a β-lactam drug appears greater than the risk of using the drug. An estimate of the risk of a fatal reaction to full-dose therapy in a skin-test-positive person is (0.50 react × 0.1 at most have anaphylaxis × 0.03 chance of a fatal reaction in skilled hands) approximately 0.15 percent or 1 in 667. The desensitization procedures appear to reduce this risk substantially. Indications for desensitization have included bacterial endocarditis, *Pseudomonas* infections, osteomyelitis, central nervous system syphilis, and syphilis in pregnancy.

An example of the kind of procedure used is presented in Table 28-3. If the agent selected for treatment is not avaiable in an oral form, oral benzylpenicillin generally is used, switching to the agent of choice when parenteral doses are given. Patients with a history of anaphylaxis are started at a hundredfold lower dose.

These doses are given at 15-minute intervals with continuous monitoring for signs of an allergic reaction. Conventional therapy then can begin.

Table 28-2 *Rationale for Oral β-Lactam Antibiotic Desensitization*

Only half of skin-test-positive patients have an acute reaction when given full-dose therapy
Most reactions are not anaphylactic
Most anaphylactic reactions are treatable
Initial doses need not be large doses
Only six reported deaths from oral β-lactam therapy
No serious acute allergic reactions in 64 patients desensitized by the oral method

Table 28-3 *Protocol for Oral Desensitization*

Dose	Units	Route
1	100	PO
2	200	PO
3	400	PO
4	800	PO
5	1,600	PO
6	3,200	PO
7	6,400	PO
8	12,500	PO
9	25,000	PO
10	50,000	PO
11	100,000	PO
12	200,000	PO
13	400,000	PO
14	800,000	PO
	Wait 30 minutes	
15	100,000	IV
16	200,000	IV
17	400,000	IV
18	800,000	IV

In one third of subjects IgE-mediated complications of the procedure and then therapy have been restricted to urticaria. No death, anaphylaxis, or other serious IgE-mediated reaction has occurred. Full courses of therapy were completed in 63 of the 64 subjects treated by this general protocol. The one patient withdrawn developed a severe immune hemolytic anemia while receiving nafcillin, a known complication of high-dose β-lactam antibiotic therapy (Sullivan, 1982). The mechanism of acute desensitization appears to be antigen-specific mast cell desensitization (Sullivan, 1982).

Patients at risk for anaphylaxis to β-lactam antibiotics can thus be identified with a considerable degree of precision. If β-lactam drugs are needed in allergic patients, acute desensitization appears to be an acceptably safe procedure for avoiding anaphylaxis (Editor's note: The protocols for penicillin skin testing and penicillin desensitization are given in Appendix 28A.)

LOCAL ANESTHETIC ALLERGY

Patients who experience untoward reactions of virtually any kind during treatment with local anesthetic agents often are told or believe that they have experienced acute allergic reactions. A careful review of the setting and nature of these reactions seldom unequivocally assigns prior reactions to IgE-mediated, pharmacologically mediated, or vasovagally mediated categories. Possible bedside immunodiagnostic methods, such as skin testing, and in vitro diagnostic methods have not been rigorously characterized and must be regarded as experimental. In general these patients must be approached as if they had experienced IgE-mediated reactions and as if they were at risk for another IgE-mediated reaction if the same or a structurally related local anesthetic agent is administered.

Analysis of apparently allergic reactions to local anesthetics and cutaneous wheal-and-flare reactions to them (de Jog, 1977) has suggested that cross-reactions are common among *p*-aminobenzoyl (PAB)-group-containing local anesthetics (Table 28-4). Reactions to local anesthetics not containing the PAB structure appear to be rare, and cross-reactions in this group appear to be rare. Vigorous efforts should be made to identify the agent associated with a prior reaction.

If the agent that provoked a reaction is known, a structurally unrelated agent can be selected. Table 28-4 presents commonly used agents according to the presence or absence of the PAB group and according to the usual sites or routes of administration. If a PAB group agent was associated with a prior reaction, an agent lacking the PAB group can be selected. If a non-PAB agent was associated with a prior reaction, a PAB agent or another non-PAB agent can be selected. If the agent implicated in a prior reaction cannot be determined, the agent or class of agent least likely to have been used is selected. Paraben preservatives in medications and procaine amide contain the PAB group and could conceivably cause a reaction in a PAB-sensitive individual.

The incomplete nature of our knowledge of allergic reactions to local anesthetics has led to the widespread use of a variety of provocative testing procedures before local anesthetics are used for anesthetic purposes (Incaudo et al., 1978). A protocol

Table 28-4 *Classification of Local Anesthetic Agents by Presence or Absence of* p-*Aminobenzoyl Group*

p-Aminobenzoyl structure present	*p*-Aminobenzoyl structure absent
Injectable Agents	
Procaine	Lidocaine
Chloroprocaine	Mepivacaine
Tetracaine	Dibucaine
	Bupivacaine
	Etidocaine
	Prilocaine
Ophthalmic Agents	
Benoxinate	Proparacaine
Topical Mucous Membrane and Cutaneous Agents	
Benzocaine	Dimethisoquine
Butamben	Cyclomethicaine
	Dyclonine
	Pramoxine
	Cocaine

Table 28-5 *Provocative Testing with Local Anesthetics*

Dose*	Concentration	Amount/Route
1	1 : 100 dilution	Prick test
2	Undiluted	Prick test
3	1 : 100 dilution	0.02 ml intradermal
4	1 : 100 dilution	0.5 ml SC
5	Undiluted	0.2 ml SC
6	Undiluted	1.0 ml SC

*The full protocol is used when the agent that provoked an allergic reaction is unknown. Doses 3, 5, and 6 are used when a structurally dissimilar agent is known. Interval between doses 15 minutes.

for provocative testing is presented in Table 28-5. If a local or systemic reaction occurs, another agent is selected, if one is available, and provocative testing is repeated. If no alternative local anesthetic agents are available, cautious use of the least reactive agent, infiltration with a weakly anesthetic H_1 antihistamine, systemic analgesic therapy, or general anesthesia should be considered in accordance with the indication for analgesia. This general approach has been successful in permitting the use of local anesthetics in patients with histories of allergic reactions to local anesthetics.

Radiocontrast Medium Reactions

Anaphylactic reactions of varying intensity occur in approximately 2 percent of all intravenous radiocontrast studies (Anonymous, 1980; Ansell et al., 1980; Gorevic & Kaplan, 1979; Greenberger et al., 1980; Lieberman et al., 1978). Recently important determinants of risk have been assessed and estimates of relative risk offered (see Table 28-6 and Ansell et al. (1980).

Patients who have experienced radiocontrast media (RCM) reactions in the past have an approximately 30 percent chance of a reaction during another RCM procedure (Greenberger et al., 1980). Premedication with glucocorticoids according to the regimen outlined in Table 28-7 reduced the reaction rate to approximately 6 percent, and most reactions have been much less severe than the initial reaction (Greenberger et al., 1980). Studies are in progress to determine whether all patients would benefit from premedication. The regimen is benign and premedication of all subjects seems reasonable, particularly those with significant risk factors (Table 28-6). Furthermore, premedication—including H_2 receptor blockade with cimetidine, ranitidine, or doxepin—is likely to be even more effective, and preliminary studies of RCM premedication seem to confirm this hypothesis. While most investigators have not detected value in low-dose intravenous pretesting with RCM (Greenberger et al., 1980), some workers advocate such a test (Sullivan et al., 1982).

Radiocontrast media reactions appear to be an example of chemically induced anaphylaxis (Anonymous, 1980) in which clear risk factors have been identified and in which premedication significantly reduced the incidence and severity of reactions.

Table 28-6 *Risk Factors for Radiocontrast Medium Reactions*

	Relative Risk			
Condition	Minor	Intermediate	Severe	Death
History of allergy	1.6	2.6	3.91	—
Asthma	1.5	2.72	5.09	—
Hay fever	1.68	1.76	2.34	—
Urticaria	1.54	4.83	2.03	—
Eczema	1.30	1.16	4.69	—
Other allergies	1.44	1.75	3.35	—
Drug reactions	1.83	1.97	3.15	—
Prior RCM* reactions	6.85	8.67	10.88	—
Cardiac disease	1.10	0.86	4.54	8.48
CHF†	1.34	0.98	5.5	53.8
CAD*‡	1.02	0.80	6.88	8.68
Arrhythmia	1.46	0.78	9.75	—

Reprinted with permission and modified from Ansell, G., Tweedie, M. C. K., West, C. R., Evans, P., & Couch, L. The current status of reactions to intravenous contrast media. *Invest. Radiol.*, 1980, *15* (6), 532.
*Radio contrast media.
†Congestive heart failure.
‡Coronary artery disease.

Table 28-7 *Protocol for Premedication to Avert Radiocontrast Medium Reactions*

Hours Before Procedure	Pharmacologic Agent	Dose
13	Prednisone (cimetidine)*	50 mg PO (300 mg PO)
7	Prednisone (cimetidine)*	50 mg PO (300 mg PO)
1	Prednisone diphenhydramine (cimetidine)*	50 mg PO 50 mg PO (300 mg PO)

*The standard protocol (Greenberger et al., 1980) for pretreatment did not include cimetidine; however, other more recent protocols, such as that used for the administration of chymopapain, recommend the use of this drug.

SUMMARY OF MANAGEMENT

Methods for detection of patients at risk for drug allergy or to avoid drug allergy are diverse and depend on the specific agent. The forces that lead to anaphylaxis are multifold, and effective avoidance measures are specific-force oriented; on the other hand, the clinical anaphylactic syndromes are similar and the treatment is similar.

Patients with histories of allergy, asthma, and cardiovascular diseases are at increased risk of experiencing some forms of drug allergy and are at increased risk of severe reactions (Ansell et al., 1980; Idsoe et al., 1968; Parker, 1980). Asthma appears to affect the mortality from anaphylaxis (Idsoe et al., 1968; Settipane et al., 1980). No clear increase in incidence of anaphylaxis has been noted in association with asthma, but asthmatic patients are roughly twice as likely to die from anaphylaxis, usually from intractable bronchial obstruction. Physicians should take special precautions to avoid anaphylaxis in asthmatics.

One recognized factor influencing the expression of anaphylaxis is beta-adrenergic blockade (Hannaway & Hopper, 1983; Jacobs et al., 1981; Newman & Schyultz, 1981). Anaphylaxis appears to be more frequent, more severe, and more difficult to treat in beta-blocked patients. Recognizing this, physicians should consider replacing beta blockers with alternative drugs such as nifedipine in patients at risk for anaphylaxis (e.g., subjects allergic to insect venom or patients receiving allergy desensitization injections).

Treatment of acute allergic reactions is addressed in detail in sections dealing with anaphylaxis, asthma, and other specific allergic manifestations. An approach to management of acute drug-induced urticaria and angioedema is summarized in Table 28-8.

Pruritus usually is the indication for treating acute urticaria. The role of tricyclic antidepressants in this context is not well defined, but these agents appear to be the most potent H_1-antihistamines now available; they also exert potent anti-H_2 actions (Richelson, 1979, 1983; Sullivan, 1982). As with other antihistamines, drowsiness is the principal side effect. The oral suspension form of doxepin is convenient since infinite flexibility in dosage is possible, in addition. The 12-hour dosage interval for 5 mg of doxepin or once daily dosage for 10 mg or higher also make this agent attractive. Patients with acute urticaria may not be responsive to epinephrine or antihistamine therapy alone. However, many of these individuals can be controlled by the combination of antihistaminics and a short course of glucocorticoid therapy. Glucocorticoids, in these moderate doses for this short interval, seldom are contraindicated if the patients' other medical problems are controlled. A similar approach may be applied to the treatment of angioedema in those patients without upper airway obstruction. (Treatment of upper airway obstruction is discussed in Chapter 11.)

If a beta-adrenergic blocking agent such as propranolol is being administered, urticaria and other allergic reactions may be particularly difficult to suppress. In patients already receiving beta-blocking drugs, the usual dose of beta agonist must be increased, and the use of combined H_1 and H_2 blockade may be considered.

Application of these principles should substantially reduce the current level of morbidity and mortality induced by drug allergy.

Table 28-8 *Pharmacologic Suppression of Acute Uncomplicated Urticaria and Angioedema in Adults**

1. Epinephrine
   (e.g., epinephrine 300 μg (0.3 ml of aqueous 1 : 1000) SC, *this may be repeated q20min for 3–4 doses if necessary*. Usually effective in the first 1–2 hours after onset but not later in course)

If this proves ineffective or is not indicated

2. Conventional H_1 antihistamines
   (e.g., chlorpheniramine 4–8 mg orally q6h or diphenhydramine 50–100 mg IM q6h)
   For emergent situations IV diphenhydramine may be used

If this proves ineffective

3. H_1 antihistamine plus H_2 antihistamine
   (H_1 antihistamines as noted above plus cimetidine 300 mg orally *or parenterally* q6h)

If this proves ineffective

4. Tricyclic antihistamines
   (e.g., doxepin 5 mg orally q12h or higher doses orally once daily)

If this proves ineffective

5. Antihistamine therapy plus short-term glucorticoid therapy
   (e.g., prednisone 40 mg orally once daily in morning for 4 days)
   For acute situations IV corticosteroids may be necessary

*Patients with acute onset of urticaria and angioedema may require vigorous therapy to avoid complications such as upper airway obstruction or hypotension. These patients may be treated as indicated in italics.

REFERENCES

Anfosso, F., Leyris, R., & Charpin, J. Drug allergy: In vitro cross-allergenicity between amoxicillin and benzyl penicillin. *Biomedicine*, 1979, *30*, 168.

Anonymous. Adverse reactions to radiocontrast media—an entire supplement of to *Investigative Radiology*, 1980, *15*, (6).

Ansell, G., Tweedic, M. C. K., West, C. R., Evans, P., & Couch, L. The current status of reactions to intravenous contrast media. *Invest. Radiol.*, 1980, *15* (6), S32.

Brown, L. A., Goldberg, N. D., & Shearer, W. T. Long term ticarcillin densensitization by the continuous oral administration of penicillin. *J. Allergy Clin. Immunol.*, 1982, *69*, 51.

Dankner, R. & H. J. Wedner. *Am. Rev. Resp. Dis.*, in press.

De Jog, R. H. *Local anesthetics* (2nd ed.) Springfield: Charles C. Thomas, 1977, pp. 272–275.

Delafuente, J. C., Panush, R. S., & Caldwell, J. R. Penicillin and cephalosporin immunogeneicity in man. *Ann. Allergy*, 1979, *43*, 337.

Gorevic, P., & Kaplan, A. P. Contrast agents and anaphylactic-like reactions. *J. Allergy Clin. Immunol.*, 1979, *63*, 225.

Green, G. R., Rosenblum, A. H., & Sweet, L. C. Evaluation of penicillin hypersensitivity: Value of clinical history and skin testing with penicilloyl-polylysine. *J. Allergy Clin. Immunol.*, 1977, *60*, 339.

Greenberger, P., Patterson, R., Kelley, J., Stevenson, D. D., Simon, R., & Lieberman, P. Administration of radiographic contrast media in high-risk patients. *Invest. Radiol.*, 1980, *15*, S40.

Grieco, M. H. Cross-allergeneicity of the penicillins and the cephalosporins. *Arch. Intern. Med.*, 1967, *119*, 141.

Hannaway, P. J., & Hopper, G. D. K. Severe anaphylaxis and drug-induced beta-blockage. *New Engl. J. Med.*, 1983, *308*, 1536.

Idsoe, O., Guthe, T., Willcox, R. R., & de Weck, A. L. Nature and extent of penicillin side-reactions with particular reference to fatalities from anaphylactic shock. *Bull. Wildlife Health Org.*, 1968, *38*, 159

Incaudo, G., Schatz, M., Patterson, R., et al Administration of local anesthetics to patients with a history of prior adverse reaction. *J. Allergy Clin. Immunol.*, 1978, *61*, 339.

Jacobs, R. L., Rake, G. W., Fournier, D. C., Chilton, R. J., Culver, W. G., & Beckman, C. H. Potentiated anaphylaxis in patients with drug-induced beta-adrenergic blockage. *J. Allergy Clin. Immunol.*, 1981, *68*, 125.

Kabins, S. A., Eisenstein, B., & Cohen, S. Anaphylactoid reaction to an initial dose of sodium cephalothin. *J. Am. Med. Assoc.*, 1965, *193*, 165.

Levine, B. B. Antigenicity and cross-reactivity of penicillins and cephalosporins. *J. Infect. Dis.*, 1973, *128*, S364.

Levine, B. B., & Zolov, D. M. Prediction of penicillin allergy by immunological tests. *J. Allergy*, 1969, *43*, 231.

Lieberman, P., Anaphylactoid reactions to iodinated contrast material. *J. Allergy Clin. Immunol.*, 1978, *62*, 174.

Newman, B. R., & Schyultz, L. K. Epinephrine-resistant anaphylaxis in a patient taking propranolol hydrochloride. *Ann. Allergy*, 1981, *47*, 35.

Parker, C. W. Practical aspects of diagnosis and treatment of patients who are hypersensitive to drugs. In M. Samter (Ed.), *Hypersensitivity to drugs*. 1972. New York: Pergamon Press, 1972, p. 367.

Parker, C. W. Drug allergy. *New Engl. J. Med.*, 1975, *292*, 511, 732, 957.

Parker, C. W. Drug allergy. In C. W. Parker, Ed., *Clinical immunology*. Philadelphia: Saunders, 1980, P. 1219.

Parker, C. W., Shapiro, J., Kern, M. & Eisen, H. N. Hypersensitivity to penicillenic acid derivatives in human beings with penicillin allergy. *J. Exp. Med.*, 1962, *115*, 821.

Petz, L. D. Immunologic cross-reactivity between penicillins and cephalosporins: A review. *J. Infect. Dis.*, 1978, *137*, S74.

Richelson E. Tricyclic antidepressants and histamine H_1 receptors. *Mayo Clin. Proc.*, 1979, *54*, 669.

Richelson E. Antimuscarinic and other receptor-blocking properties and antidepressants. *Mayo Clin. Proc.*, 1983, *58*, 40.

Rothschild, P. D., & Doty, D. B. Cephalothin reactions after penicillin sensitization. *J. Am. Med. Assoc.*, 1966, *196*, 372.

Scholand, J. F., Tennenbaum, J. I., & Cerilla, G. Anaphylaxis to cephalothin in a patient allergic to penicillin. *J. Am. Med. Assoc.*, 1968, *206*, 130.

Settipane, C, et al Anaphylactic reactions to hymenoptera stings in asthmatic patients. *Clin. Allergy*, 1980, *10*, 659.

Shapiro, J. Hypersensitivity to penicillenic acid derivatives in humans with penicillin allergy. In U.S. Department of Health, Education, and Welfare, *Proceedings of the World Forum on Syphilis and Other Treponematoses*, 1964, pp. 328–332.

Solley, G. O., Gleich, G. J., & Van Dellen, R. G. Penicillin allergy: Clinical experience with a battery of skin test reagents. *J. Allergy Clin. Immunol.* 1982, *69*, 238.

Spruill, F. G., Minette, L. J., & Sturner, W. Q. Two surgical deaths associated with cephalothin. *J. Am. Med. Assoc.*, 1974, *229*, 440.

Stevenson, D. D., Simon, R. A., & Mathison, D. A.
Aspirin sensitive asthma: Tolerance to aspirin after positive oral aspirin challenges. *J. Allergy Clin. Immunol.* 1980, *66*, 82.

Stevenson, D. D., Pleskow, W. W., Curd, J. G., Simon, R. A., & Mathison, D. A. Densensitization to acetylsalic acid (ASA) in ASA-sensitive patients with rhinosinusitis/asthma. In P. Dukor, P. Kalos, H. D. Schlumberger, & West, G. B. (Eds): *Pseudo-allergic reactions. Involvement of Drugs and Chemicals*, Basel: S. Karger, 1982, Vol. 3, p. 133.

Sullivan, T. J. Antigen-specific desensitization of patients allergic to penicillin. *J. Allergy Clin. Immunol.* 1982, *69*, 500–509.

Sullivan, T. J. Pharmacologic modulation of the whealing response to histamine in human skin: Identification of doxepin as a potent in vivo inhibitor. *J. Allergy Clin. Immunol.* 1982, *69*, 275.

Sullivan, T. J., Wedner, H. J., Shatz, G. S., Yecies, L. D., & Parker, C. W. Skin testing to detect penicillin allergy. *J. Allergy Clin. Immunol.*, 1981, *68*, 171–180.

Sullivan, T. J., Yecies, L. D., Schatz, G. S., Parker, C. W., & Wedner, H. J. Densensitization of patients allergic to penicillin using orally administered β-lactam antibiotics. *J. Allergy Clin. Immunol.*, 1982, *69*, 275–282.

Thoburn, R., Johnson, J. E., & Cluff, L. E. Studies on the epidemiology of adverse drug reactions. IV. The relationship of cephalothin and penicillin allergy *J. Am. Med. Assoc.* 1966, *198*, 345.

Van Dellen, R. G., & Gleich G. J. Penicillin skin tests as predictive and diagnostic aids in penicillin allergy. *Med. Clin. N. Am.*, 1970, *54*, 997.

Zeok, S. S., & Tseuda, K. Failure of a cephalothin test dose to produce anaphylaxis. *Anesthesia Analgesia,* 1980, *59*, 393.

H. James Wedner

Appendix 28A Adverse Reactions to Drugs

Adverse reactions to drugs represent major medical and economic problems in the United States today. It has been suggested that half of all hospital admissions may be related in one way or another to therapeutic agents. Thus, a physician must carefully weigh the therapeutic potential of any drug against the possibility of an untoward reaction, with an eye to minimizing as much as possible adverse drug reactions. This must be done with the recognition that any drug has the potential of resulting in undesirable side effects. This brief review will not attempt to catalog the numerous side effects of drugs, but will outline the types of adverse reactions which may be seen. Adverse reactions to drugs may be classified into three broad groups: dose-related toxic effects, idiosyncratic reactions, and hypersensitivity reactions.

TOXIC REACTIONS

Toxic reactions are pharmacological effects which do not relate to the primary effect of the drug and will occur to a greater or lesser extent in all patients, depending upon the quantity of the drug given. They are *normal* properties of the drug. Toxic reactions are further subdivided into *side effects* which occur within the therapeutic dose range, and *true toxicity* which occurs when blood or tissue concentrations exceed therapeutic levels. In some cases these two classifications will merge since the sensitivity of individuals to side effects can vary widely; one individual may tolerate high levels of a given drug without any observable side effects while another is unable to tolerate the drug at all. Patient perception may also be of great importance particularly where side effects are concerned. The same degree of a symptom, e.g., nausea, may be severely compromising to one patient and largely overlooked by another. A good example is the somnolence associated with antihistaminics which frequently occurs within the true therapeutic dose range; in some patients somnolence is mild while in others it may be overwhelming and necessitate discontinuance of the drug. In this case, as is true for a number of drug groups, switching from one chemical class of antihistaminic to another may allow one to maximize the therapeutic potential while minimizing the side effect (see Chapter 14). For those patients who cannot tolerate the drug, the undesirable side effects may disappear, while therapeutic potential is maintained, if the drug is continued. Alternatively, it may be possible to minimize side effects by starting at a relatively low dose and building up gradually over time. This is the case with antihistaminics, and can also be seen with such diverse groups as beta-adrenergic agonists (see Chapter 16) or antihypersensitive

ALLERGY: THEORY AND PRACTICE
ISBN 0-8089-1619-X

agents. It is important to explain to patients that there is the potential of an undesirable side effect and that it may disappear if they persevere in taking the drug.

In contrast to undesirable side effects, true toxic reactions occur at dosages which yield blood levels in excess of the therapeutic range. Adverse reactions are, none the less, intimately related to the chemical natures of the agents and amounts of drug given. Examples of toxic reactions include cardiotoxicity with digitalis, postural hypotension with antihypertensive agents and nausea, vomiting, and if, sufficient drug is given, convulsions with theophylline or its salts. The gap between therapeutic and toxic levels of a drug varies greatly and may be quite broad, giving the physician a great deal of latitude in prescribing the drug; or it may be narrow, requiring careful monitoring of blood levels to assure maximum benefit with minimum chance for toxicity. An example of this phenomenon occurs in the use of theophylline for the treatment of asthma (see Chapter 15). With theophylline the therapeutic range is 10 to 20 μg/ml, while the toxic range, beginning with mild anorexia and progressing through nausea and vomiting, generally starts between 18 and 20 μg/ml and becomes progressively worse at higher blood levels. Because theophylline biotransformation varies widely from patient to patient it is impossible to be certain that a given dose will achieve a therapeutic blood level. Therefore, it is recommended that measuring the theophylline blood level is the only way to achieve maximum therapeutic benefit while minimizing side effects. It should also be noted that with theophylline, as with a number of other drugs, some patients may experience therapeutic discomfort at blood levels which are in the low therapeutic range. In a small percentage of patients, it may be as low as 10 to 15 μg/ml. In these unusual cases one can still derive therapeutic benefit by carefully adjusting the amount and/or timing of the dose to achieve a blood or tissue level which is still therapeutic but reduces the majority of unwanted toxic effects to acceptable levels. Similar consideration to these should be taken into account with any drug where the toxic and therapeutic ranges approximate one another.

With some classes of drugs, toxic effects are related not to the absolute blood level achieved but to the total amount of drugs given. In those instances one must keep in mind the progressive amount of drug (dose × duration), and discontinue use of that particular agent prior to reaching a level associated with toxic side effects. Excellent examples of this phenomenon include gold–salt toxicity or the toxic effect of a number of antibiotics. The aminoglycoside antibiotics cause renal and ototoxicity based on the total amount of drug given; chloramphenicol also has bone marrow depression, a toxic effect also related to the total cumulative dose, although this may also be an idiosyncratic reaction (see below).

IDIOSYNCRATIC REACTIONS

Idiosyncratic reactions to drugs in general have no relation to the amount or duration of therapy. They can be seen with the initial introduction of the drug or may occur after long periods of time on an adequate therapeutic dose. They are totally unpredictable, with the exception that a patient who has had one idiosyncratic reaction to a drug is likely to have a second if the drug is reinstituted. Some idiosyncratic reactions may be relatively benign while others are life threatening. Many idiosyncratic reactions, to a greater or lesser extent, fortunately fall into the former category. One must always be aware of the potential for an idiosyncratic reaction and, in those instances where the idiosyncratic reaction may be life threatening, one must balance the potential for idiosyncratic reactions against the therapeutic benefit. This should take into account the frequency at which idiosyncratic reactions occur and the severity of those reactions. For example, although the aplastic anemia seen with chloramphenicol is disastrous, the percent of patients actually experiencing this idiosyncratic reaction is extremely small. For this reason it would be inappropriate to withhold chloramphenicol in a life-saving situation for fear of an idiosyncratic reaction. On the other hand the use of this drug in instances where an alternative, potentially less toxic antibiotic, is available would be just as inappropriate.

Toxic and idiosyncratic reactions to drugs probably have different underlying biochemical bases. In some instances, however, the result may be very similar (i.e., toxic and idiosyncratic reactions to chloramphenicol). It is important to differentiate the dose-related toxic effects from the idiosyncratic reactions. A patient who has had an idiosyncratic reaction to a drug should not be given the drug again unless the physician is faced with dire consequences. In instances where overdosages occur, however, the toxic effects can be prevented with appropriate dose regimens and thus do not prevent the patient from receiving that drug, or a drug of the same class, again.

HYPERSENSITIVITY REACTIONS

Hypersensitivity reactions (see Chapter 2) can occur with virtually any drug in the pharmacopoeia. These can be differentiated into 3 basic types: (1) immediate hypersensitivity (Type I), (2) delayed antibody mediated of the Arthus type (IgG Type II and III), and (3) cell-mediated (Type IV). Immediate (Type I) reactions may be further subdivided into anaphylactic and anaphylactoid reactions (Chapters 10, 11). Anaphylactic reactions refer to those in which the drug induces the production of IgE antibody directed against the drug or drug protein conjugates; the reaction occurs on subsequent administration of the drug following interaction of the agent with specific IgE molecules bound to tissue mast cells or circulating basophils. In contrast, anaphylactoid reactions refer to those instances where release of mast cell mediators is accomplished through a non-IgE mediated mechanism. This may be the result of direct interaction of the drug with the mast cell membrane, e.g., the release of chemical mediators by the drug polymyxin B, or it may occur secondarily, e.g., interaction of the drug with the complement system with generation of the anaphlotoxins C5a and C3a. These anaphlotoxins are capable of inducing the release of mediators from mast cells and or basophils. The net result is the same, in either case, since the mediators released are identical.

A complete discussion of the chemical mediators of anaphylaxis is presented in Chapter 3. They include a broad diversity of chemical entities including histamine, the slow-reacting substances of anaphylaxis (leukotriene C, D, and E), prostaglandin D_2, perhaps prostaglandin $F_{2\alpha}$, platelet activating factor, trypsin-like proteolytic enzymes, and a variety of other enzymes which generate potent vasoactive agents such as bradykinin, chemotactic factors for eosinophils, and neutrophils as well as heparin. These factors, alone or in combination, are responsible for the symptoms of immediate hypersensitivity reactions; skin pruritis, urticaria, angioedema, laryngeal edema, wheezing, and hypotension. The severity of the reaction will depend on the location of the activated mast cells and the number of mast cells activated. Hypersensitivity reactions may be extremely mild (hives or mild pruritus), or may be an overwhelming severe systemic allergic reaction (anaphylaxis). Immunologic reactions are the result of the generation of immunoglobulins or sensitized T cells directed against the drug. To be immunogenic, the drug must be haptenized by conjugation to tissue proteins. Thus, the ability of any drug to bind covalently (or in some cases noncovalently) to tissue proteins will be reflected in its potential for inducing Type I hypersensitivity reactions. The classic example of a Type I reaction is seen in penicillin allergic individuals, discussed in Chapter 28.

The majority of drugs which cause Type I or other hypersensitivity reactions are low molecular weight molecules which *must* react with tissue proteins to become an allergen.

Table 28A-1 *Complete Antigens*

Homologous Products
- Human plasma
- Anti henophilic globulin
- Plasma thromboplastin converting factor
- Human gamma globulin*

Heterologous Substances
- Heterologus serum (itorse serum)
- Antilymphocyte serum
- Adrenal cortical stimulating hormone
- Thyroid stimulating hormone
- Antidiuretic hormone (pituitary powder)
- Insulin
- Calgitonin
- Enzymes
- Heparin
- Ipecac
- Dextrans
- Allergen extracts

There is, however, a class of therapeutic agents that are large enough to be immunogenic (MW greater than 6,000) without conjugation. A partial list of these agents is shown in Table 28A-1. Of these the most important is insulin. Insulin induces the production of IgE antibodies in a small percentage, and IgG antibodies in a much larger but significant proportion of insulin-requiring patients. This is true of most of the biologicals shown in Table 28A-1.

Drugs are also capable of inducing IgG-type antibodies as well as IgE antibodies. In many cases these IgG anti-drug antibodies are innocuous and do not effect the bioavailability of the drug or cause any significant side reaction. Because of its high protein reactivity, greater than 90% of patients who receive parenteral penicillin will develop anti-penicillin antibodies of the IgG Type. This, does not mean that they will have any subsequent difficulties when penicillin therapy is reinstituted. Under certain circumstances, however, IgG antibodies may lead to significant drug reactions. The IgG (or IgM) reaction results, not only from antibodies which

Table 28A-2 *Procedure for Altering Protocol for Penicillin Desensitization Based on Reactions*

Type of Reaction	Alteration in Protocol
Mild local	None
Moderate local	None
Large local	Decrease dose by one-half and continue protocol from that point
Mild systemic (one or two urticaria or erythematous rash)	None
Moderate systemic (diffuse urticaria—modest decrease in blood pressure—wheezing or chest tightness	Treat with appropriate drug—decrease dose to one-tenth and begin again
Severe systemic (anaphylaxis)	Treat with appropriate drug—*STOP PROCEDURE*

Table 28A-3 *Procedures for Oral Hyposensitization*

1. Patient must be skin test positive—a history of penicillin sensitivity is *not* sufficient.
2. There must be a clear-cut need for penicillin or a penicillin derivative and the decision to use penicillin made prior to skin testing.
3. Informed consent from the patient or an appropriate relative must have been obtained.
4. A trained individual; physician, nurse or aide, *must* be *with* the patient at all times.
5. A physician *must* be on the floor at all times.
6. A patient IV must be running.
7. Injectable epinephrine 0.322 1 : 1000, diphenhydramine (Benadryl) 50 mg, and corticosteroids should be drawn up and available at the bedside.
8. Appropriate resuscitative equipment must be available.
9. All dilutions of oral and parenterol penicillin should be made up prior to beginning of procedure.

are directed to the drug haptenized on tissue proteins, but may also be the result of antibodies which are directed against proteins that have been altered by interaction with the drug. Interreaction between antibody and drug protein conjugates may yield antigen antibody complexes in the fluid phase. If these are of significant quantity and size, a serum sickness-like picture is seen. If the complex is of the appropriate size specific organs may be affected, e.g., kidneys in drug-induced lupus erythematosis or Henoch-Schoenlein purpura. Drugs may be bound (conjugated) to a specific organ-yielding reaction which are highly organ specific. Perhaps the best example of such a drug reaction results from the production of antibodies that react with quinine (quinidine) bound to platelets, and result in quinine-induced thrombocytopenia. Drugs may similarly bind to the liver, yielding a drug-induced hepatitis, or to a variety of other specific organs. These diseases may mimic other diseases in many ways, e.g., autoimmune-type phenomenon. They are generally self limited, however, and respond well simply by removal of the drug. The use of corticosteroids in these types of drug reactions is controversial since, in the majority of instances, there is rapid clearing of drug and drug protein conjugates by antibody and the use of steroids neither hinders or helps.

A variety of drugs are also associated with the development of a delayed cell mediated or delayed immunity (Type IV). In this instance the drug–protein conjugate results in the production of *effector* or cytotoxic T cells. Type IV hypersensitivity has been associated with a large number of drugs. Whether given orally, parentially, or applied to the skin, the major organ effected is the skin. When local application of the drug is the route of administration, the classic picture is a pruritic papulo-pustular eruption limited to those areas where the drug was applied (Chapter 8). In cases of a systemic reaction, the most common reaction is a generalized eczematid dermatitis: other forms include erythema multiforme and, in rare cases, erythema nodosum. Although many drugs have been implicated in Type IV reactions, the actual proof in many instances has been difficult. Reapplication of a drug to the skin (patch testing) can be done to identify reactions. On the other hand drugs given parenterally or orally may require more sophisticated studies for identification. Simple incubation of the drug with leukocytes or lymphocytes *in vitro,* however, may not yield accurate results since, as the true immunogen is already a drug-protein conjugate. In the case of a *fixed drug eruption* (a skin reaction which occurs in the same limited area of the skin each time the drug is introduced), a serum factor has been described that transforms lymphocytes, suggesting this is a Type IV reaction. Although patch testing or other laboratory studies can be performed in most instances, sophisticated laboratory studies are not necessary and sufficient information can be obtained from a careful history.

PART 1 ______________________________

Patient's Name: ______________________________

Hosp. No.: ______________ Hosp. Location: ______________

Clinic No.: ______________ Clinic Location: ______________

Private Outpatient No.: ______________________________

Patient's Address: ______________________________

Patient's Phone No.: ______________________________

Birthdate: ______________ Race: ______________ Sex: ______________

PART II: (FILL IN OR CHECK) ______________________________

Physician's Name (print) ______________________________ Date ______________

Physician's Signature ______________________________

Physician's reason for suspecting penicillin allergy ______________________________

History of previous penicillin therapy: ☐ yes ☐ no Was there a reaction? ☐ yes ☐ no

Types of previous reaction: ☐ urticaria ☐ angioedema ☐ other rash ______________
☐ serum sickness ☐ asthma ☐ anaphylaxis

Specific drug given: ______________ Route of administration: ☐ oral ☐ IM ☐ IV

Date of reaction: ______________ Patient's age at time: ______________

Other drugs used at time: ☐ none ☐ yes (specify) ______________

Other atopic diseases: ☐ rhinitis ☐ asthma ☐ eczema

Current medications: ______________________________

Diagnoses: ______________________________

PART III

	PENICILLIN G	PENICILLOYL-POLYLYSINE	PENICILLOIC ACID	OTHERS*
SCRATCH:				
control				
1 : 10,000				
1 : 100				
concentrated				
INTRADERMAL:				
control				
1 : 10,000				
1 : 100				
concentrated				

*ampicillin cephalothin carbenicillin

PART IV

Remarks:

1. Acute Reactions
2. Comments
3. If there are any questions concerning the test results, please call the DIVISION OF ALLERGY AND IMMUNOLOGY at XXX-XXXX.

Technician ______ Date ______ Time ______

Fig. 28A-1. Penicillin skin test request and testing form used at Washington University School of Medicine.

Pt. Name________________ Pt. Age______Sex________
Hospital #________________ Diagnosis________________
Physician________________ Pen. Sens.________________
(Drug used & reaction)

Penicillin derivative used for parenteral Rx________________
(Note: Phenoxymethyl penicillin used for oral doses)

#	Time	Suggested Dose, Units	Route	Actual Dose	Route	Reaction
1		100	Oral			
2		200	Oral			
3		400	Oral			
4		800	Oral			
5		1,600	Oral			
6		3,200	Oral			
7		6,400	Oral			
8		12,800	Oral			
9		25,000	Oral			
10		50,000	Oral			
11		100,000	Oral			
12		200,000	Oral			
13		400,000	Oral			
14		50,000	SC			
15		100,000	SC			
16		200,000	SC			
17		400,000	SC			
18		800,000	SC			
19		1,000,000	IM			
20		100,000	IV			
21		200,000	IV			
22		400,000	IV			
23						
24						
25						
26						
27						
28						
29						
30						
31						
32						

Fig. 28A-2. Penicillin desensitization flow sheet used at Washington University School of Medicine.

For all of the hypersensitivity reaction discussed one must remember that the degree of immunogenicity or the type of response which is stimulated depends upon the type of drug, its chemical properties, and the route of administration. For example many drugs given orally are much less immunogenic than the same drug given parenterally, as discussed in Chapter 28 for penicillin. A drug applied to the skin may induce a Type IV reaction while the same drug in oral or parenteral form is relatively nonimmunogenic. The classic example is case antihistaminic group. These are infrequent producers of hypersensitivity unless applied to the skin where they commonly produce delayed hypersensitivity reactions.

These considerations are not without practical benefit. Selection of the appropriate dosage form, avoiding those associated with the induction of hypersensitivity states, may help to prevent hypersensitivity reactions.

Table 28A-4 *Dilutions for Penicillin Hyposensitization*

1. Use Pen U.K. (phenoxymethyl penicillin) oral suspension—400,000 units/5 ml; use water for dilutions

2. Stock solution = 80,000 units/ml "A"

   Dilute

1 : 10	=	8000 units/ml	"B"
1 : 100	=	800 units/ml	"C"
1 : 800	=	100 units/ml	"D"

3. Dilute stock 1:10 = "B"
   Dilute "B" 1 : 10 = "C"
   Dilute "C" 1 : 8 = "D"

4. Volumes for oral penicillin are:

100 units	1.0 ml	"D"
200 units	2.0 ml	"D"
400 units	4.0 ml	"D"
800 units	1.0 ml	"C"
1600 units	2.0 ml	"C"
3200 units	4.0 ml	"C"
6400 units	8.0 ml	"C"
12,800 units	1.6 ml	"B"
25,000 units	3.2 ml	"B"
50,000 units	6.4 ml	"B"
100,000 units	1.25 ml	"A"
200,000 units	2.5 ml	"A"
400,000 units	5.0 ml	"A"

5. For parenterol penicillin, use units or assume 250 mg = 400,000 units

6. Dilute appropriate penicillin derivative to

1,000,000 units/ml	or	625 mg/ml	"E"
400,000 units/ml	or	250 mg/ml	"F"

7. Volumes for parenteral penicillin are

50,000 units	0.125 ml	"F"	SC	31.25
100,000 units	0.250 ml	"F"	SC	62.50
200,000 units	0.500 ml	"F"	SC	125.00
400,000 units	1.00 ml	"F"	SC	250.00
800,000 units	0.80 ml	"E"	SC	500.00
1,000,000 units	1.0 ml	"E"	IM	625.00
100,000 units	0.25 ml	"F"	IV	62.50
200,000 units	0.50 ml	"F"	IV	125.00
400,000 units	1.00 ml	"F"	IV	250.00

8. If patient tolerates 400,000 units IV he is "desensitized."

9. Assuming no complications the procedure takes 5.25 hours.

10. The procedure delivers 4,050,500 units of penicillin or 2.5 g of penicillin.

The list of drug-related adverse effects presented here, while by no means complete, does indicate the broad diversity of adverse reactions which can occur to drugs. Drugs may have side effects which represent pharmacological actions of these agents other than those which are actually desired. These toxic effects may occur at blood levels within the therapeutic range, at supra therapeutic levels, or they may be related to the cumulative dose given. The adverse reaction may be idiosyncratic in nature or may result from a hypersensitivity state. Hypersensitivity reactions of the anaphylactoid type may represent a pharmacological effect of the drug on an unknown enzyme system (e.g., aspirin), interaction with complement system, or a direct action of the drug on the surface of the mast cell or basophil. In addition, those drugs capable of conjugating to tissue proteins may generate an immune response against the drug protein complex. The immune response may be in Type I anaphylactic-type reaction by production of specific IgE, a Type II or III response due to the production of IgG, and subsequent formation of either cytotoxic antibodies or antigen–antibody complexes, or may be a Type IV cell-mediated response.

It is imperative that the physician be aware of the broad diversity of adverse reactions to drugs which can occur. In the majority of cases a careful detailed drug history will be sufficient to alert the physician to the potential of an adverse reaction to a drug and this can then be handled either by use of an alternative therapeutic modality, by appropriate treatment of the patient to block the effects of mediator release, or by appropriate desensitization procedures. It is also important that the patient as well as the physician be appraised of the potential for side effects, the nature of these side effects, and the methods which will be utilized to decrease or circumvent them. In this way the problem of drug-related adverse reactions can hopefully be minimized, and where they occur, treated appropriately. Keep in mind at all times that no drug is free of adverse effects and that as long as physicians continue to utilize drug therapy, adverse reactions will continue to be a major problem. This should not lead to therapeutic nihilism, but rather to the utilization of measures to minimize or circumvent these reactions.

SUGGEST READING

Perers, G. (ed): *Hypersensitivity to Drugs*, Pergamon Press, Ltd. 1972.

C. W. Parker. Drug Allergy, In C. W. Parker, ed., *Clinical Immunology*, Philadelphia: W. B. Saunders Co., 1980.

P. P. VanArsdel, Jr. Adverse drug reactions. In E. Middleton, Jr., C. E. Reed, E. F. Ellis, eds. *Allergy, Principles and Practice*, St. Louis, Mo: The C. V. Mosby Company, 1983.

QUESTIONS

1. Toxic reactions differ from idiosyncratic reactions in that

   a. toxic reactions are always dose related when idiosyncratic are not.
   b. A patient who experiences a toxic reaction may never receive the drug again.
   c. Idiosyncratic reactions are related to the pharmacologic properties of the drug.
   d. Idiosyncratic reactions will occur in every patient if enough drug is given.

2. The following are true of toxic reactions and side effects except:
   a. They are pharmacologic properties of the drug.
   b. They will occur in every patient if the sufficient drug is given.
   c. Once a patient has a toxic reaction he may never receive the drug again.
   d. Patient perception of the side effects varies widely.
3. Anaphylactic reactions:
   a. require the production of IgE type antibodies.
   b. release different meditors than anaphylactoid reactions.
   c. always require the agent to be "haptenized" to tissue protein.
   d. are only seen in atopic individuals.
4. A patient sensitive to penicillin would be expected to be sensitive to:
   a. ampicillin
   b. carbenicillin
   c. cephalosporins
   d. penicillium mold
5. Antihistaminics should not be used topically since:
   a. they may stimulate a Type IV hypersensitivity reaction.
   b. they are not effective in this form.
   c. they are more likely to conjugate to tissue protein and induce a Type I reaction.
   d. topically they result in IgG antibodies which block drug action.

Answers can be found in Appendix B at the end of the book.

Ronald Alan Simon, Warren W. Pleskow
Donald D. Stevenson, David A. Mathison

29

Aspirin Sensitivity

DESCRIPTION OF ASPIRIN (ASA) RESPIRATORY SENSITIVITY

Aspirin has been used as a therapeutic agent since the beginning of the century. In 1919 the first asthmatic reaction following aspirin [acetylsalicylic acid (ASA)] ingestion was reported (Cooke, 1919). Over the decades, additional reports followed, and in 1968 Samter and Beers (Samter & Beers, 1968) described in detail a clinical syndrome of hypereosinophilic nonallergic rhinitis with nasal polyps, asthma, and a unique hypersensitivity reaction to aspirin. This reaction is manifested as acute rhinorrhea, ocular injection, frequently a profound asthmatic attack, and often flushing, occurring about 1 hour following the ingestion of usual therapeutic does of aspirin. Another common feature of this syndrome is eosinophilia. These aspirin "triad" patients (asthma, nasal polyps, and aspirin sensitivity) usually have asthma and rhinosinusitis, which require regular use of corticosteroids. Despite the avoidance of aspirin and other cross-reacting substances, the respiratory disorder persists. Studies have shown that about 35% of the patients with asthma and nasal polyps-sinusitis have aspirin sensitivity, and about 8–14% of all asthmatics are aspirin sensitive (McDonald, et al., 1972; Samter & Beers, 1968; Spector et al., 1979).

Other Adverse Reactions to Aspirin

In addition to these adverse respiratory reactions to aspirin, other reactions have been described. Well known are aspirin's common side effects, and symptoms of overdosage, which are not discussed further. Urticaria and angioedema following aspirin ingestion has been reported (Szczeklik et al., 1977). It is distinctly unusual for one patient to develop both respiratory (rhinoconjunctivitis-asthma) and cutaneous (urticaria-angioedema) reactions following aspirin ingestion. This would suggest that different mechanisms are activated or that following activation of a single mechanism the reaction depends on specific target organ sensitivity. This chapter is concerned only with respiratory reactions to aspirin.

ALLERGY: THEORY AND PRACTICE
ISBN 0-8089-1619-X

MECHANISMS

The mechanisms responsible for the aspirin-sensitive reactions are unknown. Despite the clinical similarity to immediate hypersensitivity reactions, there appears to be no evidence that ASA sensitivity is IgE mediated (Schlumberger et al., 1974; Yurchak et al., 1970). Aspirin is an inhibitor of the cyclooxygenase pathway of the prostaglandin metabolism from arachidonic acid (Vane, 1971) (Fig. 29-1). It is hypothesized but difficult to conceptualize that in susceptible patients, there is a shift to production of prostaglandin $F_2\alpha$, a bronchoconstrictor, from prostaglandin E_1, a bronchodilator (Szczeklik et al., 1977; Settipane et al., 1974). Prostaglandin E_1 is also an inhibitor of mediator release (including histamine and slow-reacting substance of anaphylaxis) from the lung (Tauber et al., 1973). There are no data to support the notion that there are unique changes in prostaglandin metabolism in aspirin-sensitive asthmatics. A role for mast cell mediators in aspirin-sensitive asthma is suggested by the inhibition of aspirin provoked bronchoconstriction by H_1 antihistamines, inhaled cromolyn sodium, or oral cromolyn-like drugs such as the ketotifens (Basomba et al., 1976; Martelli, 1979; Szczeklik et al., 1977; Wuthrich, 1979).

Another, more recent hypothesis suggests that aspirin sensitivity is the result of the increased production of leukotrienes generated from arachidonic acid metabolized via the lipoxygenase pathway when the cyclooxygenase pathway is blocked by ASA (Goetzl, 1980; Hamburg & Samuelsson, 1974; Parker, 1979) (Fig. 29-2). This theory does not explain why only a subpopulation of asthmatics are aspirin-sensitive since all asthmatics would be expected to be sensitive to the increased leukotriene production.

Any hypothesis of the mechanism for aspirin sensitivity must also take into

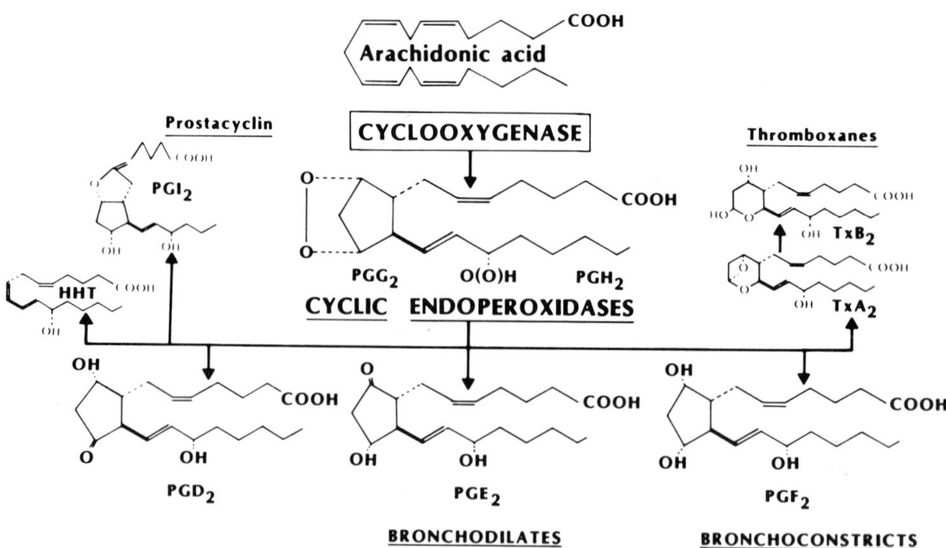

Fig. 29-1. Metabolism of arachidonic acid via the cyclooxygenase pathway to the prostaglandins.

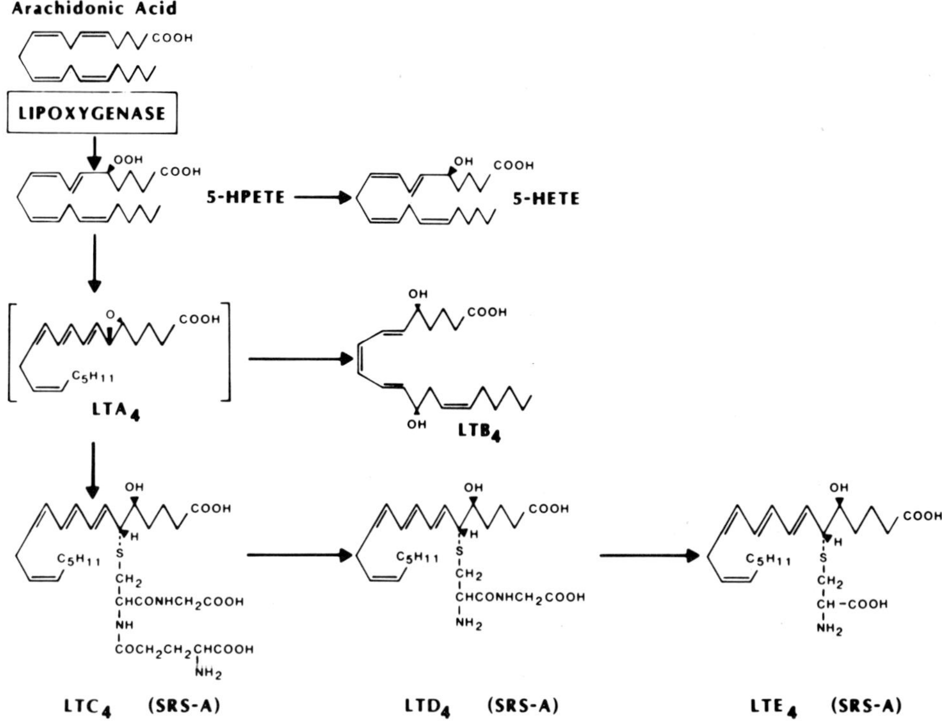

Fig. 29-2. Metabolism of arachidonic acid via the lipoxygenase pathway to the leukotrienes.

account our recent findings about the spectrum of and variation in aspirin reactions as well as aspirin desensitization and the refractory period phenomena (Pleskow et al., 1982). These phenomena are discussed in greater detail later.

One of the major arguments against IgE as the mechanism for aspirin sensitivity is the high degree of cross-reactivity between aspirin and nonsteroidal anti-inflammatory (NSAI) agents in aspirin-sensitive asthmatics (Pleskow et al., 1982). Also in support of a nonimmunologic mechanism are the facts that these agents are immunologically distinct from aspirin, and yet aspirin-sensitive patients have had adverse reactions to them following their first exposure. These agents are as follow:

Indomethacin (Indocin)
Fenoprofen (Nalfon)
Naproxen (Naprosyn)
Tolmetin (Tolectin)
Ibuprofen (Motrin)
Zomepirac (Zomax)
Sulindac (Clinoril)
Mefanamic Acid (Ponstel)

All agents such as aspirin inhibit the cyclooxygenase pathway of arachidonic acid metabolism. In fact, the degree of cross-reactivity seems to correlate with the agent's potency as a prostaglandin synthetase inhibitor (Szczeklik et al., 1977). This is in contrast to other compounds, including other salicylates like choline and sodium salicylate, which are not cyclooxygenase inhibitors and do not cross-react in aspirin-sensitive asthmatics. Likewise, since the naturally occurring salicylates in foodstuffs are not potent inhibitors of prostaglandin synthesis, it is not recommended that they be eliminated from the diet of ASA-sensitive asthmatics.

ASPIRIN CHALLENGES

Indications

Since, as noted earlier, 10–35% of all asthmatic subjects have the *potential* for being aspirin-sensitive, and since only a small number (probably less than 1%) of all asthmatics seem to improve with administration of these drugs, aspirin challenge is usually *not a routine indicated diagnostic procedure*. In addition, because a negative challenge now cannot be taken as evidence for future freedom from severe aspirin reactions, it is generally accepted that most asthmatic patients, and certainly those with nasal polyps and sinusitus, should be told to avoid these medications and use acetaminophen as an alternative analgesic-antipyretic.

Occasionally patients with asthma, have another disorder for which aspirin or other NSAI are the indicated treatment of choice. In these patients an aspirin challenge is indicated. Examples include patients with chronic rheumatologic disorders, headaches, or vascular disorders attributable to platelet dysfunction.

Challenge Procedure*

There is no standardized, generally accepted protocol for oral aspirin challenge. In addition, there is no *in vitro* assay for detection of aspirin or other NSAI respiratory sensitivity. Over the last 10 years we have performed more than 500 oral aspirin challenges, including several hundred in patients known to have respiratory sensitivity to these drugs. The following are methods that we have developed over the years:

1. Patients are challenged after obtaining a fully informed consent with emphasis placed on the possibility of a severe asthmatic reaction occurring.
2. Patients are challenged only when their asthma is in relative remission, and this often requires a period of treatment with systemic corticosteroids.
3. Patients must have the following minimum spirometric values prior to proceeding with aspirin challenge. Their best of three forced expiratory volume in one second (FEV_1) must be greater than or equal to 1.50 liters and greater than 70% of their best prior recorded value.
4. Patients continue all their regular medications, including corticosteroids and methylxanthines, but discontinue antihistamines, cromolyn sodium, and inhaled sympathomimetics 24 hours prior to the challenge. As noted earlier, there are reports in the literature that the aspirin reaction can be blocked or at least

*Modified from Pleskow, et al. (1982) and Mathison et al. (in Press).

modified and hence possibly obscured by cromolyn sodium and H_1 antihistamines (Basomba et al., 1976; Martelli, 1979; Sczceklik, et al., 1977; Wuthrich, 1979).
5. All challenges are performed in the morning in our clinical research center, or allergy laboratory, where full treatment modalities for any emergency, including full resuscitative equipment are available. A physician is always present to treat a reaction when it occurs.

We accept the possibility that continuation of corticosteroids and methylxanthines may mask a mild reaction and thereby lead to a false-negative result. However, the deterioration of asthma during a challenge when all medications are withheld may lead to false-positive results. Placebo challenges are always carried out to document the underlying stability of the asthma state during the course of the challenge.

Over the years we have developed two protocols for oral aspirin ingestion challenge that have proved safe, although they provoke a substantial asthmatic response. A 1-day challenge is performed in asthmatic patients who are unlikely to be aspirin-sensitive. This would include asthmatics who had recently tolerated the ingestion of aspirin or cross-reacting substances without adverse effects and those without a history of chronic sinusitis and polyps. The 1-day protocol is shown on Table 29-1. It involves administering 30 mg of aspirin and then 1 hour later 60 mg, followed by 150, 325, and 650 mg at 2-hour intervals. Spirometry is performed at ½-hour intervals and continued for 3 hours following the last dose or sooner if symptoms develop.

Table 29-1 *Aspirin Challenge Dosage Protocols*

One-Day

Time	ASA Dosage (mg)	Cumulativo Dosage (mg)
8:00 A.M.	30	
9:00 A.M.	60	(90)
10:00 A.M.	100	(190)
12:00 Noon	325	(495)
2:00 P.M.	650	(1145)
5:00 P.M.	End	

Two-Day

Time	Day 1 Asa Dosage (mg)	Cumulative Dosage (mg)	Time	Day 2 ASA Dosage (mg)	Cumulative Dosage (mg)
8:00 A.M.	30		8:00 A.M.	150	
11:00 A.M.	60	(90)	11:00 A.M.	325	(425)
2:00 P.M.	100	(190)	2:00 P.M.	650	(1105)
5:00 P.M.	End		5:00 P.M.	End	

A 2-day aspirin challenge is performed in those asthmatic subjects with a history of a respiratory reaction following ingestion of aspirin or cross-reacting drugs, or in those with rhinosinusitis or polyps who have not ingested ASA in the last 10 years and would be likely to be aspirin-sensitive. The 2-day protocol is also outlined in Table 29-1. An initial dose of 3 mg is administered, followed by 30 mg 1 hour later. Two hours later 60 mg is given, and if no reaction occurs, 3 hours later 100 mg is administered. Spirometry is measured every $\frac{1}{2}$ hour or sooner if symptoms occur. The next day 150 mg is administered, and then 325 and 650 mg at 3-hour intervals.

Aspirin challenges are individualized for each patient, and doses or intervals between doses may be altered at the discretion of the physician.

A lower respiratory reaction is considered to be positive if the FEV_1 value falls by greater than 25%. At this point, no additional doses of aspirin are administered, and the patient is treated with an inhaled sympathomimetic [usually isoetharine 0.5 ml delivered by an intermittent positive pressure breathing device (IPPB)]. The patient is also seen by a physician, and additional medication such as intravenous (IV) aminophylline or corticosteroids may be administered.

A challenge is considered negative if no symptoms develop, or if there is less than a 15% fall in the FEV_1. Such patients are advised that they may begin taking the drug as indicated for their conditions in usual therapeutic doses. A challenge is interpreted to be "equivocal" if the fall in FEV_1 is 15–25% or "partial" if there are nasoocular symptoms with a fall in the FEV_1 of less than 15%.

All patients considered to have a positive, equivocal, or partial reaction to aspirin challenge must have had a negative challenge to a placebo either before or more than 7 days after the aspirin challenge. Asthmatics with positive, equivocal, or partial responses to aspirin may be considered subjects for desensitization.

DESENSITIZATION TO ASPIRIN AND REFRACTORY PERIOD DETERMINATIONS

Background

The existence of a refractory period to adverse effects of aspirin in patients with aspirin sensitive asthma was first recorded in 1922 by Widal et al. (1922). This report describes a patient reacting to 100 mg of aspirin who, following the administration of increasingly larger doses of aspirin over a one month period, was able to tolerate 600 mg of aspirin without adverse effects. More recently, Zeiss & Locke (1976) reported a single patient who demonstrated a 72-hour refractory period to the adverse effects of aspirin. Bianco et al. (1977) have reported that refractoriness to the adverse effects of inhaled aspirin conjugate follows aspirin provoked bronchoconstriction by the inhaled route. We recently have also found two aspirin-sensitive asthmatic patients who were refractory to further adverse effects of aspirin following a positive oral aspirin challenge (Stevenson et al., 1980). In addition, we reported that both of these patients had improvement in their overall respiratory status as measured by symptoms and medication (corticosteroid) usage, following daily administration of aspirin over a period of almost 3 years (Stevenson et al., 1980).

Recent Investigations

Desensitization

We sought to expand these observations by attempting to desensitize a greater number of aspirin-sensitive asthmatics (Pleskow et al., 1982). In addition, we investigated the length and other clinical characteristics of the refractory period that follows desensitization to aspirin.

Following a positive aspirin reaction, further challenges were restarted when the patient's spirometric values returned to near baseline levels (usually 2–24 hours after initial reaction). Aspirin was then readministered at the dose that provoked the initial response and increased sequentially until 650 mg was tolerated or another reaction occurred. This procedure was repeated until each patient becomes unresponsive to 650 mg of oral aspirin. This was considered to be the desensitized state.

Refractory Period

After achieving the desensitized state, the patients then underwent sequential aspirin challenges at 2-, 3-, 4-, and 5-day intervals. During these intervals, aspirin was withheld. The refractory period was defined as the interval, in days, between the last ingestion of aspirin and the recurrence of a positive oral aspirin challenge.

Results

DESENSITIZATION. Over the last 3 years we have been able to desensitize all of the more than 50 aspirin-sensitive asthmatic patients whom we have studied (Fig. 29-5). The initial threshold dose provoking a positive reaction occurred between cumulative doses of 33 and 1083 mg of aspirin. About 60% of patients became desensitized after their initial aspirin reaction. In the other 40%, however, more than one aspirin-induced reaction occurred prior to reaching a densensitized state. Most of these individuals had initial aspirin reactions with very low dosages of aspirin (less than 100 mg). Figure 29-3 shows a patient who underwent five aspirin reactions prior to becoming desensitized. Initially, 33 mg of aspirin elicited a severe nasoocular and asthmatic response. When additional challenges were undertaken on the same day, continuing asthmatic responses were noted. Finally, on the third day of hospitalization, after the sixth aspirin challenge, the desensitized state was achieved. A universal finding is particularly well illustrated in this patient: following desensitization, patients are able to tolerate large doses of aspirin. (This patient received approximately 1200 mg of aspirin, which was about 34 times the initial provoking dose.)

Despite being desensitized to aspirin, the patients remain asthmatic. We have performed both methacholine and histamine inhalation challenges before and after aspirin desensitization, and the patient's hyperreactivity to both these agents are unchanged. In addition, patients maintained on aspirin, in a desensitized state, still develop asthma relapses from all of their prior provoking factors except aspirin. These include irritants, upper respiratory infection (URI), and IgE provoked mechanisms where they are relevant.

REFRACTORY PERIOD. Figures 29-3 and 29-4 are examples of how refractory periods were determined. The data for the refractory periods are noted on Figure 29-6. In

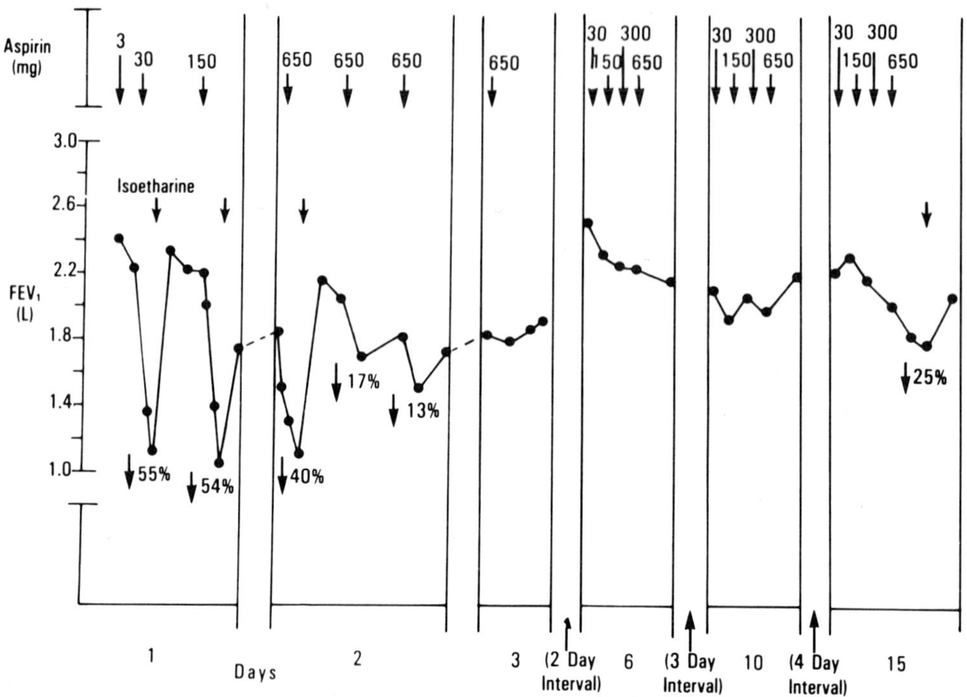

Fig. 29-3. Multiple aspirin reactions (day 1, 2) prior to aspirin desensitization (day 3), continued refractoriness to aspirin demonstrated at 2- and 3-day challenges (day 6, 10), subsequent return to aspirin sensitivity demonstrated by challenge after a 4-day interval without aspirin (day 15). From Pleskow, W. W., Stevenson, D. D., Mathison, D. A., Simon, R. A., Schatz, M., & Zeiger, R. S. *J. Allergy Clin. Immunol.*, 1982, *69*, p. 14. With permission.

general, refractory periods varied between 2 and 5 days. Typically, return to aspirin sensitivity occurred in a gradual manner, and often mild symptoms were noted during "negative" challenges (FEV_1 decline less than 25%) carried out at intervals that were shorter than the patient's refractory period. In addition, during the repeat challenges, larger doses of aspirin were often required to produce proportionately the same or even milder symptoms compared to the initial reaction. However, we recommend that in general ASA be administered at least daily to maintain the desensitized state.

CROSS-SENSITIVITY AND DESENSITIZATION

Nonsteroidal Anti-inflammatory Drugs

Further investigations established the cross desensitization of aspirin with other NSAIs having the common property of inhibiting prostaglandin synthetase. A typical patient is illustrated in Figure 29-7. This patient, as shown in Figure 29-4, had a 28% decrease in FEV_1, accompanied by symptoms of wheezing, rhinorrhea, and flushing after a cumulative dose of 133 mg of aspirin. Following resolution of the symptoms, aspirin was readministered, and the patient was found to be desensitized,

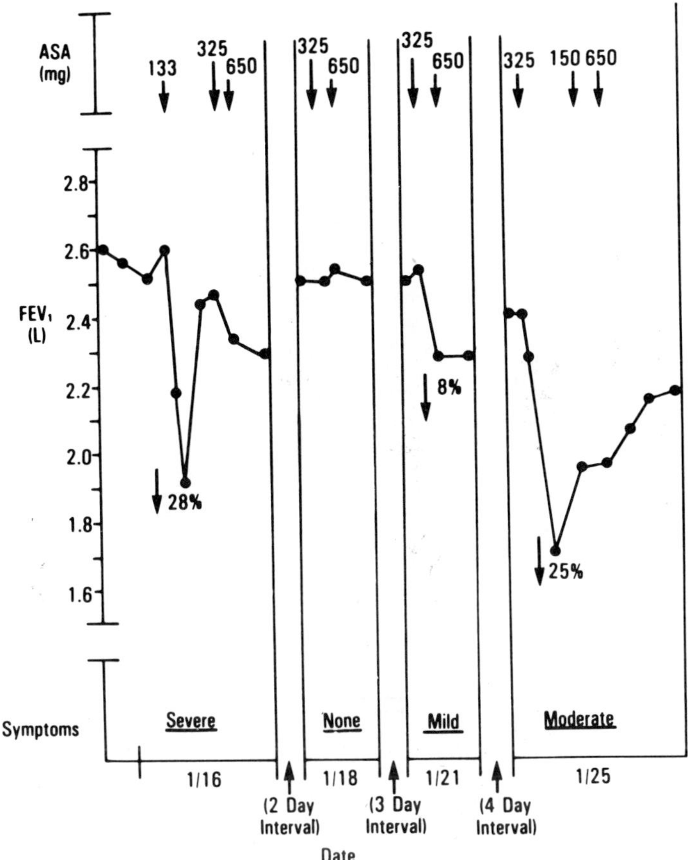

Fig. 29-4. Aspirin sensitivity and desensitization on January 16 with refractoriness at 2-day (January 18) and 3-day (January 21) intervals, but return to aspirin sensitivity on January 25 (4-day intervals). From Pleskow, W. W., Stevenson, D. D., Mathison, D. A., Simon, R. A., Schatz, M., & Zeiger, R. S. *J. Allergy Clin. Immunol.*, 1982, *69*, p. 17. With permission.

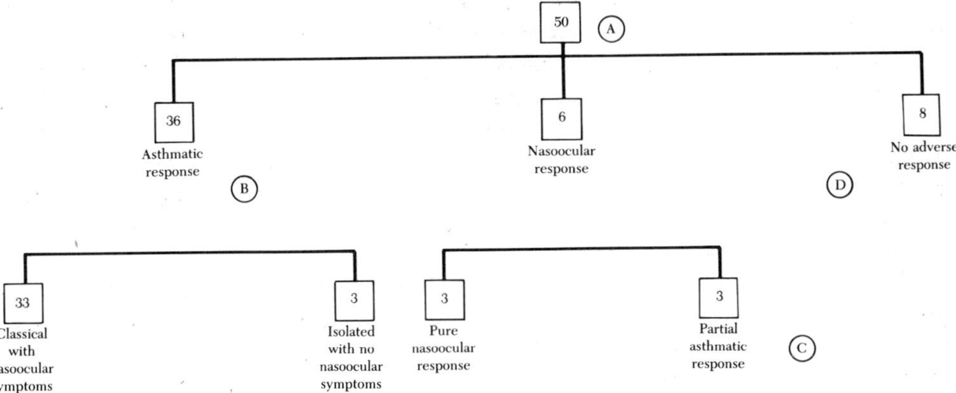

Fig. 29-5. Spectrum of respiratory responses to aspirin in 50 patients with a history of aspirin sensitivity. Legend: (A) □ = number of patients; (B) decrease $FEV_1 \geq 25\%$ from baseline; (C) decrease $FEV_1 < 15\%$ from baseline; (D) two patients had positive asthmatic reactions in prior challenges. From Pleskow, W. W., Stevenson, D. D., Mathison, O. A., Simon, R. A., Schatz, M., & Zeiger, R. S. *J. Allergy Clin. Immunol.*, 1983, *71*, 574.

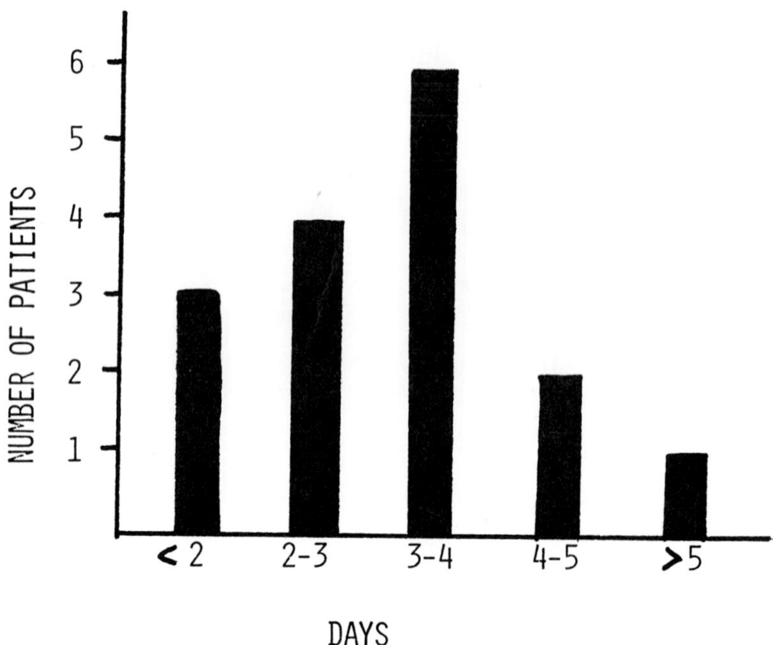

Fig. 29-6. Distribution of the refractory periods following aspirin desensitization in 16 aspirin-sensitive asthmatics. From Pleskow, W. W., Stevenson, D. D., Mathison, D. A., Simon, R. A., Schatz, M., & Zeiger, R. S. *J. Allergy Clin. Immunol.*, 1982, *69*, p. 15. With permission.

by her ability to ingest 325 mg and then 650 mg of aspirin without any symptoms or significant change in lung function. Her refractory period was determined to be 3–4 days. After a 2-day interval without aspirin, no reaction occurred following the ingestion of 650 mg. Following a 3-day interval without aspirin ingestion, there was an 8% decline in FEV_1 value accompanied by some nasal symptoms during the aspirin challenge. These mild symptoms, produced by a dose of aspirin much greater than her initial provoking dose, heralded the positive reaction, which occurred after a 4-day interval without aspirin. At that challenge, the patient's FEV_1 value declined by 32% but was accompanied by symptoms of only modest degree when compared to the initial reaction. Later that day after lung function returned to baseline, the patient was once again shown to be desensitized by her ability to ingest full doses of aspirin without reaction. Over the next 2 days 325 mg of aspirin was administered each day without adverse effect. Cross-tolerance to other NSAIs was documented by the patient's ability to ingest ibuprofen Motrin, indomethacin Indocin, and naproxen Naprosyn on consecutive days without reaction. Then, after a 6-day interval without ingesting aspirin or other NSAIs (more than 2 days beyond her established refractory period), she was rechallenged with indomethacin. The patient had a positive response to the indomethacin challenge as noted in Figure 29-7 with a fall in FEV_1 of 32% following 50 mg of indomethacin. On the following day the patient was able to tolerate 650 mg of aspirin without any symptoms. This shows refractoriness to aspirin following indomethacin desensitization.

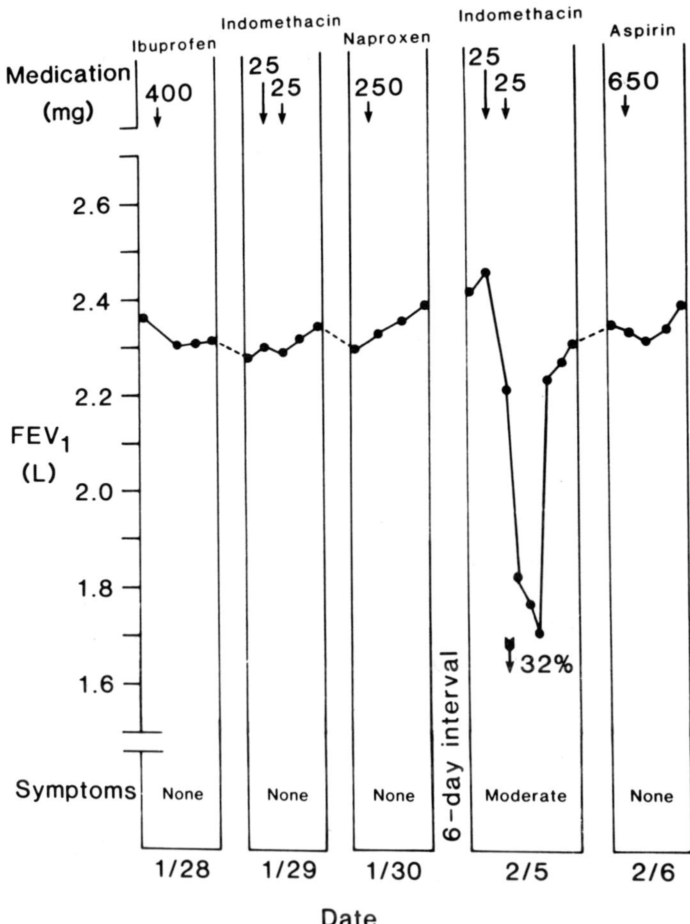

Fig. 29-7. Same patient as shown in Figure 29-4 on a consecutive day. Cross-intolerance to ibuprofen, indomethacin, and naproxen following aspirin desensitization; after a 6-day drug-free interval, sensitivity to indomethacin returned, and following desensitization with indomethacin, there was cross-tolerance for aspirin. From Pleskow, W. W., Stevenson, D. D., Mathison, D. A., Simon, R. A., Schatz, M., & Zeiger, R. S. *J. Allergy Clin. Immunol.*, 1982, 69, p. 17. With permission.

Tartrazine

Lockey first reported that tartrazine (FDC yellow dye number 5) could provoke asthma (Lockey, 1959). However, the incidence of tartrazine sensitivity in aspirin-sensitive asthmatics has not been definitely established. This is in part because data included cutaneous reactions to aspirin or required less rigorous criteria than we presently accept as sensitivity (Chafee & Settipane, 1967; Juhlin et al., 1972; Stenius & Lemola, 1976). In light of our data on the refractory period following an aspirin reaction, we wondered whether aspirin and tartrazine could cross-desensitize. If true, this might yield a false low incidence of tartrazine sensitivity in aspirin-sensitive individuals who may have had tartrazine challenges performed after a positive aspirin challenge and during their refractory periods. We therefore have begun to use tartrazine 25 mg as part of our "placebo" challenge *prior* to the aspirin challenge. The results of such challenges would indicate that tartrazine sensitivity seen in aspirin-sensitive asthma is unusual (less than 5%). We have not been able to establish whether there is cross-desensitization between aspirin and tartrazine. The low incidence and probably lack of cross-desensitization may relate to the fact that tartrazine is not a prostaglandin synthetase inhibitor (Gerger et al., 1979).

SPECTRUM OF RESPIRATORY RESPONSES TO ASPIRIN

Results of Initial Aspirin Challenges

Additional observations made by our group include the spectrum of respiratory reactions to aspirin in aspirin-sensitive individuals. In a study of 50 consecutive asthmatic patients with a history of aspirin sensitivity who underwent oral aspirin challenge, we found four types of response as illustrated on Table 29-2. Thirty-six of the 50 patients responded with a significant asthmatic reaction. Thirty-three of these 36 also developed a classic response with nasoocular complaints. Six patients who had distinct nasoocular complaints failed to meet our strict spirometric criteria for a positive asthmatic reaction to aspirin. (A fall in FEV_1 values of greater than or equal to 25%.) Three of these six patients developed asthmatic symptoms and had partial declines in FEV_1 values (falls of greater than 15% but less than 25%) and were classified as a "partial" asthmatic and nasal reactor. It should be noted that these patients failed to have a positive asthmatic response, even though their cumulative doses of aspirin exceeded 1 g. The other three patients had no significant change in FEV_1 values, despite their nasoocular complaints and well-documented asthma history.

Eight patients, despite an unequivocal history of aspirin sensitivity, had no

Table 29-2 *Results of Repeated Aspirin Challenges in 28 Aspirin-Sensitive Asthmatic Patients*

	Response(s)	
Number of Patients	Challenge 1	Challenge 2
18	Same	
3	Asthmatic-nasal	Nasal
3	Isolated asthmatic	Asthmatic-nasal
2	Asthmatic	No response
1	Asthmatic-nasal	No response—asthmatic-nasal
1	Nasal	Asthmatic-nasal—no response

discernible respiratory response whatsoever. Most interesting was the fact that two of these eight patients had previously demonstrated a positive asthmatic response to oral ingestion challenge in a double-blind placebo-controlled manner, performed at the Scripps Clinic in San Diego.

It is to be noted that in none of our aspirin challenges for asthma did we see any episodes of urticaria or angioedema.

Variability of Respiratory Response to Aspirin Following Repeat Aspirin Challenge

Twenty-eight of the 50 subjects studied have undergone two or more aspirin challenges at Scripps Clinic. Eighteen (61%) of the 28 patients had the same type of response on each aspirin challenge. The other 10 patients showed some variation in their responses on repeated challenges. Four patients went from a classic combined asthmatic and nasal response to no response at all. One of these patients later regained aspirin sensitivity on a subsequent challenge. Three patients who initially showed isolated asthmatic responses later exhibited the classic upper and lower respiratory response. One particularly interesting patient showed a full spectrum of reactions in which he had a pure nasal reaction, then a combined asthmatic and nasoocular response, and finally no response at all. We have no explanation for the variability of this phenomenon. As noted in the methods section in this chapter, we withhold antihistamines and cromolyn sodium for at least 24 hours prior to challenge. As noted earlier, we do not discontinue corticosteroids as a routine. However, we repeated the aspirin challenges in the group who became negative after an initial positive challenge, off systemic corticosteroids. At that time also there was a negative response.

We found that 25% of our patients with prior history of aspirin sensitivity later had negative aspirin challenges. It is also clear that almost all aspirin-sensitive asthmatics were able to tolerate aspirin at some time in their past (Samter & Beers, 1968).

Pure Nasal Response to Aspirin in Nonasthmatics

As noted in the beginning of the chapter, there are no generally accepted criteria for oral aspirin challenge in the diagnosis of aspirin sensitivity. Declines in FEV_1 values in the range 20–50% from baseline have been used during previous studies. We elected to consider a 25% decline in FEV_1 values as a positive response, but from the data presented, one now can recognize a respiratory reaction to aspirin in the absence of any asthmatic response when unmistakable nasoocular symptoms appear in the face of a double-blind placebo-controlled study. Furthermore, we have recently found six nonasthmatic subjects who have chronic rhinosinusitis and polyps who have no significant fall in FEV_1 values following inhalation of methacholine at up to 50 mg/ml (i.e., no bronchospastic tendency) who responded to oral aspirin challenges with dramatic nasoocular complaints, but no decline in FEV_1 values. We have proposed a broadening of the definition of respiratory aspirin sensitivity to include the purely rhinitic as well as the purely asthmatic response and classic dual reaction.

PATHOGENESIS OF ASPIRIN SENSITIVITY

Role of Mast Cell and Complement System

As noted earlier, there is no generally accepted hypothesis as to the pathogenesis of aspirin sensitivity. Although it is generally agreed that IgE mediated mechanisms are not responsible, the type of symptoms provoked and the reports of the protection from reaction afforded by inhalation of cromolyn and administration of the antihistamines have suggested a role for the respiratory mast cells. We investigated this possibility by measuring arterial and venous plasma levels of histamine, neutrophil chemotactic activity, and complement during oral aspirin challenges. Histamine and neutrophil chemotactic activities were measured as markers for mast cell activation, and complement activation was measured as a potential mechanism for activating mast cells through the anaphylatoxins C3a and C5a.

In summary, we are unable to find any evidence for activation of complement or mast cells during aspirin reactions. There were no significant levels of urinary histamine or arterial or venous plasma histamine, neutrophil chemotactic activity, or activation of complement in any of the 10 subjects tested. The inability to detect significant changes in plasma histamine or neutrophil chemotactic activity does not rule out the possibility that significant changes may have occurred at the target organ level. However, as changes in these mediators have been found in venous plasma following antigen inhalation challenge (Atkins et al., 1980; Bhat et al., 1976; Chandler et al., 1980), we feel that such an explanation is unlikely.

Role of Leukotriene (Slow Reacting Substance)

We have also investigated the possibility that aspirin sensitivity results from an overproduction of leukotrienes. This would occur from the shift in arachidonic acid metabolism from the cyclooxygenase pathway through the lipoxygenase pathway, following administration of aspirin or another NSAI, that cross-reacts with aspirin and inhibit prostaglandin synthetase activity via the cyclooxygenase pathway. We administered the agent benoxaprofen, a new NSAI that uniquely inhibits the lipoxygenase pathway (Walker & Dawson, 1979) to five aspirin sensitive asthmatics. The drug was administered in a manner which achieved plasma levels which, *in vitro*, have been shown to provide essentially 100% inhibition of leukotriene production in rat monocytes (Walker et al., 1980). Each of the aspirin-sensitive asthmatics was able to tolerate benoxaprofen administration without adverse effects. In addition, however, pretreatment with benoxaprofen did not prevent a typical nasoocular and asthmatic reaction to aspirin in any of the five patients. These data, although preliminary, would cast doubt on the theory that aspirin sensitivity results from increased production of leukotrienes, unless such metabolites can be generated from other sources or pathways that are not blocked by benoxaprofen given in this manner. Furthermore, no present mechanism can explain why only a subpopulation of asthmatics are sensitive to aspirin and why the phenomena of desensitization, refractory period, and the spectrum of responses would exist.

ASPIRIN TREATMENT OF ASPIRIN-SENSITIVE ASTHMA

We have recently reported a double blind cross-over study of the treatment with aspirin-sensitive patients with rhinosinusitis asthma (Stevenson et al., 1984). The study group of 25 ASA-sensitive patients with rhinosinusitis asthma were challenged and then desensitized to the adverse respiratory effects of ASA. The efficacy of continuous ASA administration for respiratory tract disease was compared with placebo treatment during this double blind cross-over study. The data from this group of patients indicated that desensitization to ASA followed by continuous ASA treatment appears to significantly alleviate the symptoms of two-thirds of the patients with rhinosinusitis. However, only one-half of the patients with asthma experienced evidence of improvement.

SUMMARY

Aspirin-sensitive asthmatics represent an interesting subpopulation of up to one-third of all asthmatics, depending on how they are selected. Oral aspirin challenges can provoke significant asthma, and such challenges are rarely indicated for routine diagnostic reasons. For those asthmatic patients who require treatment with aspirin or other cross-reacting NSAIs, aspirin challenge, and if positive, aspirin desensitization may be warranted. We have found that aspirin desensitization and treatment may be useful in selected patients with aspirin sensitivity.

Case History

A 38-year-old housewife, M. L., who had no history of atopic disorders such as hay fever, asthma, or eczema in childhood, first recalls the onset of nasal symptoms during one of her three pregnancies, when she was in her early twenties. At that time she developed watering of her eyes and nose, sneezing, and nasal congestion that she interpreted to be an upper respiratory infection. During that same year she developed a pruritic, dry eruption in the flexor surfaces of her arms and legs, which seemed to be exacerbated by the ingestion of fish. This cutaneous eruption has resolved.

About 2 years after the onset of her nasal symptoms, she began to notice "slight wheezing." Following the ingestion of an Alka Seltzer tablet, M. L. developed a severe asthmatic reaction that resulted in an emergency room visit. She did not correlate the asthma attack with the Alka Seltzer ingestion and took aspirin several times subsequently. It was not until she had a significant nasoocular and asthmatic reaction following the ingestion of a single pediatric aspirin tablet that she recognized aspirin did in fact precipitate rather severe episodes of asthma.

Three or four years after the onset of her nasal complaints, M. L. underwent her first nasal polypectomy. She has subsequently had an additional 15 polypectomies, the most recent 2 years ago. She has also undergone bilateral antrostomies during that procedure.

She has undergone a formal allergy evaluation on two occasions. The first, approximately 15 years ago, reportedly revealed cutaneous tests that showed significant levels of allergic antibody, although she could not remember exactly to what substances. She was given a treatment program with hyposensitization injections but after a period of about 3 years noted no improvement. Her cutaneous tests were repeated about 5 years ago, and she was informed that she had no significant reactivity.

She continues to have lower respiratory problems, but she considers her asthma difficulties only "mild." There are many days when she does not need any medication for asthma and states that only when she "does something to cause asthma" does she have difficulty. Asthma-provoking factors include exposure to nonspecific environmental irritants and exercise. She does not describe asthma difficulties following URIs.

Asthma medications include an alupent inhaler used on an as-needed (prn) basis about every 1–2 hours with severe attacks, but on most days she does not require this medication at all.

Because of her nasal complaints, she has had several 10–14-day courses of prednisone during the past year. These prednisone courses would usually begin with about 20 mg/day and taper over 1–2 weeks. Her nasal symptoms clear with prednisone but invariably recur when the steroids have been discontinued. In addition, she uses Actifed on an as-needed basis, usually up to 4 times per day. As recently as a week prior to her initial evaluation at Scripps Clinic she was placed on a topical corticosteroid spray, which she thinks is beneficial.

Her past medical history was remarkable for generalized urticaria 30 minutes following the injection of penicillin. She underwent an exploratory laparotomy in 1977 for an infected fallopian tube. Her family history was remarkable for some vague nasal complaints in her mother, but otherwise there was no family history of atopic disorders or other respiratory diseases.

Pertinent physical findings included vital signs with a temperature of 98.2°F, pulse 80 and regular, respirations 20 and unlabored, and blood pressure 140/86. She was well oriented and in no acute distress, with an obvious nasal twang to her voice. The tympanic membranes were unremarkable. Ocular examination revealed intact extraocular movements with normal fundi. The nasal mucous membranes were quite congested with profuse mucoid rhinorrhea noted. There was essentially total obstruction to airflow on the left and moderate to severe obstruction on the right. Abundant polypoid tissue was present. Sinus transilluminate again revealed adequate transillumination of both frontal sinuses but essentially no transillumination in the maxillary sinuses. The oral pharynx was unremarkable. The neck revealed no jugular venous distention, paramegaly, masses, or bruits. The lungs revealed symmetric chest expansion bilaterally with a faint forced expiratory wheeze in both lung fields. Cardiac examination revealed a regular rhythm, normal S_1 and S_2 without gallop, murmur, or rub.

Significant studies included a nasal smear that was loaded with eosinophils. Cutaneous tests for immediate hypersensitivity failed to reveal significant levels of reaginic antibodies. Lung function tests revealed a normal forced vital capacity. The FEV_1 was decreased at 2.32 liters (predicted 2.66). This increased to 2.74 following inhalation of isoetharine by IPPB. The initial forced expiratory flow at 25–75% of the forced vital capacity was 1.67 (predicted 3.07). This increased to 2.92 following inhalation of isoetharine. Paranasal sinus x-rays revealed essentially complete opacification of both maxillary sinuses. Our initial impressions were of aspirin-sensitive rhinosinusitis and asthma and history suggestive of anaphylactic sensitivity to penicillin.

The patient was placed on a course of prednisone in preparation for bilateral Caldwell-Luc antrostomies, intranasal ethmoidectomies, and polypectomies.

After recovery from surgery and a 1-month trial period of intranasal beclomethasone, M. L. entered our double-blind, placebo-controlled crossover study of aspirin treatment for aspirin-sensitive asthma.

According to the protocol outlined in this chapter, M. L. was admitted to our General Clinical Research Center and following a negative placebo challenge was given 30 mg of aspirin. There was a 27% decrease in the FEV_1 value along with typical nasoocular and chest complaints. She experienced seven reactions to 30 mg of aspirin before she was able to tolerate that dose. She then had reactions at each dose of our graded challenges and ultimately required 15 challenges before she was desensitized (able to tolerate 650 mg of aspirin without symptoms or change in FEV_1 values). She was discharged on her study medication.

REFERENCES

Atkins, P. C., Rosenblum, F., Dunsky, E. H., Coffey, R., & Zweiman, D. *J. All. Clin. Immunol.*, 1980, *66*, 478.

Basomba, A., Romer, A., Pelaez, A., Villalmanzo, I. G., & Campos, A. *Clin. Allergy*, 1976, *6*, 269.

Bhat, K. N., Arroyave, C. M., Marney, S. R., Jr., Stevenson, D. D., & Tan, E. M. *J. Allergy Clin. Immunol.*, 1976, *58*, 647.

Bianco, S., Robuschi, M., & Petrini, D. *J. Med. Sci.*, 1977, *5*(3), 129.

Chafee, F. H., & Settipane, G. A. *J. Allergy Clin. Immunol.*, 1967, *40*, 65.

Chandler, Deal, E., Jr., Waserman, S. I., Soter, N. A., Ingram, R. H., Jr., & McFadden, E. R., Jr. *J. Clin. Invest.*, 1980, *65*, 659.

Cooke, R. A. *JAMA*, 1919, *73*, 759.

Gerger, J. G., Payne, N. A., Oelz, O., Nies, A. S., & Oates, J. A. *J. Allergy Clin. Immunol.*, 1979, *63*, 289.

Goetzl, E. J. *New Engl. J. Med.*, 1980, *303*, 822.

Hamburg, M., & Samuelsson, B. *Proc. Natl. Acad. Sci (USA)*, 1974, *71*, 3400.

Juhlin, L., Michaelsson, G., & Zettersstrom, O. *J. Allergy Clin. Immunol.*, 1972, *50*, 92.

Lockey, S. D. *Ann. Allergy*, 1959, *17*, 719.

Martelli, N. A. *Am. Rev. Resp. Dis.*, 1979, *120*, 1073.

Mathison, D. A., Pleskow, W. W., Simon, R. A., & Stevenson, D. D. In S. L. Spector (Ed.), *Aspirin and chemical sensitivities and challenges in asthmatic patients*, in press.

McDonald, J. R., Mathison, D. A., & Stevenson, D. D. *J. All. Clin. Immunol.*, 1972, *50*, 198.

Parker, C. W. *J. All. Clin. Immunol.*, 1979, *63*, 1.

Pleskow, W. W., Stevenson, D. D., Mathison, D. A., Simon, R. A., Schatz. M., & Zeiger, R. S. *J. Allergy Clin. Immunol.*, 1982, *69*, 11.

Samter, M., & Beers, R. F. *Ann. Intern. Med.*, 1968, *68*, 975.

Schlumberger, H. D., Lobbeck, E. A., & Kallos, B. *Acta Med. Scand.*, 1974, *196*, 451.

Settipane, G. A., Chafee, F. H., & Klein, D. E. *J. All. Clin. Immunol.*, 1974, *53*, 200.

Spector, S. L., Wangaard, C. H., & Farr, R. S. *J. Allergy Clin. Immunol.*, 1979, *64*, 500.

Stenius, B. S., & Lemola, N. *Clin. Allergy*, 1976, *6*, 119.

Stevenson, D. D., Pleskow, W. W., Simon, R. A., Mathison, D. A., Lumry, W. R., Schatz, M., Zeiger, R. S. *J. All. Clin. Immunol.*, 1984, *73*, (4) 500.

Szczeklik, A., Gryglewski, R. J., & Czerniawslea-Mysik, G. *J. All. Clin. Immunol.*, 1977, *60*, 276

Tauber, A. I., Kaliner, M., Stechschulte, D. J., & Austen, K. F. *J. Immunol.*, 1973, *111*, 27.

Vane, J. R. *Nature New Biol.*, 1971, *231*, 232.

Walker, J. R., & Dawson, W. J. *J. Pharm. Pharmacol.*, 1979, *31*, 778.

Walker, J. R., Booe, J. R., Cox, B., & Dawson, W. *J. Pharm. Pharmacol.*, 1980, *32*, 866.

Widal, N. F., Abramin, C., & Lermoyez, J. *Press Med.*, 1922, *30*, 189.

Wuthrich, D. *Respiration*, 1979, *37*, 224.

Yurchak, A. M., Wicher, K., & Arbesman, C. W. *J. Allergy Clin. Immunol.*, 1970, *46*, 245.

Zeiss, C. R., & Lockey, R. F. *J. Allergy Clin. Immunol.*, 1976, 57, 440.

SUGGESTED READINGS

Chafee, F. H. & Settipane, G. A. *J. Allergy Clin. Immunol.*, 1974, *53*, 193.

Farr, R. S., Spector, S. L. & Wanguard, C. *Ann. Int. Med.*, 1978, *59*, 577.

Kordansky, D., Atkins, N. F., Norman, P. S. & Rosenthal, R. R. *Ann. Int. Med.*, 1978, *88*, 508.

Sczceklik, A. & Serwonska, M. *Thorax*, 1979, *34*, 654.

Smith, A. P. *Br. Med. J.*, 1971, *1*, 494.

Vedanthan, P. K., Menon, M. M., Bell, T. E. & Bergin, D. *J. Allergy Clin. Immunol.*, 1977, *60*, 8.

QUESTIONS

1. Aspirin-sensitive asthmatics are also likely to react to which of the following medications?
   a. Indomethacin
   b. Zomepirac sodium
   c. Percodan
   d. Sulindac
2. Aspirin-sensitive asthmatics can have which of the following reactions to aspirin?
   a. Asthma, rhinoconjunctivitis
   b. Rhinoconjunctivitis alone
   c. Asthma alone
   d. No reaction
   e. All of the above
3. Which of the following statements concerning aspirin-sensitive asthmatics is true?
   a. Aspirin-sensitive asthmatics should avoid dietary salicylates.
   b. By avoiding aspirin and related compounds, aspirin-sensitive asthmatics have marked clinical improvement.
   c. Aspirin sensitivity is an IgE-mediated disorder, so aspirin-sensitive asthmatics commonly have multiple other allergies.
   d. None of the above.
4. Which of the following statements concerning aspirin sensitivity are correct?
   a. Of all asthmatics, 8–14% are aspirin-sensitive.
   b. Of asthmatics with polyps and sinusitis, 35% are aspirin-sensitive.
   c. Patients with asthma, sinusitis, and polyps who have tolerated aspirin in the past may continue to take aspirin without risk.
   d. None of the above.
5. Which of the following statements concerning aspirin sensitivity are true?
   a. Aspirin challenges are safe to perform in an outpatient office setting.
   b. Following a positive aspirin reaction, most aspirin-sensitive asthmatics become refractory to further adverse effects of aspirin for a period of 2–5 days.
   c. There are nonasthmatic subjects with chronic rhinosinusitis with or without polyps who respond to aspirin with dramatic nasoocular reactions, but no asthma.
   d. None of the above.

Answers can be found in Appendix B at the end of the book.

PART 7

Pediatric Allergies

Donald B. Strominger

30

Evaluation of the "Wheezy" Infant and Child

He flung himself from the room, flung himself upon his horse and rode madly off in all directions.

Leacock

As with the approach to any disease state, the evaluation of the child with repeated bouts of respiratory distress should be meaningful and methodical. Often this patient's problem does not have an allergic basis and other underlying pathologies must be evaluated thoroughly. With our increasing understanding of the basic anatomy and physiology of the respiratory system, and the availability of sophisticated laboratory tests it is possible in a great majority of infants and children, however, to define the precise nature of the problem and treat it effectually. Since children with recurrent respiratory problems may not wheeze, this chapter includes a discussion of all conditions causing chronic and/or recurrent respiratory distress. In the small infant or child the interrelationship of (a) bronchial constriction, (b) mucus plugging, and (c) infection tends to confuse the picture. The airways are so small that any one of the three may and frequently does bring on the other two, masking the primary cause of the patient's problem. Moreover, it is also possible to be so bogged down with laboratory data that the disease or problem is not evident. This discussion deals with the variety of lesions that must be considered and sought.

ANATOMICAL

Congenital defects may occur at any level of the airway. Frequently symptoms are present from birth, although they may not become apparent until later in life when complications arise and make them more obvious.

Anomalies of the upper airway are not common but must be considered. Complete choanal atresia (Fig. 30-1) may occur and be life-threatening. Since the newborn

ALLERGY: THEORY AND PRACTICE
ISBN 0-8089-1619-X

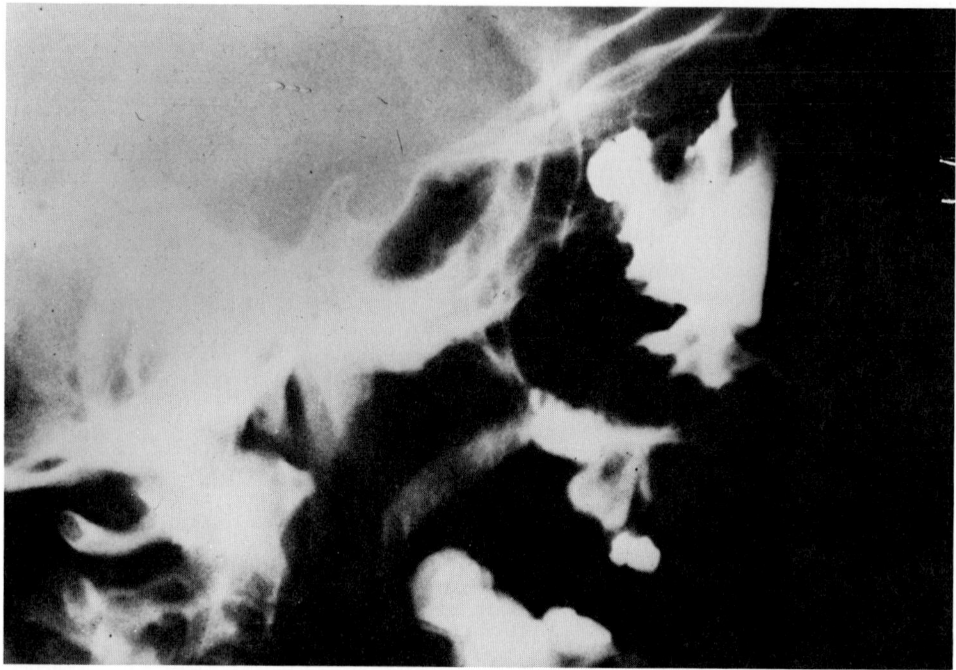

Fig. 30-1. Choanal atresia. The roentgenograph demonstrates complete choanal atresia. Radiocontrast media injected into the naris is unable to pass into the nasopharynx.

is an obligate nose breather, the mouth may have to be forced open and the tongue pressed down as an emergency measure. Partial atresia and anomalies of the nares cause almost immediate wheezing respirations. Rarely a deviated septum will cause the same problem. In this type of obstruction the wheezing is both inspiratory and expiratory.

Less dramatic but more frequent are anomalies of the palate. A cleft palate is usually diagnosed at the time of the first examination. High-arched palates may cause obstruction giving rise to symptoms similar to a partial choanal atresia. When the high-arched palate is combined with a small mandible (micrognathia) and a large tongue (macroglossia), the triad is called the *Pierre Robin syndrome*. Surgical intervention is sometimes necessary to prevent choking on the tongue. Short soft palate may give rise to problems with deglutition, resulting in chronic aspiration and causing intermittent wheezing (especially during and after meals) or intermittent aspiration pneumonia, which usually occurs in the upper lobes in infants. Conversely, an elongated uvula may give rise to a chronic cough. Malignant and benign tumors are a rare cause of upper airway obstruction. *Encephalocele* should be looked for in infants with symptoms starting at birth. Nasal polyps can be seen in infants and children and may point to cystic fibrosis (CF) as well as allergy.

Midairway lesions involve larynx, vocal cords, and trachea. Paralysis of the vocal cords may occur at birth and cause wheezing, stridor, or alterations in phonation. This can be caused by trauma directly to the larynx or injury to the recurrent laryngeal nerve. The paralysis may be unilateral or bilateral and is usually of short duration. Paralysis and/or spasm may also occur as a result of hypocalcemia (tetany of the newborn) and a variety of metabolic conditions. Laryngospasm with stridor and wheezing is not as common a manifestation as generalized irritability and tremors. Tetanus neonatorum may present in this manner, or the cause may be idiopathic hypocalcemia, hypoparathyroidism associated with DiGeorge's syndrome, high phosphate loads from improper formulas, or other conditions. Midairway obstruction can result from these lesions and may be a secondary symptom. Chest x-rays may be normal, and examination of the ears, nose, and throat may not be rewarding. If the index of suspicion is high, blood chemistries and direct laryngoscopy should be performed.

Laryngeal webs may cause varying degrees of obstruction and can also be diagnosed, usually by direct visualization. Tumors, including hemangiomas and papillomas, may occur in any area, causing varying degrees of obstructive symptoms. Rarely an anomalous bronchus (Fig. 30-2) may originate from the trachea (bronchus suis, "pig bronchus") and result in recurrent pneumonias with wheezing. In addition, the trachea may have a congenital stenosis or may be compressed by aortic arch anomalies (Fig 30-3).

Malacias (laryngomalacia, tracheomalacia, and bronchomalacia) occur in the airways as a result of delayed hardening of the cartilage and causing collapse with stridorous breathing during periods of negative pressure. The problem is present early in life and is self-limited usually by age 3 or 4. A much rarer syndrome is the

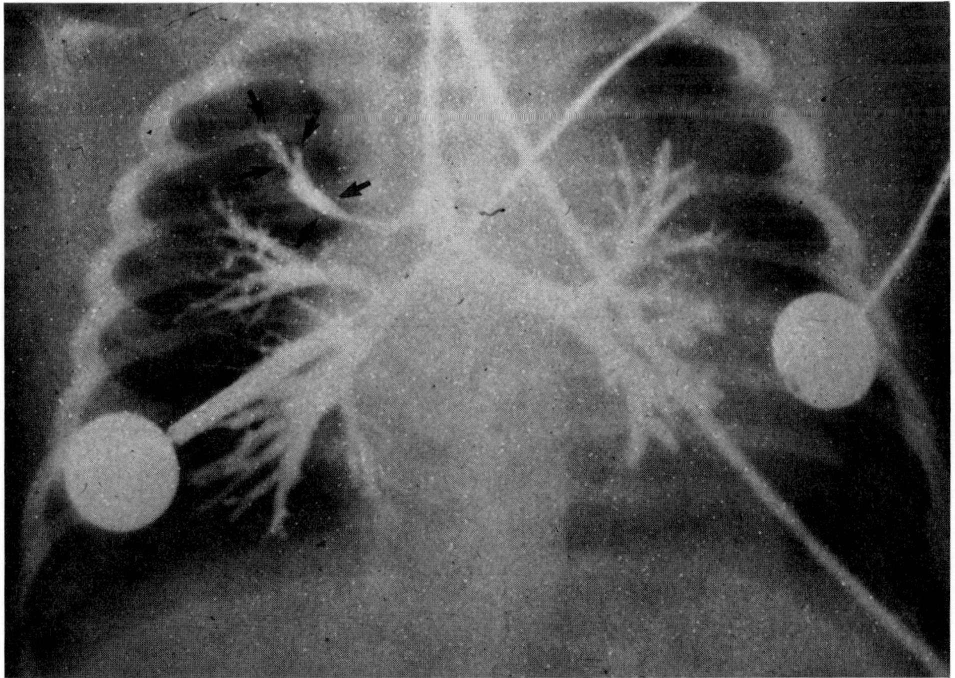

Fig. 30-2. Bronchogram of a patient with an anomalous bronchus. This patient presented with a history of episodic wheezing and recurrent pneumonias. The bronchogram demonstrated an anomalous bronchus (arrow) which originated above the origin of the right main stem bronchus.

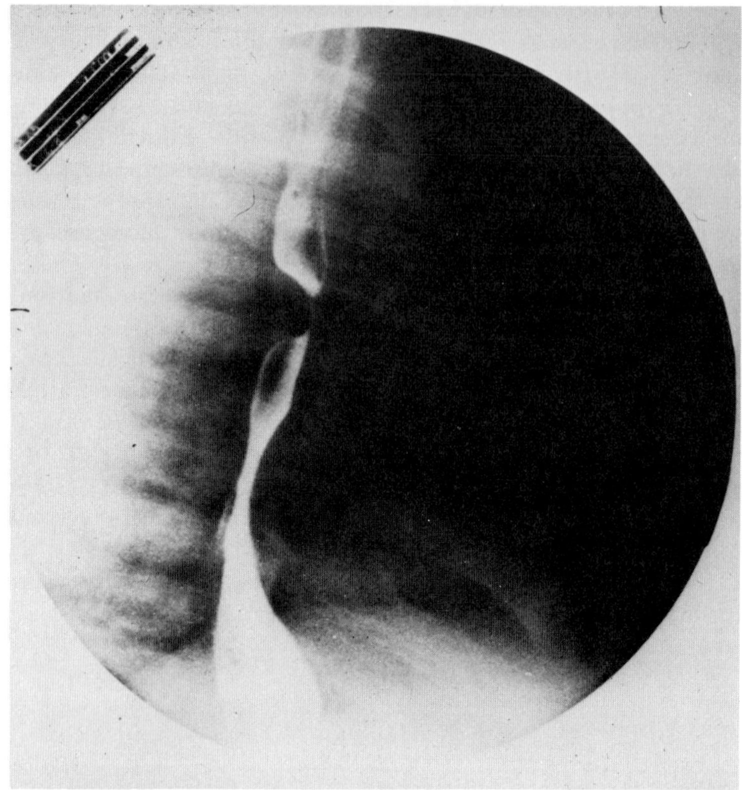

Fig. 30-3. Chest roentgenograph showing compression of the trachea in a patient with aortic arch anomalies.

complete absence of tracheal or bronchial cartilage, which has similar symptomatology.

Chondrodystrophia calcificans congenita (Conradi's disease) is a rare congential chondrodysplasia that has other dysmorphic features, with respiratory embarrassment caused by a narrow trachea and bronchus. Tracheal stenosis can be primary or in association with a tracheal esophageal (TE) fistula. These can be life-threatening when the esophagus ends in a blind pouch or there is obligate passage of food through the airway. Only in the "H"-type TE fistula may the lesion be small and cause pneumonia or intermittent respiratory distress (usually with or after feeding). This lesion may pass undetected until special radiographic techniques are employed to demonstrate a small communication between the esophagus and the trachea.

The TE fistula may be associated with anomalies of the vertebra, aortic arch, and rectum (imperforate anus); this combination is called *Vater's syndrome* and has been described with many other anomalies. Aortic arch anomalies (Fig. 30-4), whether in association with the Vater syndrome or alone, may cause extensive pressure on the trachea, or the vascular channel may be compromised, causing resultant respiratory symptoms.

Lower airways vascular abnormalities may occur in the lungs (nonpulmonary, from the aorta), giving rise to sequested lobes (Fig. 30-5). Anomalies airways (bron-

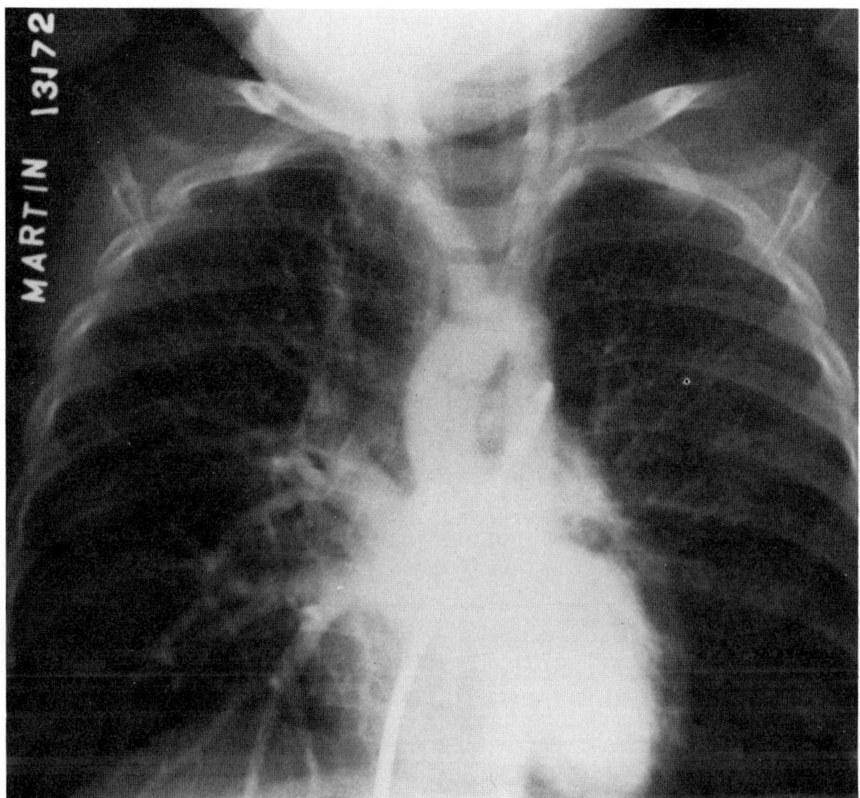

Fig. 30-4. A patient with Vater's Syndrome. This angiographic study demonstrates marked anomalies of the aortic arch.

chus suis) give rise to lung tissue and so-called tracheal lobes. Congenital cysts may rise and frequently enlarge, causing respiratory embarrassment. The argument as to whether these are penumatoceles or true congenital cysts is not germane to this discussion. It is important that they may arise in the lung parenchyma, causing compression and shift, or in the airway, causing obstructive symptoms of lobar emphysema or atelectasis. Other cysts may be in the form of bullous emphysema resulting from either traumatic (mechanical ventilation) or inflammatory origin.

Congenital lobar emphysema occurs in the left upper lobe in more than half the cases and frequently requires resection because of respiratory embarrassment. It may be associated with congenital heart diseases. Agenesis of the lung or hypoplasia may occur spuriously but more likely in association with other defects. The lesions may be silent or may be evident within several hours of birth. Acquired hypoplasia may result from a pulmonary insult early in life, causing developmental arrest.

Traumatic lesions are usually obvious, but any child who has had intubation can develop recurrent upper airway problems. Central nervous system (CNS) injury at birth when involving the respiratory center may cause immediate problems. Phrenic nerve paralysis is not uncommon.

Foreign bodies (Fig 30-6) may lodge at almost any level of the airway from the nose to the periphery. They occur most commonly in toddlers, but older children

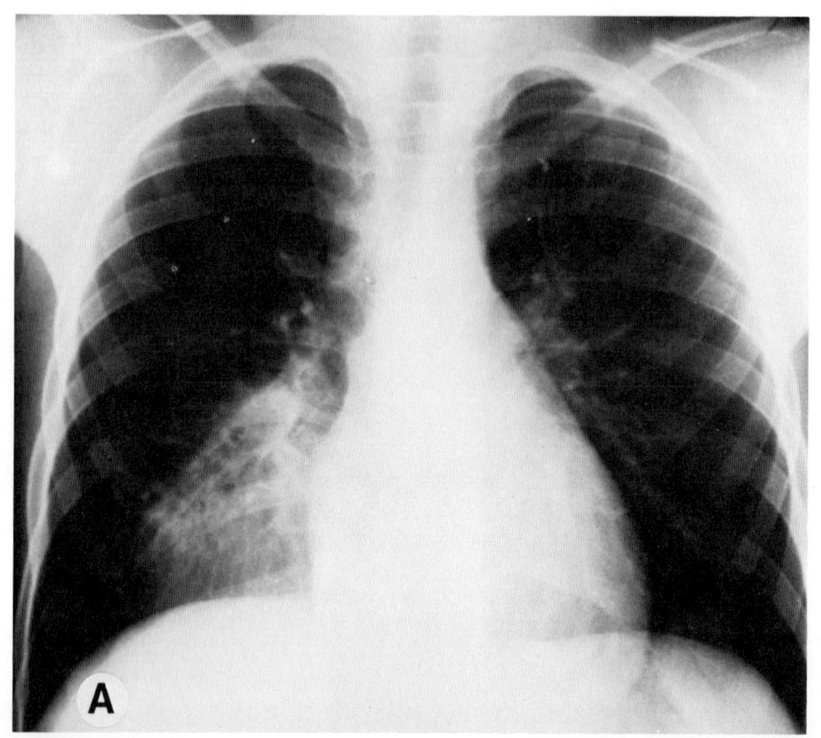
A

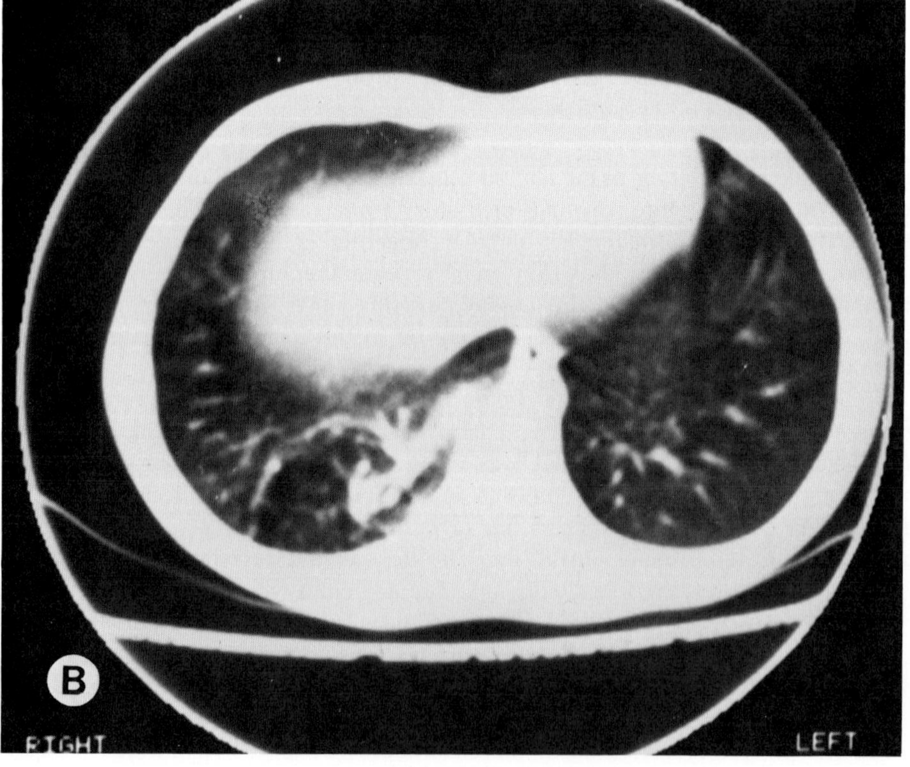
B
RIGHT
LEFT

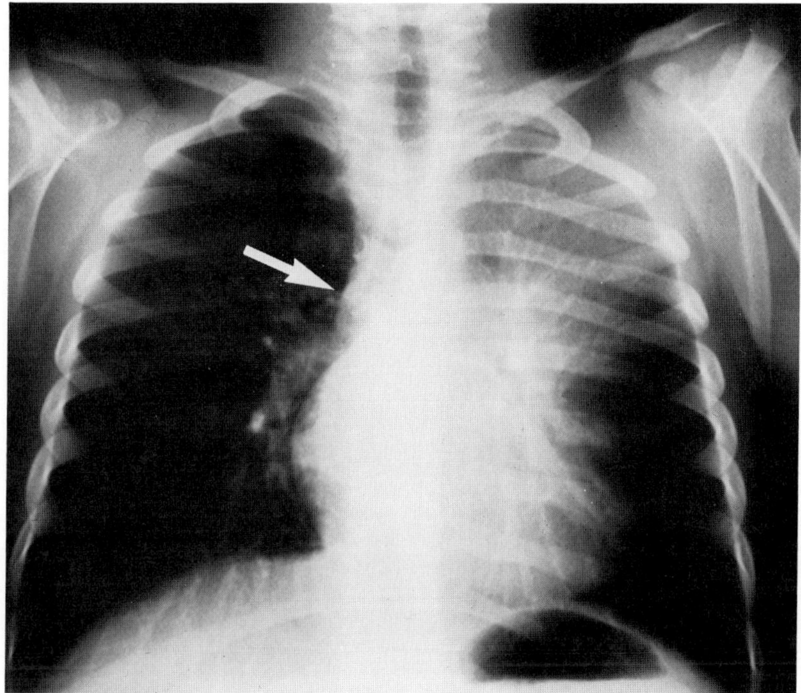

Fig. 30-6. Chest roentgenogram of a patient with a peanut lodged in the right main stem bronchus. The arrow points to the area of obstruction.

may occasionally aspirate and infants may have foreign materials poked at them by older siblings. Very rarely are they asymptomatic. Esophageal foreign bodies (Fig. 30-7) should be sought if the index of suspicion is high. Inhalation of chemicals is an ever-increasing problem and causes diffuse radiographic findings of chemical pneumonia.

INFECTIONS

Recurrence of severe bacterial infections usually have some underlying defect—anatomic, physiologic, immunologic, or biochemical. Viral infections, when caused by the respiratory syncytial virus (RSV), may recur commonly. The RSV is the most frequent cause of bronchiolitis (one-third) in the infant; thus the theories that recurrent bronchiolitis is probably asthma may not be true. Since the infant or small child may have edema and swelling of the small airway, a therapeutic trial with bronchodialators or epinephrine (Adrenalin) is not helpful when negative.

Fig. 30-5. **A,** A chest roentgenogram of a patient with lower airway vascular anomalies resulting in a sequested lobe. The patient presented with recurrent pneumonias as demonstrated in this x-ray. **B,** CAT scan of the patient seen in Figure 1 demonstrating the area of the vascular anomalies and sequested lobe.

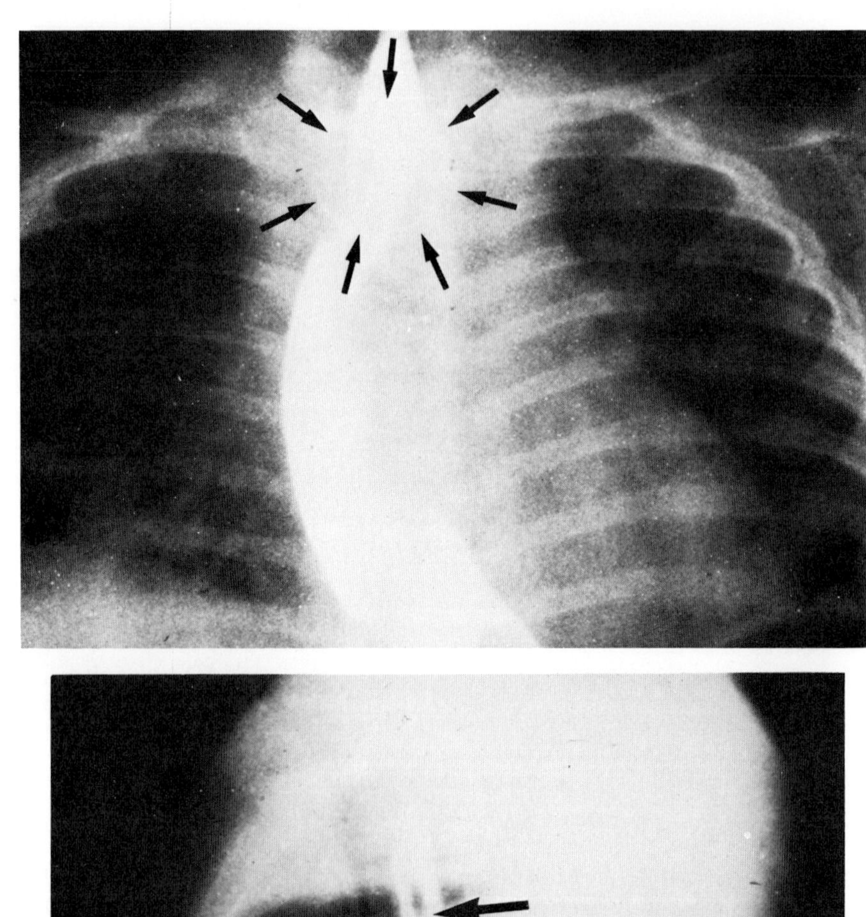

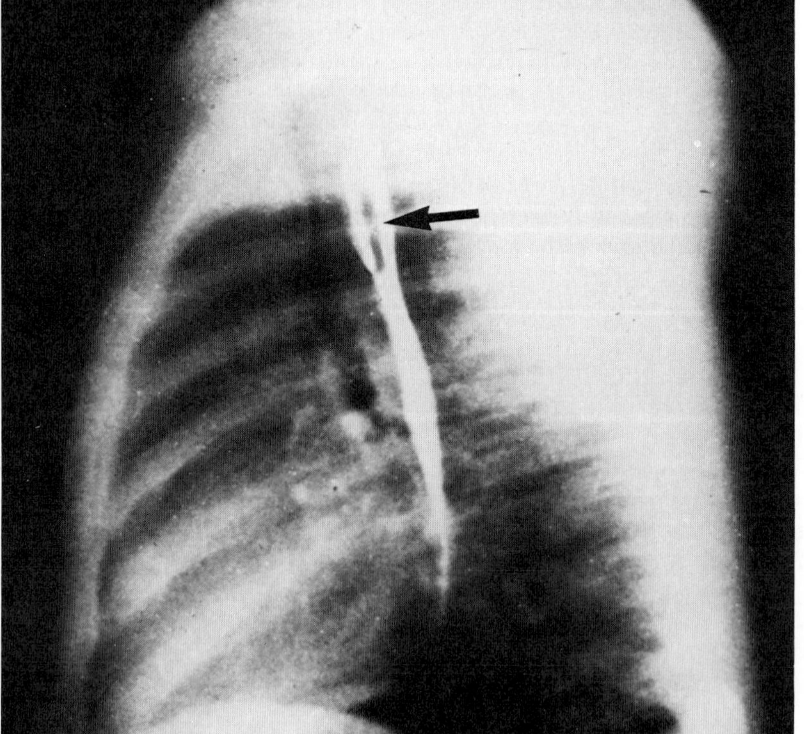

Fig. 30-7. Esophageal foreign body. P.A. (**A**) and lateral (**B**) views of a patient with a coin lodged in the esophagus.

The other myxoviruses (influenza and parainfluenza) usually give rise to croup and upper respiratory symptoms, but as with the RSV, may recur. They less commonly cause bronchiolitis. Adenoviruses are rarely recurrent but can also cause broncholitis. Possibly as a genetic or immunologic variant, adenoviral broncholitis (types 7 and 21) frequently can be fatal or produce bronchiolitis obliterans. When the process is limited to one lobe, a unilateral hyperlucent lung (Sawyer-James's syndrome) may develop.

BIOCHEMICAL

A variety of biochemical diseases may give rise to chronic lung symptoms. These usually are the result of the development of malnutrition, caused by treatment or lack thereof. Although any part of the immune system may be upset, T cells are greatly affected. As a result of the altered immune system, recurrent broncholitis and pneumonia may occur.

α_1-Antitrypsin disease, when it occurs, may be associated with infantile hepatitis

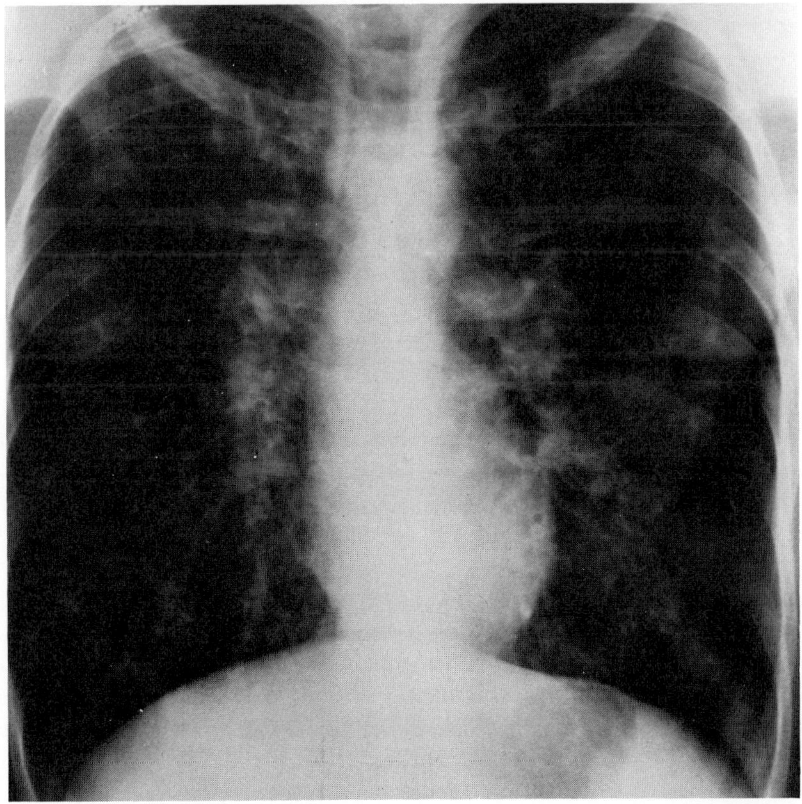

Fig. 30-8. Chest roentgenogram of a patient with cystic fibrosis. The roentgenogram demonstrates marked chronic lung disease with severe saccular bronchiectasis common in patients with cystic fibrosis.

or cirrhosis. Reports concerning the morbidity of α_1-antitrypsin heterozygotes disease have not been substantiated, but there is evidence that in some instances it may be particularly responsible for pulmonary dysfunction.

Cystic fibrosis (CF) (Fig. 30-8) is the most important genetic disease in the United States because of both frequency (1 : 20 adults are carriers, and 1 : 1600 live births are CF patients) and severity (the second leading cause of death in children). The outcome is greatly improved by early diagnosis and initiation of treatment. A properly performed sweat test by the Gibson-Cooke quantitative pilocarpine iontophoresis technique, done in a laboratory that regularly performs the test, is essential for making the diagnosis.

Cystic fibrosis may present in the first few days of life, with mild symptoms of nasal congestion or cough. The presentation may be more dramatic with pneumonia or atelectasis. Infants frequently have a severe broncholitis-like picture. In this instance steroids are life-saving. The outlook has been reported as being poor, this has not been our experience.

The usual hallmarks of malnutrition, diarrhea, and pneumonia may or may not be present. The clinician must be aware that children with CF can have excellent nutrition and only mild, intermittent wheezing. It is also important to remember that symptoms of CF may simulate those of IgE-mediated allergy, and 40% of CF patients have reactions to common allergens by skin testing. Thus a positive evaluation for allergens does not alleviate the need for a sweat test.

Hypocalcemia may occur, causing upper airway embarrassment; this has been discussed above.

PHYSIOLOGIC

In the newborn, tachypnea may result from birth injury to the phrenic nerve, causing paralysis of the diaphragm. Paradoxic respirations may occur. This condition is usually self-limited, and recovery occurs in a matter of weeks to months.

Tachycardia may cause tachypnea and shortness of breath, to some degree the result of hypoxia. The variety of cardiac malformations that might cause this is beyond the scope of this discussion. Unusually, arrhythmias may act in a similar way. With the Wolf-Parkinson-White (WPW) syndrome, intermittent symptoms may occur with each episode, and in the small child who cannot give a history, the diagnosis can be hidden.

Abnormalities of the respiratory cilia (ciliary dyskinesis) may occur. The physiologic clearing of the airway is by means of the mucociliary ladder. Debris settles on the mucous blanket in the tracheobronchial tree, and by waves of ciliary beating the mucus is slowly raised out of the airway and either swallowed or expectorated. Clearing from the peripheral airway occurs in less than 24 hours. Abnormal or absent beating occurs in the immotile cilia syndrome (ICS). Mucus remains in the airways and becomes infected, leading to bronchiectasis. Other organs that require mucous flow such as the sinuses may also be severely affected. It is thought that this rhythmic beating of the cilia *in utero* causes normal orientation of the organs in the fetus. Therefore, it would be expected that half of the patients with ICS present with Kartagener's syndrome (bronchiectasis, sinusitis, and situs inversus) (Fig. 30-9). Such patients may present early with only a chronic productive cough.

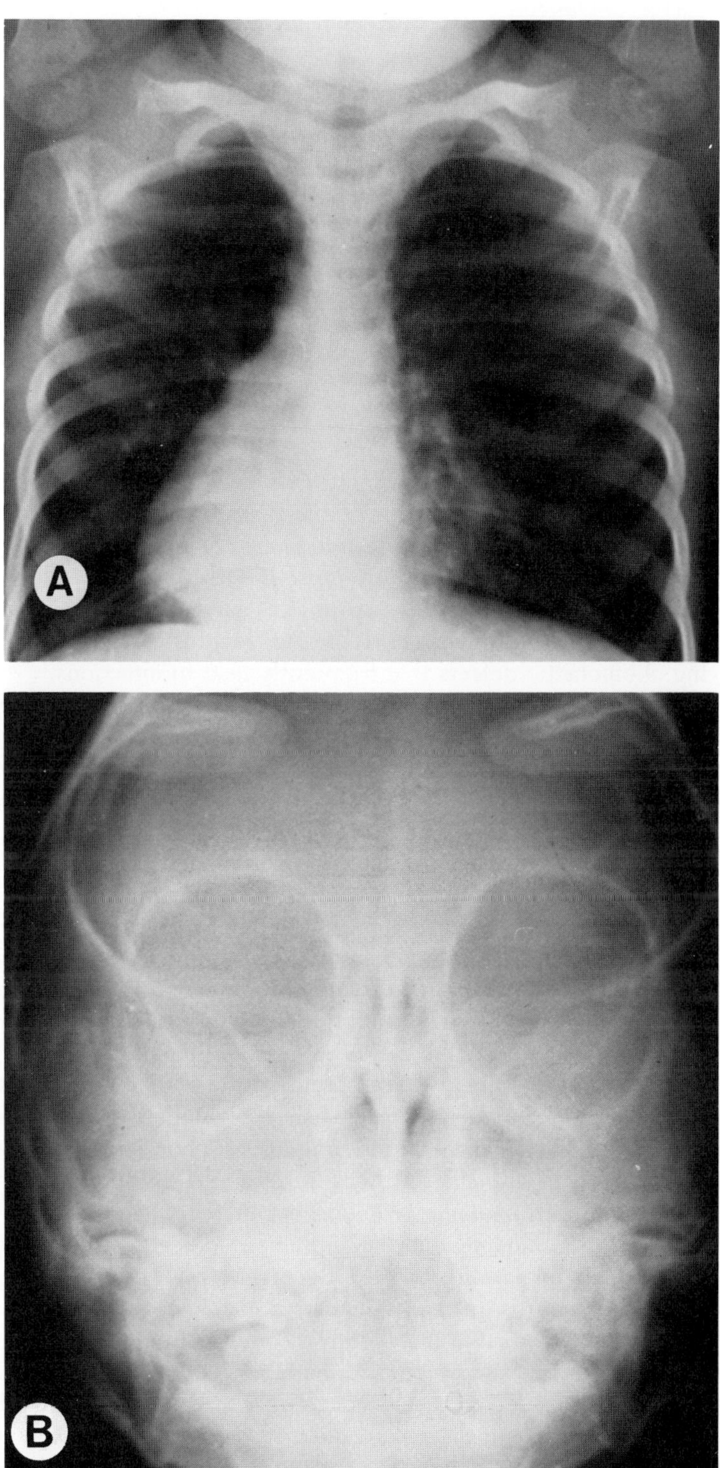

Fig. 30-9. A patient with Kartagener's syndrome. **A** demonstrates situs inversus in this young child and figure **B** demonstrates the severe sinusitis associated with this condition.

Chronic aspiration in the newborn infant or child can lead to wheezing, coughing, and pneumonia. Defects of deglutition, neurologic or anatomic, commonly cause such symptoms. Gastroesophageal reflux (GER) is common. Patients are now being recognized because of more sophisticated techniques (pH probes, esophagometry, and esophagoscopy) as well as by barium swallows. Of all these, the pH probe is the most sensitive. Patients with GER may develop recurrent pneumonia and wheezing. There is evidence that theophylline may cause GER by relaxing the gastroesophageal sphincter.

IMMUNOLOGIC

Defects of the immune system can give rise to recurrent infections; these are discussed in Chapter 31. Some may not be life-threatening and produce symptoms similar to many of the above conditions. White blood cell defects (chronic granulomas disease, chemotactic defects, etc.) usually present with relatively isolated lesions of the skin. Patients with underlying allergic problems may manifest symptoms confused with those of Buckley's syndrome, where the IgE level is extremely high, but with accompanying chemotactic defects that frequently lead to infections.

Patients with B-cell defects with abnormalities of immunoglobulins may present with repeated respiratory infections. There is a physiologic period of hypogammaglobulinemia at about 6 months when maternal IgG is disappearing and the infant's IgG has not yet developed. Children frequently develop respiratory problems at this time. Gamma globulin levels may be normal where subgroup abnormalities occur, or "blind" spots in the immune system may be present. Some adenovirus infections are not handled normally in certain genetic populations, and bronchiolitis obliterating, hypolucent lung, and a Sawyer-James-type abnormalities may occur.

Isolated IgA absence is not uncommon and has been described in association with a high incidence of circulating milk precipitins. Milk precipitins may also be found in Heiner's syndrome with increased IgA and pulmonary hemosiderosis, which also may be idiopathic and have periods of exacerbation and remission.

When the immune globulin system is completely absent (Bruton's syndrome), severe infections result, and death may occur early unless gamma globulin and antibiotics are administered. Even so, the prognosis is poor. T-cell defects in infants and children are often first diagnosed because of a severe pulmonary infection. A variety of interrelated immunologic problems occur (e.g., DiGeorge syndrome, intermittent variable immunodeficiency, complement defects) and are discussed in another section of this book (Chapter 31). Recurrent wheezing is found in various hypersensitivity pneumonitis diseases (Chapter 23).

Atopic (type I hypersensitivity) is the most common immunologic problem seen in the pediatric age group, and atopic asthma is probably the most common cause of wheezing or respiratory distress in this age group. When evaluating the patient with respiratory distress, atopic disease should be considered, but last. It is important to remember that allergy may be the predominent cause of the problem; it may be a contributory factor, or may have no role at all. Indeed, even a positive atopic evaluation does not mean that the allergy caused the problems, and it is very easy to go down the primrose path and treat a nonexistent or inconsequential allergy in a child with a more serious problem until irreversible damage has been done. Other causes of reactive airways must be ruled out before an allergy is accepted as the etiology.

Reactive airways disease including allergic asthma can be treated as a single entity since the clinical manifestations and response to medications are usually the same. The basic difference lies in whether or not immunotherapy needs to be employed. Allergic asthma may be either perennial or seasonal but often exhibits characteristic patterns. These patients will demonstrate appropriately positive skin tests and often have an elevated IgE level and a positive family history for allergic disease. A discussion of therapy and treatment of these conditions is presented in Chapter 21. It is important to note that in young children the airways are smaller (less than one-third those of an adult) and fewer (one-tenth the number of alveoli). Most of the infant's airway resistance comes from peripheral airways, but only about one-fifth of the adult resistance is peripheral. This suggests special considerations in the pediatric population since the small airways may be occluded from infection and edema, and wheezing may not always be present. In this situation responsiveness to bronchodilators may not be evident until late in the treatment sequence. The failure of the patient to respond to these agents early *does not* indicate irreversible airway disease.

It is evident now that even infrequent insults to the respiratory system of the infant and child may have life-long sequellae. Data would now indicate that reaction airways disease or bronchiolitis obliterans may occur as a result of recurrent bronchiolitis or chronic infantile "asthma." It is imperative to establish a firm diagnosis and course of therapy to prevent as much damage as possible.

QUESTIONS

1. Which of the following statements are true regarding cystic fibrosis?
   a. Cystic fibrosis is the most common genetic disease in the U.S.
   b. Nasal polyps particularly in a child should alter the physician to the possibility of C.F.
   c. Symptoms of malnutrition, diarrhea and pneumonias may be absent.
   d. No particular expertise is required in performing the sweat chloride test.
2. The differential diagnosis in children presenting with bronchiectasis should include:
   a. ciliary dyskinesia.
   b. immunodeficiency.
   c. gastroesophageal reflux.
   d. allergic asthma.
3. A toddler is noted to have persistent, recent onset, wheezing without a preceeding lower respiratory infection. The first priority of the evaluation is to:
   a. perform allergy skin test.
   b. obtain sweat chloride.
   c. exclude a foreign body in the respiratory tract.
   d. obtain arterial blood gasses.

4. A 4 year old child present with a history of bacterial/pneumonia recurring 6 times during the past 2 years. The physician should obtain:

   a. chest x-ray.
   b. quantative immunoglobulin.
   c. sweat chloride.
   d. leukocyte function study.

5. A 5 year old child is hospitalized with cough, bronchospasm, pneumonia, evidence of cirrhosis and a family history of emphysema. The most likely diagnostic possibility is:

   a. Alpha 1 anti trypsin deficiency.
   b. a respiratory syncytial viral infection.
   c. Vater's Syndrome.

Answers can be found in Appendix B at the end of the book.

James M. Corry

31

Evaluation of the Child with Recurrent Infections

Infection by a variety of microbes is a common occurrence in everyone's life. Physicians are frequently confronted by a patient whose infections are so numerous that an immunodeficiency seems possible. Despite the rarity of individual immunodeficiency diseases, an adequate evaluation is indicated in the majority of these cases. A physician must therefore be able to recognize those patients needing investigation, order tests that will adequately screen host defenses, and refer those few patients with abnormalities for further evaluation and treatment. The complexity of the immune system may intimidate many physicians, but basic knowledge of host defense mechanisms and clinical problems encountered with specific defects should provide a framework for sound clinical decisions.

NORMAL IMMUNE SYSTEM IN CHILDREN

The human body has a complex, highly developed immune system for host defense that in most instances adequately controls infections. Immunodeficiency diseases occur when a portion of this system is faulty. Often overlooked but important barriers to infection are mechanical. Disruption in the physical integrity of the skin or mucosal surfaces, obstruction in any part of the body, circulatory disorders, and foreign bodies are the most common causes of recurrent infections. Those conditions listed in Table 31-1 should be considered in cases of recurrent infection before a detailed immunologic evaluation begins.

The recently described immotile cilia syndrome is characterized by abnormal ciliary structure and movement resulting in recurrent upper respiratory infections (URIs) and pneumonias. Major manifestations include recurrent pneumonias, bronchiectasis, persistent sinusitis, and otitis media. Patients with situs inversus were previously described as having Kartagener's syndrome. The ciliary abnormalities are probably transmitted as an autosomal recessive trait with an incidence of 1 in 12,500.

ALLERGY: THEORY AND PRACTICE
ISBN 0-8089-1619-X

Table 31-1 *Common Causes of Recurrent Infections*

Foreign bodies
Ventricular shunts
Central venous catheter
Artificial heart valves
Bladder catheter
Aspirated foreign body
Obstruction
Asthma
Allergic rhinitis
Narrowed eustachian tubes
Cystic fibrosis
Immotile cilia syndrome
Smoking
Integument defects
Eczema
Burns
Skull fracture
Sinus tracts
Vascular disorders
Sickle cell anemia
Diabetes mellitus
Cardiac defects

The ciliary defects are heterogenous and affect all ciliated structures, including the spermatozoa. As a result, most males are sterile. Infection presumably results from lack of normal cleansing movement of mucus secretions produced by ciliary movement. Diagnosis is most easily made by examination of ciliated cells obtained from nasal mucosal brushings. Ciliary movement can be assessed immediately by phase-contrast microscopy. If no motion is observed. a diagnosis of immobile cilia syndrome is likely. Electron microscopic examination is necessary for definitive diagnosis.

When a microbe breeches physical barriers, a nonspecific inflammatory response is provoked with accumulation of mobile phagocytic cells from local blood vessels. Along with macrophages and neutrophils, the fluid contains vasoactive substances, complement proteins, and opsonins that attract more phagocytes and facilitate ingestion of the organisms. Many infections are halted at this stage without involving specific immune responses.

Spread of infection stimulates specific responses in the humoral or cell-mediated branches of host defense. These are discussed in Chapter 2. The normal newborn's immune response, although generally able to prevent infection, is diminished compared to that in the adult. Their peripheral blood contains B lymphocytes, which are less responsive and produce smaller quantities of antibodies with limited diversity. Subnormal responses to such pathogens as *Haemophilus influenzae* and *Neisseria meningitidis* present particularly important clinical problems. Passive maternal IgG is protective for the first 6 months of life. A gradual maturation of B-lymphocyte response then occurs with adult levels of all three immunoglobulins achieved around 10 years of age.

Cellular immunity as measured by the number of T lymphocytes, delayed skin test reactions, and response to mitogens is depressed at birth. Normal adult function is achieved within the first few years. In addition, serum levels of complement components are decreased in newborns, resulting in poor opsonization and diminished chemotaxis. Normal complement levels are attained by 1 year of age. The processes of phagocytosis and intracellular killing are below normal in early infancy but quickly improve.

HISTORIC EVALUATION

Evaluation of patients with recurring infections begins with a thorough history. Particular attention should be given to the age of onset, infecting organism, site of infection, and response to therapy. Adverse reactions to immunizations should be noted and the family history examined in detail. Previous records and pathologic specimens of family members can be extremely helpful. The patient's growth should be carefully plotted. On physical examination the presence or absence of palpable lymphoid tissue, hepatosplenomegaly, and tonsillar tissue may indicate certain immunodeficiencies. Further clues to the nature of the defect may be revealed by abnormal facies, dermatitis, subcutaneous abscesses, telangiectasias, skin pigment, or petechiae.

LABORATORY EVALUATION

Patients suspected of immunodeficiency will require laboratory evaluation. Each branch of the immune system should be investigated in an orderly manner beginning with general screening tests and progressing to more sophisticated studies in only a minority of the original patients.

Evaluation of patients suspected of antibody deficiency starts with quantitative immunoglobulins (Table 31-2). Protein electrophoresis or immunoelectrophoresis can detect gross changes but are not sensitive to individual immunoglobulin levels. All commercial laboratories can readily determine immunoglobulin levels. All values must be compared to age-adjusted controls. In general, total immunoglobulin levels less than 250 mg/dl are abnormal at all ages, and gammaglobulin treatment is indicated. Serum IgE and IgD occur in small quantities and must be measured by radioimmunoassay. In cases where secretory component deficiency is suspected, conjunctival and salivary IgA must be determined.

In most patients measures of antibody function are desirable and relatively easily obtained. Isohemmaglutinins provide a good measure of functional IgM and are present in most infants over 18 months of age. As a measure of IgG function, poliomyelitis, diphtheria, tetanus, rubella, or rubeola titers can be obtained if these immunizations have been administered. If streptococcus infection has occurred, ASO titers will be elevated. All of these titers can be obtained through local or state laboratories.

If quantitative immunoglobulins and several antibody function tests are normal, no further testing is necessary. When these tests are abnormal, referral to a major medical center for more sophisticated tests is necessary. Enumeration of peripheral

Table 31-2 *Evaluation of Humoral Immunity*

Screening tests
Quantitative immunoglobulins
Serum antibody titers (isohemagglutinins, diphtheria, polio, tetanus, rubeola, ASO)
Lateral pharyngeal x-ray
Advanced tests
Enumeration of peripheral B cells
Active immunization (typhoid, diphtheria, tetanus, meningococcus)
Secretory IgA
Immunoglobulin subclass determination
Lymph node biopsy

B lymphocytes will help further classify the immunodeficiency. B Cells with surface antibodies are usually distinguished by combination with polyvalent antiserum against human immunoglobulins. With immunofluorescent techniques, the labeled B cells can be counted. Populations of peripheral blood lymphocytes normally contain 10–20% B cells.

Specific antibody production after active immunization should also be tested. Typhoid vaccine stimulates IgG and IgM to H and O antigens, respectively. Other useful antigens include pneumococcus, diphtheria, tetanus, *N. meningitidis,* and bacteriophage X174. In doubtful cases, biopsy of a regional lymph node may be helpful. The biopsy should be performed after local intramuscular (IM) stimulation with DPT. Biopsies in antibody deficiency show a paucity of plasma cells, decreased lymphoid follicles, and absent germinal centers. Rectal biopsy will also show an absence of plasma cells. Although not readily available, difficult cases may require determination of immunoglobulin subclasses.

The evaluation of the complement system is relatively straightforward when recurrent infections are suspected. Initially blood should be sent for the total complement titer. The serum must be frozen at −70°C within 1 hour to prevent denaturation of the complement proteins. This assay tests the capacity of serum to lyse antibody-coated sheep erythrocytes, which requires the entire classic pathway. All homozygous patients will have zero capacity to lyse the erythrocytes. Therefore, a normal whole complement titer rules out a deficiency of the classic pathway as a cause of infections. If a zero value is obtained, individual component levels must be measured to determine the exact deficiency. This is usually done at medical centers and some commercial laboratories. Family members must be screened and require genetic counseling appropriate for autosomal recessive transmission. Heterozygotic family members will have normal whole complement titers despite half-normal protein levels.

Tests for alternative pathway function are not readily available but can be performed at certain medical centers. If no other cause for the infections can be found and suspicion persists, referral for alternative pathway testing should be considered.

Detailed evaluation of the cellular immune system requires sophisticated techniques available only at major medical centers. However, two screening tests are useful and can exclude most patients from further evaluations (Table 31-3). Since T cells comprise the majority of peripheral blood lymphocytes, total lymphocyte counts

Table 31-3 *Evaluation of Cellular Immunity*

Screening tests
Total lymphocyte count
Delayed hypersensitivity skin tests (SK-SD, candida, mumps, PPD, trichophyton)
Thymus x-ray
Advanced tests
T-Cell enumeration by E rossettes
Mitogen stimulation (PHA, Con A, allogeneic cells)
Lymph node biopsy
Enzyme assays—ADA, NP

will generally reflect T-cell number. The presence of lymphopenia (<2000 cells/mm) suggests a T-cell deficiency, and further evaluation is necessary. Less severe depressions are common with viral infection or malignancy. Although most patients with normal lymphocyte counts have no immunodeficiency, this does not exclude a significant defect. Delayed skin tests with a battery of antigens are generally available measures of T-cell function. The most useful antigens include candida, mumps, streptodornase-streptokinase, PPD, or trichophyton. Each is given intradermally and read at 24 and 48 hours. Unfortunately, many normal infants with inadequate infectious exposure will have negative skin tests. A normal lymphocyte count with adequate response to at least one skin test usually excludes significant cellular immunodeficiency. Further confidence can be obtained from adequate lymphoid tissue on physical examination and the presence of thymic tissue on chest x-ray.

When the above tests are abnormal or suspicion persists, referral for further evaluation should be considered (Table 31-3). Initially T cells can be enumerated by the E-rossette method. This technique makes use of natural receptors for sheep erythrocytes found on the surface of T lymphocytes. When purified lymphocytes are incubated with sheep erythrocytes, rossetting occurs with each T cell surrounded by red blood cells. The cells are then easily counted and compared to normal values of 55–75% total lymphocytes. Recently monospecific antisera directed against T cells and T-cell subsets have been produced and used to detect T cells by immunofluoretic or cytotoxic assays.

Mitogens such as phytohemagglutinin, concanavalin A (Con A), or allogeneic cells nonspecifically stimulate the majority of T cells. Stimulation causes proliferation of T cells and incorporation of radioactive thymidine from the culture media into the dividing cells. The percentage of radioactively labeled cells is then compared to corresponding controls. The *in vitro* response to mitogen remains the most sensitive technique for detecting cellular immunodeficiencies.

Detailed evaluation of phagocyte function is technically difficult. However, total and differential leukocyte counts will readily detect neutropenia (<500 cells/mm^3) and abnormal leukocyte morphology. The nitroblue tetrazolium test (NBT) will detect patients with chronic granulomatous disease. Conversion of oxygen to superoxide and other toxic products in leukocytes is required to detect the dye color, indicating a normal positive test. This test is available in many hospitals and prenatal detection can be accomplished at certain medical centers.

In vitro chemotactic assays for assessment of cell mobility are complex and only performed at major medical centers. As a screening test, however, a Rebuck inflammatory skin window can be performed in the office and abnormal patients referred for more definitive tests.

IMMUNOGLOBULIN DEFICIENCIES

The B lymphocyte plays the major role in humoral immunity. Pre-B cells can be identified in the bone marrow as cells with intracytoplasmic IgM without surface expression of IgM components (Fig. 31-1). These cells form true B cells initially expressing IgM and IgD on their surfaces. B Cells producing IgG and IgA are then formed in sequence. T-Cell help is required in B-cell development, particularly in the switch from IgM to IgG production. On combination with appropriate antigens, the B cells are activated and antibody secreting plasma cells are formed. Many of the humoral immunodeficiencies have been related to specific defects in this pathway.

As expected, deficiency in antibody production results in major problems with opsonization of bacteria. Encapsulated pyogenic bacteria including *Staphylococcus aureus*, *S. pneumococcus*, *Haemophilus influenzae*, and *Escherichia coli* are the usual infecting organisms. The major sites of infection are the middle ears, sinuses, nasal passages, lungs, gastrointestinal (GI) tract, meninges, bones, and joints. The severity of the infections varies depending on the extent of antibody deficiency. Most infections respond to antibiotic treatment, but recurrence is inevitable. Viral infections are handled normally since cell-mediated immunity is generally normal.

Transient Immunodeficiency

Transient hypogammaglobulinemia of infancy occurs when there is a delay in antibody production in the first year of life. These individuals are usually identified when low immunoglobulin levels are found during an evaluation of recurring URIs.

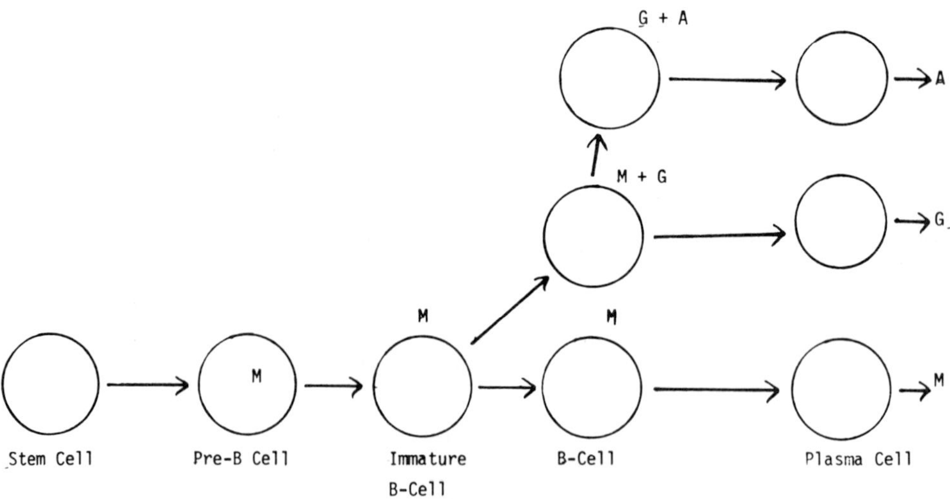

Fig. 31-1. Maturation of the B lymphocyte.

Despite low immunoglobulin levels, immunization results in normal antibody production and isohemagluttinins are present (Tiller et al., 1978). Tonsillar tissue is visible, and lymph nodes are palpable in all these patients. Immunoglobulin levels increase at 1–3 years of age, and progressive immunodeficiency does not develop. In the absence of obvious bacterial infection, gamma globulin replacement is not necessary and should be avoided.

Sex-Linked Immunodeficiency

Sex-linked agammaglobulinemia was the first immunodeficiency described and is the most severe of the humoral deficiencies. Since transplacentally transferred maternal IgG is protective for the first 6 months of life, male infants usually develop infection during the latter part of the first year. Typically they present with eczema, draining ears, purulent rhinitis, and coughing or wheezing associated with pneumonia. Several episodes of meningitis, septicemia, osteomyelitis, or arthritis are common. Lymphatic tissue is generally absent and hepatosplenomegaly is rare. The recurring pneumonias progress to bronchiectasis with chest hyperexpansion and clubbing of the nails. Chest x-rays may show scarring, fibrosis, and bronchiectasis. Sinus films are almost always opacified. Growth may be normal in the absence of significant pulmonary disease. Antibiotics offer temporary improvement, but the infections recur in the absence of gamma globulin replacement.

Recurrent viral infections are seldom a problem. Fatal hepatitis and polio virus infections have occurred in a few patients. Several cases of polio virus infection have been associated with administration of live vaccine. A persistent and fatal panencephalitis due to ECHO virus has been reported in several patients. Finally, a chronic arthritis involving large joints can be a problem but responds to gamma globulin treatment. The prognosis in agammaglobulinemia depends on the extent of bronchiectasis and the development of chronic CNS infection. With adequate treatment infections can be controlled, and patients will enter adult life.

Laboratory evaluation reveals total immunoglobulin levels of less than 250 mg/dl with IgG below 100 and IgM and IgA absent. Occasionally IgE is normal. Antibody formation does not occur with infection or immunization and isohemagluttinins are absent. Cell-mediated immunity is always normal. Patients have adequate pre-B cells in the bone marrow, but B cells are generally absent. The lack of B cells is reflected in the paucity of lymphoid tissue and depopulation of germinal follicles in lymph node biopsies. A defect in conversion of pre-B cells to B cells has been hypothesized. However, a few patients have had normal B cells in their peripheral blood.

Sex-Linked Immunodeficiency with Hyper-IgM

Patients with sex-linked immunodeficiency with hyper-IgM have infections similar to those seen in sex-linked agammaglobulinemia. The infections begin at a later age, with stomatitis and neutropenia particularly common. Lymphoid tissue is present along with hepatosplenomegaly. The prognosis is generally better than in sex-linked agammaglobulinemia. In all cases IgM is markedly elevated and may reach 1000 mg/dl; IgG, IgA, or IgE are low or absent. Total immunoglobulin levels may be normal due to the elevated IgM. B Cells containing IgM are present but do not undergo a switch to IgG or IgA production. A primary defect intrinsic to the B cells seems to be involved.

Common Variable Immunodeficiency

Common variable immunodeficiency can be sporadic or familial with equal sex involvement. Initially host defense is normal, but with advancing age a progressive decline in immune function occurs. Infections usually begin in later childhood or adulthood. Prominent clinical manifestations are recurring sinopulmonary infections with pyogenic bacteria. Bronchiectasis with rales, clubbing, and a barrel chest are common in untreated patients. Many patients are initially diagnosed in chest clinics. Sinusitis is a universal occurrence. Gastrointestinal (GI) sprue-like symptoms with steatorrhea are seen in a significant number of patients. Lactose intolerance, giardiasis, and protein-losing enteropathy are also common. Autoimmune diseases occur with increased frequency and have included hemolytic anemia, scleroderma, dermatomyositis, rheumatoid arthritis, and systemic lupus erythematous (SLE). Lymphadenopathy and hepatosplenomegaly can be seen and do not rule out the diagnosis. The prognosis has improved with gammaglobulin therapy, and most infections can be controlled.

Total immunoglobulins are generally less than 400 mg/dl with IgG below 250–300 mg/dl and IgM or IgA absent. Occasionally IgM or IgA are normal. Isohemagglutinins are depressed and antibody formation to recent immunization is lacking. Although tests of cell-mediated immunity are frequently abnormal and progressively decline, viral infections are rarely a problem.

Common variable immunodeficiency is a clinical syndrome with a heterogenous group of defects. B Cells are usually present in the peripheral blood but may be absent. *In vitro* these cells can usually be driven to secrete antibody, but the quantity is reduced, suggesting an intrinsic B-cell defect. In other instances, immunoglobulin is not formed or cannot be secreted. Many patients have T suppressor cells that inhibit antibody production by normal B cells *in vitro*. Others lack T helper cells or have a B-cell inhibitor in their sera. A complete understanding of this complex syndrome is not currently available.

Infections with Normal Immunoglobulins

Infections due to antibody deficiency can also occur with normal immunoglobulin levels. These cases are uncommon and usually sporadic. Although quantitative immunoglobulins are normal, antibody responses do not occur with infection or immunization. In a few cases, antibodies have been produced, but to a restricted group of antigens. Deficiencies of subclasses IgG_2 or IgG_4 have been reported (Schur et al., 1970). The latter deficiency results in recurrent pulmonary infections. Selective deficiency of IgG, IgM, or IgE occur in rare instances.

Selective IgA Deficiency

Selective IgA deficiency is the most common immunodeficiency, occurring in 1 out of 700 persons. Although it can be familial, most cases are sporadic. Individuals can be asymptomatic, but a significant number suffer recurrent URIs. Recent evidence suggests that many patients with IgA deficiency and recurrent infections are also deficient in IgG_2. Most infections are viral and much milder than the previous humoral deficiencies. Bronchitis, obstructive lung disease, and recurrent pneumonias can occur but are rarely debilitating. There may be an increased frequency and severity of asthma. Other associated disorders include celiac disease, intestinal nodular hyperplasia, SLE, pernicious anemia, thyroiditis, rheumatoid arthritis, and Addison's disease. This increased incidence of autoimmune disease may relate to the frequent viral infections or increased antigen load crossing the unprotected mucosal surfaces. Several instances of spontaneous recovery from IgA deficiency have been reported.

Quantitative immunoglobulins show normal IgG and IgM with IgA below 5 mg/dl. Since all IgA is produced by submucosal plasma cells, in most patients secretory IgA is also absent. Rare instances of secretory component deficiency have resulted in inability to transport IgA across mucosal surfaces while the serum IgA remains normal. (Strober et al., 1976). In most patients, IgM replaces the absent secretory IgA and provides some protection. The peripheral blood contains B cells, but the IgA B cells fail to form plasma cells. Variable abnormalities in cellular immunity have been observed in a small number of patients. The exact nature of the defect is unclear, but many patients have suppressor T cells specific for IgA B cells.

Treatment

The mainstay of treatment for humoral immunodeficiency is replacement with gamma globulin. This is accomplished with monthly injections of pooled gamma globulin (100 mg/kg monthly). More recently an intravenous (IV) immunoglobulin preparation has become available (Gamimune, Cutter Labs). This preparation obviates some of the problems of the intramuscular (IM) form but is extremely expensive. Gamma globulin injections or infusions do not effectively replace IgA and are actually contraindicated in selective IgA deficiency since anaphylactic reactions to exogenous IgA frequently result. Patients should not receive live vaccines. All infections require prompt and aggressive treatment with appropriate antibiotics. Chronic pulmonary disease necessitates a regular program of pulmonary therapy.

COMPLEMENT DEFICIENCIES

Instances of complement deficiencies have shown that intact humoral and cell-mediated immunities are not sufficient protection from bacterial infection. As previously mentioned, the complement system produces a crucial opsonin (C3b), a chemotactic factor (C5a), and terminal components capable of bacteriolysis. Absence of any of these factors results in a predilection for bacterial infections.

Deficiencies of all nine components of the classic pathway have been described. Most are hereditary with autosomal codominant mode of transmission. Each complement protein is coded at a single gene locus, and two functioning genes are necessary for normal levels. Homozygotes with no functional genes lack the corresponding complement protein. Heterozygotes have one gene and half-normal levels of that component. Despite these lower levels, the complement system functions normally.

Deficiency of the initial complement proteins (C1,C4,C2) has seldom resulted in infectious problems. Patients with combined immunodeficiency or hypogammaglobulinemia have been described with C_{1q} subcomponent deficiency. The infections seen in these patients are more likely because of their primary disorders. C_2 Deficiency has been described in over 100 individuals. Although the majority are healthy, many have had autoimmune diseases such as Henoch Schonlein purpura, dermatomyositis, SLE, and glomerulonephritis. Four C_2-deficient children have had severe recurrent infections, including pneumococcal bacteremia and meningitis (Hyatt et al., 1981). One had *Haemophilus influenzae* arthritis and bacteremia. Three of the four had alternative pathway abnormalities, which may have contributed to their infectious risk. A normal-functioning alternative pathway presumably protects the majority of these patients by permitting C3b fixation and activation of the terminal portion of the system.

As expected, homozygous patients with C3 deficiency have severe recurrent bacterial infections similar to that seen in antibody deficiency. Their sera are totally unable to produce C3b via either complement pathway, and opsonization is markedly reduced. Major infections have included meningitis, septicemia, and pneumonia. Superficial skin infections and abscesses are rarely seen. Heterzygotes have no increased frequency of infections.

Leiner's disease is a syndrome occurring in infants with severe seborrheic dermatitis, diarrhea, and recurrent infections due to gram negative organisms and *Staphlococcus aureus*. The major problem appears to be a dysfunctional C5 protein manifest as defective phagocytosis of yeast and generation of chemotactic factors. The hemolytic activity and C5 level of serum are normal. Infusions of plasma or pure C5 are helpful in preventing infections.

Absence of C5 has resulted in recurrent superficial infections in a female with SLE. Her twin was healthy. Other healthy patients have been reported, but a few have had repeated disseminated gonococcal infections. The infections were presumably due to defective generation of the chemotactic factor C5a.

Half of those patients with C6, C7, or C8 deficiency have had recurring infections with neisserial bacteria (Petersen et al., 1979). Neisserial meningitis, septicemia, or arthritis has been common along with autoimmune diseases. Their sera opsonize bacteria normally and prevent the majority of infections. However, lack of the terminal component results in defective bacteriolysis, which may be important in defense against neisserial infections.

Hereditary deficiency of alternative pathway proteins has not been reported. However, a defect in alternative pathway regulation has occurred in several patients (Abramson et al., 1971). These patients lacked C3b inactivator (Factor I), which removes C3b from bacterial surfaces. Without removal of C3b, continued destruction of C3 occurs. The resulting low C3 levels predispose patients to bacterial infections similar to C3 deficiency.

Acquired deficiencies of the complement system occur in a wide variety of disorders and are generally not associated with infections. Newborns have low levels of C3, Factor B, and early classic components that may increase their risk of infections. Abnormal alternative pathway function seen in sickle cell anemia, thalassemia, and postsplenectomy may predispose to pneumococcal septicemia.

Cell-Mediated Deficiency

Cell-mediated immunity not only provides the major defense against viral, protozoal, and fungal diseases, but T cells also influence B-cell and macrophage function. Pre-T cells arise from an unrecognized stem cell in the bone marrow (Fig. 31-2). Once in the peripheral circulation, they travel to the thymus and are converted to

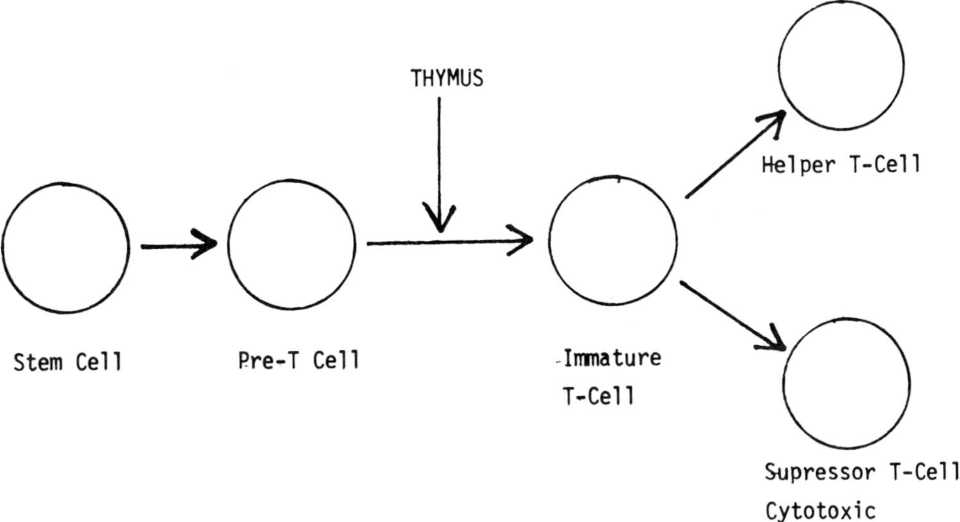

Fig. 31-2. Maturation of the T lymphocyte.

mature T cells. Complex features of the thymic microenvironment seem important for this conversion. Contact with invading microbes activates the T cells to resist infection. Defects in several of these steps have been described and result in some of the most severe immunodeficiencies known.

The majority of patients with cellular immunodeficiency suffer infections from the first few months of life. Although severe deficiencies result in devastating infections, patients with minor T-cell defects have corresponding diminished infections and may not be considered for evaluation initially. These patients have characteristic problems with viral, protozoal, and fungal infections. Pneumonias due to herpes, cytomegalovirus, *Pneumocystis carinii*, and measles are particularly common. Chronic diarrhea and fungal skin infections also suggest a cellular immunodeficiency. Many patients are first recognized with symptoms of chronic graft-versus-host reactions subsequent to blood transfusions. In these situations the transfused lymphocytes are not eliminated by the patient's T cells and attack the host tissues. Jaundice, rash, and diarrhea are the common symptoms. In addition, bacterial infections typical of antibody deficiency are usually present.

Reticular dysgenesis

Patients with congenital deficiency of the granulocytic stem cell have been described; this condition is termed *reticular dysgenesia*. These patients present in the first few days of life with failure to thrive, vomiting, diarrhea, and localized infections. All parts of host defense are lacking, and all patients reported have died within a few weeks.

DiGeorge Syndrome

The DiGeorge syndrome results from abnormal development of the third and fourth pharyngeal pouches during weeks 6–8 of embryonic life. Since the thymus forms from these pouches, thymic hypoplasia results. In addition, parathyroid gland development is absent, and certain other cardiac and facial malformations occur. Complete and incomplete forms of DiGeorge syndrome have been described.

The majority of patients present with tetany or congestive heart failure in the first few days of life. Common cardiac defects include right-sided aortic arch, aberrant left subclavian artery, right ventricular infundibular stenosis, ventricular septal defect, tetralogy of Fallot, atrial septal defect, pulmonary atresia, and hypoplastic pulmonary artery. Some patients are recognized by facial characteristics such as hypertelorism, antimongoloid slant, low-set prominent ears with notched pinna, "fish mouth," and micrognathia. Infections do not begin until later infancy. Chronic rhinitis, pneumonia, oral candidiasis, and diarrhea are particularly common. Failure to thrive is almost universal. Patients with the incomplete syndrome may lack infections and facial or cardiac problems, but all have tetany.

Laboratory studies reveal a very low calcium during active tetany. T-Cell studies vary enormously depending on the extent of the thymic abnormality. Total lymphocyte counts can be reduced or normal. T-Cell numbers are usually low and phytohemagglutinin stimulation decreased. Delayed skin tests are negative in the majority, and skin grafts have prolonged survival. Lymph node biopsy shows diminished T cells in the deep cortical areas. Despite the T-cell abnormalities, B-cell function is generally normal, although antibody deficiency has been reported.

Treatment involves early recognition of tetany and administration of calcium gluconate and vitamin D. Congestive heart failure is fatal in many cases despite vigorous treatment. If antibody function is diminished, antibiotics and gamma globulin should be given. Specific immune restoration has occurred after fetal thymus transplants. Administration of bovine thymosin has accomplished similar results.

Combined Immunodeficiency

Combined immunodeficiency is a syndrome with both cellular and humoral immune defects. Some cases are sporadic, whereas others are transmitted as an autosomal recessive trait. Although severe infections usually begin in the first few months of life, milder infections with later onset do not rule out the diagnosis.

Patients typically present with cough, wheeze, or respiratory distress due to cytomegalovirus, measles, herpes, or *Pneumocystis carinii* pneumonia. They are usually quite ill and appear wasted, particularly if chronic diarrhea has been present. Their skin may be infected with candida, microsporium, or tinea. Desquamation, seborrhea, and alopecia are common. Susceptibility to all forms of microorganisms is present. Although a few cases have lived beyond infancy, most die rapidly if immunity is not reconstituted.

Studies of cellular immunity are abnormal in all patients but can be misleading. Although most severely affected patients have lymphocyte counts less than 2000 cells/mm, some patients have no lymphopenia and normal T-cell numbers by E-rosette techniques. Since in the latter patients the T cells do not perform normally, the most sensitive methods for diagnosis are tests of T-cell function. Delayed skin tests and *in vitro* mitogen stimulation of T cells are always abnormal. In addition, immunoglobulins are low and antibody responses absent. Originally a stem cell defect was proposed as the underlying problem in combined immunodeficiency, but the presence of pre-T cells and B cells in most patients makes this less tenable. A defect in the lymphocyte maturation process seems most likely.

Although the majority of cases are fatal, bone marrow transplantation can be curative if a histocompatible donor can be found. Graft-versus-host disease (GVHD) remains a major complication. In those cases where compatible bone marrow is not available, transplants of fetal liver cells, thymus epithelium, or fetal thymus have been successful in selected patients. Special care must be given to irradiate all blood products before transfusion to avoid GVHD. Live vaccines should never be administered. While awaiting transplantation, gamma globulin injections should be given along with trimethoprim-sulfamethoxazole prophylaxis to prevent *Pn. carinni* infection.

Nezeloff's syndrome is a variant of combined immunodeficiency with normal immunoglobulin levels but no significant antibody production. Other variants occur in association with short-limbed dwarfism or cartilage hair hypoplasia. All have clinical manifestations similar to combined immunodeficiency.

Purine Salvage Pathway

Deficiency of two enzymes of the purine salvage pathway result in a syndrome similar to combined immunodeficiency. Adenosine deaminase (ADA) deficiency occurs as an autosomal recessive disorder with profound defects in cellular and humoral immunity. Severe viral and bacterial infections usually begin in the first year of life. Many patients have characteristic skeletal deformities with cupping and flaring of the ribs and abnormal transverse processes of vertebrae and scapula. Deficiency of nucleoside phosphorylase results in T-cell defects but normal B-cell function. These patients have fewer, less severe infections compared to ADA deficiency. Normal humoral immunity presumably provides some protection. It has been hypothesized that metabolites of these enzymes might be toxic to lymphocytes and prevent normal maturation. Alternatively, starvation of pyrimidine may be the major problem.

Since all cells in affected patients are enzyme-deficient, measurement of enzyme content in either erythrocytes or fibroblasts will provide the diagnosis. Diagnosis in utero has been accomplished (Hirschhorn et al., 1975). Treatment is the same as for combined immunodeficiency. In addition, several patients have improved after transfusion with erythrocytes containing ADA (Polmar et al., 1976).

Wiskott Aldrich Syndrome

Wiskott Aldrich syndrome is a sex-linked recessive disorder with recurrent infections, eczema, and bleeding due to thrombocytopenia. The initial manifestations are usually petechiae or bleeding in the first 6 months of life. Bloody diarrhea is a frequent presenting symptom. Eczema occurs early and may rapidly become superinfected. Around 6 months of age bacterial infections usually begin, with pneumonia and otitis the most common. *Haemophilus influenza, S. pneumococcus, S. aureus, Pseudamonas,* and salmonella are the most frequently isolated organisms. Although viral and protozoal infections are less common, cytomegalovirus, *Pneumocystis carinii,* varicella, and herpes infections do occur. On physical examination splenomegaly, hepatomegaly, and lymphadenopathy are the rule. Signs of chronic respiratory infection and draining ears are usually present. Intracranial hemorrhage can occur, and the incidence of malignancy is increased.

Laboratory findings are variable but abnormalities are usually found in both cellular and humoral immunity. Once present, the defects are progressive. An inability to respond to polysaccharide antigens with antibody production is the most consistent finding. As a result, most have no isohemagglutinins and fail to respond to pneumococcal, *E. coli,* or salmonella antigens. Other antibody responses to tetanus or diphtheria may be normal. Quantitative immunoglobulins show a distinctive pattern with increased IgG, low IgM, and elevated IgE and IgA. Most patients are lymphopenic and have a variable decrease in delayed skin tests, E rossettes, and T-cell mitogen responses. The platelets are small and decreased in number and have shortened survival. Although no clear etiologic mechanism has been found in this complex disorder, abnormal antigen recognition and processing by macrophages has been suggested to account for some of the immunologic findings.

Treatment begins with platelet transfusions to control bleeding. All blood products must be irradiated before use. If bleeding is uncontrollable or recurrent, splenectomy may be helpful. After splenectomy, penicillin prophylaxis is necessary to prevent pneumococcal septicemia. Pneumococcal vaccination does not produce protective antibodies. Appropriate antibiotics must be used aggressively and antiviral therapy with levamisole or arabinoside considered. Bone marrow transplantation and transfer factor has been effective in a few cases. Despite these measures, the prognosis remains poor, with early death from bleeding still common.

Ataxia Telangiectasia

Ataxia telangiectasia usually begins with ataxia during infancy followed by slow progression to disability. The gait is typically cerebellar, and mental retardation is generally present. Telangiectasias are first noticeable at 1–6 years of age, usually beginning on the bulbar conjunctiva and spreading over the face. Atopic dermatitis may also be present.

Recurrent sinopulmonary infections begin after the first few years of life. Pyogenic encapsulated bacteria are the most troublesome pathogens, and the majority of patients develop bronchiectasis despite antibiotics and gamma globulin replacement. Malignancy, CNS degeneration, and endocrinopathies develop with increasing age.

Laboratory findings are extremely variable, and no unifying etiology has been forthcoming. Lymphopenia and eosinophilia are seen along with IgA and IgE deficiency. Antibody responses are generally deficient, although autoantibodies are paradoxically increased in frequency. Cellular immunity is abnormal in 60% of patients with negative delayed skin tests, abnormal phytohemagglutinin stimulation, and decreased E rosettes. The thymus is absent on chest x-ray.

No specific treatment is available. Gammaglobulin injections, plasma infusions, and levamisole administration have not been helpful. Antibiotics remain the only effective means of therapy. Prognosis is determined by the severity of infections or the development of malignancy. Despite inadequate therapies, prolonged survival has been reported in several patients.

Mucocutaneous Candidiasis

Mucocutaneous candidiasis occurs as four clinical variants. Early onset is the most severe, with candidal infections involving the oral mucosa, nails, and extensive areas of the skin. Systemic candidiasis rarely occurs. Endocrinopathies occur in 50% of patients, including hypothyroidism, hypoparathyroidism, Addison's disease, diabetes mellitus, and pernicious anemia. The endocrine abnormalities usually appear after the onset of candidiasis.

Patients with later onset usually have milder disease involving only paronychia or the buccal mucosa. A third variant without endocrinopathies is familial with autosomal recessive transmission. Finally, patients with familial polyendocrinopathy with candidiasis suffer primarily from endocrine disease and have minimal infection.

Infections arise as a result of a specific T-cell unresponsiveness to candida. In all patients candida-delayed skin tests are negative, and T cell do not stimulate when exposed to candida *in vitro*. All other aspects of immunity are normal.

Treatment is aimed at control of candida infection and close observation for signs of endocrine disease. Intermittent IV amphotericin B has been successful in limiting infection in most people. In addition, oral clotrimazole, 5-fluorocystine, or ketoconazole have recently been shown effective. Response to transfer factor has been variable.

Defects in Chemotaxis and Phagocytosis

Orderly function of phagocytic cells is necessary to effectively remove opsonized bacteria. Initially the phagocytes are attracted and move to the site of infection by the process of chemotaxis. A properly opsonized bacterium is then ingested and intracellular killing begins. Bacterial killing is a complex event involving the conversion of oxygen to toxic metabolites. A variety of defects in the phagocytic system have been reported with characteristic patterns of infection.

When chemotaxis is abnormal mobile phagocytes do not move to the initial sites of bacterial invasion. Patients with defective chemotaxis, therefore, present with bacterial infections on body surfaces or mucosal linings. Subcutaneous abcesses, furunculosis, impetigo, stomatitis, conjunctivitis, sinusitis, and pneumonia are common. Septicemia, meningitis, and deep abcesses are much less frequent in the absence of overwhelming infection. *Staphylacoccus aureus* is the most commonly isolated organism, although other pyogenic bacteria have been isolated. Most of these defects are very rare with some occurring as isolated examples.

Chediak Higashi Syndrome

Primary cellular defects of chemotaxis result from a basic abnormality in the phagocytic cell. Chediak Higashi syndrome (CHS) is an autosomal recessive disease characterized by recurrent infections; partial loss of pigment in the skin, iris, and retina; photophobia, nystagmus; and giant granules in most granule containing cells. Infections are generally due to pyogenic bacteria, with *S. aureus*, Group A streptococcus, and *H. influenza* the most common pathogens. Usual sites of infection include the lungs, skin, subcutaneous tissue, and upper respiratory tract. The recognition of partial albinism and abnormal granules in association with recurring infections usually leads to the diagnosis.

In addition to chemotactic defects, patients have a profound neutropenia and do not develop peripheral leukocytosis when infected. Ingestion of organisms is normal, but degranulation of lysosomes is abnormal, resulting in a mild impairment in bacterial killing. The impaired chemotaxis and degranulation appears to result from defective intracellular microtubule function. Ascorbicacid improves microtubule function and has corrected defective leukocytes *in vitro* (Boxer et al., 1976).

Lazy Leukocyte Syndrome

Patients with the "lazy leukocyte" syndrome have severe neutropenia and abnormal chemotaxis. Normal numbers of neutrophil precursors are seen in the bone marrow. Clinical manifestations have included recurrent gingivitis, stomatitis, otitis media, furunculosis, and pneumonia. The patient's phagocytes do not deform easily possibly contributing to the chemotactic defect.

Actin Abnormality

A few patients have been described with defective function of actin and chemotaxis abnormalities (Boxer et al., 1974). Actin is an important contractile element in the cell and the probable basis of the chemotactic defect. Recurrent bacterial infections have been observed in each patient.

Hyper-IgE

Secondary cellular defects of chemotaxis result when an underlying disease affects the movement of the cells. Hyperimmunoglobulinemia E has been associated with depressed chemotaxis, chronic eczematous dermatitis, and recurrent staphylococcal abscesses. Other infections have included furunculosis, cellulitis, pneumonia, empyema, otitis, and rarely septicemia. Buckley's syndrome (elevated IgE, pyoderma, and depressed cellular immunity) may be related to hyper-IgE since several of the patients have had chemotactic defects. Although the elevated IgE is probably not directly involved, histamine released from IgE coated basophils can inhibit chemotaxis *in vitro*.

Miscellaneous Defects

Patients with diabetes mellitus have been reported to have abnormal chemotaxis, possibly as a result of potassium or glucose deficiency in the phagocyte. Other conditions with probable secondary cellular defects in chemotaxis include acrodermatitis enteropathica, hypophosphatemia, mannosidosis, Down's syndrome, alcoholism, cancer, malnutrition, bone marrow transplantation, and burns.

Serum deficiencies or inhibitors have been implicated in many chemotactic defects. As previously noted, C_5 deficiency results in diminished production of chemotactic factors. Normal sera contain several inhibitors of chemotaxis that are increased with certain inflammations. Many patients with glomerulonephritis, cirrhosis, Hodgkins disease, lepromatous leprosy, and sarcoidosis have had elevated levels of inhibitors detected. Recurrent infections in association with elevated IgA have been described in several patients. A role for IgA is suggested by the fact that IgA myeloma protein inhibits neutrophil chemotaxis *in vitro*. Finally, depressed monocyte chemotaxis has been described in Wiskott Aldrich syndrome as a result of cellular deactivation from supranormal levels of a lymphocyte-derived chemotactic factor.

Neutropenia

Primary cellular abnormalities of ingestion have included only the previously mentioned patients with actin dysfunction. Neutropenia can be considered as a secondary defect of ingestion since the extent of phagocytosis is markedly decreased.

Again, *S. aureus* has been the most frequent pathogen, followed by *E. coli* and *Pseudomonas*.

Splenic Dysfunction

Splenic dysfunction as seen in sickle cell anemia or postsplenectomy can also be considered a defect of ingestion. In these cases superficial infections are rare whereas septicemia and meningitis are common because of poor filtering of bacteria from the bloodstream. Pneumococcus is a particularly common pathogen.

Defects in Microbial Killing

Chronic Granulomatous Disease

Defects in killing of intracellular bacteria results in profoundly diminished host defense and subsequent infections. Chronic granulomatous disease is a syndrome of recurrent purulent infections of the skin, lymph nodes, liver, and lungs resulting from an inability to kill bacteria and fungi. Sex-linked and autosomal recessive modes of inheritance have been demonstrated. Variability in clinical severity has been described, and several molecular defects may be involved.

The onset is usually during the first year of life with pneumonitis, subcutaneous abcesses, furunculosis, osteomyelitis, conjunctivitis, stomatitis, and hepatic and perianal abscesses. Septicemia and meningitis are less common. Many patients have eczematoid or seborrheic dermatitis, persistent diarrhea, and rhinitis. The reticuloendothelial system is generally involved with lymphadenopathy and hepatosplenomegaly occurring in most patients. These tissues are engorged with unkilled bacteria crowded in phagocytes.

Staphylococcol and enteric bacteria are the usual pathogens in chronic granulomatous disease. Other organisms have included aspergillus, candida, salmonella, tuberculosis, and disseminated BCG. These organisms have the common property of not producing hydrogen peroxide. Organisms that produce hydrogen peroxide inadvertently supply the phagocyte with the means for effective intracellular killing and are seldom a problem.

During phagocytosis, CGD phagocytes do not produce microbicidal metabolites such as superoxide anion, hydrogen peroxide, or hydroxyl radical. Various enzymes such as NADH oxidase, NADPH oxidase, and glutathione peroxidase have been proposed as missing in CGD phagocytes, thereby blocking the conversion of oxygen to potent metabolites. However, no clear proof has been forthcoming. A recent finding suggests that some patients may have abnormal triggering of the killing mechanism as the result of a membrane dysfunction. Patients with glucose-6-phosphate dehydrogenase deficiency involving both erythrocytes and leukocytes have a mild form of CGD.

No specific treatment is available for CGD, but supportive care with early, frequent antibiotics and/or surgical drainage has improved the survival rate. Some patients have seemed to improve with continuous sulfonamide treatment. However, despite these measures most patients are dead by 10 years of age with only a few surviving into the fourth decade. Pulmonary disease remains the major cause of death.

Myeloperoxidase Deficiency

Patients with myeloperoxidase (MPO) deficiency are rarely subject to recurring infections. However, disseminated candidiasis and severe acne have been reported. In these patients MPO is absent from neutrophils and monocytes. Bacteria are handled normally despite the mildly impaired microbicidal activity.

Others

An ill-defined group of patients with abnormal neutrophil granules have had impaired bacterial killing. Similar abnormalities occur in Felty's syndrome, leukocyte alkaline phosphatase deficiency, neutrophil pyruvate kinase deficiency, and leukemia.

Acquired Immune Deficiency Syndrome

Adult acquired immunodeficiency syndrome (AIDS) has recently come to the forefront as a major health problem in the United States. The disease is characterized by (1) Kaposi's sarcoma or opportunistic infection in the absence of other causes of immunosuppression, (2) lymphadenopathy, (3) lymphopenia, (4) hypergammaglobulinemia, and (5) a marked decrease in the number of T helper cells with a resultant reversal in the T helper/T suppressor cell ratio. AIDS has been associated with a number of high risk groups, with the majority of patients being male homosexuals (>70%). Other groups at risk include hemophiliacs, native Haitians, female sexual contacts of homosexual or bisexual males, children of the above mentioned groups, and patients who receive blood transfusions from individuals with AIDS. Not all patients, however, fall into these categories.

Recent studies from the United States and France have identified an RNA retro virus that correlates strongly with the presence of AIDS, pre or latent AIDS (patients who do not have the full blown syndrome), and the high risk groups noted above (Shaw et al., 1984). This virus, which belongs to the class of human T cell leukemia viruses, has been designated HTLV-III and is believed to be the etiologic agent responsible for AIDS. Like the other members of this class, the virus is markedly trophic for T helper cells.

The initial evaluation of suspected AIDS patients should include a careful physical examination to determine the extent of lymphadenopathy, a white blood cell count and skin testing for cell mediated hypersensitivity. If these tests suggest AIDS then determination of the T helper/T suppressor ratio should be performed. Recently several immunological and molecular biological tests for the presence of HTLV-III have been developed. It is anticipated that these will soon be available for screening of potential AIDS patients and blood for transfusions. Treatment of the AIDS patient is largely supportive as there is no known specific therapy.

Case History

A 12-year-old male with chronic bronchiectasis, J. G. was a full-term product of a normal labor and delivery. He received routine immunizations without complications. However, at 10 months of age he was admitted to the hospital with a high fever and cough. An x-ray showed right middle lobe infiltrate with volume loss. He was begun on IV antibiotics and responded well. A blood culture subsequently grew pneumococcus. During the next year he had two episodes of pneumonia with fever that responded to oral antibiotics as an outpatient. In addition, he had frequent otitis media with rupture of the left tympanic membrane on one occasion. At 2 years of age a sweat chloride was 35 meq/l, and a barium swallow was normal.

At 2½ years of age he again developed high fever, cough, and irritability. A chest x-ray showed right upper lobe and lingular pneumonia. Nuchal rigidity was present, and a lumbar puncture produced cloudy fluid with 2500 white blood cells with 8% neutrophils. The CSF glucose was 10 mg/dl compared to a blood glucose of 75 mg/dl. Cerebrospinal fluid protein was 210 mg/dl. A gram stain of the fluid showed pleomorphic gram negative rods that were identified as *H. influenzae*. He was treated vigorously with IV antibiotics. On physical examination his height and weight were at the 25th percentile. He had purulent drainage from the left tympanic membrane. Also present was a crusted purulent nasal discharge. No tonsillar tissue was visible, nor could peripheral lymph nodes be palpated. The skin was clear. The liver and spleen were not enlarged.

An extensive evaluation for possible immunodeficiency was begun. The patient's uncle died as a child from "lung infection." No adenoidal tissue was visible on lateral neck x-rays. Sinus films showed clouding of the maxillary and ethmoid cavities. The WBC was 25,000, with 80% neutrophils. The results of quantitative immunoglobulins were IgG = 65 mg/dl with IgM and IgA undetectable. Antibody titers for polio, diphteria, and tetanus were absent. Isohemagglutinins were likewise undetectable. Peripheral blood B lymphocytes were not found by immunofluorescence. Delayed skin test for candida was positive at 48 hours. T-Cell number was normal by the E-rossette technique. A diagnosis of sex-linked agammaglobulinemia was made, and monthly IM injections of gamma globulin were begun.

He received a monthly injection for 3 years and was free of serious infections. At 6 years of age he was lost to follow-up. He returned to the hospital at 12 years of age with complaints of a chronic productive cough and a pain in his knees and elbows. Over the past 6 years he had received his gamma globulin injections sporadically since the family moved frequently. He had several episodes of pneumonia each year, many requiring hospitalization. For the past 2 years he had a chronic cough and poor exercise tolerance. For 6 months he had pain and swelling of his knees and elbows. On physical examination his height and weight had fallen to the fifth percentile. Purulent drainage from the nose was obvious. The chest had an increased antero-posterior diameter with diminished breath sounds. Early clubbing was present in all extremities. The knees and elbows were tender and swollen and had decreased range of motion. Again, no lymph nodes were palpable, and the liver and spleen were not enlarged. A chest x-ray showed panlobar infiltrates with bronciectasis. A sputum culture grew pneumococcus and *H. Influenzae*. A vigorous program of antibodies and postural drainage was begun, along with injections of gamma globulin. When last seen he continued to have a chronic cough but had been free of infection for 1 year.

REFERENCES

Abramson, N., Alper, C. A., Lachmann, P. J., Rosen, F. S., & Jandl, J. H. *J. Immunol.*, 1971, *107*, 19–26.

Boxer, L. A., Hedley-Whyte, T., & Stossel, T. P. *New Engl. J. Med.*, 1974, *291*, 1093–1099.

Boxer, L. A., Watanabe, A. M., Rister, M., Beach, H. R., Allen, J., & Baehner, R. L. *New Engl. J. Med.*, 1976, *295*, 1041–1044.

Eliasson, R., Morsberg, B., Cammer, P., Afzelius, B. The Immunology Cilia Syndrome. *New Engl. J. Med.*, 1977, *297*, 1–6.

Hirschhorn, R. Beratis, N., Rosen, F. S., Parkman, R., Stern, R., & Polmar, S. *Lancet*, 1975, *1*, 73–75.

Hyatt, A. C., Altenburger, K. M., Johnston, R. B., & Winkelstein, J. A. *J. Pediatr.*, 1981, *98*, 417–419.

Leikens, S., Parrot, R., Randoff, J. Clotrimazole treatment of chronic mucocutaneous candidiosis. *J. Pediatr.*, 1976, *88*, 864.

Oxeluis, V., Lauvell, A., Lindquist, B., Golebionska, H., Axelsson, U., Bjorkauder, J., Hanson, L. IgG subclasses in selective IgA deficiency. *New Engl. J. Med.*, 1981, *304*, 1476–1477.

Peterson, B. H., Lee, T. J., Snyderman, R., & Brooks, G. F. *Ann. Int. Med.*, 1979, *90*, 917–920.

Polmar, S. H., Stern, R. C., Schwartz, A. L., Wetzler, E. M., Chase, P. A., & Hirschhorn, R. *New Engl. J. Med.*, 1976, *295*, 1337–1343.

Schur, P. H., Borel, H., Gelfand, E. W., Alper, C. A., & Rosen, F. S. *New Engl. J. Med.*, 1970, *283*, 631–634.

Shaw, G. M., Hahn, B. H., Arya, S. K., Groopman, S. E., Gallo, R. C., Wong-Staal, F. Molecular characterization of human T-cell leukemia (lymphotropic) virus type III in the acquired immune deficiency syndrome. *Science*, 1984, *226*, 1165–1171.

Strober, W., Krakauer, R., Klarveman, H. L., Reynolds, H. Y., & Nelson, D. L. *New Engl. J. Med.*, 1976, *294*, 351–356.

Tiller, T. L., & Buckley, R. H. *J. Pediatr.*, 1978, *92*, 347–353.

Weening, R., Ross, D., Weemaes, C., Homan Muller, J., Scheik, M.: Defective initiation of the metabolic stimulation in phagocytizing granulocytes: A new congenital defect. *J. Labs. Clin. Med.*, 1976, *88*, 757–768.

SUGGESTED READINGS

Blaese, M. R. In C. W. Parker (Ed.), *Clinical immunology*. Philadelphia: Saunders, 1980, Vol. I, pp. 314–375.

Steihm, R. E., & Fulqiniti, V. A. *Immunologic disorders of infants and children*. Philadelphia: Saunders, 1980.

QUESTIONS

1. A 2-year-old patient is admitted to the hospital with *Haemophilus influenzae* meningitis. He has had two episodes of pneumococcal sepsis and pneumonia in the past. He responds to the treatment for meningitis and is normally developed. This patient is most likely deficient in which branches of his host defense?
   a. Cellular immunity
   b. Complement
   c. Humoral immunity
   d. Phagocyte function
2. Which of the following immunodeficiencies can be diagnosed *in vitro*?
   a. Chronic granulomatous disease.
   b. Combined immunodeficiency with enzyme deficiency
   c. Complement deficiency
   d. Common variable immunodeficiency
3. For which of the following immunodeficiencies is there a specific curative treatment?
   a. Ataxia telangiectasia
   b. Sex-linked agammaglobulinemia
   c. Chronic granulomatous disease
   d. Severe combined immunodeficiency
   e. DiGeorge syndrome
4. In investigation of the immunoglobulin system, which of the following tests are most appropriate and sufficient to rule out significant abnormality?
   a. B-cell enumeration by immunofluorescence
   b. Salivary IgA
   c. Quantitative immunoglobulins by radial immunodiffusion
   d. Isohemagglutinins, polio, or tetanus titers
   e. Serum protein electrophoresis
5. What is appropriate management of infants with low immunoglobulin levels and recurrent upper respiratory infections?
   a. Determination of antibody titers for specific immunizations and, if present, close observation of the patient.
   b. Begin gamma globulin injections.
   c. Start a program of antibiotic prophylaxis.

Answers can be found in Appendix B at the end of the book.

Jeffrey I. Schulman

32

Advice to Parents of the Allergic Child

In addition to making an accurate diagnosis of allergy or asthma and establishing an appropriate treatment plan, it is the physician's responsibility to thoroughly advise allergic children and their parents of the nature, therapy, and prognosis of their disease. Education and communication are among the most important factors on which successful therapy can be built.

Physician, patient, and family must all be informed in order to deal with a chronic allergic condition. It is the physician's responsibility to aid the allergic child and the immediate family in controlling the allergy or asthma, rather than allowing the illness to control the child and the family.

RECOGNIZING ALLERGY AND ASTHMA

It is disconcerting for a parent to have a child who has persistent or recurring problems for which they have no explanation. In some instances the physician can help the family deal with problems before they occur. If parents who are both allergic or asthmatic realize that their offspring have a substantial chance of developing allergy or asthma, they will be aware of problems early in their child's development and can deal with them effectively before needless frustration and anxiety accumulate. Likewise, parents should be made aware that approximately 50% of infants with eczema may subsequently develop respiratory allergy, either allergic rhinitis or asthma. Some studies would suggest that an allergy-prone or atopic infant may develop less food sensitivity if cow's milk is avoided for the first 6 months of life and allergenic foods such as egg white and citrus products until age 1 year.

ALLERGY: THEORY AND PRACTICE
ISBN 0-8089-1619-X

EVALUATION AND REFERRAL

A crucial role of the primary physician is to advise the parents of the allergic or asthmatic child regarding the need for diagnostic studies or referral to a specialist. Many factors will influence this decision. The frequency, severity, and persistence of the problem and the course of the illness are obviously important. Although allergic rhinitis is not a life-threatening illness, it can certainly be very bothersome and frustrating and have a negative effect on a child's overall function. In addition, it may cause or worsen serous otitis media and sinusitis. Therefore, it is appropriate to evaluate persistent or bothersome allergic rhinitis. Any child having recurrent or persistent lower respiratory symptoms should be thoroughly evaluated to establish a clearcut diagnosis.

Although some children do "outgrow their allergies," just as many do not and often develop worse symptoms each year (Block, 1982). There is no reason for a young child with asthma to suffer for years on the chance that the symptoms will diminish at some time in the distant future. Parents of children counseled in family asthma programs uniformly express the wish that they had been advised to see a specialist for a better understanding of the problem many years earlier.

UNDERSTANDING ALLERGY

Patients and their parents need to be informed of the basis of the allergic reaction. They should understand that an allergy is a condition in which certain individuals develop an unusual sensitivity to foreign substances or to physical conditions that are harmless to nonallergic individuals. They should know that there are multitudes of diverse substances, including animal danders, pollens, molds, house dust, mites, food, chemicals, and additives that may be responsible for initiating the allergic response.

The symptoms resulting from an allergic reaction may also vary depending on the patient's age and the anatomic location of the allergic reaction. The severity of the reaction may vary from a mild annoyance during the peak of a brief seasonal exposure to a life-threatening illness such as anaphylaxis or severe asthma. Many allergies, although not life-threatening, adversely affect a child's general emotional, intellectual, and physical well-being. If the allergic children and their parents can be helped to understand the diversity of allergic problems and variability, they will be better equipped to deal with them.

UNDERSTANDING ASTHMA

The parents of the asthmatic child should be helped to understand that the fundamental problem in asthma is the irritable or hyperactive airway. Although allergy is a common trigger of asthma, the child's parents should know that infection, irritants, and exercise may all trigger the increased secretions, edema, and bronchospasm that may cause coughing, wheezing, chest tightness, and shortness of breath. It is helpful for the child and parent to realize that asthma is the most common chronic disease of childhood, affecting five percent of children under age 15. Parents should be assured that although no cure is known for asthma, the disease can be controlled. However, the child needs to avoid significant allergens and strong irritants to the respiratory tract such as cigarette smoking in the house. Parents should be instructed in the proper use of bronchodilators. It is quite helpful if they are told in advance of the common side effects associated with a particular medication and are advised that adjustments in drugs or dosages may be needed to control a child's asthma. A broad range of medications is now available in the physician's armamentarium, so that significant side effects need not be endured in order to control the respiratory problem.

Finally, the parent should be advised that immunotherapy may be a very useful adjunct to therapy in the child whose asthma is triggered largely by immediate hypersensitivity to unavoidable aeroallergens. Control of the patient's asthma in a manner least disruptive to the child and family's lifestyle is the ideal.

ENVIRONMENTAL CONTROL

The physician should advise parents on where and when specific allergens are found, so that the child's exposure to the responsible allergens may be managed. This advice should be based on the individual child's sensitivity, not on a long list of do's and don't's presented to every allergic individual. A pet should only be removed if there is clearcut evidence that it is causing symptoms (parenthetically, parents should be advised to avoid pets in order to eliminate the necessity and trauma of removing them). Every effort should be made to individualize treatment, not destroy a child's bedroom or house because the child happens to be allergic or have asthma. However, it must be made clear to the family that making no effort to lessen exposure to significant allergens and irritants to the respiratory tract will undermine an otherwise well-designed treatment plan employing medications and/or immunotherapy.

MEDICATIONS

Effective use of pharmacologic agents in the treatment of allergic disease requires an awareness of the limitations, side effects, cost, and taste of any medication prescribed.

The school-age child should begin to assume some responsiblity for taking medication independently, depending on age and maturity. Compliance is greatly enhanced if the child understands why a pill should be taken and shares responsibility for doing so, instead of being forced to take the medication with no choice and no understanding.

IMMUNOTHERAPY

The child and parents should understand the purposes, actions, and limitations of immunotherapy. The reasons for gradually increasing doses and the fact that a systemic reaction is always possible should be clearly explained. The parents and patient should realize that improvement is not instantaneous and that immunotherapy does not help everyone. A reasonable expectation of the goals of the program and the probable duration, usually 3–4 years, should be presented.

DIET AND HYGIENE

These areas are very important for the child with chronic medical problems. Sound nutrition, adequate rest, and good hygiene are essential to helping the child cope with and overcome the illness.

ACTIVITY AND EXERCISE

Children with asthma or allergies should be just as active as their peers. Participation in exercise, sports, and other activities should be strongly encouraged. Children with exercise-induced bronchospasm triggered by sports requiring vigorous activity should be given adequate prophylaxis so that they can play on the team with their friends. Cromolyn or nebulized sympathomimetics work quite effectively for many asthmatics, so the optimal regimen to prevent exercise problems for a given child can usually be achieved. Activity, particularly swimming, helps to strengthen the chest wall musculature and improve the vital capacity.

PSYCHOLOGICAL AND EMOTIONAL CONCERNS

The role of emotions and psychological factors in causing asthma is controversial and largely unproved; however, it is clear that stress may affect many physical conditions and that any chronic illness has a significant psychological impact on the child, the immediate family, and the environment. The child with a chronic illness will often have some feelings of helplessness, overdependence, fear, anger, or guilt. The child may feel different from other children and have a negative self-image and lack of self-esteem. The physician should help in counseling the child and family to promote self-reliance, self-worth, and self-esteem along with good physical health.

In addition to the child, the parents often feel anxiety, fear, frustration, guilt, overprotectiveness, or panic; siblings may feel jealous, bitter, or resentful; and friends may feel left out and lack understanding.

The physician, through open communication and counseling, may anticipate many problems and better help the child, peers, and the family and cope with the problems in the broadest sense.

DEALING WITH THE SCHOOL

It is important that the child function in the total environment, of which school plays a prominent role. Respiratory illnesses, including allergies and asthma, are the most common cause of school absenteeism. An example of a letter addressed to the school of an asthmatic child is given in Figure 32-1.

(John Doe) has been under my care for asthma for the past _(2 years)_. Asthma is an intermittent blockage of the airways that results in coughing, wheezing, and shortness of breath. Once present, it is often worsened by exercise or significant exertion. While _(John)_ should participate fully in physical education and be encouraged to keep up with his peers, he should be allowed to cease activity if he is wheezing or short of breath.

For control of his asthma, _(John)_ takes the following medications:

1. Aminophylline 200-mg tablet every 6 hours.
2. Albuterol (Inhaler)—2 breaths no more than every 4 hours for difficulty despite the use of aminophylline. _John_ may use it for 15 minutes prior to those forms of activity that cause him difficulty.

If _(John)_ begins having difficulty at school despite his regular medications, which he should be allowed to take at school, I would recommend that he be given copious fluids to drink and be allowed to rest. For any further problems, his mother should be called, or I may be consulted.

Please let me know if I may help in any other way in allowing those at school to best help _(John)_ cope with his asthma.

Sincerely,

Al U. Pent, M.D.

Fig. 32-1. Model school letter for asthma.

Physical education may be a major problem. The teacher and school should realize that exercise is very helpful, and the child should be encouraged to participate normally in all activity, not banished, ostracised, or made to feel inferior because of respiratory problems. However, the child should be allowed to rest or take medication if problems develop, not drive to finish the race even though breathing is impossible.

The physician can markedly facilitate the child's interaction with the school by keeping the school informed about the child's condition, helping set limits, and providing information to promote better understanding of the problem. If possible, long-acting medications may be used to lessen the need for the child to take medications at school.

SOURCES OF HELP

Finally, physicians should be aware of available community resources so they may best educate the allergic children and their parents, control or prevent the symptoms, and help the children and their families cope with the illness and lead a full normal life.

Three excellent resources are:

1. The Asthma and Allergy Foundation of America (19 West 44th Street, New York, New York 10036). This organization or its closest local chapter provides infor-

mation and educational materials to the public, medical profession, and health workers. Many local chapters sponsor parent-support groups and outstanding local programs.

2. The American Lung Association (1740 Broadway, New York, New York 10019). In addition to providing a broad range of literature for the child, parent, school, and medical professional, many local associations sponsor Family Asthma Programs to teach children and their parents about asthma and how to cope with it. A new program called "Superstuff" is available on request to help elementary children and their families handle asthma.
3. U.S. Department of Health and Services. Many publications are available, including the best book for asthma and allergy sufferer, entitled *Asthma and allergies: An optimistic future* (order No. 017-044-000034-6) available for $6.50 from Superintendent of Documents, U.S. Government Printing Office, Washington, D.C. 20402.

In addition, handouts given to patients and their parents are quite beneficial. Several examples are given below.

Patient Handout: Allergy

An "allergy" is an abnormal reaction due to increased sensitivity to foreign substances (allergens) that are harmless to nonallergic individuals. The allergic reaction is essentially an overreaction of one branch of the immune system that normally protects against infection.

An allergen may be inhaled, swallowed, touched, or injected. Common allergens include pollens (grasses, trees, weeds), molds, house dust, mites, animal dander (the skin that is shed even by animals that do not shed hair), foods, medication, chemicals, insect venoms, feathers, and other household substances.

When the allergic substance enters the body, a reaction occurs in some of the white blood cells that releases chemicals (histamines and others), which cause swelling, increased secretions, and tightening of muscles in the area of the reaction. The symptoms of the allergy depend on the sensitivity of the individual, the amount of allergen exposure, and the location of the allergic reaction in the body. The same substance may cause itchy, red eyes; sneezing, congestion, and a runny nose; hives; coughing, wheezing, and shortness of breath; or abdominal pain and diarrhea. The symptoms may be seasonal if caused by certain pollens (trees and grasses in the spring, weeds in the late summer and fall in most areas) or year-round if caused by an animal, dust, or indoor mold to which one is constantly exposed.

When an allergy cannot be cured, it can be controlled. There are three general approaches to the treatment of allergy:

1. *Avoidance* of the offending substance and nonspecific irritants known to worsen most respiratory or skin conditions. This is particularly important with allergy to foods and pets.
2. *Medications* to control or prevent symptoms, used either regularly or as needed when symptoms occur.
3. *Immunotherapy* ("allergy shots") to decrease an individual's sensitivity to unavoidable allergens.

Patient Handout: Asthma

The word "asthma" is derived from the Greek word meaning "panting" or shortness of breath. Asthma is basically a tendency for the bronchial tubes to be irritable and overreact to a variety of different trigger factors. We presently do not know why some people have such sensitive bronchial tubes.

Everyone has a series of air passages in the lungs resembling an upside-down tree. The windpipe (trachea) divides into large branches to the left and right lungs, and these large branches form progressively smaller branches all the way out to the edge of the lung. Each branch (bronchus) has a thin lining blanket of mucus on the inside to help trap inhaled pollutants and germs, and each tube is surrounded by a thin layer of muscle.

In the child with asthma, three things happen in the lungs that tend to obstruct the normal flow of air out of the lungs:

1. The muscles surrounding the bronchial tubes tend to tighten, constrict, or go into spasm (bronchospasm), so the tube is narrower.
2. There is swelling (edema) of the walls of the bronchial tubes, also making them narrower for air to flow through.
3. Excessive amount of sticky mucus secretions are produced, tending to further clog the tubes.

This tendency for the sensitive bronchial tube to overreact may be triggered by a variety of factors: (a) *allergies*—generally due to inhaled substances such as animal dander, pollens, molds, or dust; (b) *infection*—usually simple viral infections such as "colds that may go into the chest"; (c) *irritants*—smoke, pollutants, strong odors, chemicals, and so on; and (d) *exercise*—activity such as running or jogging, particularly if the weather is cold.

Other possible trigger factors may include reflexes triggered by a laugh or cough or drinking an ice cold beverage, emotional stresses, sinus infection, weather changes, and reflux of food from the stomach back up the feeding tube (esophagus).

No two children with asthma are alike. One child may have only increased secretions in the smaller bronchial tubes triggered by a viral infection that leads to a pattern of persistent croupy cough with each cold, whereas another may have a sudden onset of bronchospasm triggered by exposure to a cat, manifest by sudden wheezing and shortness of breath.

Although there is no cure for asthma (we cannot eliminate the tendency for the bronchial tubes to overreact), it can be controlled.

1. The child should avoid or minimize exposure to known allergens and known irritants to the respiratory tract, such as smoke.
2. A variety of medications are available to relax the bronchial tubes and lessen secretions (bronchodilators). Some children require these only when problems begin, whereas others need medication regularly because of the nature of their disease. Children and parents should know in advance what to do if problems begin; they should be advised to take fluids, try to relax, and know what dose of which medication to take if coughing or wheezing persist. Children in whom

wheezing is triggered by infection should be given a bronchodilator at the onset of any upper respiratory illness (URI), not 2 days later when they are wheezing and short of breath. Similarly, children who are short of breath and cough with exercise should receive medication prior to beginning the exercise. Wheezing and coughing are only the tip of the iceberg; medication should be continued over several days after all symptoms cease in order to totally relieve the airway obstruction.

3. Allergy injections may reduce an allergic child's sensitivity and thus minimize one of the factors triggering the asthma.

With early diagnosis and treatment, most children with asthma can lead a very normal life and not experience chronic lung disease as adults.

Patient Handout: Environmental Control

PETS. Allergy is caused by substances in saliva and the dander (skin), not just the hair, so nonshedding dogs and animals may be major cause of difficulty. Even patients who are not allergic to pets should keep their pets far from the bedroom since the hair and dander are often quite irritating to the lining of the respiratory tract. If you are definitely allergic to a pet, and already have one, it should be kept outdoors at all times. Otherwise you will continue to have symptoms despite medications and other treatments.

HOUSE DUST. As opposed to outside dust, which is basically small particles of blowing dirt and may serve as an irritant, *house dust* is a complicated substance that may cause true allergy. It consists of breakdown products of bedding materials, rugs, curtains, human hair, animal hair and dander, molds, body parts of insects, outside dirt, and mites (microscopic animals). The best way to prevent symptoms from house dust allergy is to remove as much dust as possible from your home. It is important to pay special attention to the bedroom where much time is spent. The following suggestions will help to make the environment more comfortable.

To clean and "dust-proof" the bedroom, do this cleaning while the patient is away from the house. Initially, remove all furniture from the room. Wet mop and wet dust the room wall from top to bottom, including lights, closets, window sills, shelves, and molding. A solution of Lysol in water helps to minimize mold growth. Clean all furniture well before it is put back into the room. Wet mop and wet dust surfaces once or twice a week. Treat furnishings in the bedroom as follows:

1. Beds in the room should have wooden or metal frames. Do not use a couch, sofa, or hide-a-bed.
2. Place the mattress in a vinyl (soft plastic) cover that has a zipper. If a box spring is used, it must have a plastic cover, too. Very serviceable, zippered, plastic covers are available in many department and "dry goods" stores. More sturdy and comfortable (but also substantially more expensive) covers may be obtained from Allergy-Free Products for the Home, P.O. Box 345, 1162 W. Lynn Street, Springfield, Mo. 65801 or Allergen-Proof Encasings, 4046 Superior Avenue, Cleveland, Ohio 44103.
3. Pillows should be made of Dacron or other synthetic fiber. Do *not* use kapok, feather, or "down" pillows.

Do not use comforters, quilts, or a bedspread on the bed. Use only cotton, rayon, or synthetic fiber blankets. These should be washed often.

4. Small, washable cotton rugs may be used if washed often. If you use a rug pad, be sure that it is made of rubber. If it is impossible to remove a rug, it should be steam cleaned at least every 6 months.
5. Remove all upholstered ("stuffed") furniture, bean-bag chairs, throw pillows, stuffed toys, window drapes, and dust-catching ornaments from the bedroom.
6. Remove all stored toys, packages, and other articles from the closet. The closet should contain only the clothing in season and should be as dust-free as the room.

Close all furnace outlets in the room; otherwise, the room will become filled with dust-laden air during the operation of the furnace. An electric heater may be used to heat the room, or electric blanket may be used. The bedroom closet door and bedroom door should remain closed as much as possible.

MOLD. Mold is mildew or fungus—microscopic plants found in large quantity in nature. They are present all year round indoors and outdoors (least prevalent when the ground is covered with snow). Mold thrives under moist, humid conditions and grows on plant life or vegetation.

Suggestions for decreasing mold exposure are as follows:

1. Do not use a vaporizer. Use of vaporizers over several weeks or months often encourages mold growth in the patient's bedroom. They may seem to benefit the patient but should be avoided. Vaporizers may be used, however, for several days if medically indicated for laryngitis, severe colds, or croup. If used, they should be cleaned with half-strength Clorox or Lysol solution run through the machine for 2 hours daily. Generally a good fluid intake more effectively loosens secretions than the attempt to inhale water vapor.
2. Remove plants and stuffed animals from the patient's bedroom.
3. Regularly clean with a fungicide, such as Lysol, in water.
4. Dehumidify basement or crawl space; cross-ventilation is most helpful. Molds grow where it is damp and dark. Molds also abound in attics. Watch for household water leaks.
5. Basements and other potentially damp areas should be sealed and painted with mold-inhibiting paint; *Captan* may be added to some.
6. Since humidifiers, dehumidifiers, and air conditioners are constantly exposed to dampness, check them constantly for a musty smell and spray with a mild inhibitor such as Lysol.

IRRITANTS. Once the lining of the respiratory tract is inflamed in individuals with respiratory allergy, the nose and/or lungs are more sensitive to any potential irritants in the air. In addition to dust, mold and animal dander, smoke, chemical odors, fumes, and pollution will be very aggravating.

Smoking is harmful to everyone with asthma or respiratory allergy. There must be *no smoking* in enclosed spaces such as the house or car, or the problem will continue.

Try to minimize the patient's exposure to strong odors, such as turpentine, cooking odors, perfume, paint, and insecticide sprays, which are all potentially irritating.

Any attempt to treat asthma or respiratory allergy must begin with good environmental control and avoidance of known allergens or irritants.

Patient Handout: Immunotherapy

The most effective treatment of an allergy is avoidance of the substance that triggers the reaction. Although this is usually possible with allergy to foods or animal danders, it is obviously impractical to completely avoid house dust, molds, or pollens from grasses, trees, or weeds. Therefore, a program of immunotherapy (hyposensitization or "allergy shots") may be necessary to control the symptoms.

By injecting gradually increasing amounts of extracts of the offending allergens under the skin, an allergic individual will develop a tolerance or reduced sensitivity for those substances exposure to them.

Since, by history and skin tests, one is allergic to the substances in the injection, the most effective dose of the extract cannot be given at the onset. For safety, a very small dose is given initially and is gradually increased once or twice a week, until a maintenance dose is reached. This dose, over 1000 times greater than the initial dose, is an average protective level or the highest tolerated dose. After an optimal dose has been achieved, the interval between injections is gradually increased as tolerated, depending on the time of year and the duration of improvement following an injection.

Although rapid improvement is occasionally noted in some individuals, significant improvement usually occurs in the second 6 months of treatment. Many individuals will experience marked improvement and be able to maintain symptom-free intervals of a month between injections during the third year of immunotherapy, whereas others will continue to require more frequent injections. Those who experience adequate suppression of their allergies after 3 years may be able to discontinue the injections with permanent relief, whereas others may require treatment for longer periods of time.

REFERENCES

Bock, S. A., *J. Allergy Clin. Immunol.*, 1982, *69*, 173–177.

APPENDIX B: ANSWERS

Chapter 2

1. e. Basophils and mast cells have receptors for IgE. Activation of these cells by appropriate allergens initiates the release of histamine and other inflammatory mediators. This reaction is the basis for type I immediate hypersensitivity.

2. a. Macrophages are important phagocytic cells. They are also essential for regulation of lymphocyte function. Macrophages ingest antigens prior to presentation to specific receptors on the surface membrane of lymphocytes. Macrophages are a major cell seen in chronic inflammatory reactions.

3. c. Eosinophils release a major basic protein that is toxic to schistosomula. On the other hand, this protein may play a role in the pathogenesis of asthma since it can damage respiratory epithelial cells.

   Superoxide and hydrogen peroxide are chemicals made by neutrophils. These substances are toxic to certain microorganisms.

   B Lymphocytes differentiate in the plasma cells that secrete antibodies.

4. b,e. Allergic rhinitis and asthma are typically caused by inhaled allergens such as pollens, mold spores, house dust, and animal danders. Skin testing with extracts of these allergens induces a positive wheal-and-flare response in 15 minutes. Total serum IgE as well as specific IgE antibodies against these allergens are usually elevated. Serum immune complexes and positive patch tests are not characteristically seen in these syndromes. A lung biopsy is rarely indicated for evaluating patients with asthma; moreover, deposition of complement fragments would not be expected.

5. a–e (all). The complement system is essential for normal inflammatory responses. Complement functions in host defense include attraction of neutrophils, increased phagocytosis of bacteria by neutrophils, and direct killing of bacteria by cell lysis. Fragments created by complement activation also release histamine from blood basophils and tissue mast cells. Histamine causes leakage of fluid and cells from capillaries. In hemolytic anemia, the complement system may be activated by antibodies on the erythrocyte surface, leading to red cell lysis.

Chapter 3

1. d. Histamine is chemotactic for eosinophils but *not* for other inflammatory cells.

2. c. Platelet activating factor is an unusual phospholipid.

3. e. 5-hydroperoxyeicosatetraenoic acid (5-HPETE) is the first product in the 5-lipoxygenase pathway.

4. a. SRS is similar to histamine in many of its actions but does *not* appear to inhibit lymphocyte function.

5. b. Prostaglandin E_2 is a potent relaxer of smooth muscle. PGD_2 and $PGF_{2\alpha}$ are smooth muscle contractors.

ISBN 0-8089-1619-X

Chapter 4

1. a,c,e. Fever, sore throat, and cervical adenopathy more often are seen with respiratory tract infections, whereas sneezing and itching usually are present in patients experiencing allergic rhinitis.
2. b–d. The common seasonal mold allergens are most prevalent in the northern United States from about June until fall or after a blanketing snow. They tend to grow on dead vegetation, such as hay or fallen leaves. The inhalant allergens in *Penicillium* are different from those in penicillin.
3. c. In contrast to atopic diseases, allergic contact dermatitis is less likely to occur seasonally or in certain geographic locales (except for plant oil dermatitis). On the other hand, the distribution of the lesions (e.g., under jewelry, exposed areas, sites of makeup, perfume or hair dye application, clothing distribution, etc.) often provides valuable clues to etiology.
4. e. Asthmatics often exhibit inspiratory as well as expiratory wheezing together with increased respiratory rate. When asthma becomes severe, wheezing may cease as a result of poor ventilation, and pulsus paradoxus is common in moderate to severe asthma. However, clubbing of the digits essentially never is seen in uncomplicated asthma.
5. a,e. Hay fever usually is associated with allergic conjunctivitis, and typically the nasal mucosa is pale and swollen (although this is quite variable). In the absence of supervening infection there seldom is sinus tenderness, and nasal polyps rarely occur in children with this condition. Cobblestoning of the conjunctivae would suggest vernal conjunctivitis.

Chapter 5

1. d. Although scratch (and prick testing) are more *specific* they are less sensitive because of the smaller amount of antigen injected.
2. d.
3. c.
4. b. Whereas corticosteroid will block mast cell or basophil histamine release in the test tube, there is no evidence that this occurs *in vivo*.
5. e. A 3+ positive prick test is a highly specific reaction. No other test is needed. The skin test positivity should be correlated with this history.
6. d.

Chapter 6

1. d. Only 50% of patients with allergic rhinitis have nasal eosinophils. In patients with nonallergic rhinitis with nasal eosinophils, intranasal corticosteroids were efficacious.
2. a. In the absence of exposure to the allergen, there are no symptoms of allergic rhinitis. Answers b and d represent palliative effects only.
3. c. Skin testing is the most sensitive and cost-effective means of identifying the causative allergens.

4. d. Vasomotor rhinitis is very rarely accompanied by conjunctivitis or otitis and almost never by watery rhinorrhea.
5. a. The parasympathetic system causes nasal blood vessel dilatation, nasal obstruction, and mucus secretion.

Chapter 7

1. d. Suggest M + T. A serous effusion commonly follows an acute infection and may take weeks to resolve. Conservative therapy such as decongestants, antibiotics, Valsalva and close observation is warranted for at least 4 weeks before myringtomy and tube placement is suggested.
2. e. Young healthy infants at home are susceptible to the same common middle ear pathogens as are their older counterparts. Hospitalized infants, however, are more likely to harbor E. coli and staph aureus and should be cultured. Therefore, routine measures are indicated for cases of uncomplicated AOM. Some pediatricians require LP's in the ER to rule out meningeal infection.
3. e. The frontal sinus in children this age has not developed yet and may be misinterpreted as "opacified". Children do have ethmoid and small maxillary sinuses and these are easily evaluated on plain films for acute or chronic disease. Primary tumors of the frontal sinus are rare in children and adults.
4. d. Rhinitis medicamentosa presents in two forms—a rebound congestion or atrophic mucosal changes depending on the body's response to chronic sympathetic stimulation and vasoconstrictors. The treatment is to stop all decongestants and use topical steroid sprays for their antiinflammatory effect.
5. f. Chronic sinusitis is a result of longstanding mucosal irritation due to allergic, mechanical and infection agents. Medical therapy is generally adequate to control symptoms; surgery is recommended in those cases where symptoms persist despite medical therapy due to permanent mucosal changes.

Chapter 8

1. True. The majority of patients with atopic eczematous dermatitis have a personal or family history of asthma, hayfever, allergic rhinitis, or atopic eczema. However, 20 percent of the patients have neither a personal nor a family history of atopy.
2. False. Skin biopsies of allergic eczematous contact dermatitis reveal mainly nonspecific changes characteristic of an eczematous dermatitis, but with no clue to an etiologic diagnosis. Patch testing with appropriate materials is the best diagnostic test presently available. Standard test trays are available and additional materials can be tested if properly prepared.
3. False. Allergic eczematous contact dermatitis is due to a type IV immune reaction, i.e., a delayed type hypersensitivity. At present, there is no consistently effective immunotherapy. Treatment is symptomatic and is individualized depending upon the distribution and severity of the eruption.
4. e. All of the above statements are correct regarding associated disorders and complications related to atopic eczematous dermatitis. There are numerous other associated findings which are covered in the text.

5. b. The pattern and distribution of the skin lesions is quite helpful in diagnosing an allergic eczematous contact dermatitis. The linear pattern of the lesions and restricted distribution to the arms is quite characteristic of various plant resin contact reactions. This can also be helpful when similar lesions appear restricted to the facial area, characteristic of certain cosmetic allergies.

Chapter 9

1. e. Despite a thorough evaluation, the etiology of chronic urticaria and angioedema in about two-thirds of the cases is not found. However, it does not appear to be caused by the other possibilities listed as answers to this question.
2. d. Although urticaria and angioedema may be the presenting complaint of rheumatic diseases and malignancies, it is uncommon, and the underlying disease usually is manifest by 6 months. Patients are aware of this possibility and are quite concerned that "something else is wrong."
3. a. Epinephrine is immediately indicated for these life-threatening problems.
4. c. As is well illustrated in the case report, antihistamines do little other than perhaps reduce the itching once the lesions are present.
5. d. There is no convincing evidence that emotions or anxiety-provoking situations can cause hives. Vitamin deficiency or vitamin excesses are not related (curative) to acute or chronic urticaria and angioedema. Interpretative skin testing for foods and aeroallergens must be conservative. A positive skin test for coconut, chocolate, or bananas does not necessarily mean that the cause of the swelling has been uncovered. When a large battery of food skin tests are applied, many normal individuals will react with a positive test to certain foods. This may be an irritative phenomenon or an IgE-mediated reaction. Only resolution of the swelling with elimination of the putative offending food is strong evidence for an etiologic role.

Chapter 10

1. a. Subcutaneous epinephrine that exerts multiple antianaphylactic effects including decreasing edema and vascular permeability, increasing cardiac output, bronchodilation and inhibition of further mast cell release. Although helpful in preventing late onset and recurrent anaphylaxis, steroids are not considered necessary in initial resuscitation efforts. Vasopressors of course would not help airway obstruction secondary either to bronchospasm or edema.
2. c. Intravenous contrast material seems to induce mast cell release by a direct or pharmacological mechanism, whereas b and d are examples of IgE-mediated and a, of immune-complex-mediated processes.
3. d. Sulfa allergy. The only drugs for which skin testing accurately detects allergic sensitivity include penicillin and some other B-lactam antibiotics and certain hormones including insulin and antisera of heterologous animal origin such as horse serum.
4. d. Oral challenge may be dangerous and in general should be avoided. Skin testing or RAST may be performed instead.
5. d. Each of these actions will help to prevent anaphylactic reactions.

Chapter 11

1. b. Physicians commonly make the error of administering an antihistamine alone as their first line of therapy for histamine-related events, and then waiting to see if this will be effective. The therapy that is appropriate for *acute* reversal of histamine effect is epinephrine, although an antihistamine such as Benadryl should be administered simultaneously in therapy of ongoing histamine release. Delay in administration of epinephrine can be potentially dangerous, given the accelerated nature of many anaphylactic or anaphylactoid reactions.

2. e. Though loss of consciousness is an infrequent complication of anaphylaxis or anaphylactoid reactions, it can be seen as a sequela of hypotension. Loss of consciousness from other etiologies, such as hypoglycemic coma or vasovagal syncope, is not associated with respiratory distress. Respiratory distress can be seen in myocardial infarction, arrhythmias, and pulmonary emboli due to acute cardiac failure and/or inability to oxygenate the blood. The respiratory distress of anaphylaxis or anaphylactoid reactions is generally due to laryngea edema and/or bronchospasm. In this patient with loss of consciousness preceded by respiratory distress, we are not informed regarding the presence of stridor, urticaria, or angioedema. Hence it is difficult to distinguish whether this was a primary cardiopulmonary versus histamine-related event.

3. e. Prausnitz-Kustner transfer and RAST testing are measures of skin-sensitizing, reaginic antibody. They are positive in anaphylactic reactions and negative in anaphylactoid reactions and thus can distinguish the two. Provocative challenging by the oral or inhaled routes may be positive in both anaphylactic and anaphylactoid reactions and thus cannot distinguish the two.

4. b. The mechanism of RCM reactions, for the majority of cases, is probably anaphylactoid. Evidence for an immunologically mediated reaction is lacking. No skin tests are available to predict the likelihood of such reactions. In patients with a history of previous ARs to radiographic contrast, the incidence of a repeat reaction is much higher than in those without such a history. Repeat reactions may be less severe, as severe, or more severe than the initial event. Reactions may indeed be life-threatening, and deaths have been reported. Hence the decision to embark on a radiographic contrast material study should be made after careful consideration of its necessity. If the study is an important diagnostic adjunct to the patient's evaluation, premedication with steroids and diphenhydramine can quite significantly diminish the severity and frequency of repeat reactions.

5. d. Patients with IgA deficiency may receive blood as washed red cells, by autotransfusion, and from IgA-deficient donors. Washed red cells are probably the most convenient blood source and can be prepared by three serial manual washes of red cells in saline, or serial washes through a mechanical washer, which leaves an approximate 1% level of residual plasma. Although packed cells contain less serum than whole blood, there is still sufficient IgA present to cause a severe anaphylactoid reaction.

Chapter 12

1. c. The patient is obviously allergic to house dust mite and feather antigen and environmental control is the treatment of choice. Increasing humidity is counterproductive, the psychiatrist's opinion is suspect because chronic allergic diseases may mimic depression, and immunotherapy and switching drugs are not appropriate as initial measures.

2. c. Quarternary ammonium compounds are found in numerous fabric softeners which are used in clothes dryers.

3. b. Very likely antigens involved in causing the patient's asthma are cockroach antigen, and mouse and rat dander. These allergens must be investigated. Smoke antigens are not reliable and should not be tested, although smoke should be avoided. Other measures (a and d, above) would probably provide only minor benefits.

4. e. Sodium metabisulfite, MSG, cigarette smoke, and cockroach antigen have all been clearly implicating as triggers of asthma attacks.

Chapter 13

1. d. Studies have not yet provided that DGL ragweed is effective in humans. Coseasonal injections are often administered once or twice weekly with increasingly stronger concentrations of extract being given and a high rate of large local and systemic reactions. Sublingual immunotherapy has never proved to be effective. Perennial immunotherapy with aqueous ragweed extract is safe and effective if gradually increasing doses are administered, building up to approximately 2500 PNU per injection every 2–4 weeks.

2. c. Persons with mold sensitive asthma may wheeze after eating blue cheese or slightly moldy bread, or drinking beer fermented with yeast. Hives in association with blue cheese is no indication for mold immunotherapy. Mold-sensitive asthma usually occurs in the damp months of the year (March through early November) and not in winter. Farmers with acute hypersensitivity pneumonitis secondary to thermophilic fungi are treated symptomatically and advised to avoid incriminating allergens, since immunotherapy to thermophiles is of no benefit. Although immunotherapy to molds has not definitely been shown to be effective in isolated double-blind placebo-controlled studies, a course of immunotherapy for persons with difficult-to-control asthma worsened by the moldy surroundings of damp grass, leaves, and basement is indicated.

3. e. There are no specific immunologic criteria that can predict successful immunotherapy.

4. c. Large local reactions need only be treated with an ice pack and perhaps an antihistamine. Local epinephrine is unnecessary unless the reaction is becoming systemic. Elevating the arm and applying heat may increase the absorption, effecting a systemic reaction. The onset of action of oral corticosteroids is too prolonged to benefit a large local reaction.

5. e. Long-term studies of aqueous immunotherapy have not found any increased incidence of malignant, immune complex mediated, or local diseases.

Chapter 14

1. c. Recent studies have demonstrated that the combination of H_1 and H_2 receptor antagonists is effective in the management of chronic urticaria patients unresponsive to conventional therapy. Cimetidine alone is unlikely to be effective.
2. c. The major complaints of drowsiness and persistent nasal stuffiness are most likely to benefit from the addition of a sympathomimetic decongestant.
3. d. The patient most likely has ethylenediamine sensitivity but may take antihistamines from classes other than ethylenediamine and piperazine.
4. b. Brompheniramine has been associated with increased teratogenic effects. A trial of antihistamine would be justified if symptoms are not severe.
5. b. All other answers are incorrect here.

Chapter 15

1. d. Theophylline is not a cerebral vasoconstrictor.
2. d.
3. a.
4. b. Intravenous aminophylline is clearly indicated. A constant infusion without a loading dose or a small loading dose is generally reserved for patients already taking oral theophylline.
5. a. Decrease
   b. Decrease
   c. Decrease
   d. No change
   e. Decrease

Chapter 16

1. c.
2. c.
3. d.
4. c.
5. d.

Chapter 17

1. c. Cromolyn has little or no actions except its effect on the mast cell or basophil.
2. e. Cromolyn is an effective inhibitor of mediator release from mast cells irrespective of the stimulus.
3. b. Beta-adrenergic agents prevent the early phase whereas corticosteroids inhibit the late phase; only chromolyn is capable of inhibiting both.
4. d. Cromolyn is a prophylactic drug and cannot be used in wheezing patients who cannot activate the spinhaler.

Chapter 18

1. c. Administration of either long-acting steroids (a) or a second late-afternoon or evening dose of short-acting steroid (b and d) results in hypothalamic-pituitary-adrenal suppression.

2. a. An ADA of even 80 mg doses of prednisone does not suppress the tuberculin reaction.

3. c. The primary consideration is the withdrawal of steroids based on clinical evidence that the remaining therapeutic program is sufficient to control the patient's asthma. Answer a is based on an unlikely presumption and risks an exacerbation, whereas answers b and d initiate programs not likely to be required because of the patient's short-term exposure to steroids and absence of past steroid dependancy.

4. d. Based on current evidence, only d is correct.

5. a. An exacerbation of asthma in a previously steroid-dependent patient transferred to BDA requires a prompt temporary return to systemic steroids. There is concern regarding this patient's likely adrenal insufficiency in addition to the problem of asthma control.

Chapter 19

1. d. It is generally recognized that immunotherapy be maintained without increasing the dose using the same time interval between injections, as long as this dose does not produce untoward reactions. There is no evidence that immunotherapy has a deleterious influence on pregnancy and that it may reduce the need for medication. It would be inappropriate to risk reactions by increasing the dose. It should not be initiated because of the uncertainty of patient tolerance to immunotherapy generally.

2. b. Brompheniramine is reported to have had teratogenic effects and is unsafe. Prednisone is safe, and it, along with prednisilone, is blocked to a significant degree by the placenta. If corticosteroids are required, there should be no hesitation to use them with rapid changeover to prednisone or prednisilone as soon as the condition allows. The iodide in potassium iodide is taken up by the fetal thyroid, and increases of TSH production occur with development of goiter and with possible respiratory complications. Tetracycline is contraindicated because of effects on the infant's teeth.

3. c. Theophylline may be administered during pregnancy. Theophylline is an effective medication for administration to the pregnant asthmatic as it appears to have minimal evidence of toxicity, except when given in excessive amounts. Theophylline levels should be monitored in the mother as they would be in nonpregnant individuals at a dose similar to that in terms of mg/kg of someone of equal body lean weight.

4. a. Oxytocin appears to have no effect on the asthmatic process, even though it causes uterine contraction. Prostaglandin F_2 alpha is a potent bronchoconstrictor and is contraindicated in the asthmatic. Demerol is a respiratory depressant and is not recommended in patients with asthma for this reason. Diethylether is not in itself bronchospastic but will produce bronchial irritability. Halothane is the anesthetic of choice when a general anesthetic is required.

5. d. Pregnancy may worsen or improve and indeed seems to have less of an effect on preexisting asthma. When there is improvement, it tends to be noted in the first

trimester with exacerbation after parturition. The common rule is the more severe the asthma, the more severe the problem will be during pregnancy.

Chapter 20

1. c. Significant abnormalities are present and demonstrable by spirometry long after the patient begins to improve subjectively.
2. d. Left ventricular preload does not change and it may decrease.
3. c. While mild to moderate hypoxemia may be seen in moderate asthma, severe hypoxemia is only seen in very severe asthma. It is a bad sign.
4. d. Pulmonary vascular resistance increases rather than decreases.
5. c. Changes in arterial blood gases and pulsus paradoxus are late signs and indicate significant worsening. Expiratory flow rates give an accurate reflection of asthma from mild to severe.
6. c. Ventilatory drive is increased in acute asthma.

Chapter 21

1. False. Emotions may be a contributory factor and may cause exacerbations of asthma but are not included in an etiologic classification.
2. False. Although many mild asthmatics will require only one drug, it is wise to prescribe, for most asthmatics, several drugs. This will diminish the overreliance on one drug and thereby decrease the possibility of abuse of that drug.
3. False. Although they require careful patient instructions and they should not be given to children (but if indicated to their parents for use in the children), they may be extremely useful.
4. d. Dehydration, arrhythmias, and acidosis may lead to death, but mucus impaction of the airways is the usual root cause of fatalities in asthma.
5. True. One expects to find a low P_{CO_2} in mild asthma because of alveolar hyperventilation. A normal or slightly elevated P_{CO_2} may be a premonitory sign of impending hypercapbia.

Chapter 22

1. a. False. He would have job-related symptoms only if he inhaled enough TMA to produce irritation of the respiratory tract. Even then, they would occur while he was at work.

   b. True. Anti-TM-HSA antibodies have been found in all workers who have developed "TMA flu".

   c. False. The finished product of epoxy resin doesn't cause immunologic reaction.

   d. True. The "TMA-flu" syndrome is caused by interaction of antiTMA-HSA IgG antibodies and inhaled TMA.

2. a. True. Peak expiratory flow recordings can be made by the employee and will corroborate symptoms of occupational asthma whenever it occurs.

   b. True. Polyurethane varnish contains TDI.

c. False. Toluene diisocyanate antibodies have rarely been detected.

d. True. Once a person is "sensitized" to TDI, symptoms will recur with even minimal exposure.

3. a. Flour sensitivity has developed after as much as 17 years employment.

b. True. Wheat flour is a complete antigen that stimulates production of IgE antibodies; therefore, it will yield positive immediate skin test reactions and positive bronchial challenge results.

c. True. Apparently, the allergen in raw flour is destroyed during the process of baking.

d. False. They are all true.

4. a. False. Much information is needed about threshold limit values for many substances.

b. True. Both management and labor unions have resisted collection of such data for various reasons.

c. True. That is the definition of an "irritating substance."

d. False. Even with funding and personnel at 1980 levels, only a few of the biggest manufacturing plants could be surveyed.

5. a. No. Oak and mahogany have rarely been reported to provoke bronchial constriction.

b. Yes.

c. No. Skin test reactions with woods, even western red cedar, occur rarely.

d. Yes. By preventing mediator release by bronchial mast cells.

Chapter 23

1. c. Farmer's lung, bagassosis, and pigeon breeder's lung are all examples of extrinsic allergic alveolitis due to inhalation of organic dust. Silicosis does not affect the alveoli and does not seem to represent a hypersensitivity response to an organic dust.

2. c. Answers a, b, and d are all true; c is false because serum precipitating antibody is simply an indication of exposure to the organism and an appropriate immune response. Significant numbers of asymptomatic individuals may have a serum precipitating antibody to organic dust antigen.

3. c. Answer a is false in that the classic signs and symptoms of hypersensitivity pneumonitis appear 4–6 hours after exposure to the offending antigen; b is wrong for the same reason. Answer d is incorrect in that hypersensitivity pneumonitis does not involve an immediate IgE anaphylactic-like picture. Answer c is correct in that the progressive dyspnea, cough, and weight loss may classically be associated with chronic hypersensitivity pneumonitis.

4. b. Allergic bronchopulmonary aspergillosis is associated in 100% of cases with a strong, positive, immediate skin test reaction. Another immunologic hallmark is a positive precipitating antibody to *A. fumigatus*. Finally, the *A. fumigatus* growing in the respiratory tract is a potent stimulus to the manufacture of IgE.

5. b. Allergic bronchopulmonary aspergillosis can be considered to be a complication of asthma. It is uniformly found in atopic individuals, the vast majority of whom have a history of antecedent asthma.

Chapter 24

1. c. Gaps in the pollen wall.
2. b. *Ambrosia hispida* (coastal ragweed) may be found flowering in southern Florida year round.
3. a.
4. b.
5. c. And also the closely allied *Cannabis sativa* (marihuana).

Chapter 25

1. c.
2. b.
3. d.
4. d.
5. d.

Chapter 26

1. b. Rice is rarely, if ever, allergenic. Metabisulfites generally cause wheezing, not urticaria. Also, other foods commonly sprayed with metabisulfites, such as salads, should elicit symptoms. Crab is a crustacean, and he is probably allergic to it as well. Clams, oysters, abalone, and fish are not crustaceans, and he is probably not allergic to them.
2. c. Milk is the most likely etiology of increased mucus production, although it is not known whether IgE is involved in the pathogenesis. Symptoms will be eliminated by avoidance of milk and milk products. Other procedures (b and d) are not indicated. Persistent problems to this degree are rarely psychosomatic.
3. d. Chocolate (especially chocolate chips and unsweetened chocolate used in cakes) contains large quantities of phenylethylamine, which may produce headaches many hours later or the next morning. Other foods such as pretzels may contain phenylethylamines or tyramine. She is not "allergic" to chocolate; in fact, she may tolerate milk chocolate. Mold-containing foods might exacerbate rhinitis, but not this type of headache. "Tension headache" should not be considered unless easily remediable causes such as phenylethylamine, caffeine withdrawal, and cooling of neck muscles during sleep are ruled out. Furthermore, patients with tension headache do *not* awaken with headache.
4. d. Influenza shots may produce severe (even fatal) reactions.
5. a. Elimination of the most likely causes is the procedure of choice. Occult infections are less commonly found. Diaries are inappropriate for frequent symptoms, and RAST testing to all available food antigens is prohibitively expensive. Adjustment of medications is appropriate only if etiology cannot be determined.

Chapter 27

1. b. Answers a, c, and d are also causes of death but account for smaller percentages.
2. c. Answers a, b, and d are ancillary measures that may be helpful, but are not a substitute for appropriate doses of epinephrine given when there is the slightest suspicion of anaphylaxis.
3. b,c. Whereas increasing local reactions may be an indication of increased risk (a), this risk is felt to be minimal, and not an indication for immunotherapy. The reaction (d) may be toxic or nonimmunologically mediated. It is also possible that it represents decreased sensitivity with time or reaction to venom antigens not present in the standard battery. This patient should be retested after any subsequent sting because of the possibility of an anamnestic response to specific IgE.
4. b,c. Answer a is incorrect. Sting challenges confirm that venom RAST levels do not predict the clinical risk or the severity of a reaction. They only indicate the presence or absence of sensitization. The venom skin test is more sensitive than RAST (d). False-positive and false-negative results occur in 15–20% of patients relative to skin tests. A fall in specific IgE and a rise in IgG is generally associated with clinical protection (e). However, there is no absolute level or ratio that can be accepted in any individual as proof of that person's state of immunity sufficient to recommend discontinuing immunotherapy.
5. a–d. Inhalant allergy to hymenoptera antigens is the only acceptable indication for immunotherapy with WBE. Low levels of venom antigens in WBE mixtures make skin testing unreliable. Treatment with WBE does not increase IgE levels nor protect from a challenge sting. Previous treatment with WBE may result in sensitization to vespid body antigens. Some confusion then may exist when venom containing body proteins is used for skin testing. Weakly positive vespid reactions should be interpreted cautiously in this situation.

Chapter 28

1. a. This is perhaps the *key* difference.
2. c. Because toxic reactions are dose-related the patient may receive the drug again, avoiding the toxic level.
3. a. All other forms with minor exceptions (Chapter 11) are anaphylactoid.
4. a. This is a common fallacy.
5. a.

Chapter 29

1. a–e. All of the above. Indomethacin, zomepirac sodium, and sulindac are all prostaglandin synthetase inhibitors. Aspirin-sensitive asthmatics show cross-sensitivity (and cross desensitization) to all of these agents in the proportion to their degree of prostaglandin synthetase activity. Percodan contains aspirin as one of it's components.
2. e. All of the above. See section on variability of response to aspirin following repeat aspirin challenge earlier in chapter.

3. None of these statements is correct. Dietary salicylates are not prostaglandin synthetase inhibitors and do not seem to cross-react with aspirin in aspirin-sensitive subjects. Avoidance of dietary salicylates does not seem to ameliorate the course of an aspirin-sensitive asthmatic. Despite avoiding aspirin and related compounds, patients with aspirin-sensitive asthma continue to have profound respiratory difficulties. Aspirin sensitivity has not been shown to be an IgE-mediated phenomenon; therefore, the incidence of other allergies in the aspirin-sensitive group is no different from the general population. Our current theories concerning the pathogenesis of aspirin sensitivity include alterations in arachidonic acid metabolism produced by aspirin unique to aspirin-sensitive asthmatics as well as abnormalities of respiratory mast cells.
4. a,b. Studies have shown that 8–14% of all asthmatics challenged with aspirin have positive reactions. In the group of asthmatics with polyps and sinusitis, this number increases to 35%. Because of the spectrum and variability of responses to aspirin, there is reason to propose that all asthmatics should avoid aspirin and substitute acetaminophen as an antipyretic analgesic. Because the group of asthmatics with polyps and sinusitis have a 35% chance of being aspirin-sensitive at any particular time, this group should clearly avoid aspirin.
5. b,c. Aspirin-provoked asthmatic reactions can be quite severe. Graded-dose challenges beginning with as little as 30 mg of aspirin have, in our hands, provoked profound falls in FEV_1 values. If one does consider aspirin challenges, therefore, it should be done in a hospital setting, where emergency equipment for treatment of severe asthma and even resuscitation are available. Most patients do become refractory to further adverse effects of aspirin following a single aspirin reaction. However, a number of patients require more than one challenge with a positive response before they become desensitized. We have seen one individual who had 7 reactions to a 30-mg dose and ultimately 16 reactions in total before she was able to tolerate 650 mg of aspirin without any adverse effect. The refractory period following aspirin desensitization is 2–5 days. The return to aspirin sensitivity is a gradual one. For an explanation of answer c, see section on pure nasal response to aspirin in asthmatics in this chapter.

Chapter 30

1. a,b, and c are true. D is incorrect because the sweat chloride test should be preformed by a laboratory that does them on a regular basis by means of quantitative pilocarpine ionophoresis.
2. a and b. Although gastroesophageal reflux can cause wheezing and recurrent pneumonia it does not cause bronchitis. Uncomplicated asthma will not cause bronchiectasis.
3. c. New onset of bronchospasm in a toddler required that the physician exclude the possibility of a foreign body by obtaining chest roentenogram, lung scan or CAT scan and if necessary bronchoscopy.
4. All of the above. Recurrent bacterial chest infections usually have a detectable etiology which may be anatomic, physiologic, immunologic or biochemical in origin.
5. The child most likely has homozygous alpha-1-antitrypsin deficiency.

Chapter 31

1. b,c. Patients with complement or immunoglobulin deficiency typically suffer systemic infection with pyogenic encapsulated bacteria. Sepsis, meningitis, and pneumonia are very common. These patients rarely have problems with viral, protozoal or fungal organisms as seen in cellular immune defects. Abscesses and skin infections are also less common and occur more frequently with phagocyte abnormalities. Many patients with humoral or complement deficiency grow normally until severe pulmonary disease develops.

2. a,b. Chronic granulomatous disease and combined immunodeficiency with enzyme deficiency can be diagnosed *in vitro,* but the techniques are available only at a few medical centers.

3. b,d,e. Sex-linked agammaglobulinemia can be effectively treated with gamma globulin injections or plasma infusions at monthly intervals. Strict compliance with this program will prevent most severe bacterial infections. Transplantation of histocompatible bone marrow has resulted in complete immunologic reconstitution in patients with severe combined immunodeficiency. In other related cases the use of fetal thymus, fetal liver cells, or thymus epithelium has also been successful. Patients with DiGeorge syndrome have been effectively treated with fetal thymus transplants or thymosin infusions. At this time no specific treatments are available for ataxia tetangiectasia or chronic granulomatous disease.

4. c,d. Quantitative immunoglobulins can be determined most easily by radial immunodiffusion. A normal value will generally rule out significant abnormality. Serum protein electrophoresis is not sensitive to low levels of individual immunoglobulin classes and will fail to detect some abnormalities. To detect those patients with normal levels of nonfunctioning immunoglobulins, antibody function tests should be performed. Isohemagglutinins are IgM antibodies, whereas polio and tetanus are predominantly IgG. Further testing is not necessary if the level and function of antibodies are normal.

5. a. The majority of infants with low immunoglobulin levels respond normally to antigenic stimulation and injection. If they have evidence of antibody formation determination by isohemagglutinins, polio, or tetanus titers, gamma globulin injections are not recommended. The infant should be followed closely and immunoglobulin levels determined at regular intervals. Only if there is evidence for bacterial infection of a severe nature, gamma globulin injections should be considered.

Index

A

B

C

D

E

F

G

H

I

J

K

L

M

N

O

P

Q

R

S

T

U

V

W

X–Y